Kremkau's

SONOGRAPHY

Principles and Instruments

Kremkau's

SONOGRAPHY

Principles and Instruments

Flemming Forsberg, PhD

Professor of Radiology
Thomas Jefferson University
Philadelphia, Pennsylvania

ELSEVIER

11TH EDITION

Elsevier
3251 Riverport Lane
St. Louis, Missouri 63043

KREMKAU'S SONOGRAPHY: PRINCIPLES AND INSTRUMENTS, ELEVENTH EDITION ISBN: 978-0-443-26129-9

Senior Content Strategist: Luke Held
Content Development Manager: Danielle M. Frazier
Publishing Services Manager: Deepthi Unni
Project Manager: Surya Narayanan Jayachandran
Design Direction: Amy Buxton

Printed in India

Last digit is the print number: 9 8 7 6 5 4 3 2 1

To my children, Mark and Anya, with all my love!!

On a professional level, I would like to dedicate this edition to Barry B. Goldberg, MD, Professor Emeritus of Radiology, Thomas Jefferson University, and to Fredrick W. Kremkau, PhD, Professor Emeritus of Radiologic Sciences, Wake Forest University School of Medicine, for their impact on the field of ultrasound imaging in general, over so many years, and for their guidance and advice to me personally.

PREFACE

IMPORTANT NOTE FOR READERS, INSTRUCTORS, AND STUDENTS

This 11th edition of the textbook introduces a major change in its approach to understanding and applying the principles of sonography—namely, a new author and, therefore, a new style and viewpoint, albeit based on the existing editions and pedagogical principles. This is discussed in "New to this Edition" in this Preface.

This book is intended for sonography students, allied-health personnel, and physicians who seek an understanding of the principles and instruments of diagnostic sonography. Applying these underlying principles in practice improves the quality of medical care involving ultrasound imaging. The best sonographers and physicians understand these principles and apply them in their practice.

The purpose of this book is to explain how contemporary diagnostic ultrasound works. It serves as a textbook on sonographic principles in educational programs and helps readers scan safely and effectively, handle artifacts skillfully, and prepare for registry and board examinations. The content of the book is driven by my assessment of contemporary technology in the field (as the author), and it is also based on my 30+ years of experience in teaching material like this in medical schools and at conferences and seminars.

Although this latest edition includes newer developments in the field (e.g., Chapter 6), the emphasis is still on the fundamentals. For the sake of beginners, the text is simplified, yet at the same time it (hopefully) maintains its usefulness for more experienced users. Although the book is designed for nonphysicists and nonengineering readers, understanding the material will require some effort. Admittedly, the material can still come across as being difficult. It simply cannot be made easy for everyone and still maintain the necessary level of expertise for appropriate application in practice. However, my years of lecturing and publication experience have convinced me that the material can be understood with reasonable preparation and effort on the part of the student. Topics not covered in this textbook include photoacoustic imaging, therapy applications, investigational techniques, the historical development of sonography, how to perform diagnostic examinations, and how to interpret the results. Other books cover these topics.

DIFFERENCES RELATIVE TO EARLIER EDITIONS AND NATIONAL EXAMINATIONS

Each new edition is different from earlier editions as well as from the current content of registry and specialty board examinations. That is because this text is up to date with current technology, whereas examinations change much more slowly because of the thorough and time-consuming process required to update certifying exams (lots of practice tests and surveys, committee decisions, as well as the review and approval of new questions). Outdated descriptions of technology and instrument features that are no longer widely present in the field are mainly eliminated with each new edition (although occasionally such concepts have been retained to allow students to gather the perspective required to comprehend and pass registry exams). Nonetheless, the book changes more rapidly than the examinations. The philosophy of the book has always been to be as consistent as possible with prevailing, contemporary ultrasound technology and usage, and I have strived to maintain this in the current edition (even as the new author on the block).

FEATURES

- Comprehensive coverage of the principles of sonography
- Preparation for the ARDMS SPI examination
- Latest developments in commercially available ultrasound technology
- Introduction of the current principles of system operation as they relate to narrow or broad transmit beam functions
- Hundreds of color illustrations and images
- Hundreds of exercises with answers
- Comprehensive multiple-choice examination with annotated answers
- Consistent pedagogy, including learning objectives, chapter outlines, and key terms
- Key points set off by icons
- Advanced concepts are included at appropriate locations in the text and in Chapter 6, more specifically
- Math and physics reviews, videos, and an interactive exam on the Evolve website
- Descriptive subheadings
- Boxes and tables
- Glossary

NEW TO THIS EDITION

- Normally, each new edition of this textbook, which appears every 4 or 5 years, involves including new features or technologies that have appeared (e.g., elastography) and/or removing those that have disappeared (e.g., the replacement of the cathode-ray tube with the flat-panel display). The 10th edition introduced a major change in ultrasound technology by recognizing that there are two principles of operation available in modern ultrasound systems. However, time (and a new author) has allowed those two concepts to be described more as different transmit strategies (using narrow or broad transmit beams), admittedly resulting in fundamentally different processing approaches for focusing, etc.
- Reorganizing the 10 chapters by folding the concepts of narrow and broad transmit beams (referred to in the 10th edition as *principle 1* and *principle 2*) into the expanded

Chapters 4 and 5 on imaging of anatomy and of flow and motion.
- New Chapter 6 dedicated to advanced ultrasound technologies and maintaining the expansion of former Chapter 7 into current Chapters 8 and 9.
- The ever-expanding incorporation of AI into ultrasound systems is certainly adding to the "black box" feel of diagnostic ultrasound. However, as long as we are sending ultrasound into the body and receiving ultrasonic echoes, these will be sonographic systems. But what we do with the retuning echoes will be radically different depending on the processing principles applied.
- New illustrations and images demonstrating the latest and best images from the newest equipment.
- Expanded content on volume imaging, elastography, contrast-enhanced ultrasound imaging, and point-of-care ultrasound, keeping students up to date with the latest technology.
- The latest instrument output data and official safety statements.
- Alignment with the JRC-DMS National Education Curriculum and the ARDMS examination specifications, making this a useful text for preparing for the SPI examination.

PERSONAL NOTE

When Fred Kremkau first approached me to take over his "baby", I was both honored and terrified. Trying to shepherd such a successful textbook, which has been around for over 40 years, reaching a 10th edition in 2020, onward is a daunting task. But here we are! I am pleased that Elsevier will keep the book going beyond Fred and, of course, thrilled that it has been renamed from *Sonography: Principles and Instruments* to *Kremkau's Sonography: Principles and Instruments*. The fundamental aim remains the same: to describe the latest in diagnostic ultrasound and sonographic technology in terms useful to the clinical personnel applying it to the benefit of patients, and I trust it will be valuable to you as you pursue your career in this exciting and rewarding field.

That being said, I really don't think I will manage to produce 10 editions… But I'll worry about that tomorrow.

FOR THE STUDENT

The chapters within this book should be read sequentially, because each chapter builds on material presented previously. Key terms are listed at the beginning of each chapter, are highlighted in blue in the chapter, and are defined in the Glossary at the back of the book.

The following resources are available at http://evolve.elsevier.com/Kremkau/sonography/:
- Companion, instructional videos on the following:
  - Ultrasound (Chapter 2)
  - Transducers (Chapter 3)
  - Instruments for Imaging Anatomy (Chapter 4)
  - Instruments for Imaging Flow (Chapter 5)
  - Advanced Techniques (Chapter 6)
  - Artifacts (Chapter 7)
  - Quality Assurance (Chapter 8)
  - Safety (Chapter 9)
- Mathematics review
- Physics review
- Lists of mathematical symbols
- Compilation of mathematical equations
- Compilation of boxes and tables
- Demonstration videos on the following:
  - Use of a sonographic phantom as a patient surrogate
  - Effect of frequency on attenuation and penetration
  - Image formats of various transducer types
  - Impact of output and gain controls on the image
  - Color Doppler displays and control effects
  - Spectral Doppler displays and control effects
  - Aliasing artifact and ways to correct it

After studying this text, the student should be able to:
- Describe what an ultrasound is
- Describe the pulse-echo principle
- Compare narrow and broad transmit beam systems
- Explain how ultrasound is sent into the body
- Explain how ultrasound detects and locates anatomic structures
- Discuss how echoes are received from the body and processed in the instrument
- Describe how anatomic information is presented on the display
- Explain how ultrasound detects and measures tissue motion and blood flow
- List the ways motion and flow information are presented using either narrow or broad transmit beams
- Explain how flow detection is localized to a specific site in tissue
- List the common artifacts that can occur in diagnostic sonography
- Discuss how the performance of ultrasound scanners is tested
- Describe the risk and safety issues associated with diagnostic ultrasound

FOR THE INSTRUCTOR

The following resource is available at http://evolve.elsevier.com/Kremkau/ultrasound:

Instructor's Electronic Resource containing an instructor's manual, PowerPoint slides, a test bank, and an image collection.
- The instructor's manual includes outlines and summaries of textbook chapters, visual learning exercises, lab and learning assignments, and review questions.
- The PowerPoint presentation includes notes for instructors.
- The test bank includes over 400 questions.
- The image collection can be downloaded in PowerPoint or as JPEG files.

Also, note under For the Student, there is a series of instructional videos on the following topics:
- Ultrasound (Chapter 2)

- Transducers (Chapter 3)
- Instruments for Imaging Anatomy (Chapter 4)
- Instruments for Imaging Flow (Chapter 5)
- Advanced Techniques (Chapter 6)
- Artifacts (Chapter 7)
- Quality Assurance (Chapter 8)
- Safety (Chapter 9)

ACKNOWLEDGMENTS

I would like to thank the following people for help with this book:

D. P. Bahner, MD, A. Berggrein, V. Berghella, MD, M. Bonet Vazquez, MPH, L. Brames, PMP,
J. D'Amico, RDMS, C. DeStefano, RDMS, K. Dickie, BS, T. Erpelding, PhD,
J. B. Fowlkes, PhD, S. Guenther, CRGS, A. Gurung, PhD, F. W. Kremkau, PhD,
O. Kripfgans, PhD, T. Lopez, RDMS, P. Machado, MD,
S. McAleavey, PhD, M. E. McDonald, DHSc,
K. Nam, PhD, L. Needleman, MD,
P. O'Kane, MD,
M. Perkovic, BS, RDMS,
W. T. Shi, PhD, C. Shields, RDMS, K. Wager, RDMS,
K. Wallace, PhD, C. E. Wessner, MS, RDMS, M. A. Wheatley, PhD, A. Wilkinson, MS, RDMS

representing Butterfly Network, Canon Medical Systems USA, Clarius, Drexel University, GE HealthCare, Philips Medical Systems, Siemens Healthineers, Thomas Jefferson University, University of Michigan, University of Rochester, Wake Forest University School of Medicine

For their cooperation and assistance, thank you to:
Danielle Frazier and Luke Held at Elsevier Inc.

CONTENTS

1

Sonography: A Window into the Human Body

LEARNING OBJECTIVES

After reading this chapter, the student should be able to do the following:

- Explain the pulse-echo principle used in ultrasound imaging.
- List the differences between narrow and broad transmit beam imaging.
- Describe the image formats used in ultrasound imaging.
- Explain how the Doppler effect is applied in diagnostic ultrasound.
- List the ways in which Doppler information is presented.

CHAPTER OUTLINE

Sonography—Narrow and Broad Transmit Beam Imaging

Doppler Ultrasound—Detecting and Displaying Motion and Flow

KEY TERMS

Broad transmit beams
Color flow imaging
Doppler effect
Doppler ultrasound
Four-dimensional (4D) imaging
Grayscale image
Image
Linear scan
Narrow transmit beams
Pulse-echo technique
Scan line
Sector scan
Sonography
Spectral Doppler
Transducer
Three-dimensional (3D) imaging
Two-dimensional (2D) imaging
Ultrasound
Volume imaging

Bats, dolphins, and other animals used **ultrasound** naturally long before we humans adopted it for our needs. These animals use ultrasound to detect, locate, determine the motion of, and capture prey; to avoid obstacles; to detect and avoid predators; and to court their mates. One early use we humans made of ultrasound techniques was for the detection of icebergs, which became very popular on the North Atlantic shipping routes in the aftermath of the sinking of RMS Titanic (in April 1912). **Sonography** or more commonly diagnostic ultrasound imaging is the use of ultrasound in medical anatomical and flow imaging (i.e., Doppler ultrasound). Doppler ultrasound modes include the detection, quantification, and evaluation of tissue motion and specifically blood flow by using the **Doppler effect** with ultrasound. This chapter presents an overview of the principles of diagnostic ultrasound imaging including Doppler ultrasound. Here, we are introducing the concepts. In the subsequent chapters, we will dive into the details.

SONOGRAPHY—NARROW AND BROAD TRANSMIT BEAM IMAGING

Diagnostic ultrasound or sonography is medical **two-dimensional (2D) and three-dimensional (3D)** anatomical and flow **imaging** using ultrasound. *Ultra* is a prefix that means *beyond*. Thus ultrasound is sound that is higher in pitch than the range of human hearing. Unlike some of the other medical imaging techniques, ultrasound imaging is not a passive push-button activity. Rather, it is an interactive process that involves a patient being examined by a sonographer (acquiring the images) yielding a **transducer** (also called a probe) transmitting ultrasound, and an instrument or scanner (also called a system) for analyzing and displaying images as well as, finally, a physician/radiologist who interprets the images (occasionally referred to as a sonologist). Understanding and application of the underlying physical and electronic principles presented in this book strengthen the expertise of the sonographer and the radiologist and improve the quality of medical care involving diagnostic ultrasound that patients receive.

> Medical imaging with ultrasound is called *diagnostic ultrasound imaging* or *sonography*.

An **image** is a reproduction, representation, or imitation of the physical form of a person or object. An ultrasound image is the visible counterpart of an invisible object, produced in an electronic instrument by the interaction of ultrasound with the object. Ultrasound provides a noninvasive way of looking inside the human body (Fig. 1.1) to image otherwise hidden anatomy. Anatomic imaging with ultrasound is accomplished with the **pulse-echo technique**. Pulses of ultrasound generated by a transducer are sent into the patient, where they produce echoes at organ boundaries and within biological tissues. These echoes return to the transducer, where they are detected and presented on the display of an ultrasound scanner. A transducer (Fig. 1.2) generates the ultrasound pulses and receives the returning echoes. Diagnostic ultrasound requires knowledge of the origin of each echo and its strength as it returns from the patient. An ultrasound system (Fig. 1.3) processes the echoes and presents them as visible dots, which form the anatomic image on the display. The brightness of each dot corresponds to the echo strength, producing what is known as a **grayscale image**. The location of each dot corresponds to the anatomic location of the echo-generating structure.

Traditionally, the underlying operating principle for all ultrasound systems throughout the 50+ year history of changing technologies in diagnostic ultrasound imaging has been based around **narrow** focused **transmit beams**. Now with improved computing and processing power, the field of diagnostic ultrasound is moving toward transmitting **broad** (unfocused or minimally focused) **transmit beams**, which has major implications for various characteristics and features of these scanners. This book recognizes this transition and will illuminate the differences throughout the chapters.

When using (traditional) narrow transmit beams, positional information is determined by knowledge of the direction of the pulse when it enters the patient and by measuring the time it takes for each echo to return to the transducer. The proper location to show the echo can then be determined from a starting point on the display (usually at the top). With knowledge of the sound speed, the ultrasound system uses the echo arrival time to determine the depth of the structure that produced that echo.

> Diagnostic ultrasound is accomplished with the pulse-echo technique.

> Echoes from tissue interfaces and other anatomical structures map these structures in an ultrasound image.

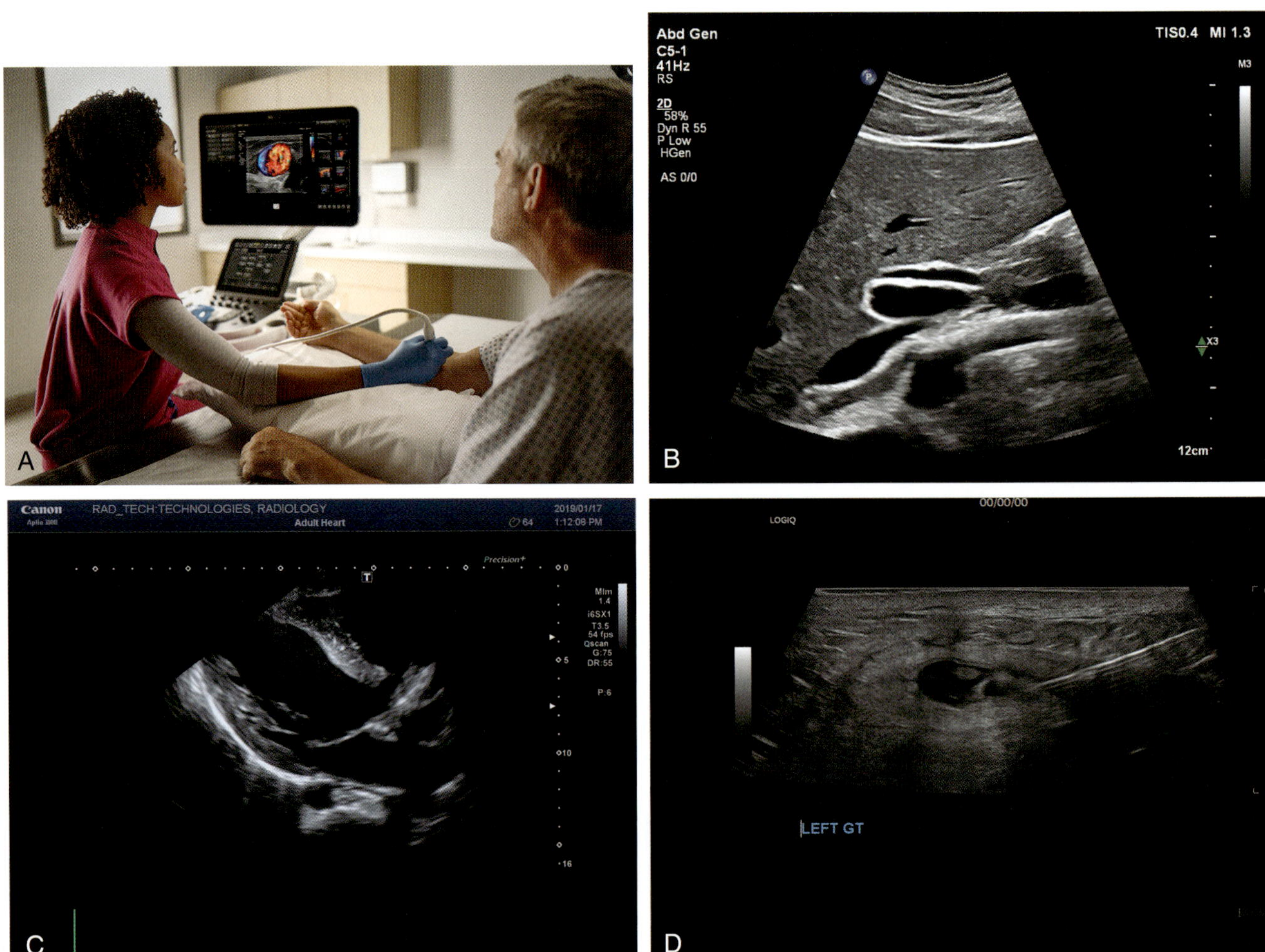

Fig. 1.1 **A**, Ultrasound provides a window into the human body, allowing us to see what would otherwise be hidden from view. Images shown are as follows: **B**, abdominal; **C**, cardiac; **D**, Muscoloskeletal imaging guiding a hip injection. (**A–B**, Courtesy Philips Medical Systems; **C**, Courtesy Canon Medical Systems USA; **D**, Courtesy GE HealthCare.)

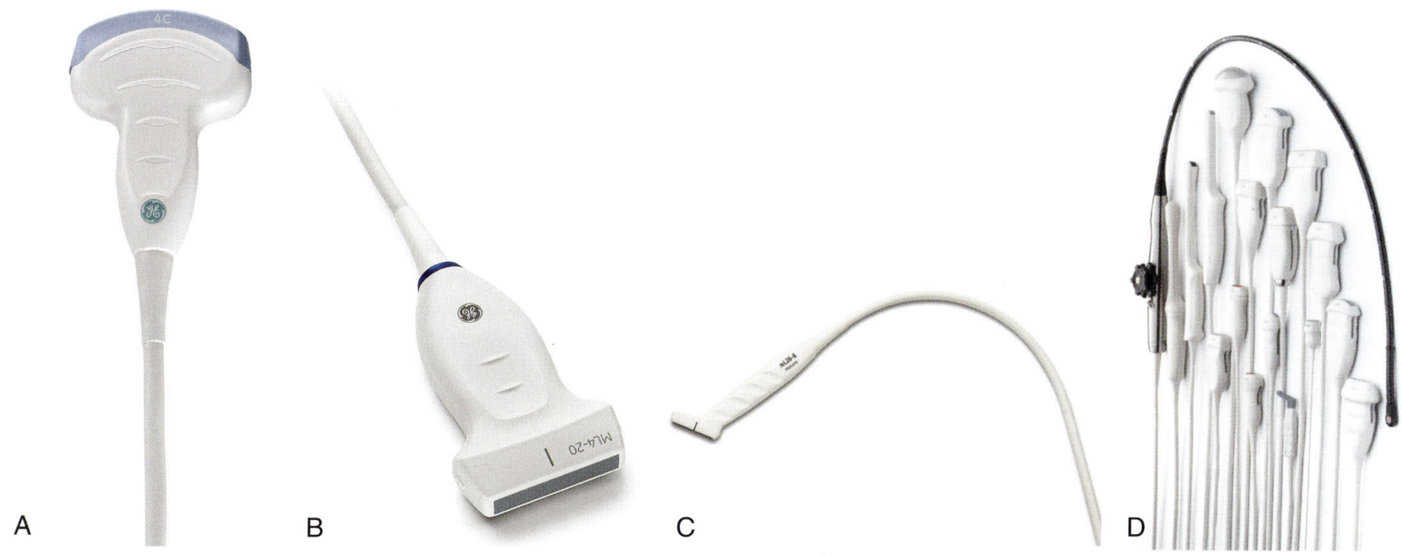

Fig. 1.2 (**A–D**) Transducers.

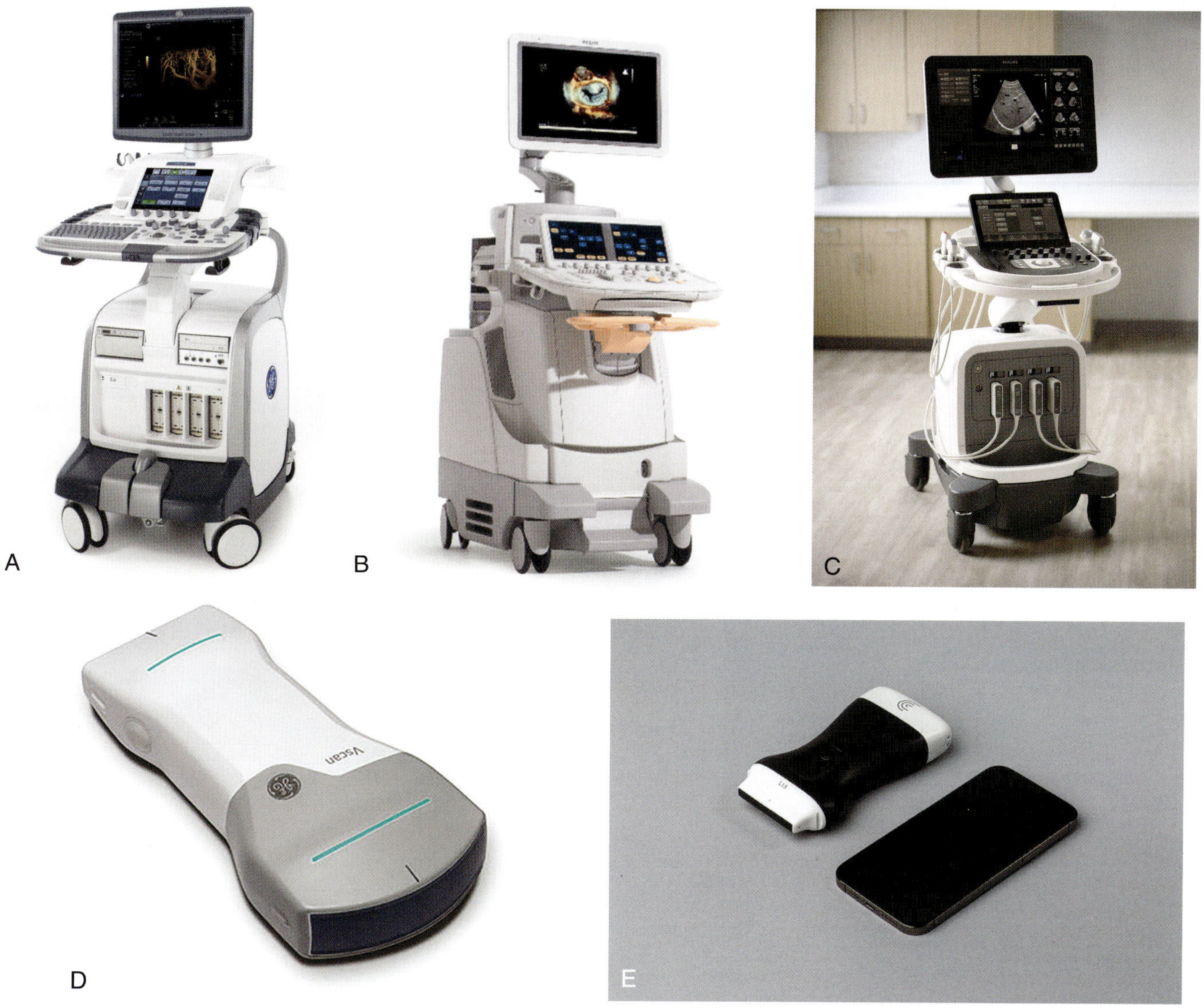

Fig. 1.3 **A–C**, Ultrasound scanners on carts for traditional radiology applications; **D and E**, smaller handheld systems for point-of-care ultrasound applications. (**A and D**, Courtesy GE HealthCare; **B–C**, Philips Medical Systems; **E,** Clarius).

If one pulse of ultrasound is sent into tissue, a series of dots (one line of echo information, specifically, an echo line, data line, or scan line) is displayed (Fig. 1.4). Not all of the energy in an ultrasound pulse is reflected back from any one structure. Rather, most of the original pulse continues to be reflected back from deeper structures. The echoes from one pulse appear as one **scan line** (see Fig. 1.4, E–F). When the process is repeated, with different starting points for each subsequent pulse, a cross-sectional image of the underlying anatomy is constructed (Fig. 1.5). Pulses that travel in the same direction from different points yield vertical parallel scan lines and a rectangular image, as shown in Fig. 1.6. These cross-sectional images are produced with vertical parallel scan lines that are so close together that they cannot be identified individually. The rectangular display resulting from this procedure is often called a **linear scan**, or **linear image**, referring to the linear array transducer that is used to produce it. A second approach to sending ultrasound pulses through the body being imaged is shown in Fig. 1.7. In this method, each pulse originates from the same starting point, but subsequent pulses travel in slightly different directions. This approach results in a **sector scan**, or **sector image**, which has a shape similar to a slice of pie or a fan (Fig. 1.8). Fig. 1.9 shows a format that is a combination of the two techniques just described; that is, pulses (and scan lines) originate from different starting points (as in a linear image), and each pulse (and scan line) travels in a slightly different direction from that of the previous one (as in a sector image). In this example, the starting points form a curved line across the top of the scan, rather than a straight line, as in the linear scans shown in Fig. 1.6, and this is considered a **curvi-linear sector image**.

> Ultrasound images are composed of many (hundreds) of scan lines.

When using a few broad transmit beams (in the ultimate implementation a single plane wave), these pulses of ultrasound travel through the anatomical cross-section to be imaged, but they do not produce a one-for-one correspondence between transmitted pulse and displayed scan line. Instead, all the echo information throughout the imaged cross-section is collected, and then a massive computational process determines the location and strength of each echo at a given location in the anatomy. This approach is used in newer, more sophisticated ("high-end") instruments and produces improved image quality compared with traditional narrow beam scanners. More detail on both approaches will be presented in Chapters 4 and 5.

A 2D scan format is commonly limited to three types: (1) linear, (2) sector, and (3) a combination of the two (most commonly a curvi-linear format, although other formats exist). Occasionally, other formats altogether may be used, but in any case, what is required is that the ultrasound pulses are sent through all portions of the anatomy that are to be imaged. Traditionally, each pulse

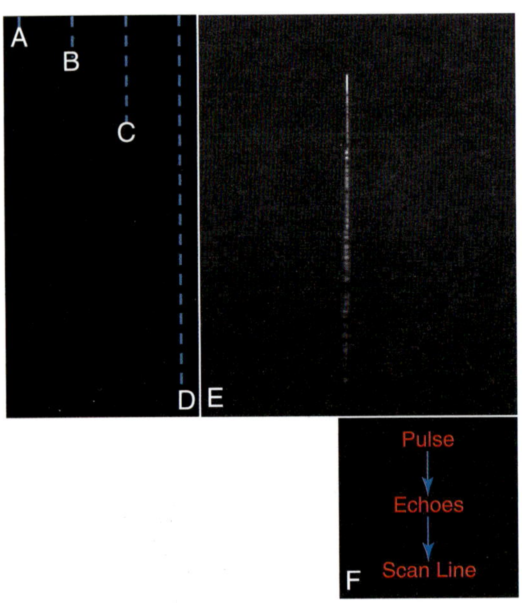

Fig. 1.4 One pulse of ultrasound generates a single scan line (series of echoes) as it travels through tissue. Echoes are presented in sequence on a scan line while they return from tissue during pulse travel. **A**, The first echo is displayed. **B**, The second echo is added. **C**, Three more echoes are added. **D**, All the echoes from a single pulse have been received and displayed as a completed scan line. **E**, A complete scan line results from one emitted pulse. In practice, this is accomplished in less than one one-thousandth of a second. **F**, According to the pulse-echo imaging principle, one pulse traveling through tissues produces a stream of echoes that become one scan line on the display.

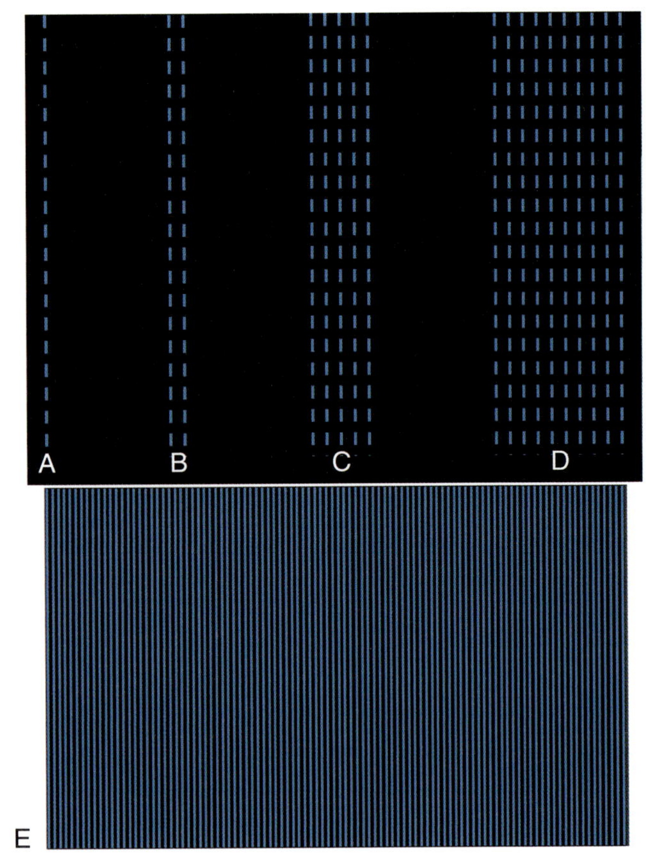

Fig. 1.5 A single rectangular image or scan (also called a frame) is composed of many vertical parallel scan lines. Each scan line represents a series of echoes returning from a pulse traveling through the tissues. **A**, One scan line from one pulse, as generated in Figure 1.4. **B**, A second scan line is added. **C–D**, Five and ten scan lines, respectively. **E**, A complete frame consisting of (in this example) 100 scan lines.

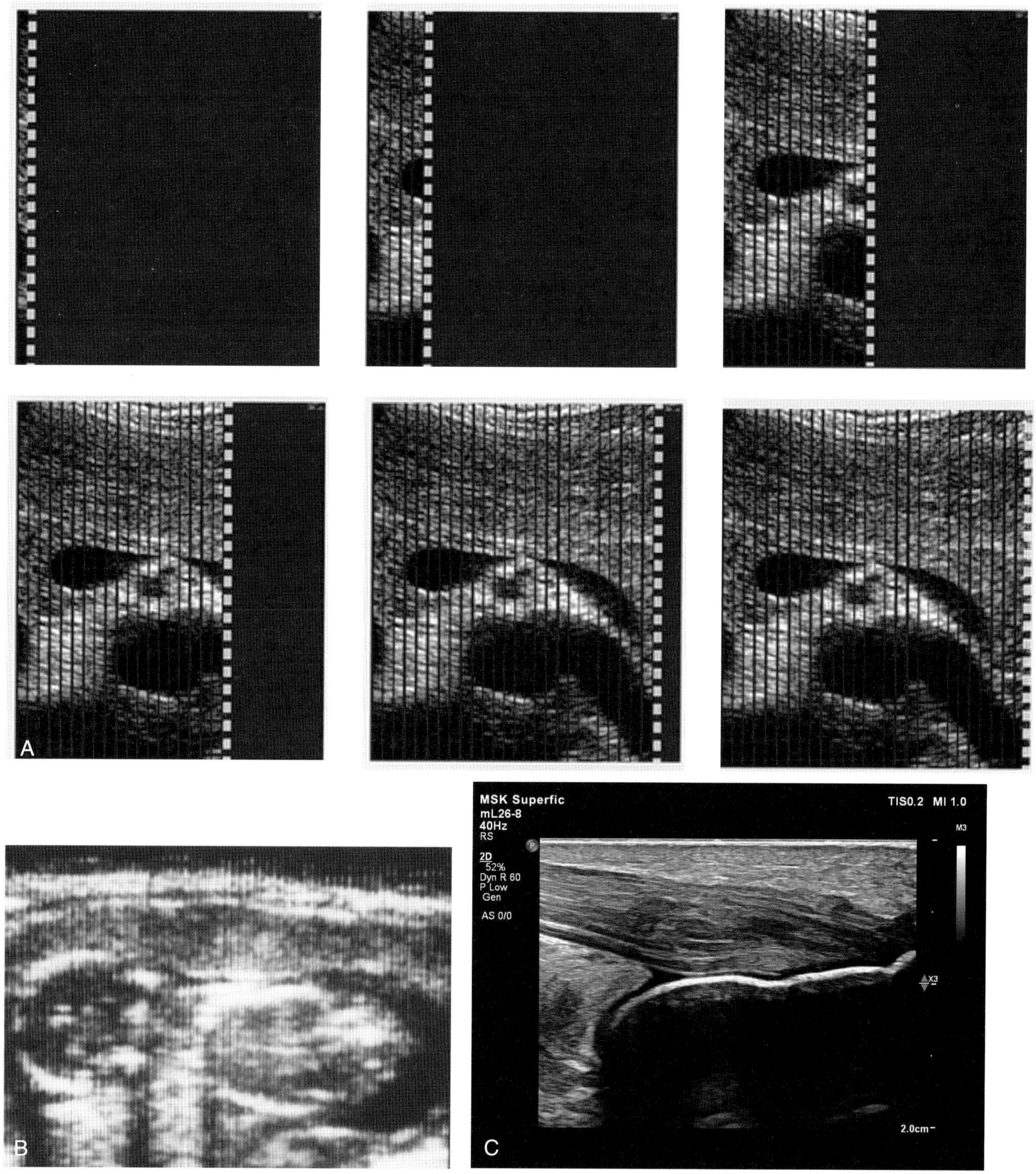

Fig. 1.6 **A**, Ultrasound scan lines sent sequentially through a thin rectangular volume of tissue produces a rectangular image, commonly called a *linear image or linear scan.* **B**, Fetal image from the late 1970s, revealing the 120 vertical parallel scan lines of which it is composed. **C**, Clinical linear (rectangular) scan of the Achilles tendon. (Courtesy Philips Medical Systems.)

generates a series of echoes, resulting in a series of dots (a scan line) on the display, and the resulting cross-sectional image is composed of many (typically 96–256) of these scan lines. The scan format determines the starting points and paths for individual scan lines, according to the starting point and path for each pulse used to generate each scan line. With broad transmit beams, the retrospective computational virtual beam-forming process determines the echo information displayed at each location in the scan. The clinical cross-sectional grayscale images produced are sometimes called *B scans.* This term implies that the images are produced by scanning the ultrasound through the imaged cross-section (i.e., sending pulses through all regions of the cross-section) and converting the

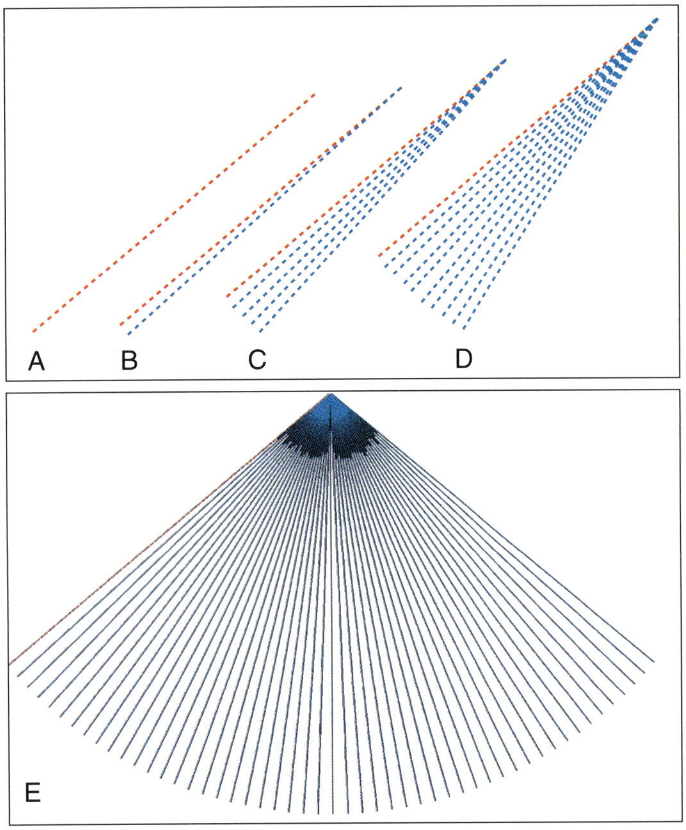

Fig. 1.7 A single sector frame is progressively built up with 1 (**A**), 2 (**B**), 5 (**C**), 10 (**D**), and 100 (**E**) scan lines in sequence. All originate from a common origin and travel out in different directions.

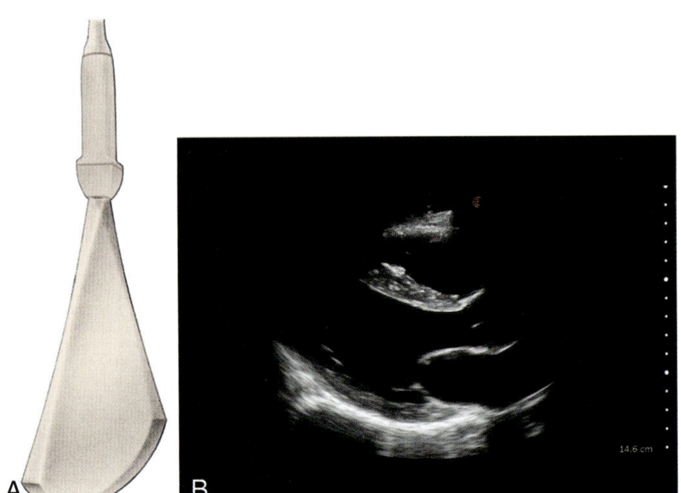

Fig. 1.8 **A**, Ultrasound sent through a thin pie slice–shaped volume of tissue produces an image commonly called a sector *image or sector scan.* **B**, Sector scan of adult heart (Courtesy Clarius.)

echo strength into the brightness of each represented echo on the display (hence, *B* [brightness] scan). The terms *B scan* and *grayscale scan* have the same meaning.

> A 2D ultrasound image is presented in linear (rectangular) or sector forms.

For decades, diagnostic ultrasound was limited to 2D cross-sectional scans (or "slices" or "imaging planes") through the

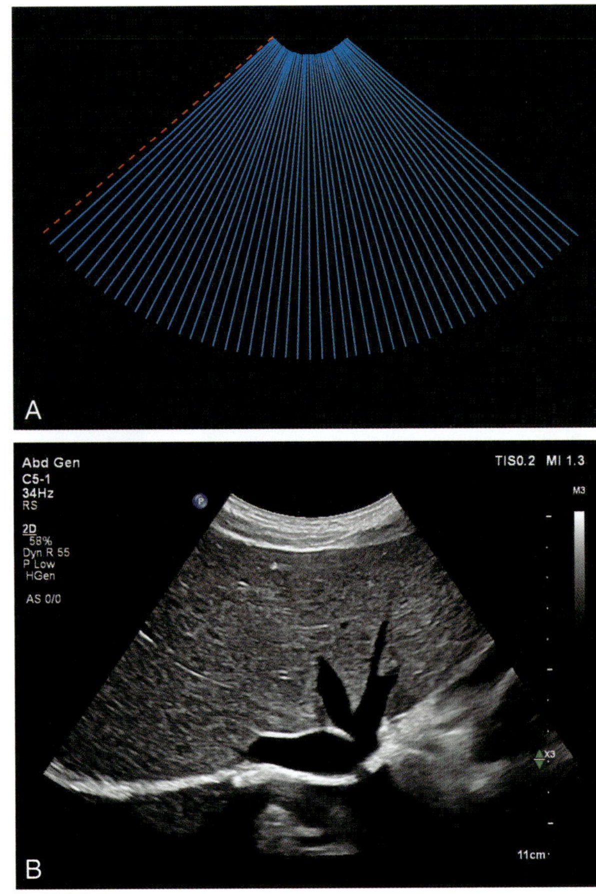

Fig. 1.9 **A**, A modified form of a sector scan is produced when pulses and scan lines originate from different points across the curved top of a sector display. **B**, Abdominal scan using the scan format shown in **A**. (Courtesy Philips Medical Systems).

anatomy. Today, 2D imaging has been extended to 3D scanning and imaging, also called **volume or 4D imaging** (3D imaging over time being marketed as 4D imaging). This method requires scanning the ultrasound through many adjacent 2D tissue cross-sections to form a 3D volume of echo information similar to a loaf of sliced bread (Fig. 1.10). This 3D volume of echoes can then be processed and displayed to present 2D images or 3D volumes of the anatomy.

> Ultrasound images can be displayed in 2D, 3D, or 4D formats.

DOPPLER ULTRASOUND—DETECTING AND DISPLAYING MOTION AND FLOW

Echoes produced by moving objects have frequencies that are different from that of the pulses generating that echo. This phenomenon is called the Doppler effect, which is put to use in medical ultrasound to detect and measure tissue motion and blood flow and in astronomy to measure the motion of stars and galaxies. The Doppler effect is named after Christian Andreas Doppler, the Austrian physicist who first described this phenomenon in a lecture in 1842 in Prague.

The use of Doppler radar in weather forecasting, aviation safety, and vehicle speed detection (police radar) has made *the*

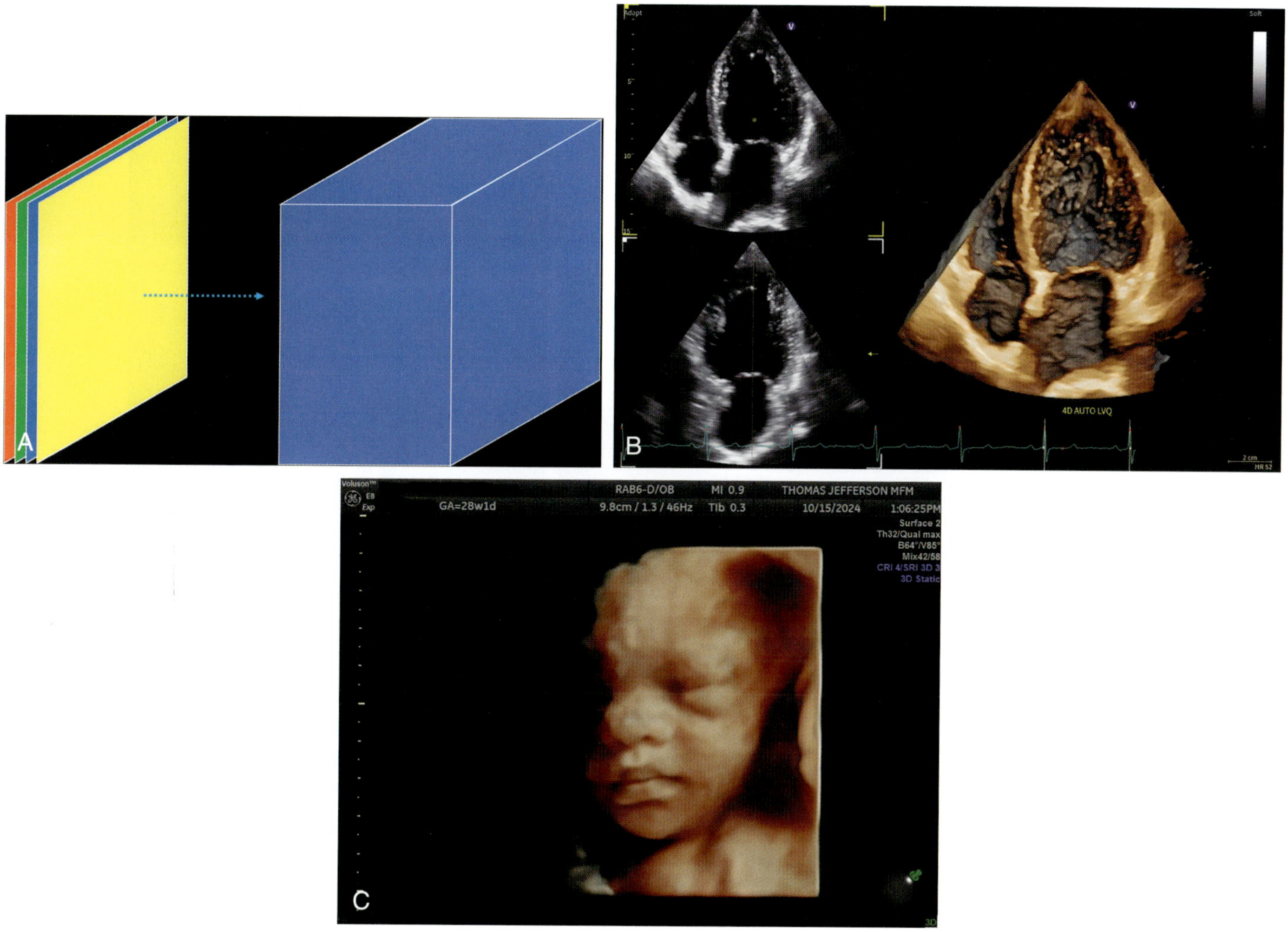

Fig. 1.10 Three-dimensional (volume) sonographic images. **A**, Three-dimensional echo data acquired by obtaining many two-dimensional sections of echo information (*colored slices*) from the imaged anatomy, forms a three-dimensional volume of stored echo information (*blue box*). **B**, Cardiac four-chamber view. **C**, Fetal head. (**B**, Courtesy GE HealthCare; **C**, Courtesy Colleen Shields & Vincenzo Berghella, Thomas Jefferson University Hospital.)

Doppler effect a household term (Fig. 1.11). In addition to its observation in everyday life (as demonstrated by the changing pitch of a siren or horn heard as a vehicle passes by), the Doppler effect has been applied to automatic door openers in public buildings, burglar alarms, and other motion-detecting devices.

> The Doppler effect is a change in frequency caused by objects moving relative to each other.

Doppler ultrasound has been used in diagnostic medicine for many decades. Long-standing applications include monitoring the fetal heart rate during labor and delivery as well as evaluating blood flow in the heart and in the arteries and veins of the circulation. Rapid scanning, acquisition, and processing of Doppler data enable color-coded 2D, 3D, and 4D presentations of Doppler information (**color flow imaging** displays) to be superimposed on grayscale (i.e., anatomical) images (Fig. 1.12). Doppler information is applied to loudspeakers for audible evaluation and to **spectral Doppler** displays for quantitative analysis (Fig. 1.13). The spectral Doppler mode can include anatomical imaging to guide and select the location(s) from which the spectral information is acquired (Fig. 1.14).

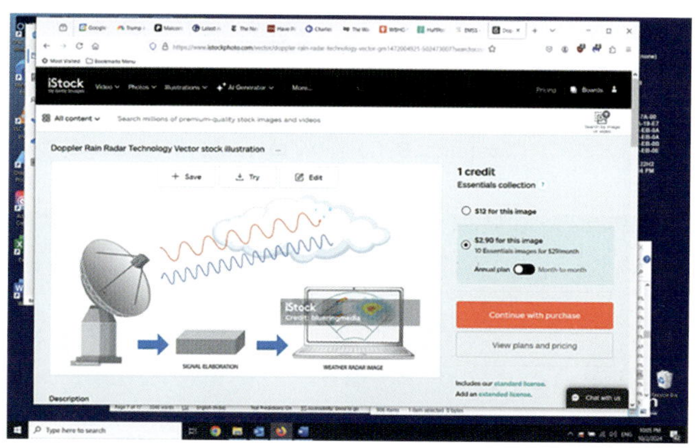

Fig. 1.11 Doppler radar for weather forecasts.

> Doppler information is presented in audible, color flow (color or power Doppler imaging), and spectral Doppler forms.

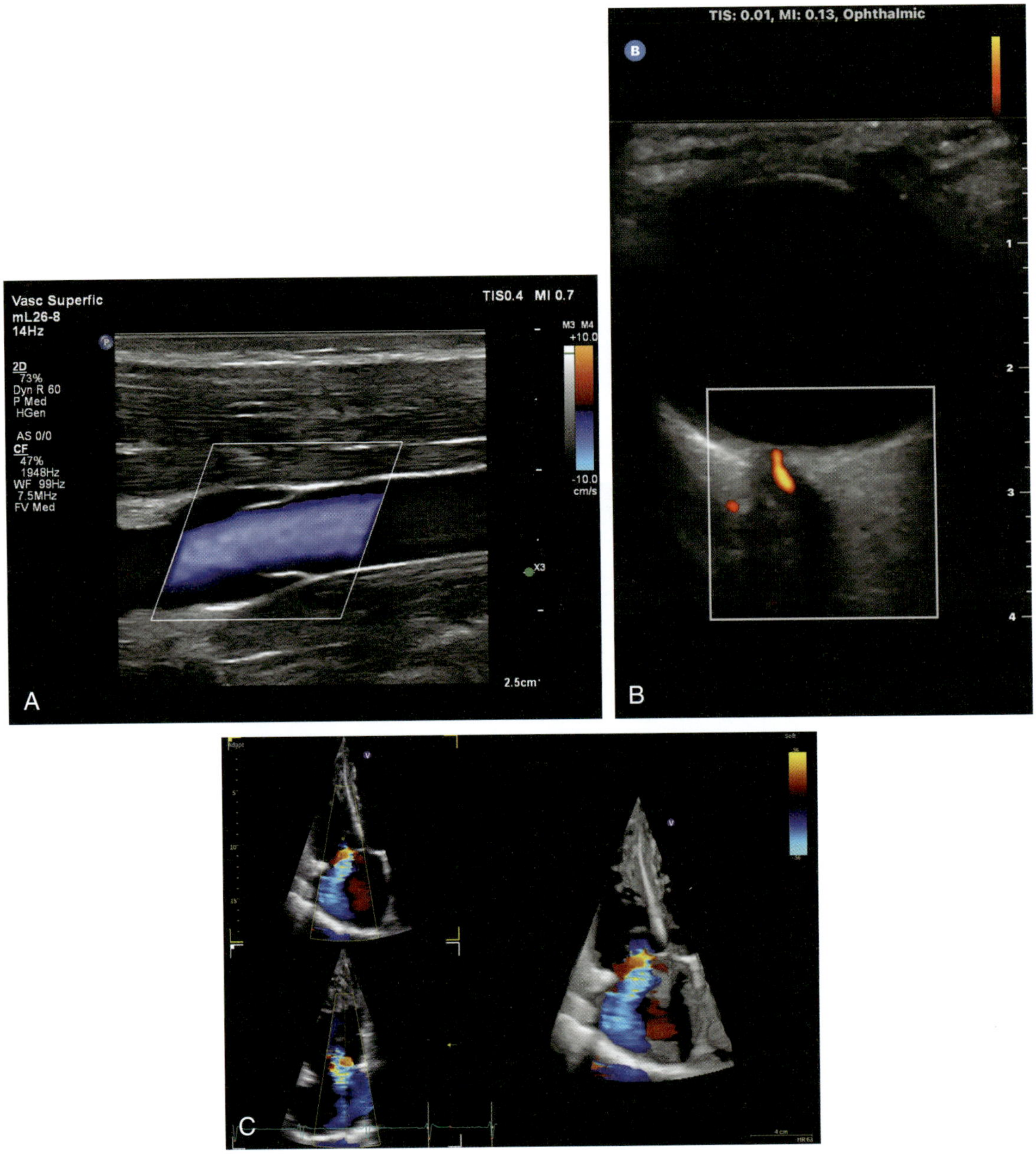

Fig. 1.12 Color flow imaging displays of blood flow. Presented in forms called (A) color Doppler imaging, (B) power Doppler imaging, and (C) three-dimensional (3D) color Doppler imaging. (**A**, Courtesy Philips Medical Systems; **B**, Courtesy the Butterfly Network; **C**, Courtesy GE HealthCare.)

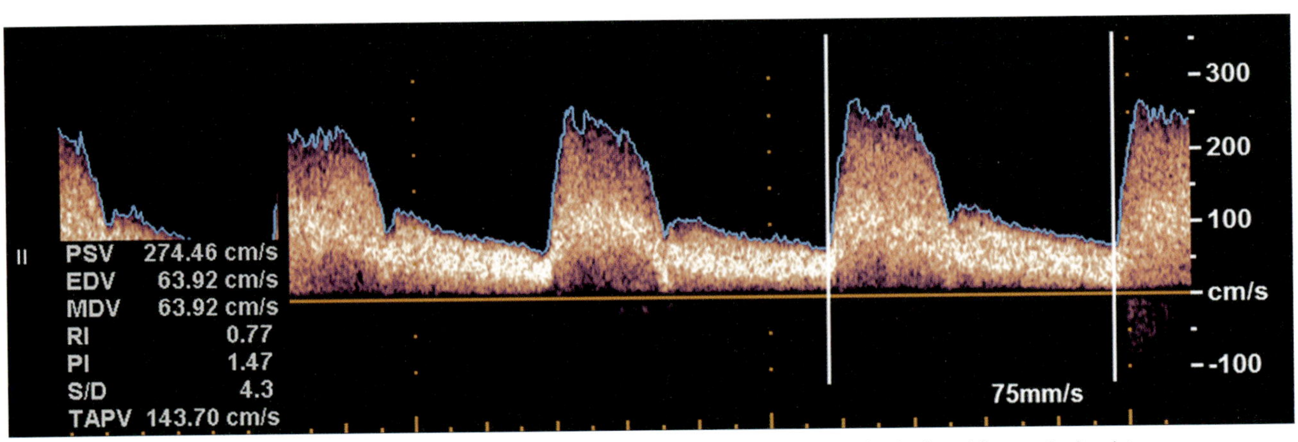

Fig. 1.13 Spectral-Doppler display of arterial blood flow with presentation of calculated flow velocity data.

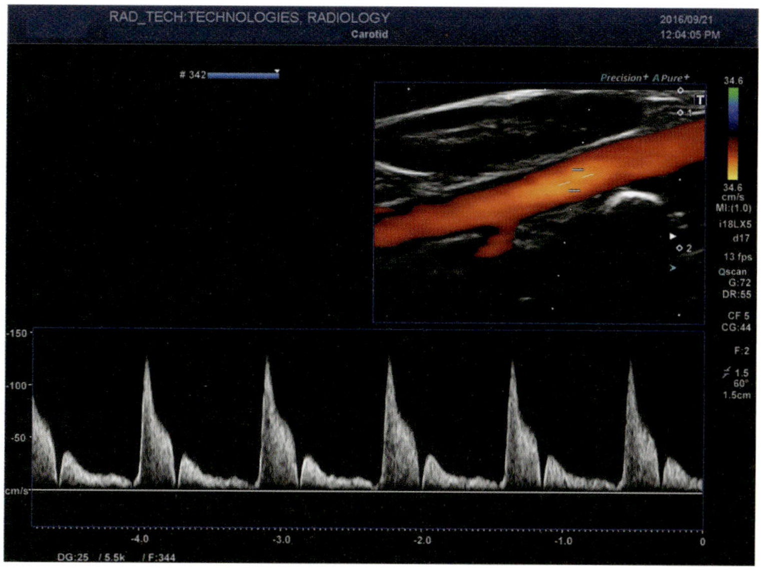

Fig. 1.14 Spectral-Doppler display of blood flow in the carotid artery. The anatomical image shows the direction (*dotted line*) and specific location (*small horizontal lines on top of dotted line*) from which the spectral-Doppler information was acquired.

REVIEW

The following key points are presented in this chapter:

- Medical imaging with ultrasound is called diagnostic ultrasound imaging or sonography.
- Diagnostic ultrasound is accomplished with the pulse-echo technique.
- Echoes from tissue interfaces and other anatomical structures map these structures in an ultrasound image.
- Ultrasound images are composed of many (hundreds) of scan lines.
- Two principles of operation are present in the variety of current, commercially available, sonographic systems.
- A 2D ultrasound image is presented in linear (rectangular) or sector forms.
- Ultrasound images can be displayed in 2D, 3D, or 4D formats.
- The Doppler effect is a change in frequency caused by objects moving relative to each other.
- Doppler information is presented in audible, color flow (color or power Doppler imaging), and spectral Doppler forms.

EXERCISES

Answers appear in the Answers to Exercises section at the back of the book.

1. The diagnostic ultrasound imaging (sonography) method has two parts:
(1) Sending ____________ of ____________ into the body and (2) using ____________ received from the anatomy to produce a(n) ____________ of that anatomy.
a. packs, sound, information, listing
b. pulses, frequencies, echoes, description
c. ultrasound, scans, power, image
d. pulses, ultrasound, echoes, image

2. Ultrasound grayscale scans are ____________-____________ images of tissue cross-sections and volumes.
a. pulse-echo
b. virtual-anatomic
c. pseudo-gray
d. artificially presented

3. The brightness of an echo, as presented on the display, represents the ____________ of the echo.
a. strength
b. location
c. origin
d. frequency

4. A linear scan is composed of many ____________, ____________ scan lines.
a. horizontal, parallel
b. horizontal, curved
c. vertical, parallel
d. vertical, curved

5. A sector scan is composed of many scan lines with a common ____________.
a. length
b. brightness
c. origin
d. direction

6. A linear scan has a ___________ shape.
   a. linear
   b. round
   c. square
   d. rectangular
7. The shape of a sector scan is similar to a ___________ of ___________.
   a. slice, pie
   b. slice, bread
   c. scoop, pudding
   d. loaf, bread
8. A sector scan can have a(n) ___________ or a ___________ top.
   a. angled, straight
   b. pointed, curved
   c. normal, inverted
   d. curved, angled
9. Fig. 1.15 is an example of an image in which the scan lines do not originate at a common _______.
   a. amplitude
   b. disease
   c. origin
   d. time

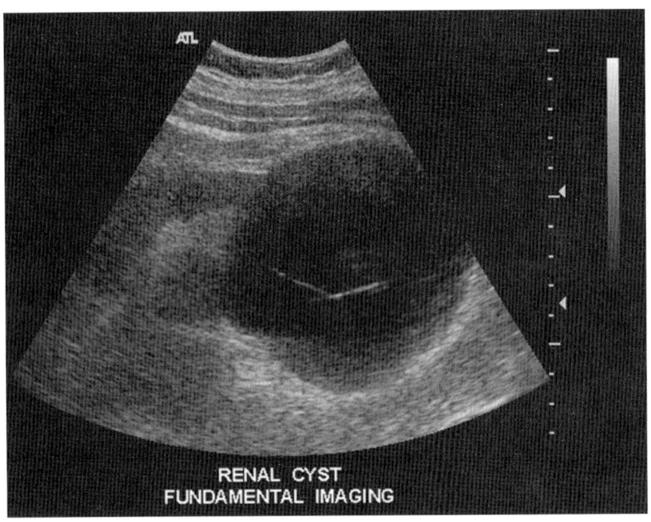

Fig. 1.15 Illustration to accompany Exercise 9.

10. Sonography is accomplished by using a pulse-echo technique. The important information gained from this technique includes the ___________ from which each echo originated and the ___________ of each echo. From this information, the instrument can determine the echo ___________ and _________ on the display.
    a. location, strength, location, brightness
    b. location, frequency, frequency, color
    c. anatomy, time, delay, color
    d. anatomy, strength, delay, brightness
11. The ___________ is the interface between the patient and the instrument.
    a. sonographer
    b. Doppler
    c. transducer
    d. display
12. Transducers generate ultrasound ___________ and receive returning ___________.
    a. pulses, echoes
    b. waves, images
    c. echoes, pulses
    d. images, echoes
13. Echo information in 3D is presented on ___________ displays.
    a. TV
    b. 2D
    c. 3D
    d. 4D
14. Acquisition of a 3D echo data volume requires scanning the ultrasound through several tissue ___________.
    a. angles
    b. orientations
    c. types
    d. cross-sections
15. The Doppler effect is a change in echo ___________.
    a. amplitude
    b. intensity
    c. impedance
    d. frequency
    e. arrival time
16. The change referred to in Exercise 15 is a result of ___________.
    a. pathology
    b. motion
    c. pulses
    d. echoes
17. The motion that produces the Doppler effect is that of the ___________.
    a. transducer
    b. sound beam
    c. display
    d. reflector
18. In medical applications, the flow of ___________ is commonly the source of the Doppler effect. Doppler information is applied to ___________ for audible evaluation and to ___________ for visual analysis.
    a. urine, loudspeakers, computers
    b. blood, earphones, computers
    c. lymph, earphones, displays
    d. blood, loudspeakers, displays

19. The visual display of Doppler information can be in the form of a ___________Doppler display or a ___________ Doppler display.
   a. color, spectral
   b. grayscale, color
   c. linear, sector
   d. static, temporal
20. Color flow Doppler displays can present Doppler-___________ and Doppler-___________ information in color.
   a. frequency, shift
   b. frequency, pressure
   c. shift, power
   d. bandwidth, shift
21. Fig. 1.16 shows a___________.
   a. 2D linear image
   b. 2D sector image
   c. modified sector image
   d. 3D grayscale image
   e. spectral display

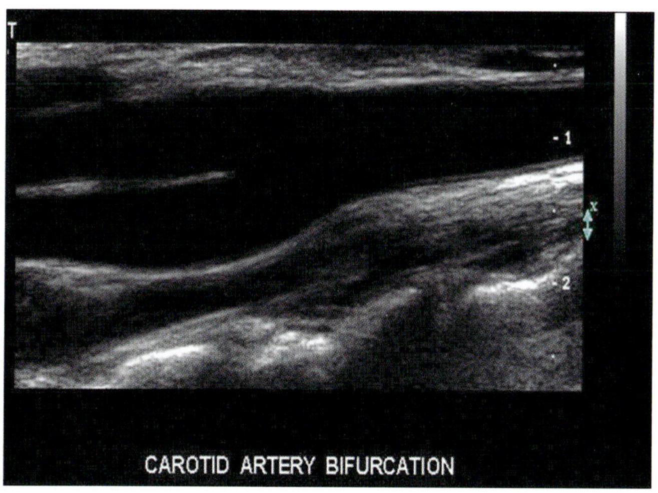

Fig. 1.16 Illustration to accompany Exercise 21.

22. Fig. 1.17 shows a ___________.
   a. 2D linear image
   b. 2D sector image
   c. modified sector image
   d. 3D volume scale image
   e. spectral display

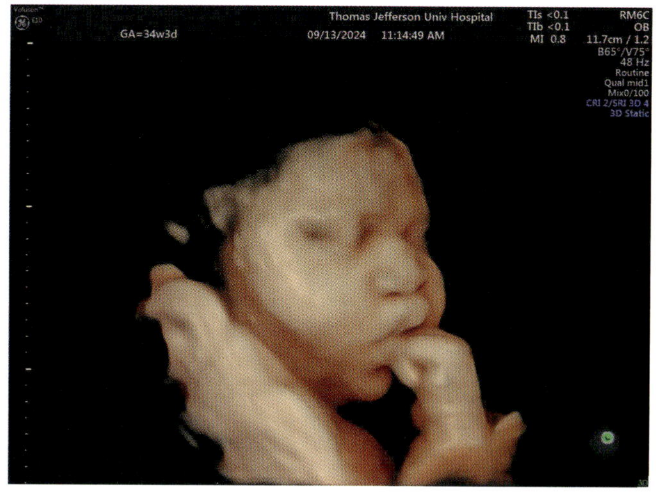

Fig. 1.17 Illustration to accompany Exercise 22. (Courtesy Corinne DeStefano & Vincenzo Berghella, Thomas Jefferson University Hospital.)

23. Fig. 1.18 shows a ___________.
   a. 2D linear image
   b. 2D sector image
   c. modified sector image
   d. 3D gray-scale image
   e. spectral display

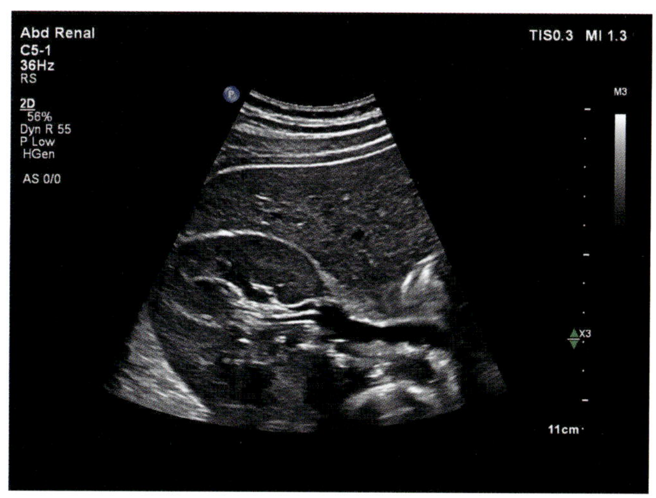

Fig. 1.18 Illustration to accompany Exercise 23.

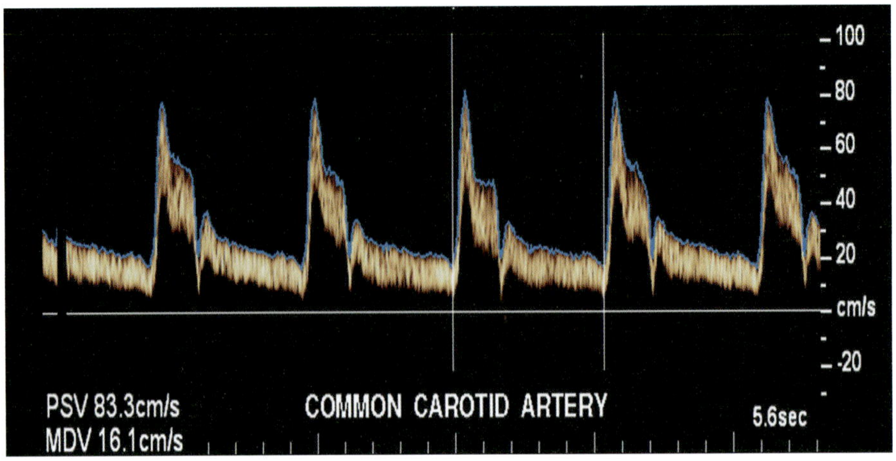

Fig. 1.19 Illustration to accompany Exercise 24.

24. Fig. 1.19 shows a ___________.
    - **a.** 2D linear image
    - **b.** 2D sector image
    - **c.** modified sector image
    - **d.** 3D gray-scale image
    - **e.** spectral display
25. Fig. 1.20 shows a ___________.
    - **a.** 2D linear image
    - **b.** 2D sector image
    - **c.** modified sector image
    - **d.** 3D gray-scale image
    - **e.** spectral display

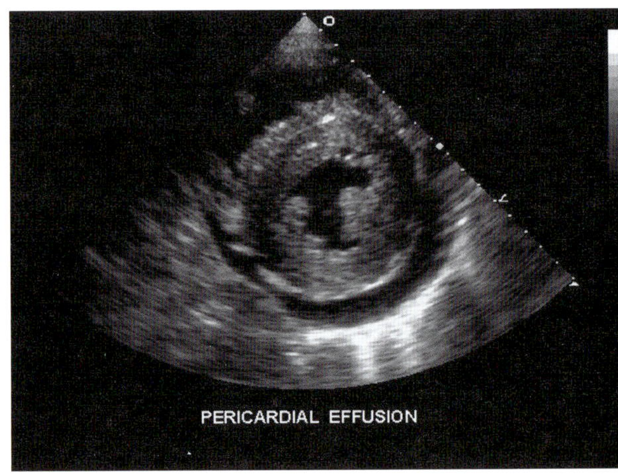

Fig. 1.20 Illustration to accompany Exercise 25.

2

Ultrasound: Sound We Don't Hear

LEARNING OBJECTIVES

After reading this chapter, the student should be able to do the following:

- Explain the concept of frequency and its importance in diagnostic ultrasound.
- Define ultrasound and describe its behavior.
- Discuss how harmonics are generated.
- Compare continuous and pulsed ultrasound.
- Describe the weakening of ultrasound while it travels through tissue.
- Discuss the generation of echoes in tissue.
- Define detail resolution.
- Discuss three aspects of detail resolution (axial, lateral, and elevational).
- Differentiate among resolution.
- List the factors that determine detail resolution.

CHAPTER OUTLINE

Sound
Pulsed Ultrasound
Attenuation
Echoes
Detail Resolution

KEY TERMS

Absorption
Acoustic
Acoustic variables
Amplitude
Attenuation
Attenuation coefficient
Axial
Axial resolution
Backscatter
Bandwidth
Compression
Constructive interference
Continuous wave
Coupling medium
Cycle
Decibel
Density
Destructive interference
Detail resolution
Duty factor
Echo
Elevational resolution
Energy
Fractional bandwidth
Frequency
Fundamental frequency
Harmonics
Hertz
Impedance
Incidence angle
Intensity
Intensity reflection coefficient
Intensity transmission coefficient
Interference
KiloHertz
Lateral
Lateral resolution
Longitudinal wave
Medium
MegaHertz
Nonlinear propagation
Oblique incidence
Penetration
Period
Perpendicular
Perpendicular incidence
Power
Pressure
Propagation
Propagation speed
Pulse
Pulse duration
Pulse-repetition frequency
Pulse-repetition period
Pulsed ultrasound
Range equation
Rarefaction
Rayl
Reflection
Reflection angle
Reflector
Refraction
Resolution
Scatterer
Scattering
Shear wave
Sound
Spatial pulse length
Speckle
Specular reflection
Stiffness
Strength
Transmission angle
Transverse wave
Ultrasound
Wave
Wavelength

Sound is defined in two primary ways—by our experience (what we hear with our human auditory system) and by the physical principle. The physical concept describes what travels from the source of the sound to the listener or receiver, and this forms the cornerstone of our understanding of diagnostic ultrasound. Ultrasound is similar to the ordinary sound we hear except that it is beyond the range of human hearing (i.e., its frequency is too high as discussed later in this chapter). While ultrasound travels through the human body, it interacts with the anatomy in ways that enable its use in diagnostic imaging. In this chapter, we consider what ultrasound is, how it is described, and how it travels through and interacts with human anatomy. After digesting this material, you will be prepared to learn in subsequent chapters how ultrasound is generated, received, and processed to produce anatomic, ultrasound images and to detect and present motion and flow information.

SOUND

Waves

Diagnostic ultrasound imaging uses ultrasound to produce images of the internal anatomy, tissue motion, and blood flow. Ultrasound is a form of sound. Through our sense of hearing, we experience sound daily. Nonetheless, the physical principle of sound is less evident. In spoken communication, sound is produced by a speaker and is heard by a listener. Sound travels from the speaker to the listener, so it is something that travels (i.e., propagates) through a medium such as air. But what is this sound that is traveling through air? Sound is a traveling variation in pressure (Fig. 2.1, A). When the speaker speaks, variations in pressure are produced in the throat and mouth. These pressure variations travel through air to the listener, where they stimulate the auditory response in the ear and brain.

In more general terms, we can say that sound is an acoustic wave. A wave is a traveling variation in one or more quantities called wave variables. For example, a water wave is a traveling variation in water surface height. Dropping a pebble into a pond disturbs the surface of the water, causing it to move up and down. These up-and-down movements then travel across the surface of the pond so that motion, similar to that generated where the pebble entered the water, eventually occurs at the far shore. Similar to water waves, sound involves mechanical motion in the medium through which it travels. The pressure variations in the sound wave cause the particles of the medium to vibrate back and forth.

> A wave is a traveling variation of a quantity or quantities called wave variables.

Associated with pressure variations in a sound wave, density variations also exist. Density is the concentration of matter (mass per unit volume). Pressure, density, and particle vibration are called acoustic variables, because they are quantities that vary in a sound wave. While sound travels through a medium, pressure and density go through cycles of increase and decrease, and particles of the med ium oscillate in motion. At any point in the medium, pressure and density increase and decrease in repetitive cycles while the sound wave moves through (or travels past) that point. Regions of low pressure and density are called rarefactions, and regions of high pressure and density are called compressions. Compressions and rarefactions travel through a

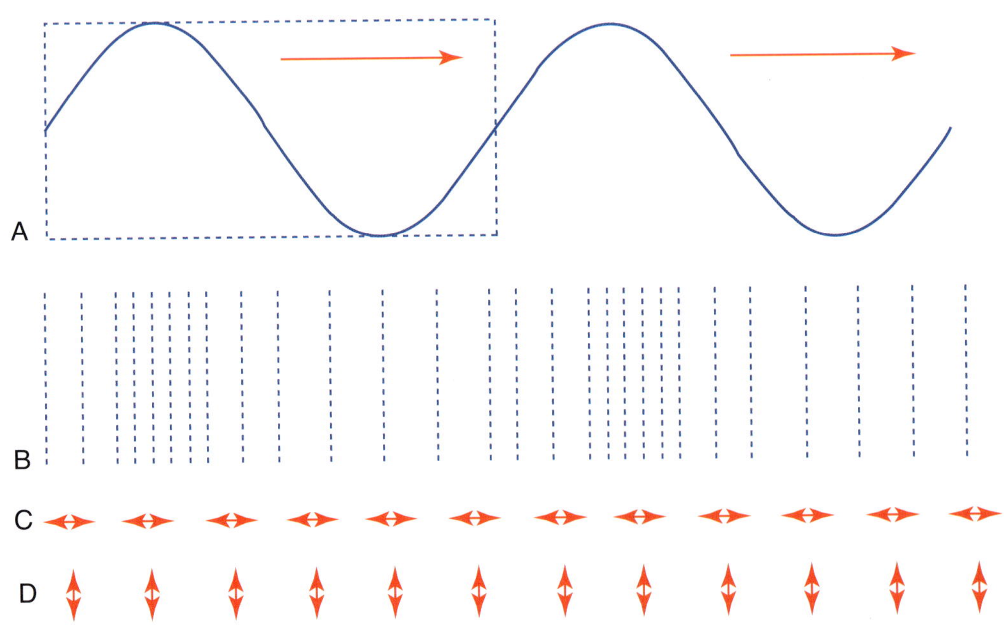

Fig. 2.1 A, Sound is a traveling pressure variation. The box encloses one cycle of pressure variation. The pressure wave in this example is traveling to the right, as indicated by the arrows. **B,** Sound is also a traveling density variation. Regions of compression (high density) and rarefaction (low density) travel along with the high- and low-pressure regions of the wave. **C,** Particles vibrate back and forth in a sound wave. This vibratory motion is parallel to the direction of travel of the wave. Such a wave is called a longitudinal wave. Thus sound is a longitudinal, compressional pressure wave. **D,** A transverse (shear) wave involves motion perpendicular to the direction of wave travel.

medium with a sound wave (see Fig. 2.1, B). Sound requires a physical medium through which to travel; that is, it cannot pass through a vacuum. Sound is a mechanical, compressional wave in which back-and-forth particle motion is parallel to the direction of wave travel (see Fig. 2.1, C). Such a wave is called a **longitudinal wave** or compressional wave.

The up-and-down motion of a water surface is **perpendicular** to the direction the wave travels in. This type of wave is called a **transverse wave** or **shear wave** (see Fig. 2.1, D). Electromagnetic waves such as light, radio, x-rays, and microwaves are transverse waves of electric and magnetic fields that involve no particle motion. The particle motion of sound waves contains both wave elements that are parallel to the direction of wave travel (a longitudinal wave, which is what is commonly used in ultrasound imaging), and waves that travel perpendicular to the direction of wave travel (rarely used in diagnostic ultrasound except in the case of shear-wave elastography; discussed in Chapter 6).

> Sound is a traveling variation of acoustic variables.

> Acoustic variables include pressure, density, and particle motion.

Sound is described by terms that are used to describe all waves. These terms include *frequency*, *period*, *wavelength*, *propagation speed*, *amplitude*, and *intensity*.

Frequency

Frequency (f) is a measurement of how often something happens. For example, there are 365 days in a year and 24 hours in a day. Frequency, as it relates to sound, is a count of how many complete variations (cycles) of pressure (or any other acoustic variable) occur in 1 second. As shown in Fig. 2.1, A, pressure starts at its normal (undisturbed) value. This would be the pressure in the medium if no sound were traveling (or propagating) through it. While a sound wave travels through a medium, the pressure at any point in the medium increases to a maximum value, returns to normal, decreases to a minimum value, and returns to normal. This is a description of a complete cycle of variation in pressure as an acoustic variable.

> A cycle is one complete variation in pressure or another acoustic variable.

The positive and negative halves of a pressure cycle correspond to compression and rarefaction, respectively. In other words, when the pressure is higher, the medium is denser (more tightly packed), and when the pressure is lower, the medium is less dense (spread more out). While a sound wave travels past a point in the medium, this cycle of increasing and decreasing pressure and density is repeated over and over. The number of times it is repeated in 1 second is called *frequency* (Fig. 2.2). Thus frequency is the number of cycles that occur per second. Frequency units include **Hertz** (Hz), **kiloHertz** (kHz), and **megaHertz** (MHz). One Hertz is one cycle per second. One kiloHertz equals 1000 Hz. One megaHertz equals 1,000,000 Hz.

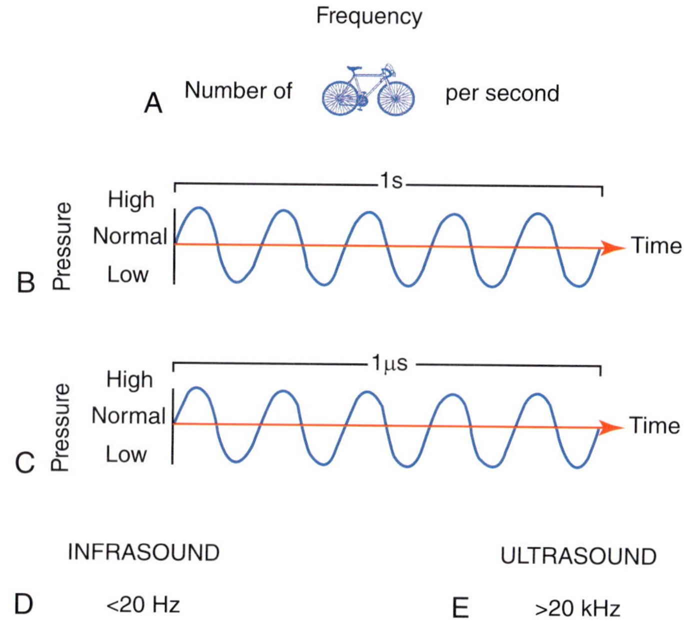

Fig. 2.2 A, Frequency is the number of complete variations (cycles) that an acoustic variable (pressure, in this case) goes through in 1 s. **B,** Five cycles occur in 1 s; thus the frequency is five cycles per second, or 5 Hz. **C,** If five cycles occur within one-millionth of a second, also known as a microsecond (1 μs) (i.e., 5 million cycles occurring in 1 s), the frequency is 5 MHz. **D,** Infrasound is sound that human beings cannot hear because the frequencies are too low (less than 20 Hz). **E,** Ultrasound is sound that human beings cannot hear because the frequencies are too high (greater than 20 kHz).

> Frequency is the number of cycles in a wave that occur in 1 second.

> One Hertz equals one cycle per second. The abbreviation for Hertz is *Hz*.

> One kiloHertz equals 1000 cycles per second. The abbreviation for kiloHertz is *kHz*.

> One megaHertz equals one million cycles per second. The abbreviation for megaHertz is *MHz*.

Human hearing operates in a frequency range of approximately 20 to 20,000 Hz (or 20 kHz), although great variation exists on the upper frequency limit in individuals. Sound with a frequency of less than 20 Hz is called *infrasound*, because its frequency is too low for human hearing. Sound with a frequency of 20,000 Hz or higher is called *ultrasound*, because its frequency is too high for human hearing. Frequency is important in diagnostic ultrasound, because of its impact on the **resolution** and **penetration** of ultrasound images. Frequency is controlled by the choice of transducer and by the ultrasound scanner.

> Infrasound is sound of a frequency too low for human hearing.

> Ultrasound is sound of a frequency too high for human hearing.

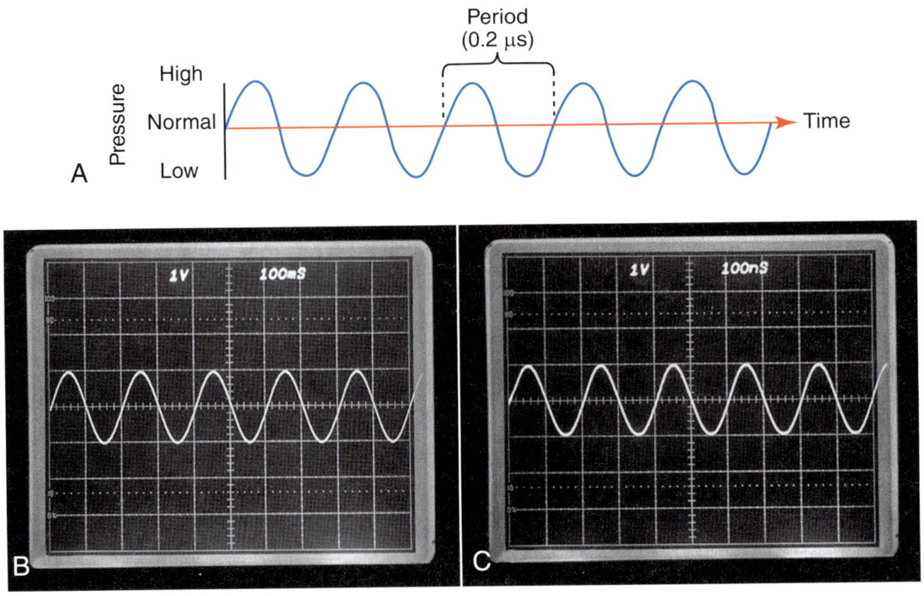

Fig. 2.3 Period is the time it takes for one cycle to occur. **A,** Each cycle occurs in 0.2 μs, so the period is 0.2 μs. If one cycle takes 0.2 (or one-fifth) millionths of a second to occur, it means that 5 million cycles occur in 1 s, so the frequency is 5 MHz. **B,** Photograph of a tracing of a 5-Hz wave. The total screen width represents 1 s. One can see that five cycles occur in 1 s and that each cycle takes one-fifth (0.2) of a second to occur (period). If this were a pressure wave, it would be an example of infrasound (frequency is 5 Hz, i.e., less than 20 Hz). **C,** In this tracing, the total screen width is 1 μs. If five cycles occur in 1 μs, the period is 0.2 μs, and the frequency is 5 MHz, as in **A**. If this were a pressure wave, it would be an example of ultrasound (frequency greater than 20 kHz).

Period

Period (T) is the time that it takes for one cycle to occur (Fig. 2.3). In ultrasound, the common unit for period is the microsecond (μs). One microsecond equals one-millionth of a second (0.000001 second). For example, the period for 5 MHz ultrasound equals 0.2 μs. Because 5 MHz ultrasound contains 5 million cycles in a second, each cycle has only one-fifth of a millionth of a second (0.2 μs) to occur. The importance of the period will become apparent when **pulsed ultrasound** is considered in the next section. Table 2.1 lists common periods. Period decreases while frequency increases because, when more cycles are packed into 1 second, there is less time for each one. Indeed, period equals 1 divided by frequency.

$$T(\mu s) = \frac{1}{f(MHz)}$$

> Period is the time that it takes for one cycle to occur.

> If frequency increases, period decreases.

Wavelength

Wavelength (λ) is the length of space that one cycle occupies (Fig. 2.4). If we could stop a sound wave, visualize it, and measure the distance from the beginning to the end of one cycle, the measured distance would be the wavelength of the sound wave. Wavelength is the length of a cycle from "front" to "back."

TABLE 2.1 Common Ultrasound Periods and Wavelengths in Tissue

Frequency (MHz)	Period (μs)	Wavelength (mm)[a]
2.0	0.50	0.77
3.5	0.29	0.44
5.0	0.20	0.31
7.5	0.13	0.21
10.0	0.10	0.15
15.0	0.07	0.10

[a]Assuming a (soft tissue) propagation speed of 1.54 mm/μs (1540 m/s).

More precisely, it could be called *cycle length*, but traditionally it has been called *wavelength*. For ultrasound, wavelength is commonly expressed in millimeters. One millimeter (1 mm) is one-thousandth of a meter (0.001 m). The importance of wavelength will be evident when **detail resolution** of images is considered. Table 2.1 lists common wavelengths in sonography.

> Wavelength is the length of a cycle in space.

Propagation Speed

Propagation speed (c) is the speed with which a wave moves through a medium. For sound, **propagation** speed is the speed at which a particular value of an acoustic variable moves (Fig. 2.5), at which a cycle moves, and at which the entire wave moves. All of these are the same speed. Relevant propagation

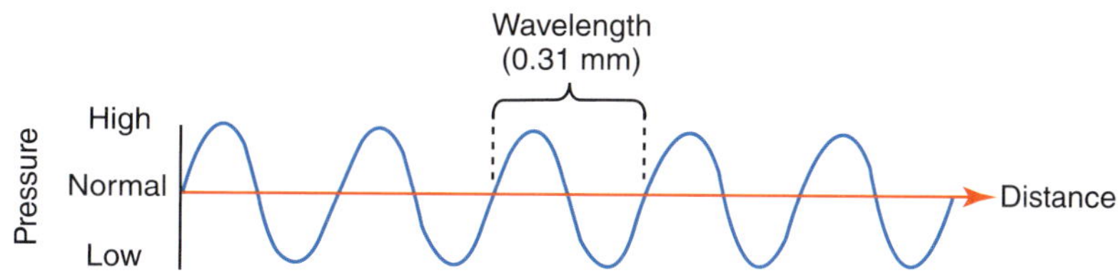

Fig. 2.4 Wavelength is the length of space over which one cycle occurs. In this figure, each cycle covers 0.31 mm. Thus the wavelength is 0.31 mm. This figure differs from Figs. 2.2 and 2.3 in that the horizontal axis represents distance rather than time. For a propagation speed of 1.54 mm/μs and a frequency of 5 MHz, the wavelength is 0.31 mm.

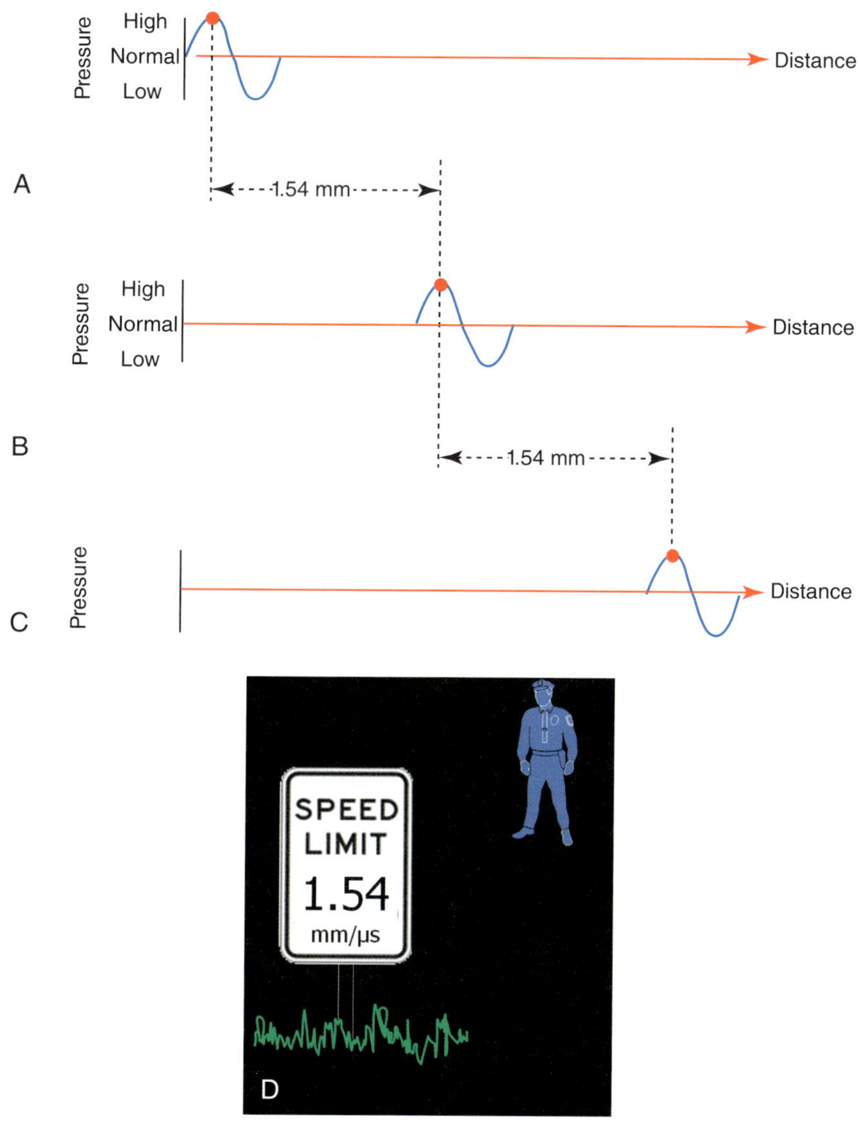

Fig. 2.5 Propagation speed is the speed with which a particular value of an acoustic variable (also the rest of the cycle and, indeed, the entire wave) travels through a medium. **A,** The movement of a maximum (identified by the *red dot*) is shown in this figure. **B,** 1 μs after A. **C,** 1 μs after B and 2 μs after **A**. The maximum (dot) moves 1.54 mm in 1 μs and 3.08 mm in 2 μs. The propagation speed is 1.54 mm/μs. The propagation speed in this figure (1.54 mm/μs), when divided by the frequency in Figure 2.3, C (5 MHz), equals the wavelength in Figure 2.4 (0.31 mm). **D,** Propagation speeds in soft tissue average 1540 m/s, or 1.54 mm/μs.

speed units include meters per second (m/s) and millimeters per microsecond (mm/μs).

ADVANCED CONCEPT

Speed is the rate of change of position of an object. Speed is often called velocity, although, strictly speaking, velocity is defined as speed with direction of motion specified. An example of wind speed might be 25 miles per hour (mph), but its velocity would be 25 mph out of the northwest.

Propagation speed is the speed at which a wave moves through a medium.

Wavelength depends on frequency and propagation speed. The relationship between the three is that wavelength is equal to propagation speed divided by frequency.

$$\lambda(\text{mm}) = \frac{c\ (\text{mm}/\mu\text{s})}{f\ (\text{MHz})}$$

This equation shows that wavelength will decrease when frequency increases, which is confirmed in Table 2.1. Later we will see that detail resolution improves with increasing frequency because of the decrease in wavelength.

> If frequency increases, wavelength decreases.

An example of the relationship among frequency, wavelength, and propagation speed is seen by comparing Figs. 2.3, C; 2.4; and 2.5. In these figures, frequency is 5 MHz, wavelength is 0.31 mm, and propagation speed is 1.54 mm/μs (or 1540 m/s) given the following equation:

$$\lambda(\text{mm}) = \frac{c\ (\text{mm}/\mu\text{s})}{f\ (\text{MHz})} = \frac{1.54\ \text{mm}/\mu\text{s}}{5\ \text{MHz}} = 0.31\ \text{mm}$$

Propagation speed is determined by the medium, primarily its stiffness (hardness). **Stiffness** is the resistance of a material to compression. Stiffness is the inverse of compressibility; that is, a compressible material such as a sponge has low stiffness, and a stiff (hard) material such as a rock has low compressibility. Stiffer media have higher sound speeds. Thus propagation speeds are lower in gases (which are highly compressible), higher in liquids, and highest in solids (which are nearly incompressible). The average longitudinal propagation speed in soft tissues is 1540 m/s, or (in more relevant units for our purposes) 1.54 mm/μs. Values for soft tissues range from 1.44 to 1.64 mm/μs. These values are similar to those for liquids such as water, which is not surprising, since soft tissue is mostly water. Shear waves travel much more slowly than longitudinal waves. Shear wave propagation speeds in tissues range from 0.5 to 10 m/s.

> Propagation speeds are highest in solids and lowest in gases.

> The average propagation speed of sound in soft tissues is 1.54 mm/μs.

In the bowel, because it contains gas, the propagation speed of sound is much lower than in other soft tissues. However, this difference is not important because ultrasound does not penetrate air-filled bowels well enough for imaging. In bone, because it is a solid, propagation speeds are higher (3–5 mm/μs) than in soft tissues. Soft tissue propagation speeds are within a few percent of the average, so the average can be assumed for all soft tissues with relatively little error. Fat is farthest from the average, about 6% lower. Nonetheless, propagation speed is important, because ultrasound scanners use it to place echoes on the display. Hence, more and more systems do estimate sound speed variations throughout the image and compensate for any discrepancies in object location.

ADVANCED CONCEPT

The propagation speed in any medium depends on the density (ρ) and stiffness of the medium. By density, we mean *mass density,* which is the mass per unit volume. The stiffness is the resistance to compression, also called the hardness or the bulk modulus of elasticity (B). The reciprocal of bulk modulus is the compressibility of a medium. Specifically, propagation speed depends on the bulk modulus-density ratio:

$$c(\text{m/s}) = \left[\frac{B(\text{N/m}^2)}{\rho(\text{kg/m}^3)}\right]^{1/2}$$

This relationship predicts that an increase in bulk modulus increases propagation speed and that an increase in density decreases propagation speed. If we compare gases, liquids, and solids, we find that generally more dense materials have higher propagation speeds, not lower. The reason is that higher-density materials generally have higher stiffness also, and the stiffness differences between materials are generally greater than the density differences. Thus the stiffness differences dominate the effect on the propagation speed so that, in general, solids have higher propagation speeds than liquids, and liquids have higher speeds than gases.

Harmonics

The dependence of propagation speed on pressure causes strong sound (pressure) waves to change shape while they travel (Fig. 2.6), because the higher pressure portions of the wave travel faster than the lower pressure portions. This movement changes a wave that originally has a smooth curve shape (called *sinusoidal*; illustrated in Fig. 2.6, A) and it will progress toward a saw-tooth nonsinusoidal shape (see Fig. 2.6, C). Propagation in which speed depends on pressure and the shape of the wave changes is called **nonlinear propagation**. A continuous (not pulsed) sinusoidal waveform is characterized by a single frequency (equal to the number of cycles per second). Any other wave shape contains additional frequencies that are even and odd multiples of the original frequency. The original

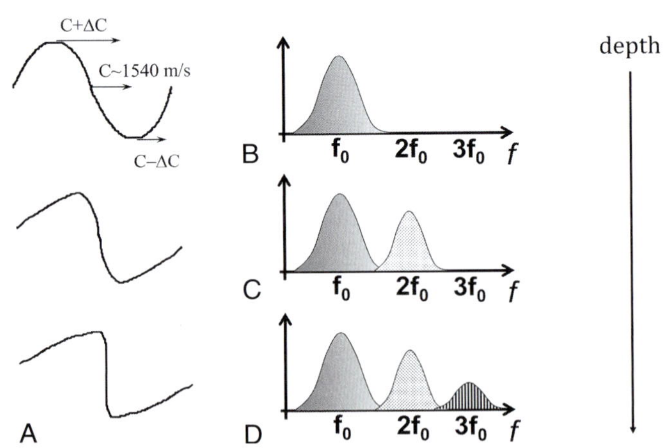

Fig. 2.6 In nonlinear propagation, propagation speed depends on pressure and compression. **A,** Higher-pressure portions of the wave travel faster than the lower-pressure portions, because the molecules are closer together (compressed). **B–C,** Thus the wave changes shape while it travels deeper. **D,** This change from the initial sinusoidal shape introduces harmonics that are even and odd multiples of the fundamental frequency.

frequency is called the **fundamental frequency.** The even and odd multiples are called *even* and *odd* **harmonics**, respectively. A frequency analysis of the wave in Fig. 2.6, A would yield a single (fundamental) frequency such as 2 MHz. Analysis of parts B and C would reveal, in addition to fundamental frequency, harmonics at 4, 6, and 8 MHz. While the shape becomes less sinusoidal, the harmonics become stronger. Therefore they are stronger in part C than in part B. The use of harmonic frequency echoes (so called tissue harmonic imaging) improves the quality of ultrasound images and will be discussed in more detail in Chapter 6.

> Harmonics are even and odd multiples of the fundamental frequency.

PULSED ULTRASOUND

Thus far we have discussed terms (*frequency*, *period*, *wavelength*, and *propagation speed*) that are sufficient to describe **continuous wave** (CW) ultrasound in which cycles repeat indefinitely. However, most ultrasound, imaging uses pulsed ultrasound rather than CW. Pulsed ultrasound is not on continuously but rather consists of a few cycles of ultrasound (i.e., a pulse). **Pulses** are separated in time with gaps of no ultrasound. Ultrasound pulses are described by some additional parameters that we will now discuss.

> With CW ultrasound, cycles repeat indefinitely. Pulsed ultrasound consists of pulses separated by gaps in time. A pulse is a few cycles of ultrasound.

Pulse-Repetition Frequency and Period

The term *frequency* is the number of cycles occurring per second for in CW mode. For a pulsed wave, it is the number of cycles per second within the transmitted pulse. Similarly, the **pulse-repetition frequency** (PRF) is the number of *pulses* that occur in 1 second (Fig. 2.7). Diagnostic ultrasound typically involves a few thousand pulses per second, so PRF is commonly expressed in kHz. One kHz equals 1000 Hz. Frequency (the number of cycles per second) and PRF (the number of pulses per second) are independently controlled by operator (sonographer) of the ultrasound scanner or by the scanner itself.

The term *period* refers to the time for one cycle to occur, whereas **pulse-repetition period** (PRP) refers to the time from the beginning of one pulse to the beginning of the next (Fig. 2.8). Its common units are milliseconds (ms, or one-thousandth of a second). The PRP is the reciprocal of PRF. Hence, the PRP decreases as the PRF increases because, when more pulses occur in a second, the time between them decreases.

$$\text{PRP(ms)} = \frac{1}{\text{PRF(kHz)}}$$

PRF is controlled automatically by the scanner to satisfy requirements that are discussed later. With Doppler techniques, the operator controls PRF, which is also described in later chapters. PRF is important because it determines how quickly images are generated. For example, with a PRF of 5 kHz, 5000 pulses are produced each second, generating 5000 scan lines per second when using narrow (typically focused) transmit beams. If, for example, each image has 100 scan lines, 50 images will be produced per second. This is also called *frame*

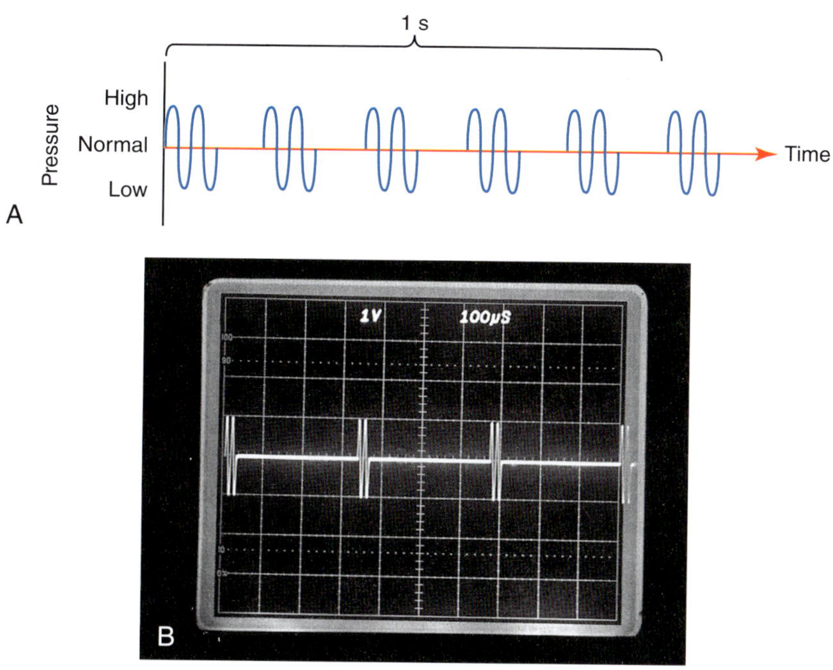

Fig. 2.7 Pulse-repetition frequency (*PRF*) is the number of pulses that occur in 1 s. **A,** Five pulses (containing two cycles each) occur in 1 s; thus the PRF is 5 Hz. **B,** In this photograph, three pulses occur in 1 ms (or one-thousandth of a second); thus the PRF is 3 kHz. The total scaled screen width is 1 ms.

rate, and it will determine how well rapidly moving structures can be followed.

PRF is the number of pulses that occur in 1 second.

PRP is the time from the beginning of one pulse to the beginning of the next one.

If PRF increases, PRP decreases as they are inversely proportional.

Pulse Duration

Pulse duration (PD) is the time that it takes for one pulse to occur (see Fig. 2.8). PD is equal to the period (T, the time for one cycle) times the number of cycles in the pulse (n) and is expressed in microseconds. Grayscale imaging pulses are typically two or three cycles long. Compared with longer ones, shorter pulses improve the (axial) resolution of the images (i.e., the ability to resolve closely spaced scatterers in an image). Doppler ultrasound pulses are typically 5 to 32 cycles long.

$$PD(\mu s) = n \times T(\mu s)$$

Diagnostic ultrasound pulses are typically two or three cycles long. Doppler pulses are typically 5 to 32 cycles long.

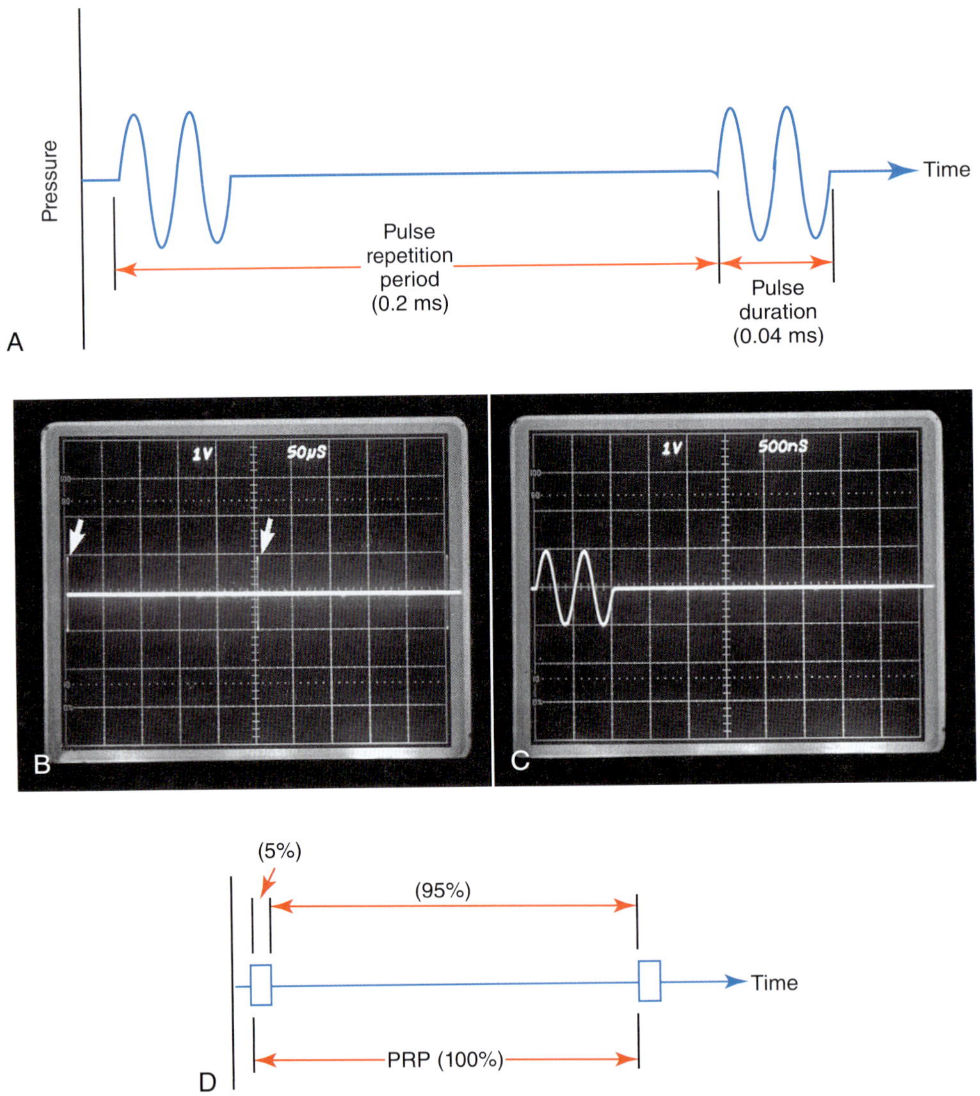

Fig. 2.8 The pulse-repetition period *(PRP)* is the time from the beginning of one pulse to the beginning of the next. **A,** The PRP is 0.2 ms (200 μs). Therefore the pulse-repetition frequency is 5 kHz. The pulse duration (PD) is the time that it takes for one pulse to occur. The PD is equal to the period multiplied by the number of cycles in the pulse. The PD is 40 μs. The duty factor (DF) is the fraction of time that sound is on. The DF is 40/200, which equals 0.2, or 20%. **B,** This photograph shows that the PRP is 0.25 ms (the pulse-repetition frequency is 4 kHz). The period is 0.5 μs, as shown expanded in **C,** and the PD is 1 μs. From one pulse to the next (PRP of 0.25 ms, or 250 μs), the sound is on (PD) for 1 μs. The DF in this example is 0.004, or 0.4%. The screen width is 0.5 ms in **B** and 5 μs in **C**. **D,** The DF is the fraction of time that pulsed ultrasound is actually on. In this example, the PRP represents 100% of the time from the start of one pulse to the start of the next one. Of this time, the sound is on 5% of the time (PD divided by PRP) and off 95% of the time.

PD decreases if the number of cycles in a pulse is decreased or if the frequency is increased (reducing the period). In general terms, the operator of the ultrasound system chooses the imaging frequency.

> PD is the time for a pulse to occur.

> If frequency is increased, period is decreased, reducing PD. If the number of cycles in a pulse is reduced, PD is decreased. Shorter pulses improve the axial resolution of ultrasound images.

Duty Factor

Duty factor (DF) is the fraction of time that pulsed ultrasound is on (see Fig. 2.8, D). CW ultrasound is on 100% of the time (hence, the name). Pulsed ultrasound, by definition, is not on all of the time. The DF indicates how much of the time the ultrasound is on. Longer pulses increase the DF because the sound is on more of the time.

> DF is the fraction of time that pulsed ultrasound is on.

DF is the fraction of the PRP that the sound is on. The remainder of the time to the next pulse is the time for receiving echoes that will form a scan line on the instrument display. Higher PRFs increase the DF because there is less listening time between pulses. Thus the DF increases with increasing PD or PRF. DF has no units because it is a fraction with time in both the numerator and denominator. Thus the DF is simply expressed as a decimal, such as 0.10 or 0.25, or more often as a percentage, such as 10% or 25%. The importance of the DF will become evident when intensities and safety issues are discussed later. The DF is equal to PD divided by the PRP, because PD represents the amount of time that sound is on, and the PRP is the time from one pulse to the next. Thus the ratio of the two represents the fraction of time that pulsed ultrasound is on.

$$DF = \frac{PD(\mu s)}{PRP(\mu s)} = \frac{PD(\mu s) \times PRF(kHz)}{1000(kHz/MHz)}$$

The factor of 1000 converts kilohertz to megahertz to be consistent with microseconds of PD. Multiplying the DF by 100 expresses it as a percentage. For example, if the PD is 2 μs and the PRP is 250 μs, then

$$DF = \frac{2}{250} = 0.008 \text{ or } 0.8\%$$

A range of DFs is encountered in diagnostic ultrasound because of the various conditions chosen by the instrument and the operator. Typical DFs are in the range of 0.1% to 1.0%. For Doppler ultrasound, because of longer PDs, the range of typical DFs is 0.5% to 5.0%.

> If the PD increases, the DF increases.

> If PRF increases, PRP decreases and DF increases.

Spatial Pulse Length

If we could stop a pulse, visualize it, and measure the distance from its beginning to its end, the measured distance would be spatial pulse length (SPL). **SPL** is the length of a pulse from front to back (Fig. 2.9, A). SPL is equal to the length of each cycle times the number of cycles in the pulse. The length of each cycle is a wavelength. Hence, SPL increases with wavelength and increases with the number of cycles in the pulse.

> SPL is the length of space occupied by a pulse.

Because wavelength decreases with increasing frequency, SPL decreases with increasing frequency (Fig. 2.9, B–C). Units for SPL are in millimeters (mm). SPL is an important quantity when considering detail resolution because shorter pulse lengths improve resolution.

> If the number of cycles in a pulse increases, SPL increases. If frequency increases, wavelength and SPL decrease.

> Shorter pulses improve detail resolution of ultrasound images.

Frequency

Frequency expresses the number of cycles in a wave that would occur in 1 second if the ultrasound lasted for an entire second. This is obviously the case for CW ultrasound; however, in pulsed ultrasound, there are gaps between pulses. For example, in 5 MHz CW ultrasound, there are actually 5 million cycles transmitted in 1 second. So what about 5 MHz pulsed ultrasound? The frequency, 5 MHz, indicates the number of cycles per second within the pulse being transmitted. The actual number of cycles that occur in 1 second for pulsed ultrasound depends on the DF. Say the DF is 0.01, or 1%, then the ultrasound is on (or present) only one-hundredth of the time, and the actual number of cycles per second is 50,000 (1% of 5 million). The quiet time between pulses eliminates 99% of the cycles in this example, even though the frequency implies that there are 5 million cycles per second. Nonetheless, the frequency for pulsed ultrasound is still given as 5 MHz, because the behavior of the pulses (regarding period, wavelength, propagation speed, and other characteristics such as attenuation) is identical to that of 5 MHz CW ultrasound.

Bandwidth

In contrast to CW ultrasound, which can be described by a single frequency, ultrasound pulses contain a range of frequencies

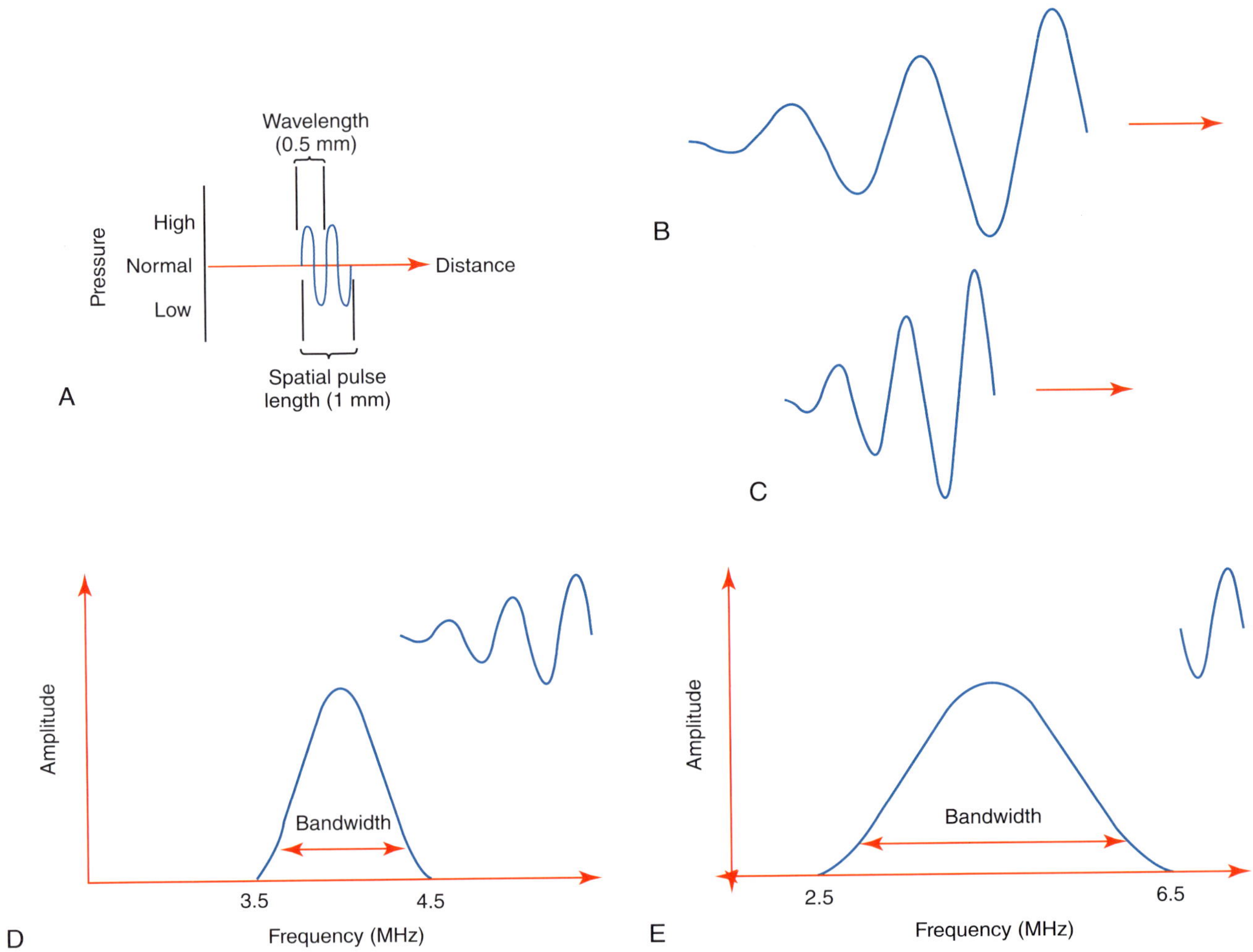

Fig. 2.9 **A,** Spatial pulse length (SPL) is the length of space over which a pulse occurs. SPL is equal to wavelength multiplied by the number of cycles in the pulse. In this figure, the wavelength is 0.5 mm, there are two cycles in each pulse, and the SPL is 0.5 × 2, or 1 mm. This figure differs from Figs. 2.7, A and 2.8, A in that the horizontal axis represents distance rather than time. **B–C,** Three-cycle damped (decreasing in amplitude) pulses of ultrasound traveling to the right. **B,** Lower-frequency pulse with longer wavelength and SPL. **C,** Higher-frequency pulse with shorter wavelength and SPL. **D–E,** Plots of the frequencies and the amplitude of each frequency component present in two ultrasound pulses. Bandwidth is the range of frequencies present. Compare the bandwidth for a narrow band, longer pulse **(D)** with the bandwidth for a broadband, shorter pulse **(E)**.

referred to as the **bandwidth** (Fig. 2.9, D–E). The shorter the pulse (the fewer the number of cycles), the higher the number of frequencies it contains (broader bandwidth), since time and frequency are inversely proportional. **Fractional bandwidth** is bandwidth divided by operating frequency and is unit-less. It describes how large the bandwidth is compared to the operating frequency.

> Bandwidth is the range of frequencies contained in a pulse.

Frequency is the number of cycles per second. Frequency determines the resolution and penetration achievable in ultrasound images, as discussed later. PRF is the number of pulses produced per second. It determines the number of scan lines produced per second and the number of images produced per second (the frame rate, which is discussed later).

ADVANCED CONCEPT

Bandwidth is specified by some definition of where in the frequency range it starts and stops. For example, a 6-dB bandwidth refers to the range of frequencies that includes those that have half or greater the amplitude (≥ one-fourth the power) of the strongest frequency component, which is the operating frequency. A 20-dB bandwidth includes amplitudes that are one-tenth or greater of the strongest (one-hundredth or greater the power). Clearly, a 20-dB bandwidth is greater than a 6-dB bandwidth even though they are describing the same pulse.

The reciprocal of fractional bandwidth is called *quality factor* (Q). The quality factor is given by operating frequency divided by bandwidth. Shorter pulses (with their broader bandwidths) have lower Qs. This may seem like a contradiction because we stated previously that shorter pulses produce better resolution. So how could this be a lower quality? In the early days of electronics, for example, in radio, narrow bandwidth was good (e.g., in radio, to tune in one station and, at the same time, to tune out another station that is nearby on the frequency dial). However, in much of modern electronics (including, e.g., the internet), broad bandwidth is good, being associated with, for example, high-fidelity sound and video and high information transmission rates. Thus it is best to forget that Q originally stood for "quality" and simply to think of it as "Q," since in many cases, including diagnostic ultrasound, low Q is good Q. In clinical practice, the Q term is not used very often. Fig. 2.10 gives two examples.

Bandwidth is often mentioned in connections with the internet. Broader bandwidth connections permit faster information transfer and thus cost more. To achieve higher information transmission rates, a higher bit rate is required. Bits (and gaps) must be shorter in temporal length to be transmitted at a higher bit rate. Shorter bits have broader bandwidth just as shorter ultrasound pulses do. Thus higher bit rates require broader bandwidth connections to accomplish.

ATTENUATION

We now consider the magnitude of the cyclic variations in a continuous or pulsed ultrasound wave. **Amplitude** and **intensity** are indicators of the **strength** of the sound. They are related to how loud the sound would be if it could be heard. Ultrasound, however, cannot be heard, so loudness is irrelevant. Nevertheless, amplitude and intensity are important indicators of how strong, or "intense," the ultrasound is.

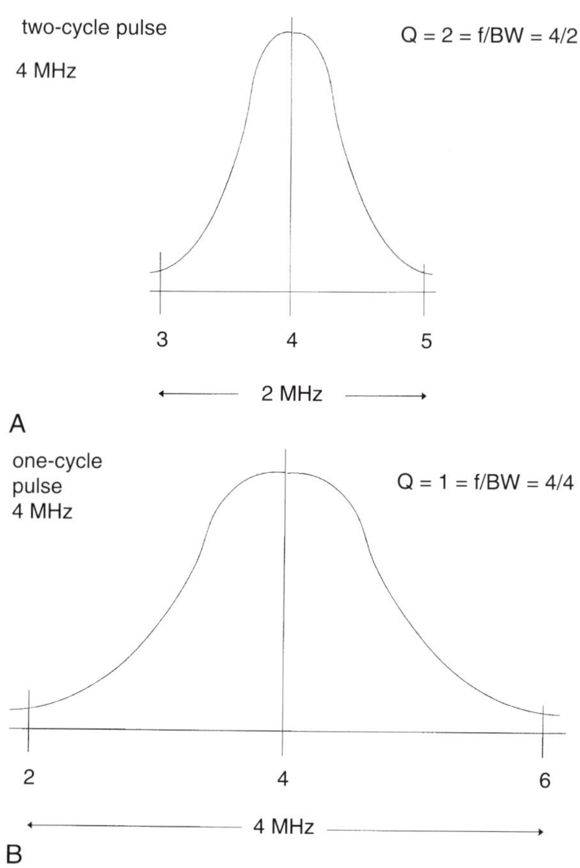

Fig. 2.10 A, A 4-MHz, two-cycle pulse has a Q factor of approximately 2, and therefore a bandwidth of approximately 2 MHz (from 3 to 5 MHz). **B,** A 4-MHz one-cycle pulse has a Q factor of approximately 1, and therefore a bandwidth of approximately 4 MHz (from 2 to 6 MHz). Shorter pulses have broader bandwidths and lower Qs.

Amplitude

Amplitude is the maximum variation that occurs in an acoustic variable. Amplitude is a measure of how far a variable gets away from its normal, undisturbed value (its value if there were no sound present). Amplitude is the maximum value minus the normal (undisturbed or no-sound) value (Fig. 2.11, A). Amplitude is expressed in units that are appropriate for the acoustic variable considered. For example, megapascals (MPa) are the units that express pressure amplitude.

Intensity

Energy is the ability to accomplish work. Heat, light, x-rays, microwaves, and mechanical motion are forms of energy. Sound is a form of mechanical energy that can do work. For example,

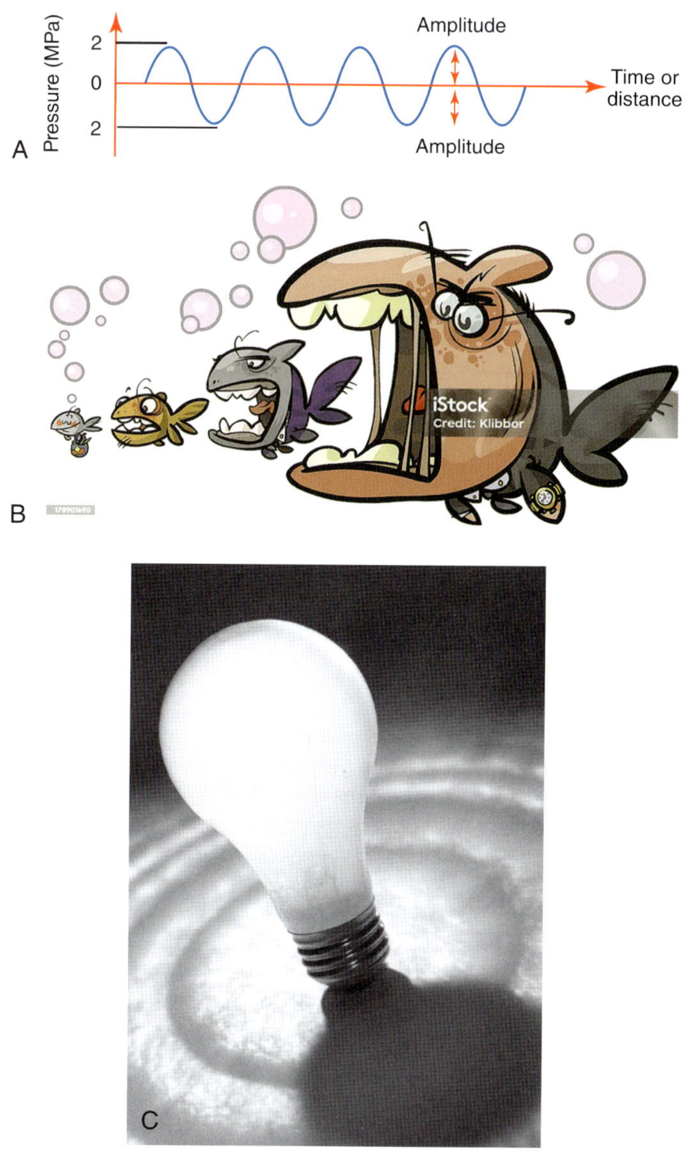

Fig. 2.11 A, Amplitude is the maximum amount of variation that occurs in an acoustic variable (pressure, in this case). In this figure, the amplitude is 2 megapascals (MPa). **B,** Intensity is the power divided by the area over which the power is distributed (as in the big fish or the beam area in ultrasound).

it can vibrate objects in its path or raise the temperature of a medium through which it is traveling. **Power** is the rate at which energy is transferred from one part of a system to another (e.g., a lamp plugged into a wall outlet) or from one location to another (e.g., energy that travels along a laser or ultrasound beam). Power is energy transferred divided by the time required to transfer energy, that is, the transfer rate. Power units include watts (W—as on light bulbs) and milliwatts (mW). One milliwatt is one-thousandth of a watt.

Intensity (*I*) is the rate at which energy passes through a unit area. It is equal to the power in a wave divided by the area (*A*) over which the power is distributed (see Fig. 2.11, B). Ultrasound is generated by transducers in the form of beams, somewhat similar to laser beams, but as sound instead of light. Beam area is expressed in centimeters squared (cm^2). Intensity units include milliwatts per centimeter squared (mW/cm^2) and watts per centimeter squared (W/cm^2). The average intensity of a sound beam is the total power in the beam divided by the cross-sectional area of the beam.

$$I(mW/cm^2) = \frac{P(mW)}{A(cm^2)}$$

An increase in power increases intensity. An increase in area decreases intensity because power is less concentrated. A decrease in area (focusing) increases intensity because power is more concentrated.

> If the power within an ultrasound beam increases, intensity increases. If beam area decreases (focusing), intensity increases (and *vice versa*, obviously).

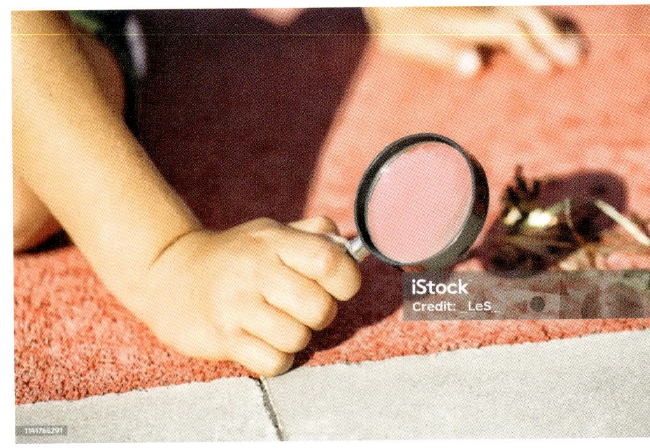

Fig. 2.12 Sunlight does not normally ignite a fire, but when the sunlight is focused, intensity increases, and ignition can occur.

Intensity is an important quantity in describing the sound that is transmitted into the body by a transducer and in discussing potential bioeffects and safety. An analogy may be made to the effect of sunlight on dry kindling (Fig. 2.12). Sunlight normally will not ignite the kindling, but if the same light power from the sun is concentrated into a small area (increased intensity) by focusing it with a magnifying glass, the kindling can be ignited. In this example, increasing intensity produces an effect, even though power remains the same. The beam area is determined by the transducer, in particular how (or if) it focuses the transmitted beam. Intensity is proportional to amplitude squared. Thus if amplitude is doubled, intensity is quadrupled. If amplitude is halved, intensity is quartered.

ADVANCED CONCEPT

Several different intensities (or rather different aspects of the beam intensity) can be measured in diagnostic ultrasound. Reasons for this are as follows:

1. Like a flashlight beam, intensity is not constant across a sound beam but is usually highest in the center and falls off near the periphery (Fig. 2.13).
2. In the case of pulsed ultrasound, intensity varies with time (Fig. 2.14), that is, the intensity is some value during each pulse but is zero between pulses.
3. Intensity is not constant within pulses (Fig. 2.15) but rather starts out high and then decreases toward the end of the pulse.

For spatial considerations, the spatial peak (SP) and spatial average (SA) values are used. SP is the greatest intensity found across the beam, usually at the center. SA is the average for all values found across the beam, including the larger values found near the center and the small values near the periphery.

For temporal (time) considerations, temporal average (TA), pulse average (PA), and temporal peak (TP) values are used. TP is the greatest intensity found in the pulse at any time point. PA is the average for all values found in a pulse, including the larger values found at its beginning and the small values found near the end. TA includes the "dead" time between pulses where there is zero intensity. Thus TA is the lowest value, TP is the highest, and PA is somewhere in between for a given pulsed beam. PA and TA values are related by the DF. TA intensity (I_{TA}) is equal to the PA intensity (I_{PA}) multiplied by the DF.

$$I_{TA} = I_{PA} \times DF$$

Hence, if the DF is 0.01 (meaning the sound is on or present 1% of the time), the TA intensity (or I_{TA}) will be one-hundredth the PA intensity. The greater the DF, the greater the I_{TA} will be. If the sound is continuous instead of pulsed, the DF is equal to 1, and the PA intensity and TA intensity are identical.

The pulses shown in Figs. 2.14 and 2.16 have constant amplitude and, therefore, intensity within each pulse. Pulses used in diagnostic ultrasound, however, are more like those shown in Fig. 2.15. The peak intensity occurring within each pulse is called the TP intensity (or I_{TP}). The intensity averaged over the PD is called the PA intensity (or I_{PA}). For constant-amplitude pulses, I_{TP} and I_{PA} are equal. Six intensities result from these spatial and temporal considerations:

1. SA-TA (I_{SATA})
2. SP-TA (I_{SPTA})
3. SA-PA (I_{SAPA})
4. SP-PA (I_{SPPA})
5. SA-TP (I_{SATP})
6. SP-TP (I_{SPTP})

SA-TA averages spatially across the beam and temporally, yielding the lowest value for a given beam. SP-TP is the spatial as well as TP, so it is the highest intensity value.

ADVANCED CONCEPT—cont'd

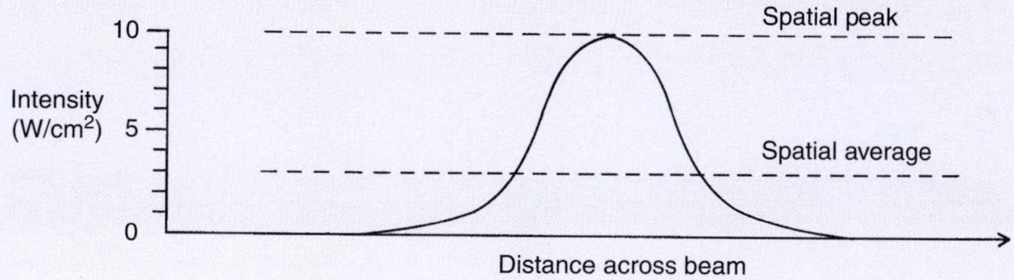

Fig. 2.13 Intensity varies across the beam. In this figure, the spatial peak intensity (at the beam center) is 10 W/cm², and the spatial average is 3 W/cm². In addition to varying across the beam, intensity varies along the direction of beam travel because of focusing and attenuation.

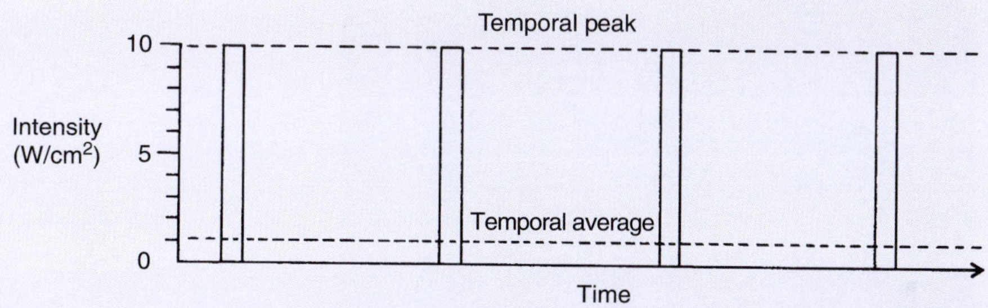

Fig. 2.14 Intensity versus time for pulsed ultrasound. Temporal peak intensity (10 W/cm²) is the intensity when the sound is actually on. Temporal average intensity (1 W/cm²) is the intensity that is averaged over time. In this figure, the duty factor is 0.1. This figure assumes constant intensity within pulses. Sonographic pulses are depicted more accurately in Figure 2.15.

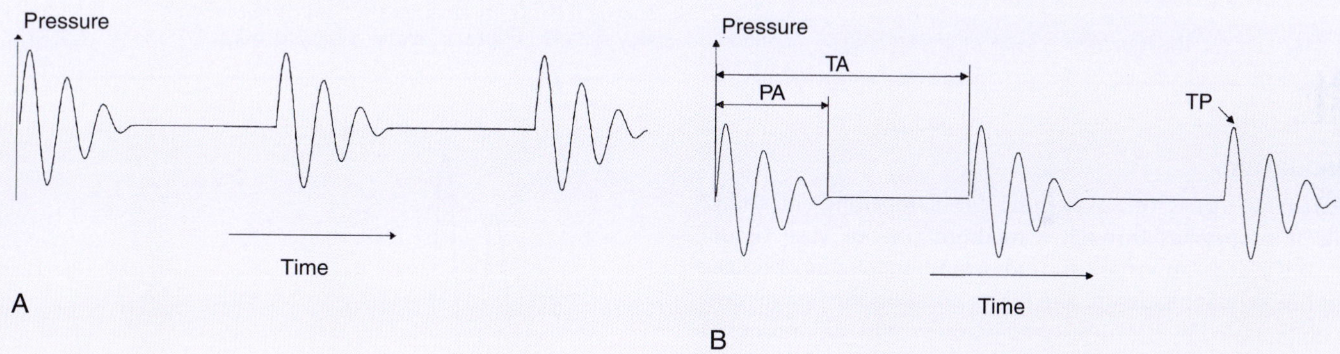

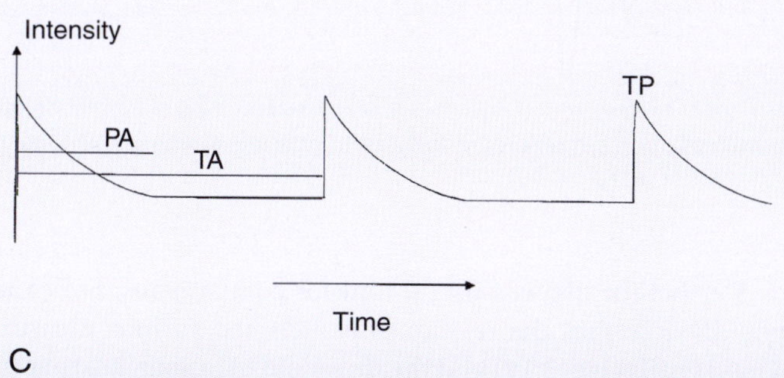

Fig. 2.15 **A,** The ultrasound pulses used in sonography have cycles of differing pressure amplitudes within each pulse. They are called damped pulses. **B,** The relevant times for three intensities are shown. Temporal average *(TA)* intensity is averaged over the pulse-repetition period; pulse average *(PA)* intensity is averaged over the pulse duration; and temporal peak *(TP)* intensity is not averaged over time. **C,** Intensity versus time for the pressure waveforms of **A** and **B.** The values for TP, PA, and TA intensities are shown. Temporal peak is the largest value (no averaging). Pulse average is smaller because it is averaged over pulse duration (including the portions with lower intensities). TA is smallest because it is averaged over the pulse-repetition period (including the time with no intensity).

Example 2.1

The SP-PA intensity is 500 mW/cm², and the DF is 2% (0.02). Calculate SP-TA.

$$I_{SPTA} = I_{SPPA} \times DF = 500 \times 0.02 = 10\ \text{mW/cm}^2$$

Example 2.2

The SP-TP and SP-PA intensities are 6 and 2 W/cm², respectively. Calculate SP-TA if the DF is 1%.

$$I_{SPTA} = I_{SPPA} \times DF = 2 \times 0.01 = 0.020\ \text{W/cm}^2 = 20\ \text{mW/cm}^2$$

Continued

ADVANCED CONCEPT—cont'd

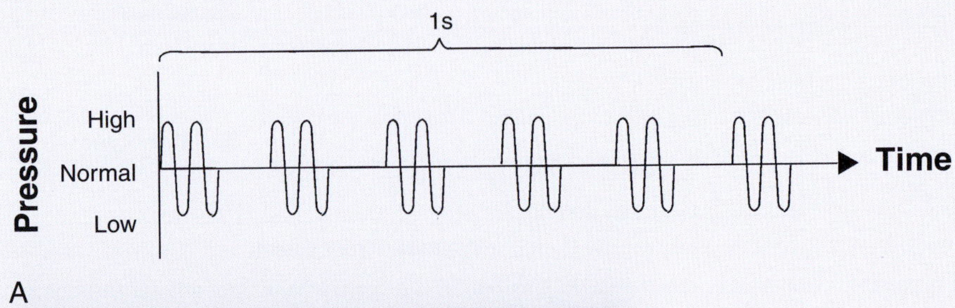

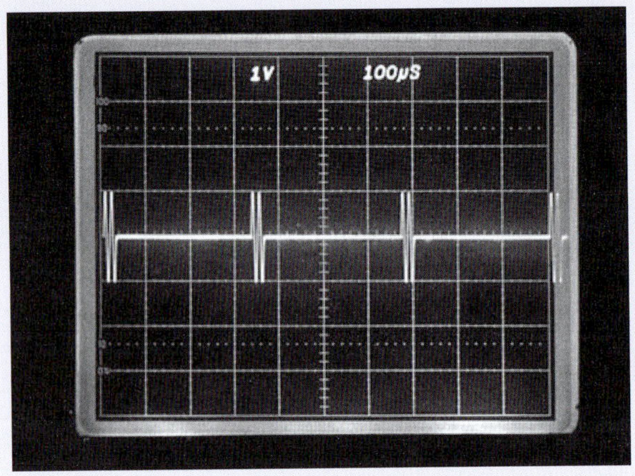

Fig. 2.16 Pulse-repetition frequency is the number of pulses occurring in 1 s. **A,** Five pulses (containing two cycles each) occur in 1 s; thus the pulse-repetition frequency is 5 Hz. **B,** Three pulses occur in 1 ms (or one-thousandth of a second); thus the pulse repetition frequency is 3 kHz. The total screen width is 1 ms.

Attenuation

Attenuation (a) is the weakening (or dampening) of sound while it propagates through a medium (in our case tissue) (Fig. 2.17). It is important to understand attenuation because (1) it limits imaging depth, and (2) its effect on the image must be compensated by the ultrasound scanner. With an unfocused beam in any medium, such as tissue, amplitude and intensity will decrease as the sound travels through the medium. This reduction in amplitude and intensity as sound travels is called *attenuation* (Fig. 2.18). Attenuation encompasses a number of phenomena: absorption of sound (conversion of sound to heat) while it travels as well as reflection and scattering of the sound (echoes) as the beam crosses tissue interfaces and travels through heterogeneous tissues. Absorption is the dominant factor that contributes to attenuation of ultrasound in soft tissues. The generation of echoes by the reflection and scattering of sound is crucial to ultrasound imaging but contributes relatively less to attenuation in most cases. Decibel is the unit used to quantify attenuation. The attenuation coefficient (α) is the attenuation that occurs with each centimeter the sound wave travels: As the attenuation coefficient also depends on frequency (higher frequencies means more vibrations and more energy converted to heat, i.e., absorption), the unit for α is decibels per centimeter per MHz (dB/cm MHz). The farther (i.e., deeper) the sound travels, the greater the attenuation.

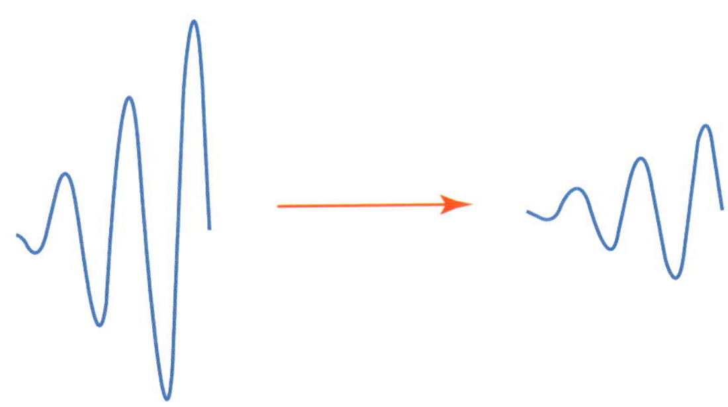

Fig. 2.17 An ultrasound pulse is weakened (reduction of amplitude) as it travels through a medium (in this case, from left to right). This weakening is called *attenuation*.

Decibel (or dB) is a useful unit for comparisons. For example, dB describes the relationships between various measured sound levels (Fig. 2.19) and the threshold of human hearing (the weakest sound we can hear). Table 2.2 gives examples of various values. Decibels are calculated as the logarithm of the ratio of two powers or intensities. In the case of attenuation, they are the intensities before and after attenuation has occurred. Two decibel values are particularly useful: 3 dB corresponding to an intensity ratio of one-half, that is, an intensity reduction of 50%; and 10 dB corresponding to an intensity ratio of one-tenth, that is, an intensity reduction of 90% (see Figs. 2.18 and 2.20).

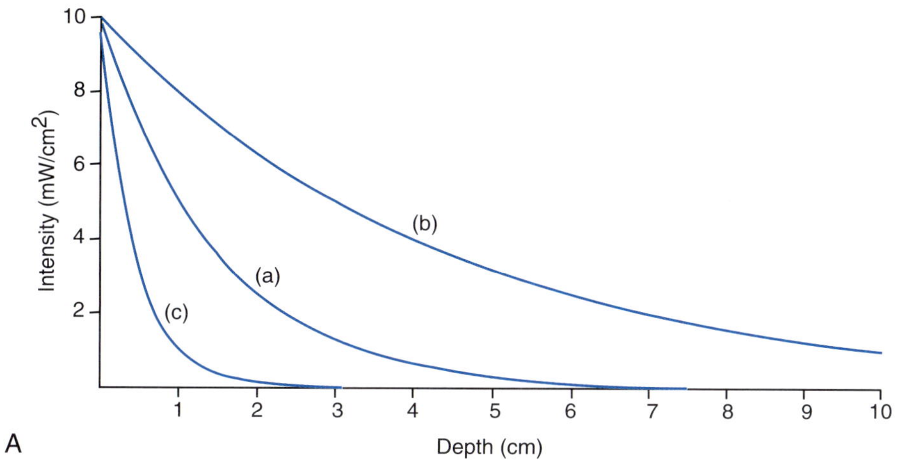

3 dB → 1/2

B 10 dB → 1/10

Fig. 2.18 Attenuation of sound while it travels through a medium. **A,** *(a)*, The intensity decreases by 50% for each 1 cm of travel. This corresponds to an attenuation coefficient of 3 dB/cm. In *(b)*, the attenuation coefficient is 1 dB/cm, whereas in *(c)*, the attenuation coefficient is 10 dB/cm. **B,** Two easy-to-remember values for decibels and their corresponding intensity reductions are (1) a 3-dB attenuation corresponds to an intensity reduction (50%) to one-half the original value, and (2) a 10-dB attenuation corresponds to an intensity reduction (90%) to one-tenth the original value.

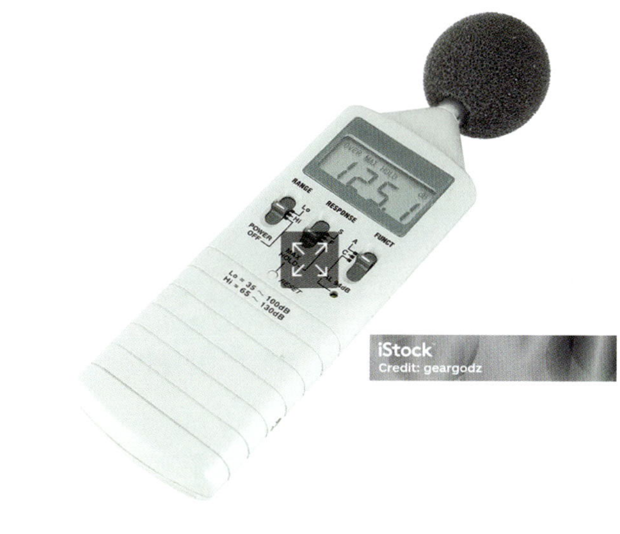

Fig. 2.19 A sound level meter based on decibels.

Example 2.3

Compare the following two intensities in decibels.

$$I_1 = 20\ \text{mW/cm}^2,\ I_2 = 10\ \text{mW/cm}^2$$

I_2 is one half of I_1. Therefore I_2 is 3 dB less than I_1.

Example 2.4

Compare (in decibels) I_2 with I_1, where I_1 = 10 mW/cm² and I_2 = 0.01 mW/cm².

Each factor of 10 is equivalent to 10 dB. I_1 is 1000 times I_2, so I_2 is 30 dB less than I_1.

TABLE 2.2 Sound Levels

Sound	Level (dB)
Pain threshold	130
Rock concert	115
Chain saw	100
Lawn mower	90
Vacuum cleaner	75
Normal conversation	60
Whisper	30
Hearing threshold	0

Example 2.5

While a 1 MHz sound wave passes through tissue, its intensity at one point is 1 mW/cm². At a point 10 cm farther along, it is 0.1 mW/cm². What are the attenuation and attenuation coefficient values?

Because intensity is reduced to one-tenth from the first point to the second, attenuation is 10 dB. The attenuation coefficient is attenuation divided by the separation between the two points as a function of frequency. In this case,

$$\alpha = \frac{10\ \text{dB}}{10\ \text{cm} \times 1\ \text{MHz}} = 1\ \text{dB/cm MHz}$$

Table 2.3 lists various values of intensity ratio and percentage values with corresponding decibel values of attenuation (assuming a 1-MHz pulse). To determine attenuation in decibels, multiply the attenuation coefficient by the sound path length (L) (how far the sound has traveled) in centimeters at a given frequency.

$$a(\text{dB}) = \alpha(\text{dB/cmMHz}) \times L(\text{cm}) \times f(\text{MHz})$$

If the attenuation coefficient increases, attenuation increases.

If the path length increases, attenuation increases.

Attenuation increases with increasing frequency. Persons who live in apartments or dormitories experience this fact when they hear mostly the bass notes through the wall from a neighbor's sound system (or from a neighbor/sound system located in another building). In soft tissues, there is approximately 0.5 dB of attenuation per centimeter for each megaHertz of frequency (practical range of 0.3–0.7 dB/cm MHz; Table 2.4) for a longitudinal, compressional sound wave (transverse, shear waves have significantly greater values of attenuation—by a factor of 10,000). In other words, the average attenuation coefficient in decibels per centimeter in soft tissues is approximately equal to one-half the frequency in megaHertz. To calculate the attenuation in decibels, multiply one-half of the frequency in megaHertz by the path length in centimeters.

$$a(dB) = 1/2(dB/cmMHz) \times f(MHz) \times L(cm)$$

If frequency increases, attenuation increases.

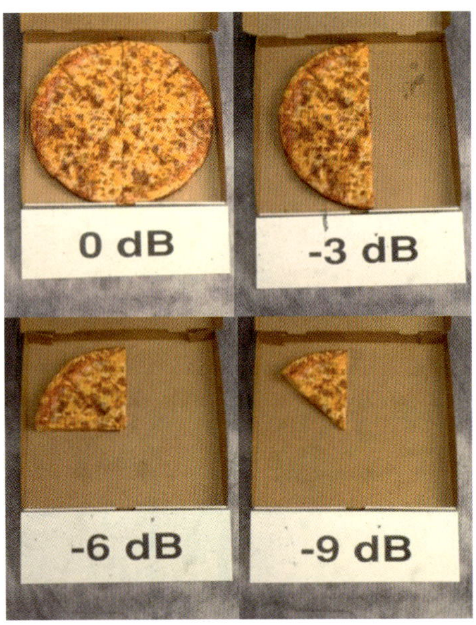

Fig. 2.20 Each reduction of 3 dB corresponds to removing half of the pizza.

The intensity ratio corresponding to the number of decibels may be obtained from Table 2.3. This ratio is equal to the fraction of the intensity that remains at the end of the travel distance relative to that at the beginning. If the intensity at the beginning is known, the intensity at the end may be found by multiplying the beginning intensity by the intensity ratio. The following is a summary of this four-step process:

1. Multiplying the frequency by one-half yields the approximate attenuation coefficient.
2. Multiplying the attenuation coefficient by the path length yields attenuation (remember echoes travel both there and back, i.e., a factor of 2).

TABLE 2.3 Attenuation for Various Intensity Ratios

Attenuation (dB)	Intensity Ratio	Percent Intensity Ratio
0	1.00	100
1	0.79	79
2	0.63	63
3	0.50	50
4	0.40	40
5	0.32	32
6	0.25	25
7	0.20	20
8	0.16	16
9	0.13	13
10	0.10	10
15	0.032	3.2
20	0.010	1.0
25	0.003	0.3
30	0.001	0.1
35	0.0003	0.03
40	0.0001	0.01
45	0.00003	0.003
50	0.00001	0.001
60	0.000001	0.0001
70	0.0000001	0.00001
80	0.00000001	0.000001
90	0.000000001	0.0000001
100	0.0000000001	0.00000001

The intensity ratio is the fraction of the original intensity remaining after attenuation.

TABLE 2.4 Average Attenuation Coefficients in Tissue

Frequency (MHz)	Average Attenuation Coefficient for Soft Tissue (dB/cm)	Intensity Reduction in 1-cm Path (%)	Intensity Reduction in 10-cm Path (%)
2.0	1.0	21	90
3.5	1.8	34	98
5.0	2.5	44	99.7
7.5	3.8	58	99.98
10.0	5.0	68	99.999

3. The intensity ratio is then determined for the decibel value calculated in step 2 (by using Table 2.3). This is the fraction of the original intensity that remains at the end of the path.
4. Multiplying the intensity ratio by the intensity at the start of the path yields the intensity at the end of the path.

Example 2.6

If 4-MHz ultrasound with 10 mW/cm^2 intensity is applied to a soft tissue surface, what is the intensity 1.5 cm into the tissue?

Step 1: Multiply frequency by one-half to yield an attenuation coefficient of 2 dB/cm.

Step 2: Multiply the attenuation coefficient (2 dB/cm) by path length (1.5 cm) to yield an attenuation of 3 dB.

Step 3: From Table 2.3 as a reference, an attenuation of 3 dB corresponds to an intensity ratio of 0.5. Thus 50% of intensity remains after the sound travels through this path.

Step 4: Multiply the intensity ratio (0.5) by the intensity at the beginning of the path (10 mW/cm^2) to yield the intensity at the end of the path. The result is 5 mW/cm^2. (Note that in pulse echo mode where echoes travel back to a transducer, another 50% of intensity will be lost so only 2.5 mW/cm^2 arrives at the transducer.)

Attenuation is higher in the lung than in other soft tissues because of the air present in this organ. Attenuation is higher in bones than in soft tissues.

ADVANCED CONCEPT

A clarification regarding the distance L (in centimeters) in the equation [a (dB) = ½ (dB/cm-MHz) × f (MHz) × L (cm)] is useful. In this equation, L is the distance (path length) the sound has traveled. For ultrasound imaging, the sound must make a round trip from the transducer to the reflector and back. Thus the distance that the sound travels to image an object is *twice* the distance to the object. Thus if imaging *depth* is being considered, rather than sound *travel distance*, the attenuation is approximately 2 × 0.5 dB/{[cm (depth)] MHz} rather than 0.5 dB/{[cm (travel distance)] MHz}.

A practical consequence of attenuation is that it limits the depths of images (penetration) that can be obtained. Penetration decreases, while frequency increases (Fig. 2.21). Table 2.5 lists attenuation coefficients and typical imaging depths for various frequencies in soft tissue.

> If frequency increases, penetration decreases.

The depths needed to reach various parts of human anatomy determine the frequencies used in diagnostic ultrasound, which range from 1 to around 30 MHz for most applications. Within this range, lower frequencies are used for deeper penetration, and higher frequencies are used for superficial applications and invasive transducers (rectal, vaginal, and esophageal) with the very highest frequencies being used in dermatological applications (e.g., melanoma). Even higher frequencies (as high as 70 MHz) are used for some specialized applications, including ophthalmologic imaging and intravascular imaging with catheter-mounted transducers. Frequencies less than 2 MHz are used in cardiology and for some large-animal applications.

ECHOES

Ultrasound is useful as an imaging tool because of the reflection and scattering of sound waves at organ and tissue interfaces and scattering within heterogeneous tissues. The reflected and scattered sound waves produce the **echoes** that is necessary for diagnostic pulse-echo imaging with ultrasound. These phenomena are considered in this section. We consider two cases, perpendicular and **oblique incidence**. Perpendicular, considered first, is the simpler case, whereas oblique is in practice the more common case.

Perpendicular Incidence

Perpendicular incidence denotes a direction of travel of the ultrasound wave perpendicular to the boundary between two media (Fig. 2.22). The incident sound may be reflected back into the first medium or transmitted into the second medium; most often, both occur. When there is perpendicular incidence, the reflected sound (i.e., the echo) travels back along the same path the incident pulse traveled through the first medium (i.e., the reflected sound returns in a direction opposite to the incident sound). In the case of perpendicular incidence, the transmitted sound continues to move through the second medium and does not change direction. The intensities of the reflected sound (the echo) and the transmitted sound depend on the incident intensity at the boundary and the impedances of the media on either side of the boundary.

Impedance

Impedance (z) determines how much of an incident sound wave is reflected (back into the first medium) and how much is transmitted into the second medium. Impedance is equal to the density (ρ) of a medium, multiplied by the propagation speed in it. Impedance increases if density increases or if propagation speed increases. Impedance is measured in **rayls** or kg/(m^2 s). The average soft tissue impedance is 1,630,000 rayls.

$$z(\text{rayls}) = \rho(\text{kg/m}^3) \times c(\text{m/s})$$

> Impedance increases if density increases or if propagation speed increases.

Dividing the reflected (echo) intensity by the incident intensity yields the fraction of the incident intensity that is reflected. This fraction is called the **intensity reflection coefficient** (IRC) or just the **reflection coefficient**. For example, if the incident intensity (Ii) is 10 mW/cm^2 and the reflected, intensity (Ir) or echo is 1 mW/cm^2, the IRC is one-tenth, or 0.1. In this case, one-tenth (10%) of the incident sound is reflected. Dividing the transmitted intensity (It) by the incident intensity yields

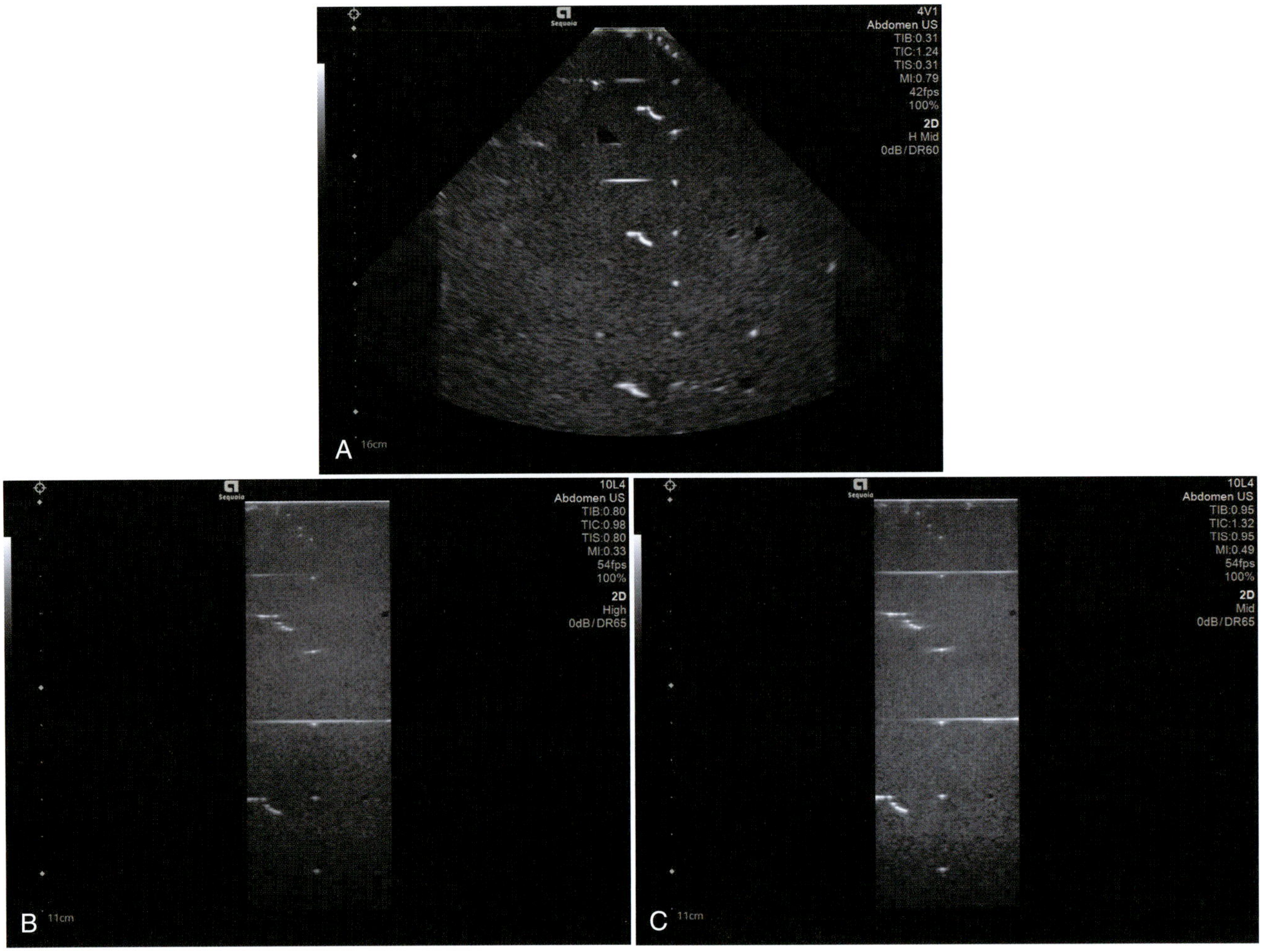

Fig. 2.21 Examples of penetration in a tissue-equivalent phantom at 2–3 MHz, a depth in excess of 16 cm **(A)**, 6–8 MHz a depth of about 11.5 cm **(B)**, and 8–10 MHz a depth of around 9.5 cm **(C)**. Penetration decreases while frequency increases.

TABLE 2.5 Typical Values for Attenuation Coefficient and Depth Penetration

Frequency (MHz)	Attenuation Coefficient (dB/cm)	Penetration (cm)
2.0	1.0	30
3.5	1.8	17
5.0	2.5	12
7.5	3.8	8
10.0	5.0	6
15.0	7.5	4

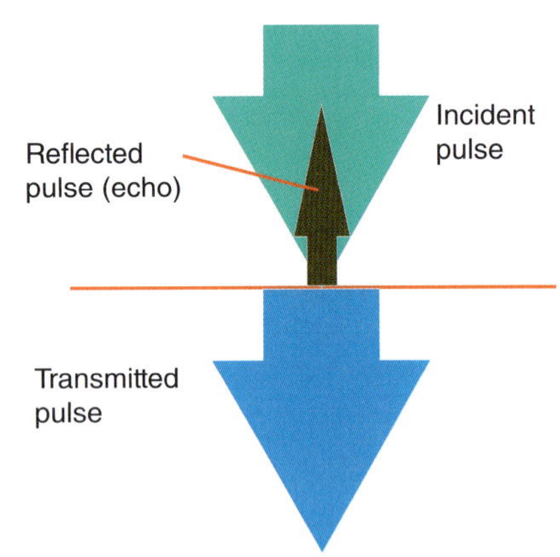

Fig. 2.22 Reflection and transmission at a boundary with perpendicular incidence. The incident pulse is partially reflected (echo) with the remainder (transmitted pulse) continuing into the second medium. The strengths of the reflected and transmitted pulses are determined by the impedances of the two media at the boundary.

the fraction of the incident intensity that is transmitted into the second medium. This fraction is called the **intensity transmission coefficient** (ITC) or just the **transmission coefficient**. For example, if the incident intensity is 10 mW/cm^2 and the transmitted intensity is 9 mW/cm^2, the ITC is nine-tenths, or 0.9. In this case, nine-tenths (90%) of the incident sound is transmitted into the second medium. The sum of the reflection and transmission coefficients must equal 1 (i.e., 100%) to account for all the incident sound intensity (what is not reflected at the boundary must be transmitted into the second medium). The two previous examples are really the same example, because if 10% of the sound is reflected back into the first medium, then

90% is transmitted into the second medium; that is, 100% of the incident sound arriving at the boundary is accounted for.

For perpendicular incidence, the reflection coefficient depends on the impedances as follows:

$$\mathrm{IRC} = \frac{I_r(\mathrm{W/cm^2})}{I_i(\mathrm{W/cm^2})} = \left[\frac{(z_2 - z_1)}{(z_2 + z_1)}\right]^2$$

From this relationship between the reflection coefficient and the impedances, we see that the coefficient depends on the difference between the impedances. The greater the difference between the impedances, the stronger the echo. The greater the similarity of the impedances, the weaker the echo. If the media impedances are the same, the difference between them is zero, and there is no echo.

> If the difference between the impedances increases, the intensity reflection coefficient (and echo intensity) increases.

The transmission coefficient depends on the reflection coefficient as follows:

$$\mathrm{ITC} = \frac{I_t(\mathrm{W/cm^2})}{I_i(\mathrm{W/cm^2})} = 1 - \mathrm{IRC}$$

Because the coefficients must add up to 1 (100%), larger reflection coefficients mean smaller transmission coefficients, and vice versa. As you would expect, if more of the incident sound is reflected (stronger echo), less remains to travel into the second medium.

> If IRC increases, then the ITC decreases.

If the impedances are equal, there is no echo, and the transmitted intensity is equal to incident intensity. This is what we expect: if no sound is reflected at a boundary, then all of it travels into the second medium meaning there was in reality no boundary. Conversely, we can see that if there is no reflection, the media impedances must be equal. If the impedances are equal, then there is no echo (i.e., no boundary), and the transmitted intensity equals the incident intensity.

If a large difference exists between the impedances, there will be nearly total reflection (an IRC close to 1, and an ITC close to 0). An example of this is an air-soft tissue boundary. For this reason, a gel **coupling medium** is used to eliminate any air between the transducer and the skin providing a good sound path from the transducer into the body.

Example 2.7

For impedances of 40 and 60 rayls, determine the intensity reflection and transmission coefficients.

$$\mathrm{IRC} = \left[\frac{(60-40)}{(60+40)}\right]^2 = \left(\frac{20}{100}\right)^2 = 0.2^2 = 0.2 \times 0.2 = 0.04$$

$$\mathrm{ITC} = 1 - 0.04 = 0.96$$

In Example 2.5, the IRC can be expressed as 4% and the ITC as 96%. The sum of the two coefficients is 100%, emphasizing the fact that all of the incident intensity must be reflected or transmitted.

If the incident intensity is known, the reflected and transmitted intensities can be calculated by multiplying the incident intensity by the IRC and the ITC, respectively.

Example 2.8

For Example 2.7, if the incident intensity is 10 mW/cm², calculate the reflected and transmitted intensities.

From Example 2.7, the intensity reflection and transmission coefficients are 0.04 and 0.96, respectively, thus

$$I_r = 10 \times 0.04 = 0.4\ \mathrm{mW/cm^2}$$
$$I_t = 10 \times 0.96 = 9.6\ \mathrm{mW/cm^2}$$

The coefficients give the fractions of the incident intensity that are reflected and transmitted. By multiplying the coefficients by 100, these fractions are expressed in percentages. Their sum must always equal 1 (or 100%). In Example 2.7, all of the incident intensity is accounted for (0.4 mW/cm² reflected, 9.6 mW/cm² transmitted, for a total of 10 mW/cm², or 100% of the incident intensity).

ADVANCED CONCEPT

Reflection and transmission of ultrasound at a boundary can also be expressed in amplitude terms. For a plane wave, pressure amplitude and intensity are related as follows:

$$I = \frac{p^2}{z}$$

That is, intensity depends on pressure amplitude squared. Intensity reflection and transmission coefficients then depend on the square of the amplitude coefficients. Amplitude coefficients are slightly more involved because amplitudes can be positive or negative, whereas intensities are always positive. The amplitude reflection coefficient (ARC) is as follows:

$$\mathrm{ARC} = \frac{p_r}{p_i} = \frac{(z_2 - z_1)}{(z_2 + z_1)}$$

where p_r is reflected pressure amplitude and p_i is incident pressure amplitude.

If z_2 equals z_1, there is no reflection (ARC = 0). If z_1 is greater than z_2, p_r is negative. The amplitude transmission coefficient is as follows:

$$\mathrm{ATC} = \frac{p_t}{p_i} = \frac{2z_2}{(z_2 + z_1)}$$

where p_t is transmitted pressure amplitude.

If z_2 equals z_1, then ATC equals 1; that is, p_t equals pi. If z_1 is greater than z_2, then p_t is less than pi.

The ITC in terms of impedances is as follows:

$$\mathrm{ITC} = \frac{4z_1z_2}{(z_2 + z_1)^2}$$

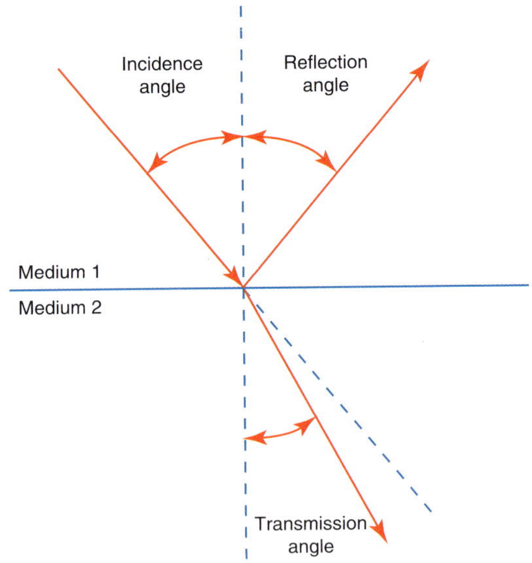

Fig. 2.23 Reflection and transmission at a boundary with oblique incidence. Incidence and reflection angles are equal. The transmission angle depends on the incidence angle and the media propagation speeds.

Oblique Incidence

Oblique incidence denotes a direction of travel of the incident ultrasound that is not perpendicular to the boundary between two media (Fig. 2.23). This situation is by far the most common in diagnostic ultrasound. The direction of travel with respect to the boundary is given by the **incidence angle** (θ_i), as shown in Fig. 2.23. In geometry, angles are measured from a line perpendicular to the surface. For perpendicular incidence, the incidence angle is zero. The reflected and transmitted directions are given by the **reflection angle** (θ_r) and **transmission angle** (θ_t), respectively. The reflection angle always equals the incidence angle.

$$\theta_i\,(\text{degrees}) = \theta_r\,(\text{degrees})$$

This phenomenon is also observed in optics (e.g., a laser beam reflecting off a mirror). The transmission angle depends on the propagation speeds in the media. Note that for oblique incidence, the reflected sound does not return to the transducer but travels off in some other direction.

Refraction

If the direction of sound changes when it crosses a boundary, it means that the transmission angle is different from the incidence angle. A change in the direction of sound when it crosses a boundary is called **refraction**. If the propagation speed in the second medium is greater than in the first medium, then the transmission angle is greater than the incidence angle and vice versa (Fig. 2.24).

$$\text{If } c_1 < c_2, \text{ then } \theta_i < \theta_t. \text{ If } c_1 > c_2, \text{ then } \theta_i > \theta_t$$

The changes caused by refraction are approximately proportional. For example, if the speed increases by 1% when the sound enters the second medium, the transmission angle will be approximately 1% greater than the incidence angle. Similarly, if the speed in the second medium is less than in the first, the transmission angle is less than the incidence angle. No refraction occurs if the propagation speeds are equal. Also, if the incidence angle is zero (perpendicular incidence), there is no refraction, even though there may be different propagation speeds in the media. Thus the two requirements for refraction to occur are:

1. Oblique incidence
2. Different propagation speed on either side of the boundary

Refraction is important because when it occurs, lateral position errors (refraction artifacts) can occur in the image.

Example 2.9

If the incidence angle approaching a boundary is 20 degrees, the propagation speed in the first medium is 1.7 mm/μs, and the propagation speed in the second medium is 1.6 mm/μs, then what are the reflection and transmission angles? The incidence and reflection angles are always equal; thus the reflection angle is 20 degrees. The ratio of the media speeds is 1.6/1.7, which is equal to 0.94. This result indicates a 6% reduction in speed when the sound crosses the boundary. Because the speed decreases by 6%, the transmission angle is approximately 6% less than the incidence angle, that is, 94% of the incidence angle ($0.94 \times 20 = 19$ degrees).

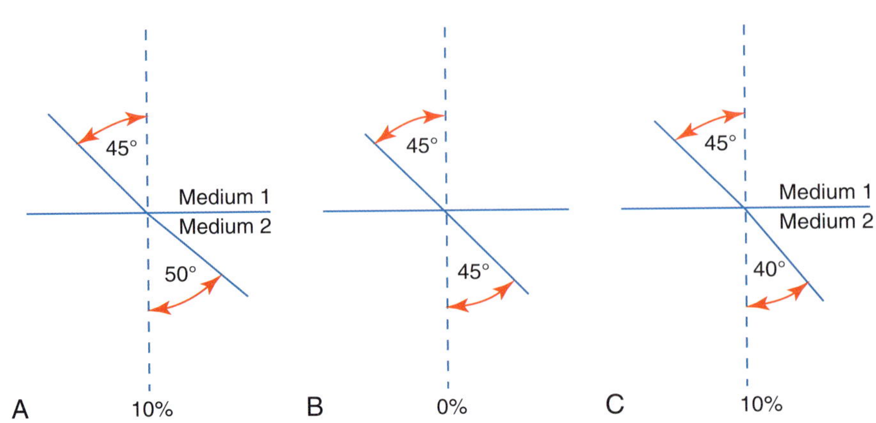

Fig. 2.24 Transmission angles for an incidence angle of 45 degrees and propagation speeds through medium 2 that are 10% greater than **(A)**, equal to **(B)**, and 10% less than **(C)** the propagation speed through medium 1.

Refraction occurs with light, sound, and any other type of wave. It is the principle upon which lenses operate. Refraction is also the cause of the distorted view of objects seen in a fishbowl or swimming pool. As with sound, when light crosses a boundary obliquely and a change in the speed of the light occurs, the direction of the light changes.

ADVANCED CONCEPT

The exact relationship between the incidence and transmission angles is known as Snell's law:

$$\left[\frac{\sin(\theta_i)}{\sin(\theta_t)}\right] = \frac{c_1}{c_2}$$

where c_1 and c_2 are the propagation speeds in media 1 and 2, respectively, in Fig. 2.25. This equation can be rearranged to yield the transmission angle:

$$\left[\theta_t = \sin^{-1}\left\{\frac{c_1}{c_1}\left[\sin(\theta_t)\right]\right\}\right]$$

The meaning of "$\sin^{-1}$ (S)" is the angle the sine of which is S.

Under the right conditions, there can be an angle at which there is *no* reflection (complete transmission into the second medium).

Because Snell's law involves ratios of sines and speeds, a good approximation allows the use of the ratio of the angles rather than the sines. This is why the angle ratio is approximately equal to the speed ratio, as discussed previously. If Snell's law is used in Fig. 2.25, the calculated incidence angle is 18.8 degrees, confirming validity of using the angles, rather than the sines, as an approximation.

For oblique incidence, the reflection equation involves angles in addition to impedances:

$$ARC = \frac{(z_2\cos\theta_i) - (z_1\cos\theta_t)}{(z_2\cos\theta_i) + (z_1\cos\theta_t)}$$

If c_2 is greater than c_1, then there is a critical incidence angle (θ_c) beyond which there is *total* reflection (no transmission into the second medium):

$$\theta_c = \sin^{-1}\left(\frac{c_1}{c_2}\right)$$

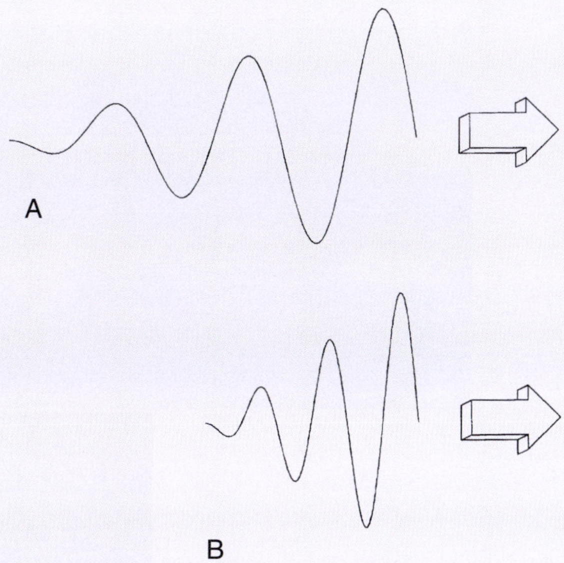

Fig. 2.25 **A–B**, Three-cycle damped (decreasing in amplitude) pulses of ultrasound traveling to the right. **A,** Lower-frequency pulse with longer wavelength and spatial pulse length. **B,** Higher-frequency pulse with shorter wavelength and spatial pulse length.

Scattering

The discussion thus far has assumed that a boundary is large (relative to the pulse wavelength), flat, and smooth. The resulting reflections are called *specular* reflections. If, however, the size of the reflecting object is comparable with that of the wavelength or smaller, or if a larger object does not have a smooth surface, the incident sound will be scattered in all directions (so called spherical waves). Scattering is the redirection of sound in many directions by rough surfaces (sometimes called diffuse scattering) or by heterogeneous media (Fig. 2.26), such as (cellular) tissues, or particle suspensions, such as blood (called Raleigh scattering). These cases are analogous to light in which **specular reflections** occur in mirrors. But with rougher surfaces, such as a white wall, light is scattered at the surface and mixed up while it travels back to the viewer's eyes. Therefore an observer does not see his or her reflected image when facing a wall. When light passes through fog, which is a suspension of water droplets in air, it is also scattered. This effect limits the viewer's ability to see through fog. Although scattering inhibits vision (we cannot see ourselves reflected in a wall, and we cannot see well through fog), it is of great benefit in ultrasound imaging. Scattering benefits the goal of ultrasound, which is to see the "wall" (tissue interface) itself, not the reflection of "oneself" (the transducer in this case). The sonographer also desires to see the "fog" (tissue parenchyma) itself, not just the objects beyond it.

Backscatter (sound scattered back in the direction from which it originally came) intensities from rough surfaces and heterogeneous media vary with frequency and **scatterer** size. Normally, scatter intensities are less than boundary specular-reflection intensities, and they increase with increasing frequency. The intensity received by the sound source from specular reflections is highly angle dependent. Scattering from boundaries helps make echo reception less dependent on incidence angle. Unlike the reflection from specular boundaries, scattering permits ultrasound imaging of tissue boundaries that are not necessarily perpendicular to the direction of the incident sound (Fig. 2.27, A–B). Scattering also allows for imaging of tissue parenchyma (Fig. 2.21, C) in addition to organ

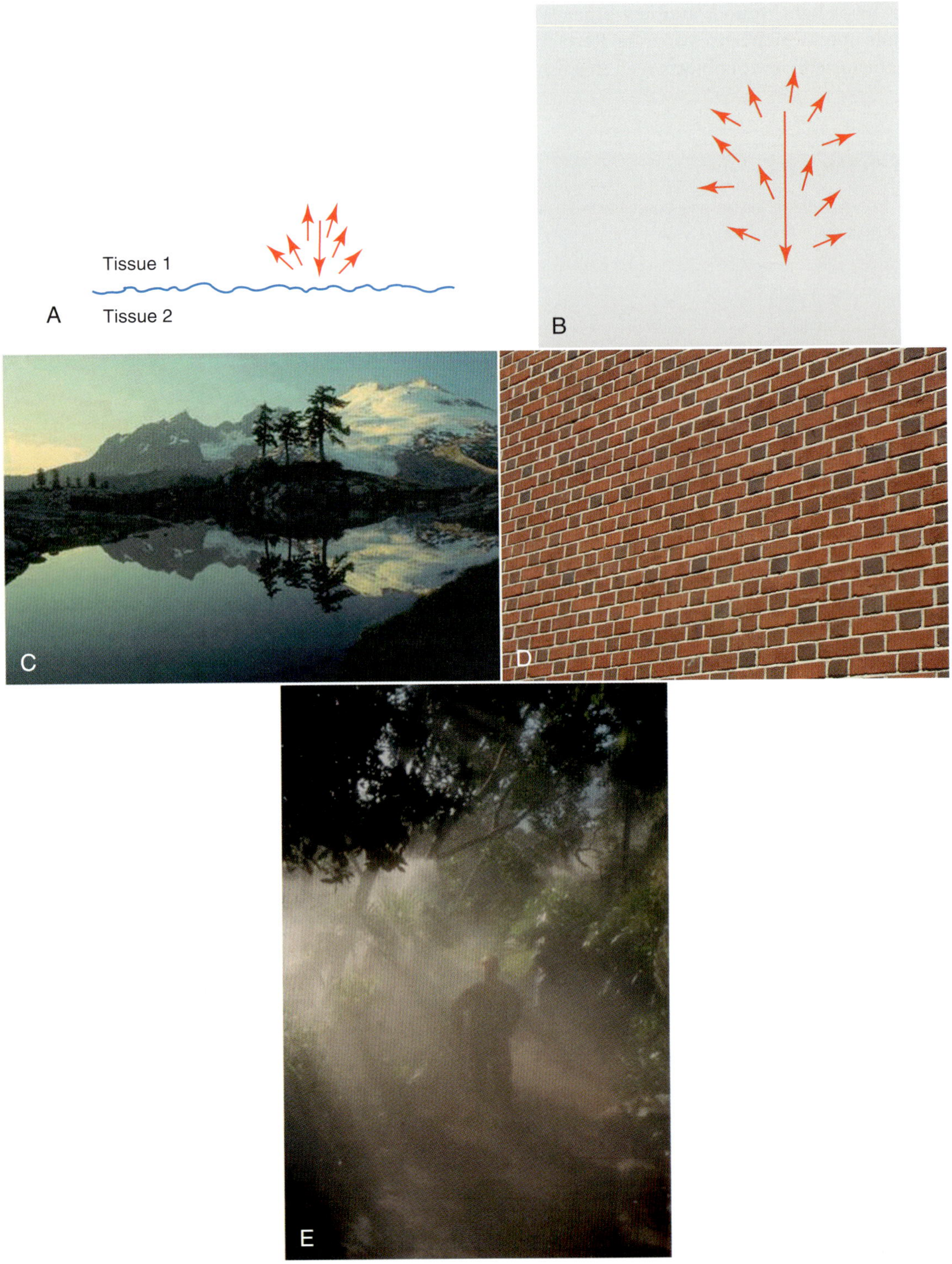

Fig. 2.26 A sound pulse may be scattered by a rough boundary between tissues **(A),** or within tissues because of their heterogeneous character **(B).** The differences between a specular surface (smooth lake) **(C),** a scattering surface (brick wall) **(D),** and a scattering medium (fog) **(E)** are illustrated.

boundaries. Scattering is relatively independent of the direction of the incident sound and therefore is more characteristic of the scatterers. Most surfaces in the body are rough for imaging purposes. Reflections from smooth boundaries (e.g., vessel intima) depend not only on the acoustic properties at the boundaries but also on the angles involved.

Speckle

An ultrasound pulse, with its finite length and width, simultaneously encounters many scatterers at any instant in its travel. Thus numerous echoes (i.e., spherical waves) are generated simultaneously within the pulse while it interacts with these scatterers. The echoes may arrive at the transducer in such a way that they

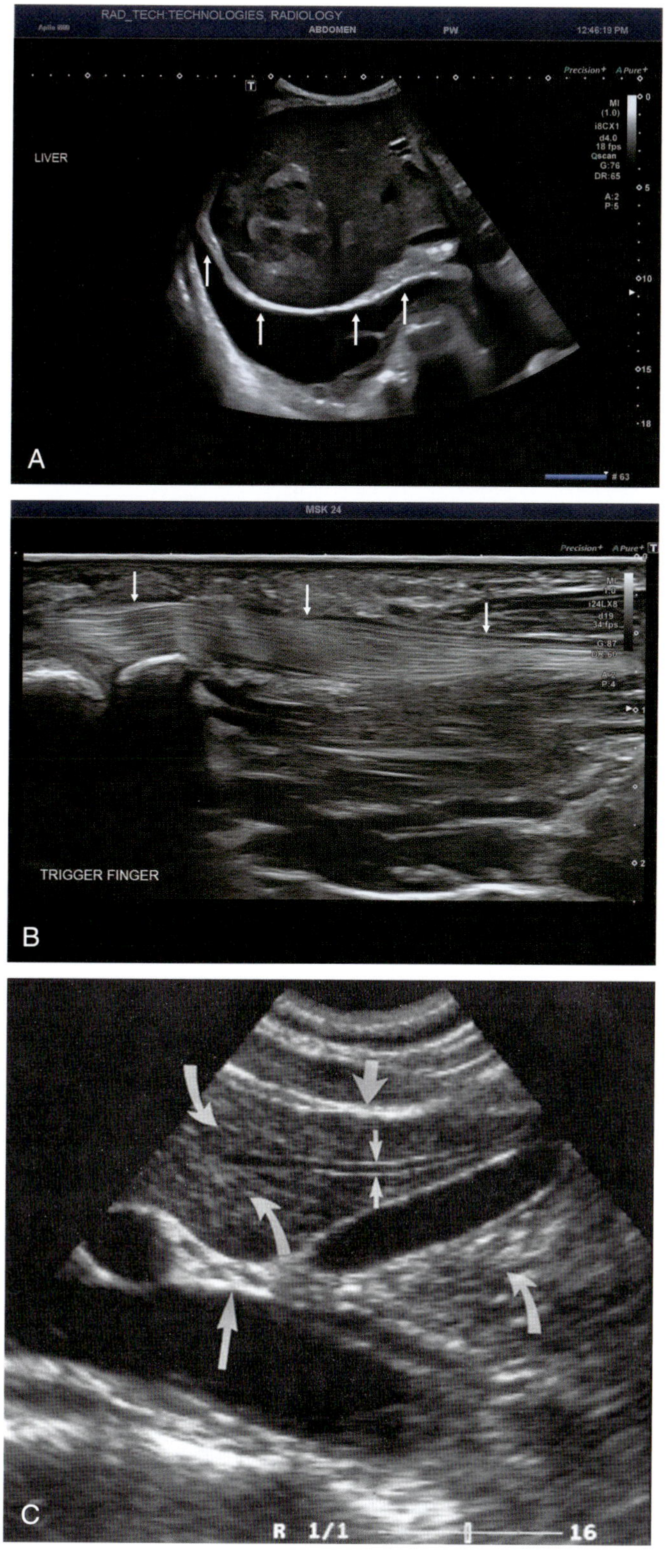

Fig. 2.27 **A,** Longitudinal abdominal scan in which the diaphragm is imaged, even where it is not *(arrows)* perpendicular to the beam and scan lines. **B,** Strong echoes *(arrows)* from a tendon associated with trigger finger. **C,** Abdominal scan showing echoes from tissue boundaries *(straight arrows)* and regions of scattering from within tissues *(curved arrows)*, allowing parenchymal imaging.

reinforce (**constructive interference**) or partially or totally cancel (**destructive interference**) each other out (Fig. 2.28, A–B). While the ultrasound beam is moved through the tissues, with scatterers moving into and out of the beam, the **interference** alternates between being constructive and being destructive, resulting in a displayed dot pattern—a grainy appearance like oatmeal porridge was flung at the display—that does not directly represent scatterers but, rather, represents the interference pattern of the scatterer distribution scanned. This phenomenon is called *acoustic speckle* (**speckle** for short) and is similar to the speckle observed with lasers (see Fig. 2.28, C). Although speckle is a deterministic phenomenon, it is often treated as a form of acoustic noise in diagnostic ultrasound imaging.

Range Determination

Now that sound propagation, reflection, and scattering have been considered, we can discuss an critical aspect of diagnostic ultrasound: the determination of the distance (range) from the transducer to an echo-generating structure and thus the appropriate location for each echo's placement on the display. To position the echoes properly, the following two items of information are required:

1. The direction from which the echo came (which, in traditional narrow transmit beam imaging, is assumed to be the direction in which the transmitted pulse is launched).
2. The distance to the **reflector** or scatterer where the echo was produced.

With regard to point 2, the scanner cannot measure distance directly; rather, it measures travel time and determines the distance from it. Similarly, directly measuring the distance between two cities would be inconvenient (a long measuring tape would be required), but we could determine the distance by asking someone to drive from one city to the other and observe the time required. Of course, we would not know when the person arrived at the other city if we were not a passenger in the car, so we would instruct the driver to return immediately after arriving at the destination (Fig. 2.29) to give us that information. Let us say that the round trip took exactly 4 hours. What was the distance traveled? We, of course, cannot determine the answer unless we know the speed traveled. If the driver was traveling at a speed of exactly 50 mph for the entire round trip (a difficult achievement), then we can determine that the distance traveled was 200 miles (50 mph × 4 hours). Therefore the distance to the city is 100 miles. Note that the total distance was halved because round-trip travel time was used to determine the one-way distance.

Similarly, in ultrasound imaging, the distance (d) to a reflector is calculated from the propagation speed and pulse round-trip travel time (t) according to the following **range equation**:

$$d(\text{mm}) = \tfrac{1}{2}[c(\text{mm}/\mu\text{s}) \times t(\mu\text{s})]$$

> As reflector distance increases the round-trip time increases.

To determine the distance from the source to the reflector, the propagation speed in the intervening medium must be known or assumed, and the pulse round-trip time must be

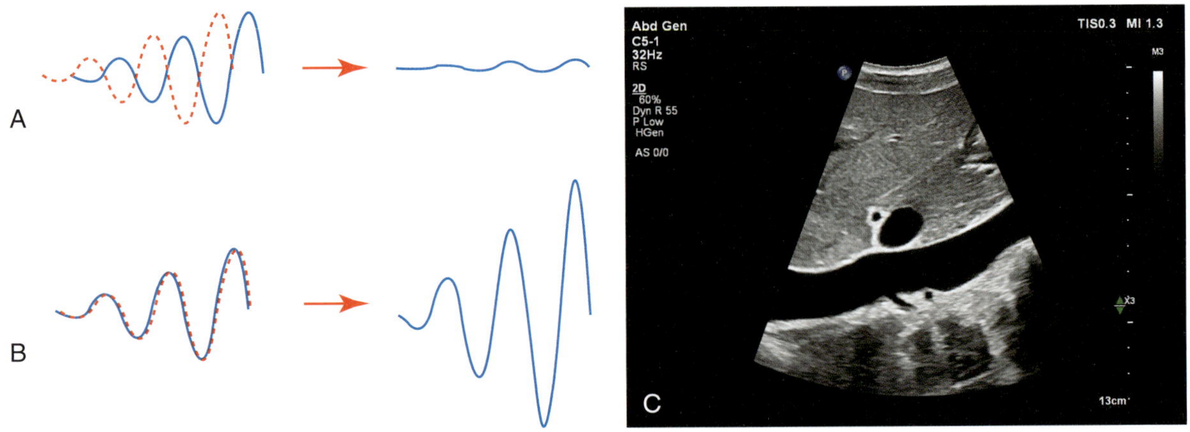

Fig. 2.28 **A,** Two similar echoes with slightly different arrival times sum to a nearly zero amplitude (destructive interference). **B,** Two similar echoes arriving nearly simultaneously sum to nearly double amplitude (constructive interference). **C,** Speckle, the grainy appearance of the tissues, is seen in this image.

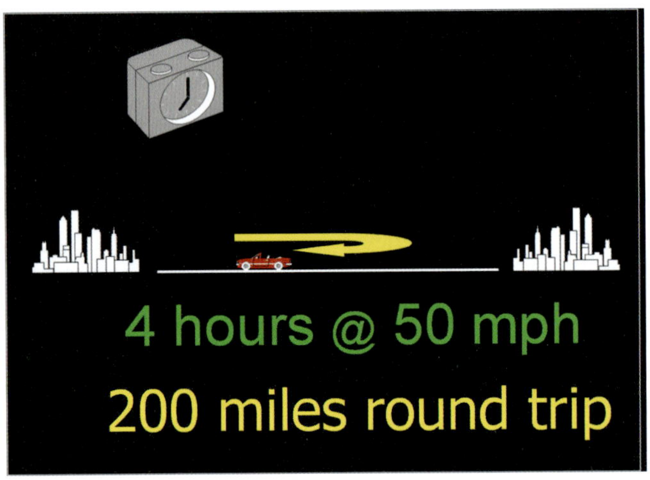

Fig. 2.29 The distance between two cities can be determined by making a round trip by car. Multiplying the speed of travel by one-half of the round-trip travel time yields the distance between the cities. If the speed is 50 mph and the round-trip travel time is 4 h, the distance between the cities is 100 miles. In this example, the round-trip distance traveled is 200 miles, obtained by multiplying the speed (50 mph) by the elapsed travel time (4 h).

measured. The reason that the factor one-half appears is that the round-trip time is the time for the pulse to travel to and return from the reflector. However, only the distance to the reflector is the desired information. The average propagation speed in soft tissue (1.54 mm/μs or 1540 m/s) is assumed in using the range equation. Because multiplying 1.54 by one-half yields 0.77, the distance (in millimeters) to the reflector can be calculated by multiplying 0.77 by the round-trip time (in microseconds).

In the problem that involves determining the distance between cities, 50 mph is equivalent to 0.83 mile/min or 1.20 min/mile. Thus at this speed, 2.4 minutes of round-trip travel are required for each mile of distance separating the cities. Similarly, sound speed in tissue is 1.54 mm/μs, so 0.65 μs is required for each millimeter of travel (6.5 μs are required for 1 cm of travel). Therefore 13 μs of round-trip travel time are required for each centimeter of distance from the transducer to the reflector.

TABLE 2.6 Pulse Round-Trip Travel Time for Various Reflector Depths

Depth (cm)	Travel Time (μs)
0.5	6.5
1	13
2	26
3	39
4	52
5	65
10	130
15	195
20	260

To confirm this, substitution of 13 μs for t in the foregoing range equation yields a reflector distance of 10 mm (1 cm).

$$d = 1/2(c \times t) = 1/2(1.54 \times 13) = 1/2(20) = 10\text{ mm} = 1\text{ cm}$$

All of this information leads to the important 13 μs/cm rule: the pulse round-trip travel time is 13 μs for each centimeter of distance from source to reflector (Table 2.6; Fig. 2.30). Fig. 2.31 illustrates the correspondence between echo arrival time and reflector depth.

Example 2.10

If an echo returns 104 μs after a pulse was emitted by a transducer, at what depth is the echo-producing structure located?

With the range equation:

$$d(\text{mm}) = 0.77\text{ mm/μs} \times 104\text{μ/s} = 80\text{ mm} = 8.0\text{ cm}$$

With the 13 μs/cm rule:

$$d(\text{mm}) = \frac{104\text{ μs}}{13\text{ μs/cm}} = 8\text{ cm}$$

Table 2.7 provides common values for several acoustic parameters, while Table 2.8 summarizes how various parameters change with frequency.

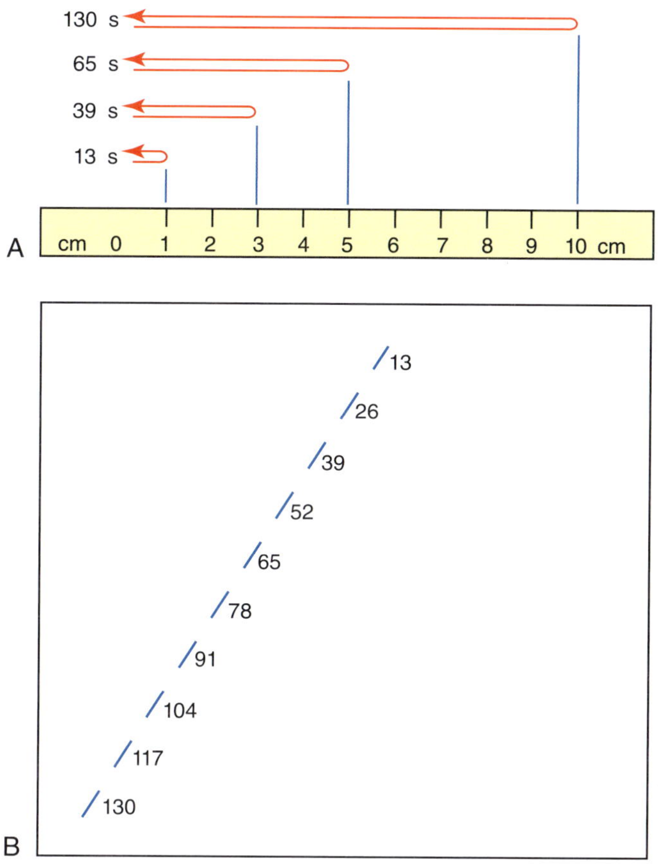

Fig. 2.30 **A,** Echo arrival times for 1, 3, 5, and 10 cm reflector distances. **B,** Echoes from 1, 2, 3, 4, 5, 6, 7, 8, 9, and 10 cm depths arrive at the times indicated (in microseconds).

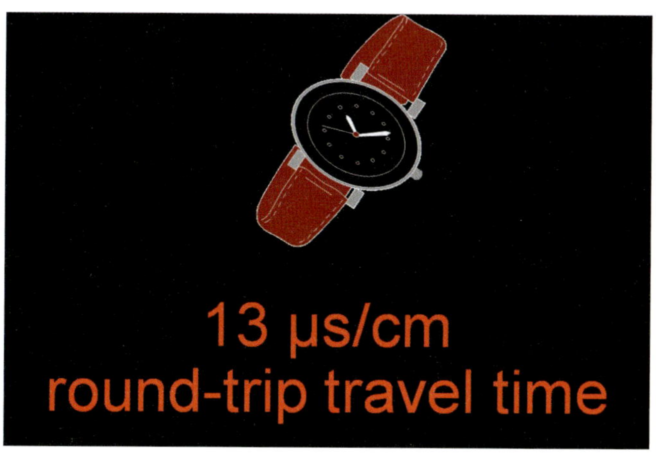

Fig. 2.31 Substituting the average speed of sound in soft tissues into the range equation yields the 13-µs/cm round-trip travel time rule.

DETAIL RESOLUTION

Imaging resolution has three aspects:

- Detail
- Contrast
- Temporal

Contrast and temporal resolutions relate more directly to instruments and are discussed in Chapters 4 and 5. Detail resolution (Fig. 2.32) relates more directly to the ultrasound pulse and is discussed in this chapter. If two reflectors are not separated sufficiently, they produce overlapping (not distinct) echoes that are not separated on the instrument display. Rather, the echoes merge together and appear as one. Thus the echoes are not resolved. If distinct (separated by a gap) echoes are not generated initially in the anatomy, then the reflectors will not be separated on the display. In ultrasound imaging, detail resolution has two aspects, **axial** and **lateral**, which depend on the length and width of ultrasound pulses, respectively, as they travel through tissues.

TABLE 2.7 Acoustic Parameters in Tissue

	SYMBOL OR RANGE OF PARAMETER	
	Abbreviation	**Common Values**
Frequency	F	2–30 MHz
Period	T	0.05–0.5 µs
Wavelength	Λ	0.08–0.8 mm
Propagation speed	C	1.44–1.64 mm/µs
Impedance	Z	1,300,000–1,700,000 rayls
Pulse-repetition frequency	PRF	4–15 kHz
Pulse-repetition period	PRP	0.07–0.25 ms
Cycles per pulse	N	1–3
Pulse duration	PD	0.1–1.5 µs
Spatial pulse length	SPL	0.1–2.5 mm
Duty factor	DF	0.1–1%
Pressure amplitude	P	0.1–4 MPa
Intensity[a]	I_{SPTA}	0.01–100 mW/cm²
Attenuation coefficient	α_c	1–10 dB/cm

[a]Spatial-peak, temporal average.

TABLE 2.8 Dependence of Various Factors on Increasing (↑) Frequency

Symbol or Dependence Parameter	Abbreviation	↑ Increase ↓ Decrease
Period	T	↓
Wavelength	λ	↓
Pulse duration	PD	↓
Spatial pulse length	SPL	↓
Attenuation	α	↑
Penetration	pen	↓

Axial Resolution

Axial resolution (AR) is the minimum reflector separation required along the direction of sound travel (along the scan line) to produce separate echoes (Fig. 2.33). The important factor in determining AR is SPL. AR is equal to one-half of the SPL.

$$AR(mm) = \frac{SPL(mm)}{2}$$

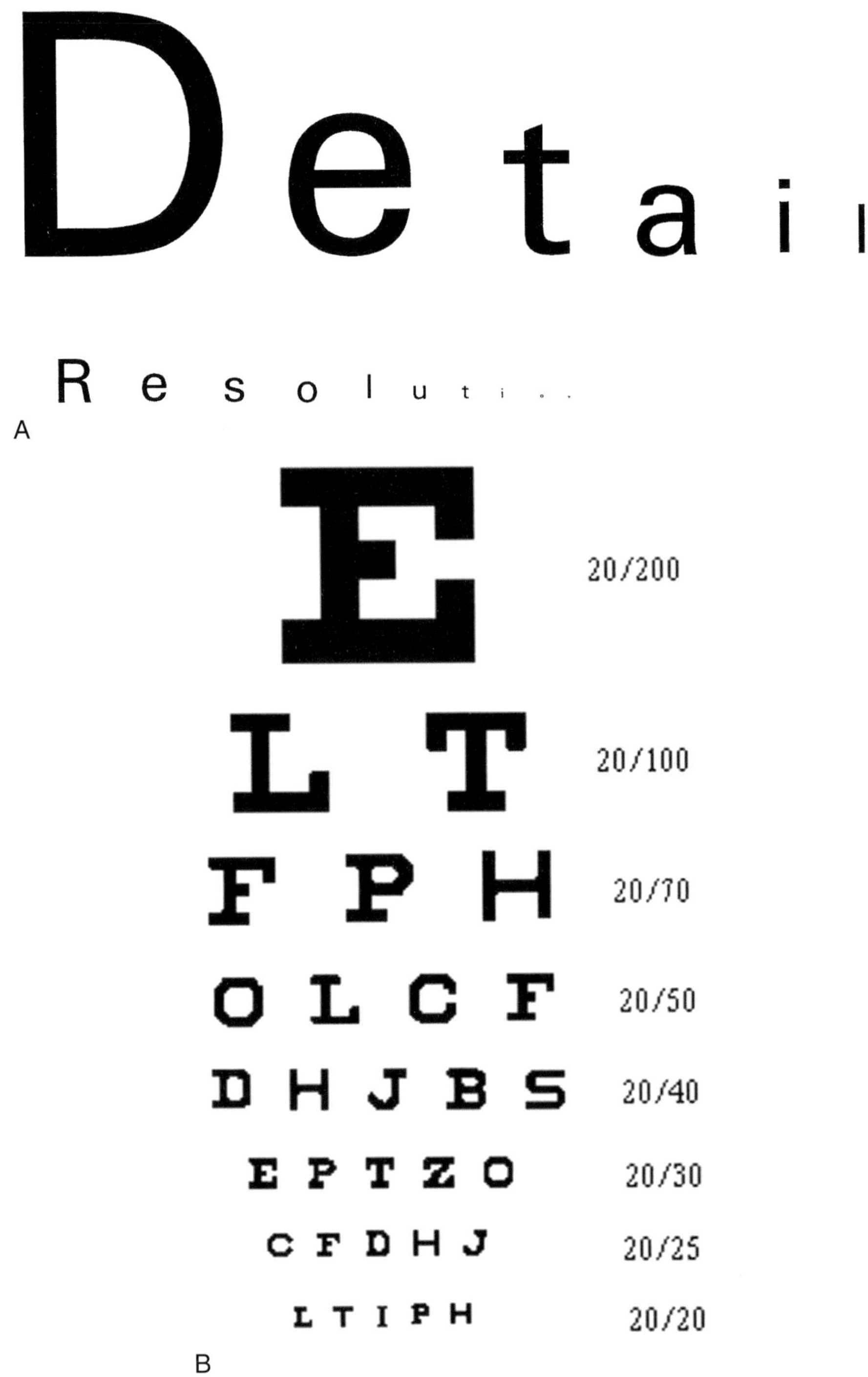

Fig. 2.32 **A,** Excellent detail resolution is the ability to image fine detail. Smaller is better; that is, tinier details can be discerned. **B,** Snellen vision testing chart.

> AR is the minimum reflector separation necessary to resolve reflectors along scan lines. AR equals SPL (in mm) divided by 2.

Note that the axial (and indeed detail resolution) decreases as frequency increases; smaller is better for resolution. The smaller the AR, the finer the detail that can be displayed; thus the two reflectors can be closer along the sound path and still be seen distinctly, thereby allowing tinier objects or finer detail to be displayed. To improve AR, SPL must be reduced. Because SPL is wavelength multiplied by number of cycles in the pulse, one or both of these factors must be reduced. Wavelength is reduced by increasing frequency. The number of cycles in each pulse is controlled by the ultrasound scanner. Because the number of cycles per pulse has been reduced to a minimum (one to three) by transducer design, the only way the instrument operator can improve AR further is to increase frequency. With an increase in frequency, however, comes a reduction in penetration (imaging depth)

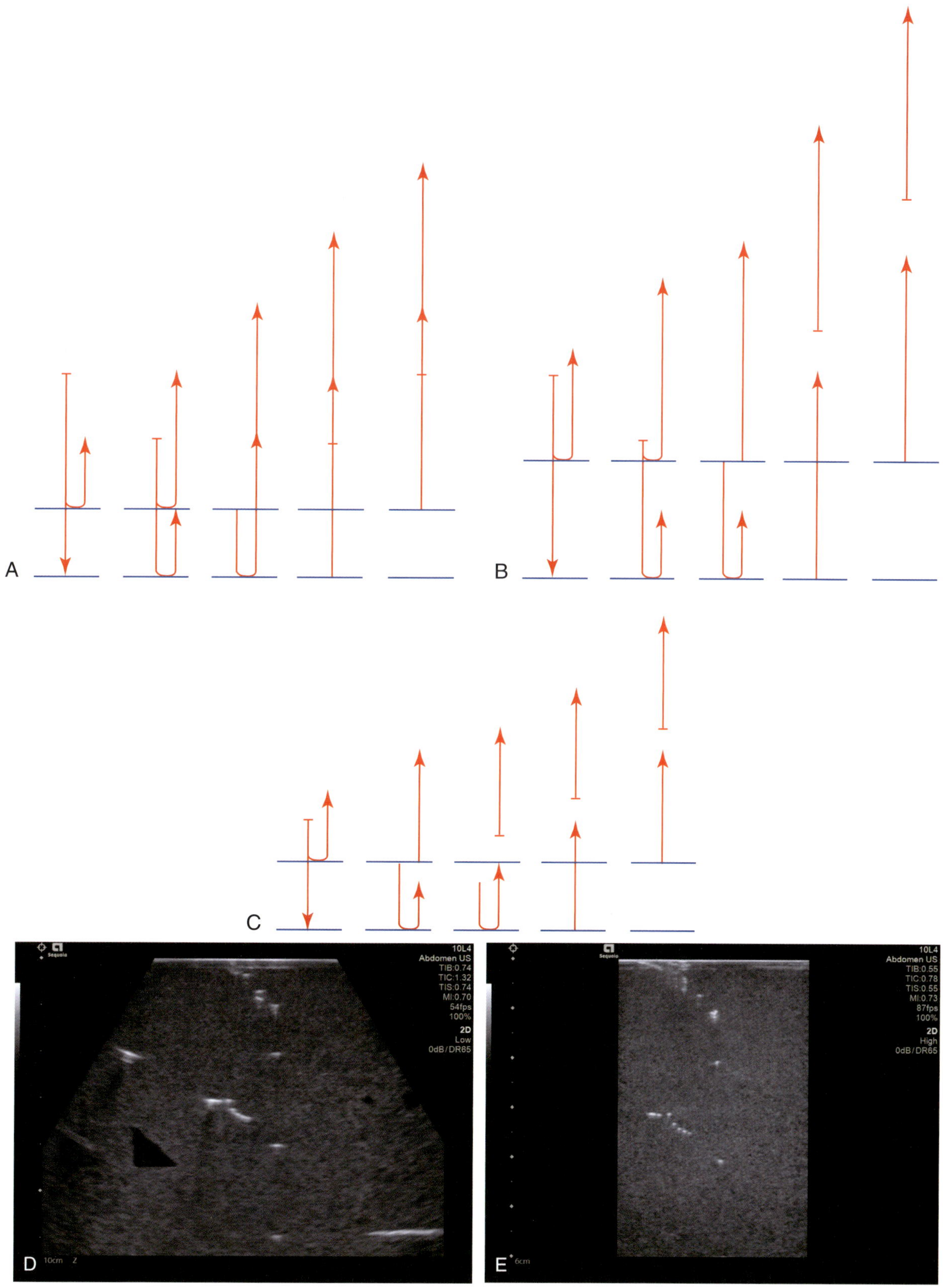

Fig. 2.33 Axial resolution. Action proceeds in time from left to right in each part of the figure. **A,** The separation of the reflectors is less than half of the spatial pulse length and thus echo overlap occurs. Separate echoes are not produced. The reflectors are not resolved on the display. **B,** The reflector separation is increased so that it is greater than half of the spatial pulse length. Echo overlap does not occur. Separate echoes are produced, and the reflectors are resolved on the display. **C,** The reflector separation is the same as in **A,** but resolution is achieved by shortening the pulse to yield separate echoes. Axial resolution improves while frequency increases: **D,** 4–5 MHz, with a resolution of 3.0 mm; **E,** 8–10 MHz, with a resolution below 1.0 mm.

because attenuation increases while frequency increases. Consequently, diagnostic ultrasound imaging revolves around the tradeoff between resolution and penetration with changing frequency.

Lateral Resolution

Lateral resolution (LR) is the minimum reflector separation in the direction perpendicular to the **beam** direction (i.e., the width of the pulse across scan lines) that can produce two separate echoes when the beam is scanned across the reflectors (Fig. 2.34). LR is equal to the beam width (w_b) or pulse width in the scan plane.

$$LR(mm) = w_b(mm)$$

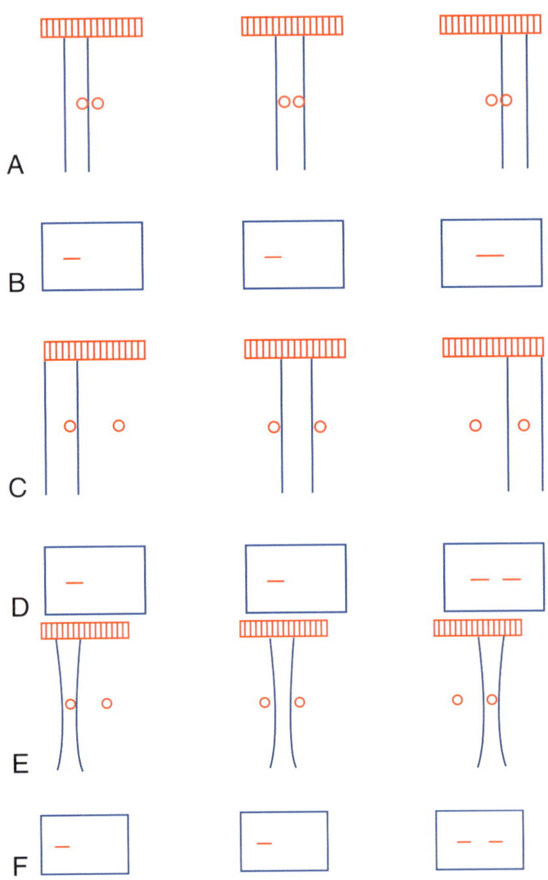

Fig. 2.34 Lateral resolution. Reflector separation (perpendicular to beam direction) is less than beam diameter in **A** and **B,** whereas in **C** and **D,** reflector separation is greater than the beam diameter. Action proceeds in time from left to right in each part of the figure. **A,** The beam first encounters the left reflector, then is reflected by both reflectors, and finally is reflected by the right reflector. **B,** This scanning sequence results in continual reflection from one or both reflectors. Separate echoes are not produced, and the reflectors are not resolved. **C,** The beam encounters the left reflector, then fits between both reflectors (yielding no echo), and, finally, is reflected by the right reflector. **D,** Separate echoes are produced, and the reflectors are resolved on the display. **E,** Two separate echoes are generated when the beam is focused and narrower than the reflector separation. **F,** The two reflectors are resolved on the display.

> LR is the minimum reflector separation necessary to resolve reflectors across scan lines. LR equals beam (or pulse) width (in mm).

As with AR, smaller LR is better. A smaller value indicates an improvement (finer detail and the ability to image tinier objects). Beam width varies with the distance from the transducer (described in more detail in Chapter 3), and so does LR. If the lateral separation between two reflectors is greater than the pulse diameter, two separate echoes are produced when the beam is scanned across them. Thus the echoes are resolved, or detected, as separate reflectors.

> For detail resolution, smaller is better.

> If frequency increases, detail resolution improves, but penetration decreases.

Diagnostic ultrasound transducers often have better AR than LR, although the two may be comparable in the focal region of strongly focused beams. Fig. 2.35 shows examples of detail resolution.

Elevational Resolution

Section thickness (i.e., pulse thickness as a function of depth) can be considered a third aspect of detail resolution and is therefore sometimes called **elevational resolution**. Elevational resolution contributes to section thickness artifact, also called *partial-volume artifact*. This artifact is a filling in of what should be anechoic structures, such as cysts. This filling in occurs when

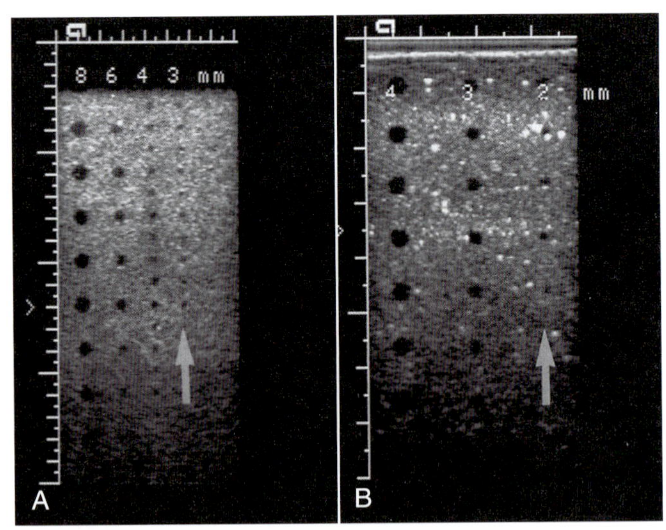

Fig. 2.35 A, An image of a resolution penetration phantom that contains circular anechoic regions ("cysts") in tissue-equivalent material. From left to right, the cysts are 2, 4, and 8 mm in diameter at 3 cm in depth. Close examination reveals that the 3-mm cysts are the smallest that can be resolved. This image was produced with a 3.5-MHz transducer. **B,** The same phantom is imaged with a 7-MHz transducer. In this instance, the 2-mm cysts can be seen. Note the loss of penetration compared with that shown in **A** (8 cm vs. 20 cm). Detail resolution can be improved by increasing the frequency of the ultrasound beam, but at the expense of decreasing the imaging depth.

the section thickness is larger than the size of the structure. Thus echoes from outside the structure are included in the image, and the structure appears to be echoic. The thinner the section, the less its negative effect on sonographic images. Focusing in the section thickness plane reduces section thickness artifacts.

The effect of elevational resolution is different from that of AR and LRs. They cause axial and lateral smearing of small structures, whereas section thickness brings structures into the image that should be outside. Section thickness artifact is discussed and illustrated in Chapter 7.

REVIEW

The following key points are presented in this chapter:

- Sound is a wave of pressure and density variations and particle vibration.
- Ultrasound is sound that has a frequency greater than 20 kHz.
- Frequency denotes the number of cycles occurring in 1 second.
- Harmonic frequencies are generated while sound travels through tissue.
- Wavelength is the spatial length of a cycle (i.e., its physical dimension in space).
- Propagation speed is the speed of sound through a medium.
- The medium determines propagation speed.
- The average propagation speed of sound through soft tissue is 1.54 mm/μs.
- Pulsed ultrasound is described by PRF, PRP, PD, DF, and SPL.
- Amplitude and intensity describe the strength of sound.
- Attenuation is the weakening of sound caused by absorption, reflection, and scattering.
- Attenuation increases with frequency and path length (i.e., depth).
- The average attenuation coefficient for soft tissues is 0.5 dB/(cm MHz).
- Imaging depth decreases as frequency increases.
- Impedance is the density of a medium multiplied by propagation speed.
- When sound encounters boundaries between media with different impedances, part of the sound is reflected, and the remainder is transmitted further into the second medium.
- With perpendicular incidence, and if the two media have the same impedance, there is no reflection.
- The greater the difference in the impedances of the media at a boundary, the greater is the intensity of the echo that is generated at the boundary.
- With oblique incidence, the sound is refracted at a boundary between media for which propagation speeds are different.
- Incidence and reflection angles at a boundary are always equal.
- Scattering occurs at rough media boundaries and within heterogeneous media.
- Pulse-echo round-trip travel time (13 μs/cm) is used to determine the distance to a reflector.
- AR is equal to one-half of the SPL.
- LR is equal to beam width.

EXERCISES

Answers appear in the Answers to Exercises section at the back of the book.

1. A wave is a traveling variation in quantities called wave ___________.
 a. lengths
 b. variables
 c. cycles
 d. periods

2. Sound is a traveling variation in quantities called ___________ variables.
 a. wave
 b. pressure
 c. density
 d. acoustic

3. Ultrasound is sound with a frequency greater than ___________ Hz.
 a. 2
 b. 15
 c. 20,000
 d. 1540

4. Acoustic variables include ___________, ___________, and particle motion.
 a. stiffness, density
 b. hardness, impedance
 c. amplitude, intensity
 d. pressure, density

5. Which of the following frequencies is in the ultrasound range?
 a. 15 Hz
 b. 15,000 Hz
 c. 15 kHz
 d. 30,000 Hz
 e. 0.004 MHz

6. Which of the following is not an acoustic variable?
 a. pressure
 b. propagation speed
 c. density
 d. particle motion

7. Frequency is the number of ___________ an acoustic variable goes through in a second.
 a. cycles
 b. amplitudes
 c. pulse lengths
 d. Duty factors

8. The unit of frequency is ___________, which is abbreviated as ___________.
 a. hertz, Hz
 b. megahertz, MHz
 c. kilohurts, khts
 d. cycles, cps

9. Period is the ___________ that it takes for one cycle to occur.
   a. length
   b. amplitude
   c. time
   d. height
10. Period decreases while ___________ increases.
   a. wavelength
   b. pulse length
   c. frequency
   d. bandwidth
11. Wavelength is the length of ___________ over which one cycle occurs.
   a. time
   b. space
   c. propagation
   d. power
12. Propagation speed is the speed with which a(n) ___________ moves through a medium.
   a. wave
   b. particle
   c. frequency
   d. attenuation
13. Wavelength is equal to ___________ ___________ divided by ___________.
   a. propagation speed, frequency
   b. media density, stiffness
   c. pulse length, frequency
   d. wave amplitude, period
14. The ___________ and ___________ of a medium determine propagation speed.
   a. amplitude, intensity
   b. wavelength, period
   c. impedance, attenuation
   d. density, stiffness
15. Propagation speed increases if ___________ is increased.
   a. amplitude
   b. frequency
   c. density
   d. stiffness
16. The average propagation speed in soft tissues is ___________ m/s or ___________ mm/ms.
   a. 10, 3
   b. 1540, 1.54
   c. 3, 10
   d. 1.54, 1540
17. Propagation speed is determined by the _________.
   a. frequency
   b. amplitude
   c. wavelength
   d. medium
18. Place the following classifications of matter of increasing sound propagation speed.
   a. gas, solid, liquid
   b. solid, liquid, gas
   c. gas, liquid, solid
   d. liquid, solid, gas
19. The wavelength of 7-MHz ultrasound in soft tissues is ___________ mm.
   a. 1.54
   b. 0.54
   c. 0.22
   d. 3.33
20. Wavelength in soft tissues ___________ while frequency increases.
   a. is constant
   b. decreases
   c. increases
   d. weakens
21. It takes ___________ ms for ultrasound to travel 1.54 cm in soft tissue.
   a. 10
   b. 0.77
   c. 154
   d. 100
22. Propagation speed in bone is ___________ that in soft tissues.
   a. lower than
   b. equal to
   c. higher than
   d. 10 m/s greater than
23. Sound travels fastest in ___________.
   a. air
   b. helium
   c. water
   d. steel
24. Solids have higher propagation speeds than liquids because they have greater ___________.
   a. density
   b. stiffness
   c. attenuation
   d. propagation
25. Sound travels most slowly in ___________.
   a. gases
   b. liquids
   c. tissue
   d. bone
26. Sound is a ___________ ___________ wave.
   a. mechanical expressional
   b. electromagnetic transverse
   c. electromagnetic longitudinal
   d. mechanical longitudinal
27. If propagation speed is doubled (a different medium) and frequency is held constant, the wavelength is ___________.
   a. decreased
   b. doubled
   c. halved
   d. unchanged
28. If frequency in soft tissue is doubled, propagation speed is ___________.
   a. decreased
   b. doubled
   c. halved
   d. unchanged

29. If wavelength is 2 mm and frequency is doubled, the wavelength becomes ___________ mm.
    a. 4
    b. 1
    c. 2.5
    d. unchanged
30. Waves can carry ___________ from one place to another.
    a. information
    b. density
    c. impedance
    d. speed
31. From given values for propagation speed and frequency, ___________ can be calculated.
    a. amplitude
    b. impedance
    c. wavelength
    d. intensity
32. If two media have different stiffnesses, the one with the higher stiffness will have the higher propagation speed. True or false?
33. The second harmonic of 3 MHz is ___________ MHz.
    a. 2
    b. 3.2
    c. 6
    d. 9
34. Odd harmonics of 2 MHz are ___________ MHz.
    a. 1, 3, 5
    b. 2, 4, 6
    c. 6, 9, 12
    d. 6, 10, 14
    e. 10, 12, 14
35. Even harmonics of 2 MHz are ___________ MHz.
    a. 1, 3, 5
    b. 2, 4, 6
    c. 4, 8, 12
    d. 6, 10, 14
    e. 10, 12, 14
36. Nonlinear propagation means that ___________.
    a. the sound beam does not travel in a straight line
    b. propagation speed depends on frequency
    c. harmonics are not generated
    d. the waveform changes shape while it travels
37. In nonlinear propagation, additional frequencies appear that are ___________ and ___________ multiples of the fundamental frequency. They are called ___________.
    a. double, triple, harmonics
    b. double, triple, subharmonics
    c. odd, even, harmonics
    d. odd, even, subharmonics
38. If the density of a medium is 1000 kg/m^3 and the propagation speed is 1540 m/s, the impedance is ___________ rayls.
    a. 1540
    b. 2540
    c. 540
    d. 1,540,000
39. If two media have the same propagation speed but different densities, the one with the higher density will have the higher impedance. True or false?
40. If two media have the same density but different propagation speeds, the one with the higher propagation speed will have the higher impedance. True or false?
41. Impedance is ___________ multiplied by ___________.
    a. density, propagation speed
    b. frequency, oblique incidence
    c. wavelength, propagation speed
    d. attenuation, PD
42. The abbreviation CW stands for ___________.
    a. corrected waveform
    b. continuous window
    c. continuous wave
    d. contrast waveform
43. PRF is the number of ___________ occurring in 1 second.
    a. cycles
    b. pulses
    c. periods
    d. wavelengths
44. Pulse-repetition ___________ is the time from the beginning of one pulse to the beginning of the next.
    a. frequency
    b. time
    c. duration
    d. period
45. The PRP ___________ while PRF increases.
    a. increases
    b. decreases
    c. is unchanged
    d. is undetermined
46. PD is the ___________ it takes for a pulse to occur.
    a. frequency
    b. time
    c. duration
    d. period
47. SPL is the ___________ of ___________ that a pulse occupies while it travels.
    a. length, time
    b. length, space
    c. amount, amplitude
    d. intensity, energy
48. ___________ is the fraction of time that pulsed ultrasound is actually on.
    a. Pulse duration
    b. Pulse intensity
    c. Duty factor
    d. Duty frequency
49. PD equals the number of cycles in the pulse multiplied by ___________.
    a. frequency
    b. period
    c. wavelength
    d. amplitude

50. SPL equals the number of cycles in the pulse multiplied by ___________.
    a. frequency
    b. period
    c. wavelength
    d. amplitude
51. The DF of continuous wave sound is ___________.
    a. 1
    b. undefined
    c. 1540
    d. 10
52. If the wavelength is 2 mm, the SPL for a three-cycle pulse is ___________ mm.
    a. 6
    b. 0.6
    c. 0.4
    d. 1
53. The SPL in soft tissue for a two-cycle pulse of frequency 5 MHz is ___________ mm.
    a. 6
    b. 0.6
    c. 0.4
    d. 1
54. The PD in soft tissue for a two-cycle pulse of frequency 5 MHz is ___________ ms.
    a. 6
    b. 0.6
    c. 0.4
    d. 1
55. For a 1-kHz PRF, the PRP is ___________ ms.
    a. 6
    b. 0.6
    c. 0.4
    d. 1
56. For Exercises 54 and 55 together, the DF is ___________.
    a. 0.0004
    b. 0.004
    c. 0.04
    d. 0.4
57. How many cycles are there in 1 second of continuous wave 5-MHz ultrasound?
    a. 5
    b. 500
    c. 5000
    d. 5,000,000
    e. None of the above
58. How many cycles are there in 1 second of pulsed 5-MHz ultrasound with a DF of 0.01 (1%)?
    a. 5
    b. 500
    c. 5000
    d. 5,000,000
    e. None of the above
59. In Exercise 58, how many cycles did pulsing eliminate?
    a. 100%
    b. 99.9%
    c. 99%
    d. 50%
    e. 1%
60. For pulsed ultrasound, the DF is always ___________ 1.
    a. less than
    b. greater than
    c. equal to
61. ___________ is a typical DF for sonography.
    a. 0.1
    b. 0.5
    c. 0.7
    d. 0.9
62. Amplitude is the maximum ___________ that occurs in an acoustic variable.
    a. time
    b. variation
    c. distance
    d. frequency
63. Intensity is the ___________ in a wave divided by ___________.
    a. amplitude, power
    b. area, power
    c. power, amplitude
    d. power, area
64. A unit for intensity is ___________.
    a. mW/cm^2
    b. MHz/cm^2
    c. cm/MHz
    d. mm/cm^2
65. Intensity is proportional to ___________ squared.
    a. mW
    b. watts
    c. attenuation
    d. amplitude
66. If power is doubled and area remains unchanged, intensity is ___________.
    a. unchanged
    b. halved
    c. doubled
    d. quadrupled
67. If area is doubled and power remains unchanged, intensity is ___________.
    a. unchanged
    b. halved
    c. doubled
    d. quadrupled
68. If both power and area are doubled, intensity is ___________.
    a. unchanged
    b. halved
    c. doubled
    d. quadrupled
69. If amplitude is doubled, intensity is ___________.
    a. unchanged
    b. halved
    c. doubled
    d. quadrupled

70. If a sound beam has a power of 10 mW and a beam area of 2 cm^2, the spatial average intensity is ___________ mW/cm^2.
   a. 10
   b. 2
   c. 20
   d. 5
71. Attenuation is the reduction in ___________ and ___________ as a wave travels through a medium.
   a. amplitude, intensity
   b. amplitude, wavelength
   c. intensity, speed
   d. amplitude, speed
72. Attenuation consists of ___________, ___________, and ___________.
   a. amplitude, intensity, power
   b. amplitude, wavelength, power
   c. absorption, reflection, scattering
   d. scattering, amplitude, speed
73. The attenuation coefficient is attenuation per ___________ of sound travel.
   a. second
   b. centimeter
   c. cycle
   d. wavelength
74. Attenuation and the attenuation coefficient are given in units of ___________ and ___________, respectively.
   a. dB, dB/cm MHz
   b. mW/cm^2, mW/cm MHz
   c. dB, dB/cm^2
   d. dB^2, mW/dB MHz
75. For soft tissues, there is approximately ___________ dB of attenuation per centimeter for each megahertz of frequency.
   a. 1.54
   b. 3
   c. 5
   d. 0.5
76. For soft tissues, the attenuation coefficient at 3 MHz is approximately ___________.
   a. 15 dB/cm
   b. 3 dB
   c. 1.5 dB/cm
   d. 15 dB
77. The attenuation coefficient in soft tissue _______ while frequency increases.
   a. increases
   b. decreases
   c. weakens
   d. decelerates
78. For soft tissue, if frequency is doubled, attenuation is ___________. If path length is doubled, attenuation is ___________. If both frequency and path length are doubled, attenuation is ___________.
   a. doubled, doubled, quadrupled
   b. doubled, doubled, doubled
   c. doubled, quadrupled, quadrupled
   d. quadrupled, quadrupled, quadrupled
79. If frequency is doubled and path length is halved, attenuation is ___________.
   a. doubled
   b. halved
   c. quadrupled
   d. unchanged
80. Absorption is the conversion of ___________ to ___________.
   a. energy, amplitude
   b. heat, sound
   c. sound, heat
   d. sound, intensity
81. Absorption can be greater than attenuation in a given medium at a given frequency. True or false?
82. Attenuation is higher in bone than in soft tissue. True or false?
83. The imaging depth (penetration) ___________ while frequency increases.
   a. increases
   b. decreases
   c. is unchanged
   d. is undetermined
84. If the intensity of 4-MHz ultrasound entering soft tissue is 2 W/cm^2, the intensity at a depth of 4 cm is ___________ W/cm^2.
   a. 0.16
   b. 0.32
   c. 0.48
   d. 0.64
85. If the intensity of 40-MHz ultrasound entering soft tissue is 2 W/cm^2, the intensity at a depth of 4 cm is ___________ W/cm^2.
   a. 0.00002
   b. 0.000002
   c. 0.0000002
   d. 0.00000002
86. The depth at which half-intensity occurs in soft tissues at 7.5 MHz is ___________ cm.
   a. 0.6
   b. 0.7
   c. 0.8
   d. 0.9
87. When ultrasound encounters a boundary with perpendicular incidence, the ___________ of the tissues must be different to produce a reflection (echo).
   a. impedances
   b. densities
   c. speeds
   d. hardnesses
88. With perpendicular incidence, two media ___________ and the incident ___________ must be known to calculate the reflected intensity.
   a. impedances, amplitude
   b. amplitudes, impedance
   c. impedances, intensity
   d. amplitudes, intensity

89. With perpendicular incidence, two media ___________ must be known to calculate the intensity reflection coefficient.
  a. densities
  b. speeds
  c. hardnesses
  d. impedances
90. For an incident intensity of 2 mW/cm^2 and impedances of 49 and 51 rayls, the reflected intensity is ___________ mW/cm^2, and the transmitted intensity is ___________ mW/cm^2.
  a. 0.8, 1.2
  b. 0.08, 1.92
  c. 0.008, 1.992
  d. 0.0008, 1.9992
91. If the impedances of the media are equal, there is no reflection. True or false?
92. With perpendicular incidence, the reflected intensity depends on the ___________.
  a. density difference
  b. impedance difference
  c. impedance sum
  d. b and c
  e. a and b
93. Refraction is a change in ___________ of sound when it crosses a boundary. Refraction is caused by a change in ___________ ___________ at the boundary.
  a. speed, sound direction
  b. direction, propagation speed
  c. amplitude, media impedance
  d. direction, media attenuation
94. Under what two conditions does refraction not occur?
  a. perpendicular incidence or equal media propagation speeds
  b. oblique incidence or equal media propagation speeds
  c. perpendicular incidence or unequal media propagation speeds
  d. oblique incidence or unequal media propagation speeds
95. The low speed of sound in fat is a source of image degradation because of refraction. If the incidence angle at a boundary between fat (1.45 mm/ms) and kidney (1.56 mm/ms) is 30 degrees, the transmission angle is ___________ degrees.
  a. 28
  b. 30
  c. 32
  d. 33
96. Reflection of sound in many directions while it encounters rough media junctions or particle suspensions (heterogeneous media) is called __________.
  a. specular
  b. refraction
  c. propagation
  d. scattering
97. Backscatter helps make echo reception less dependent on incident angle. True or false?
98. What must be known to calculate the distance to a reflector?
  a. Attenuation, speed, and density
  b. Attenuation and impedance
  c. Attenuation and absorption
  d. Travel time and speed
  e. Density and speed
99. No reflection will occur with perpendicular incidence if the media ___________ are equal.
  a. impedances
  b. speeds
  c. densities
  d. attenuations
100. Scattering occurs at smooth boundaries and within homogeneous media. True or false?
101. Axial resolution is the minimum reflector separation required along the direction of the ___________ ___________ to produce separate ___________.
  a. scan lines, echoes
  b. sound travel, amplitudes
  c. double reflectors, lines
  d. scan lines, amplitudes
102. Axial resolution depends directly on ___________ ___________
  a. the peak amplitude
  b. spatial echo distance
  c. spatial pulse length
  d. spatial pulse width
103. Smaller axial resolution is better. True or false?
104. If there are three cycles of a 1 mm wavelength in a pulse, the axial resolution is ___________ mm.
  a. 1.0
  b. 1.5
  c. 2.5
  d. 3.0
105. For pulses traveling through soft tissue in which the frequency is 3 MHz and there are four cycles per pulse, the axial resolution is ___________ mm.
  a. 1.0
  b. 1.5
  c. 2.5
  d. 3.0
106. If there are two cycles per pulse, the axial resolution is equal to the ___________. At 5 MHz in soft tissue, this is ___________ mm.
  a. wavelength, 5.0
  b. wavelength, 0.3
  c. duration, 1.54
  d. duration, 0.2
107. Doubling the frequency causes axial resolution to be ___________.
  a. doubled
  b. increased
  c. degraded
  d. halved
108. Doubling the number of cycles per pulse causes axial resolution to be ___________.
  a. doubled
  b. increased
  c. degraded
  d. halved
109. When studying an obese subject, a higher frequency likely will be required. True or false?
110. If better resolution is desired, a lower frequency will help. True or false?

111. If frequencies less than ___________ MHz are used, axial resolution is not sufficient.
   a. 0.1
   b. 2
   c. 5
   d. 20
112. If frequencies higher than ___________ MHz are used, penetration is not sufficient for most applications.
   a. 0.1
   b. 8
   c. 15
   d. 30
113. Increasing frequency improves resolution because ___________ is reduced, thus reducing ___________
   a. attenuation, depth of penetration
   b. attenuation, spatial pulse length
   c. wavelength, spatial pulse length
   d. wavelength, depth of penetration
114. Increasing frequency decreases penetration because ___________ is increased.
   a. reflection
   b. heating
   c. speed
   d. attenuation
115. Lateral resolution is the minimum ___________ between two reflectors at the same depth such that when a beam is scanned across them, two separate ___________ are produced.
   a. separation, propagations
   b. amplitude, propagations
   c. separation, echoes
   d. amplitude, echoes
116. Lateral resolution is equal to ___________ ___________ in the scan plane.
   a. beam width
   b. pulse length
   c. beam length
   d. pulse height
117. Lateral resolution does not depend on ___________.
   a. frequency
   b. aperture
   c. phasing
   d. depth
   e. damping
118. For an aperture of a given size, increasing frequency improves lateral resolution. True or false?
119. Lateral resolution varies with distance from the transducer. True or false?
120. For a given frequency, a smaller aperture always yields improved lateral resolution. True or false?
121. Lateral resolution is determined by ___________. (There is more than one correct answer to the question.)
   a. damping
   b. frequency
   c. aperture
   d. number of cycles in the pulse
   e. distance from the transducer
   f. focusing
122. A two-cycle pulse of 5 MHz ultrasound produces separate echoes from reflectors in soft tissue separated by 1 mm. True or false?
123. Because diagnostic ultrasound pulses are usually two or three cycles long, axial resolution is usually equal to ___________ to ___________ wavelengths.
   a. 2, 3
   b. 4, 6
   c. 1, 3.5
   d. 1, 1.5
124. What are the axial resolutions in Fig. 2.36, A–B?
   a. 5 mm, 4 mm
   b. 4 mm, 3 mm
   c. 3 mm, 2 mm
   d. 2 mm, 1 mm

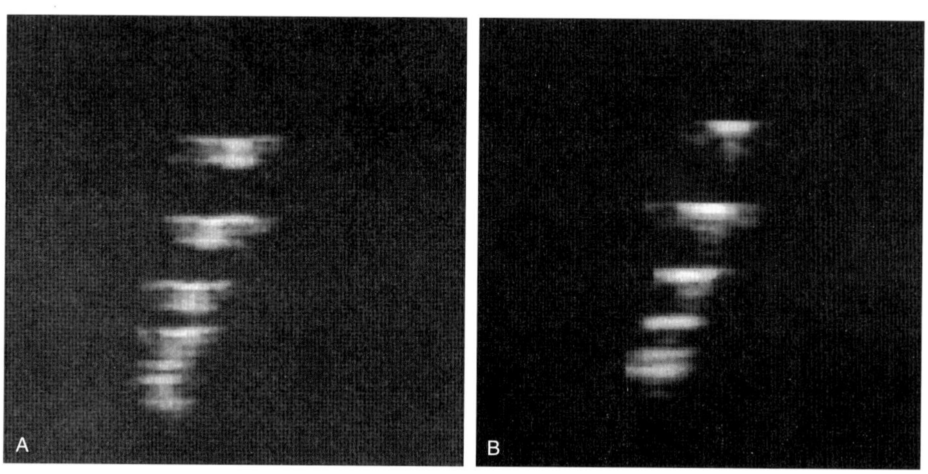

Fig. 2.36 Illustration to accompany Exercise 124. **A,** An image of a set of six rods in a test object. They are separated by 5, 4, 3, 2, and 1 mm from top to bottom. This scan was made with a transducer that produces 3.5-MHz ultrasound. The first three rods have been separated, whereas the images of the last three rods have merged. This image also shows small reverberation echoes behind each rod. **B,** The same rods imaged with a 5-MHz transducer. Higher-frequency transducers produce shorter pulse lengths and therefore provide improved axial resolution.

3

Transducers: Transmitting and Receiving

LEARNING OBJECTIVES

After reading this chapter, the student should be able to do the following:

- Describe the construction of a simple transducer and the function of each part.
- Explain how a transducer generates ultrasound pulses.
- Explain how a transducer receives echoes.
- Describe a sound beam and list the factors that affect it.
- Discuss how sound beams are focused and automatically scanned through anatomy.
- Compare linear, convex, phased, and vector arrays.

CHAPTER OUTLINE

KEY TERMS

Aperture
Apodization
Array
Beam
Composite
Convex array
Crystal
Curie point
Damping
Disk
Dynamic aperture
Dynamic focusing
Element
Far zone
Focal length
Focal region
Focal zone
Focus
Grating lobes
Lead zirconate titanate
Lens
Linear
Linear array
Linear phased array
Linear sequenced array
Matching layer
Natural focus
Near zone
Operating frequency
Phased array
Phased linear array
Piezoelectricity
Point of care ultrasound
Probe
Resonance frequency
Scanhead
Sector
Sensitivity
Side lobes
Sound beam
Source
Transducer
Transducer assembly
Ultrasound transducer
Vector array

This chapter describes transducers, the devices that generate, transmit, and receive ultrasound. Transducers form the connecting link between the ultrasound-tissue interactions described in Chapter 2 and the ultrasound systems described in Chapters 4 and 5, The sound produced by these transducers is confined in beams (or scan-lines) rather than traveling in all directions away from the **source**. These beams can be focused and are automatically scanned through tissue by the transducers.

CONSTRUCTION AND OPERATION

A **transducer** converts one form of energy to another. **Ultrasound transducers** (Fig. 3.1) convert electric energy into mechanical energy (i.e., ultrasound), and vice versa. The electric voltages applied to transducers are converted to ultrasound. Ultrasound echoes received by the transducers produce electric voltages. Airpods (Fig. 3.2A), microphones (see Fig. 3.2B), and loudspeakers accomplish similar functions with audible sound.

Some transducers include parts of the electronics that otherwise used to be located in the scanner internally, in the transducer handle. Some transducers, typically used for point-of-care ultrasound (**POCUS**), even include *all* the electronics necessary for imaging except the display within the probe itself. They can be attached to a smartphone or tablet (see Fig. 3.1C) for control and display.

Piezoelectric Element

Ultrasound transducers operate according to the principle of **piezoelectricity** originally discovered by Pierre Curie and his brother Jacques in 1880. This principle states that some materials, when deformed by an applied pressure, produce a voltage. Conversely, piezoelectricity also results in the production

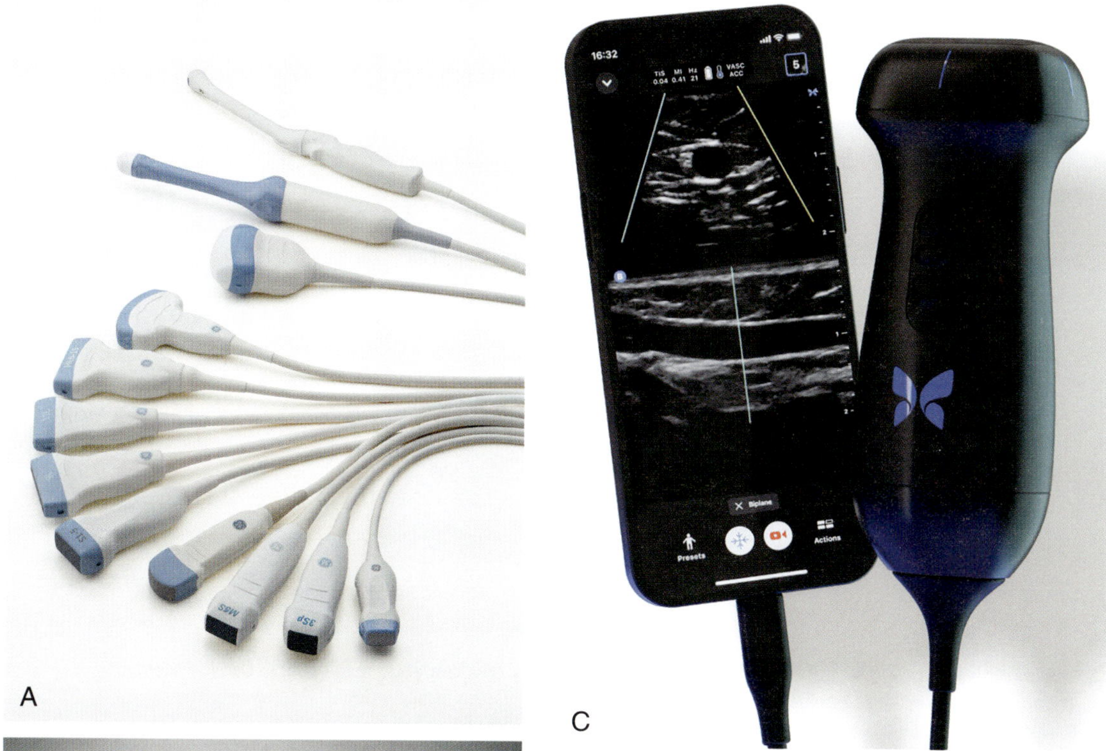

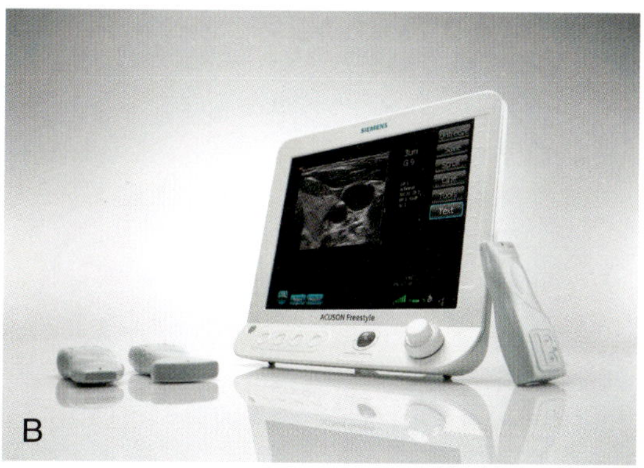

Fig. 3.1 **A,** Transducers of various types. **B,** Cable-free transducers are commercially available. **C,** Transducer that include all the electronics necessary for direct attachment to a smart phone or tablet for control and display. (**A,** Courtesy GE Healthcare. **B,** Courtesy Siemens Healthineers. **C,** Courtesy Butterfly Network.)

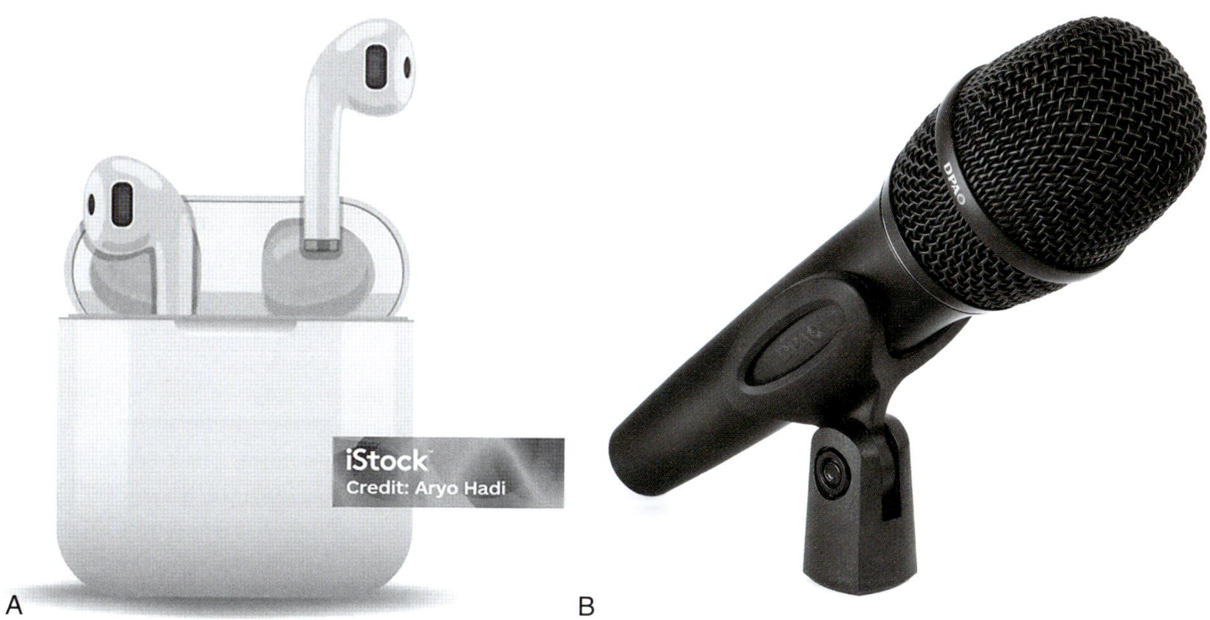

Fig. 3.2 **A,** Airpods. **B,** Microphone. (**B,** Courtesy DPA Microphones)

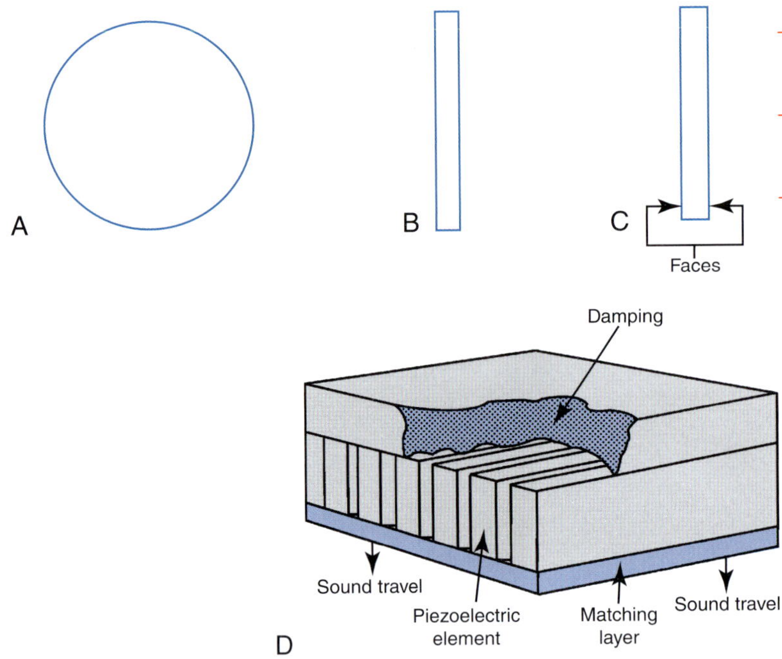

Fig. 3.3 **A,** Front view of a disk transducer element. **B,** Front view of a rectangular element. **C,** Side view of either element with no voltage applied to faces (normal thickness), with voltage applied (increased thickness), and with opposite voltage applied (decreased thickness). **D,** The internal parts of a transducer assembly (scanhead or probe). The damping (backing) material reduces pulse duration, thus improving axial resolution. The matching layer improves sound transmission into the tissues. Not included in this illustration are a lens and a protective/insulating layer that commonly are attached to the front of the assembly.

of a pressure when an applied voltage deforms these materials. Various formulations of **lead zirconate titanate** (designated PZT) were commonly used as materials in the production of ultrasound transducer **elements**. Ceramics such as these are not naturally piezoelectric. They are made piezoelectric during their manufacture by being placed in a strong electric field while they are above a critical temperature (the **Curie point**), which rearranges the dipoles within the material. In this case, dipoles are molecules that have separate positive and negative electrical charges at either end/side (see Fig. 3.3C). These ceramics often are combined with a nonpiezoelectric polymer to create materials called *piezo-composites*. These **composites** have lower impedance and improved bandwidth, **sensitivity**, and **resolution** and are used in most modern ultrasound transducers.

> Piezoelectric elements convert electric voltages into ultrasound pulses (mechanical energy) and convert returning echoes back into voltages.

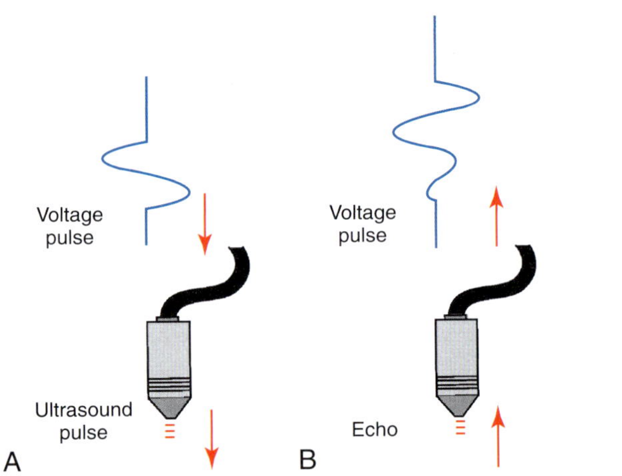

Fig. 3.4 A transducer converts electric voltage pulses into ultrasound pulses **(A)** and converts received echoes into electric voltage pulses **(B)**.

Single-element transducers take the form of disks (Fig. 3.3A) and are only used for in vitro studies. **Linear array** transducers contain numerous elements, each having a rectangular shape (see Fig. 3.3B). When an electric voltage is applied to the faces of either type, the thickness of the element increases or decreases, depending on the arrangement of the internal dipoles and, thus, the polarity of the voltage (see Fig. 3.3C). The term *transducer element* (also called piezoelectric element, active element, or crystal) refers to the piece of piezoelectric material (see Fig. 3.3D) that converts electricity to ultrasound and vice versa. Elements, with their associated case and **damping** and matching materials (see Fig. 3.3E), are called a transducer assembly, probe, scanhead, array, or, simply, a *transducer*.

Transducers typically are driven by one cycle of alternating voltage for diagnostic ultrasound imaging. This single cycle–driving voltage produces a two- or three-cycle ultrasound pulse. Longer driving voltages, typically 5 to 32 cycles, are used in Doppler modes. This operation produces an alternating pressure wave that propagates from the transducer as a sound pulse (Fig. 3.4A). The frequency of the sound produced is equal to the frequency of the driving voltage, which must be reasonably near the **operating frequency** (f_o) of the transducer for operation with acceptable efficiency. The operating frequency (also referred to as the **resonance frequency** of the transducer

TABLE 3.1 Transducer Element Thickness for Various Operating Frequencies

Frequency (MHz)	Thickness (mm)
2.0	1.0
3.5	0.6
5.0	0.4
7.5	0.3
10.0	0.2

[a]Assuming an element propagation speed of 4 mm/μs.

element) is the preferred, or center, or natural, frequency of operation for the element. Operating frequency is determined by the following:

- The propagation speed of the element material (ct).
- The thickness (th) of the transducer element.

Operating frequency is such that the thickness of the element corresponds to half a wavelength in the element material. Typical diagnostic ultrasound elements are 0.2 to 1 mm thick (Table 3.1) and have propagation speeds of 4 to 6 mm/μs. Since wavelength decreases as frequency increases, thinner elements yield higher frequencies (Fig. 3.5). This is analogous to smaller bells producing higher-pitched sounds (see Fig. 3.5C–D). The transducer converts the returning echo into an alternating voltage pulse (see Fig. 3.4B).

$$f_0\,(\text{MHz}) = \frac{c_t\,(\text{mm}/\mu\text{s})}{2 \times \text{th}(\text{mm})}$$

Thinner elements operate at higher frequencies.

ADVANCED CONCEPT

When a ceramic crystal is raised beyond the Curie point (about 350°C for PZT ceramics), the molecules in the crystal lattice can reorient with respect to each other. The molecules are normally oriented randomly, yielding no piezoelectric properties. If raised beyond the Curie point while in a strong electric field, the molecules (which are tiny electric dipoles) line up with the electric field. When the crystal is cooled below the Curie point while in the field, the crystal lattice is locked into the molecular structure that piezoelectric crystals naturally have, with the molecular dipoles lined up parallel to each other. Now if a voltage is applied to the front and rear faces of the element, it will get thicker or thinner as the dipoles together rotate toward or away (depending on the polarity of the voltage) from parallelism with the electric field produced by the voltage (see Fig. 3.3C). If a polarized ceramic element is heated above the Curie point while not in an electric field, the molecules reorient randomly, and the element loses its piezoelectric properties.

With wide-bandwidth transducers (e.g., those having a fractional bandwidth of at least 70%), voltage excitation can be used selectively to operate the same transducer at more than one frequency (Fig. 3.6). The transducer is driven at one of two or three or more selectable frequencies by voltage pulses with the selected frequency. The two or three frequencies must fall within the transducer bandwidth. Choosing the higher frequency yields better **detail resolution**. If the resulting penetration is not sufficient for the study at hand, however, a lower frequency can be selected (resulting in some degradation in detail resolution). Manual or automatic frequency switching is quicker, more convenient, and more cost-effective than physically changing transducers.

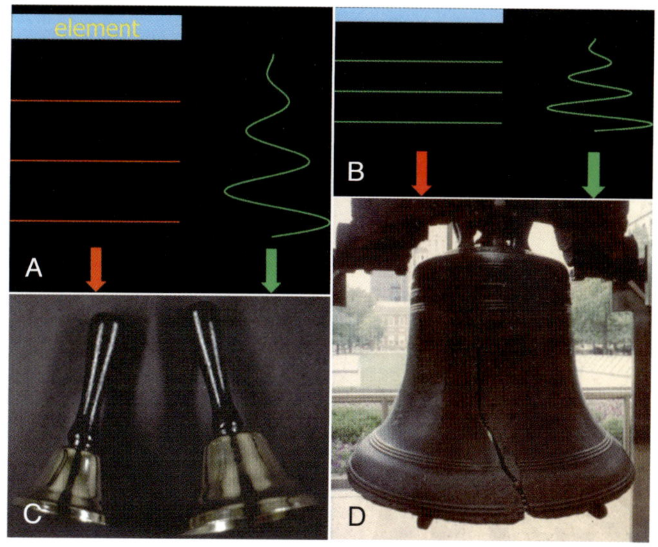

Fig. 3.5 **A,** Thicker elements operate at lower frequencies. **B,** Thinner elements operate at higher frequencies. **C–D,** Smaller and larger bells ring with higher and lower pitches, respectively.

Damping Material

Ultrasound pulse repetition frequency (PRF) is equal to the voltage PRF. This is the number of voltage pulses sent to the transducer each second, which is determined by the instrument driving the transducer. Pulse duration is equal to period multiplied by number of cycles in the pulse. Damping (also called *backing*) material, a mixture of metal powder and a plastic or epoxy resin, is attached to the rear face of the transducer elements to reduce the number of cycles in each pulse (see Figs. 3.3E and 3.7). Damping reduces pulse duration and spatial pulse length, which improves resolution but reduces probe sensitivity. This method of damping is analogous to packing foam rubber around a bell that is rung by a tap with a hammer. The rubber reduces the time that the bell rings after the tap. The rubber also reduces the loudness of the ringing. In the case of ultrasound transducers, the damping material additionally reduces the ultrasound amplitude and thus decreases the efficiency and sensitivity (ability to detect weak echoes) of the system (an undesired effect). This is the price paid for reduced spatial pulse length (a desired effect resulting in improved detail resolution) with damping. Typically, pulses of two to three cycles are generated with (damped) diagnostic ultrasound transducers. Reducing the number of cycles in the pulses broadens their bandwidth. Typical bandwidths for modern transducers range from 50% to 100%. An example of a 100% bandwidth is a 5-MHz operating frequency with a bandwidth of 5 MHz, that is, from 2.5 to 7.5 MHz.

Composites and damping material shorten pulses and improve detail resolution but reduce probe sensitivity.

Transducers intended for continuous wave Doppler ultrasound use are not damped because pulses are not used in this application. These transducers have higher efficiencies (or sensitivity) because energy is not lost to the damping material.

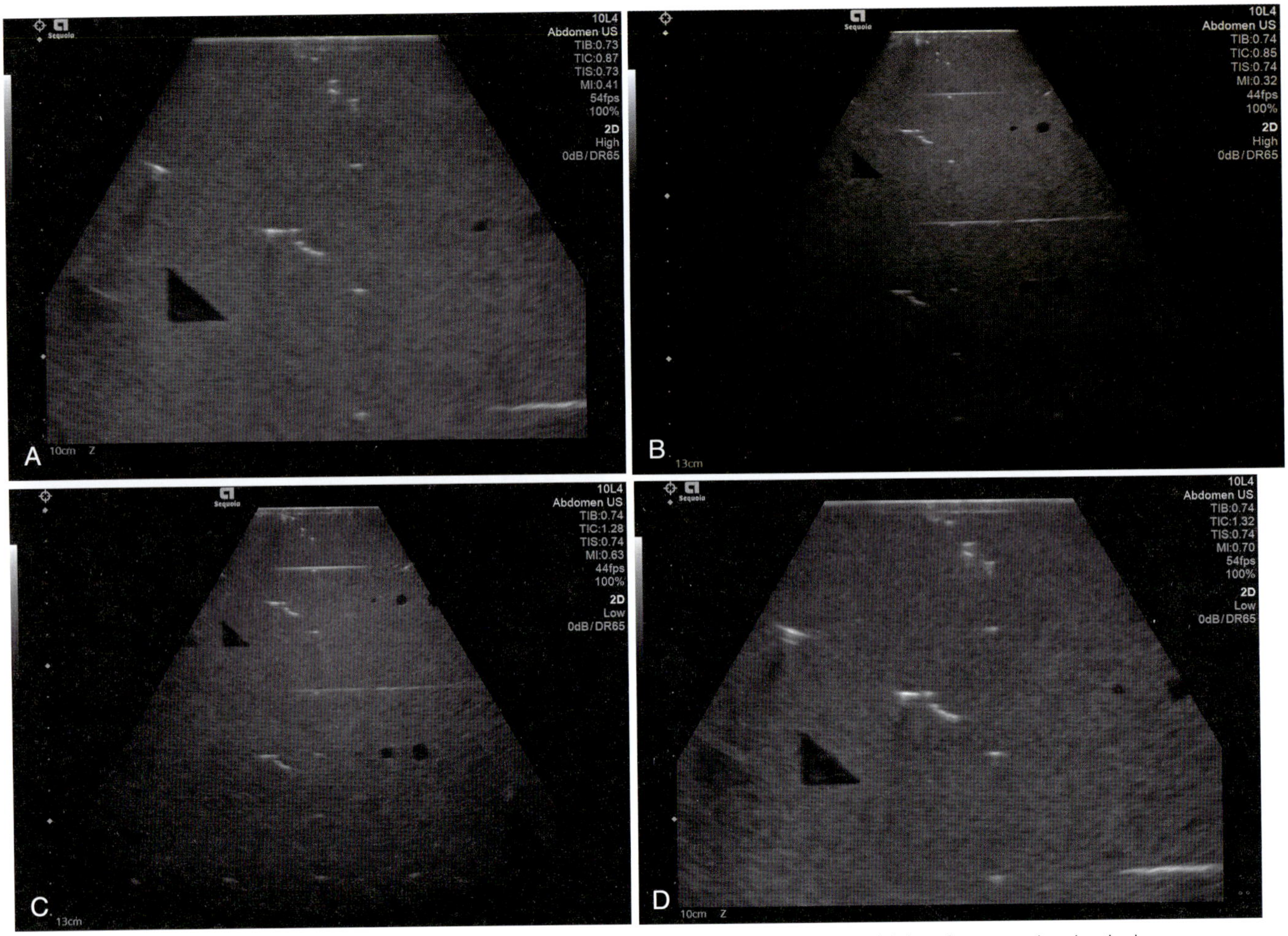

Fig. 3.6 Multiple-frequency operation allows the transducer to provide (at a higher frequency) selectively better detail resolution **(A)** with reduced penetration **(B)** or (at a lower frequency) deeper penetration **(C)** with some degradation of resolution **(D)**.

Matching Layer

Because transducer elements are solid (having high density and sound speed), the impedance is approximately 20 times that of tissues. Without compensation, this factor would cause approximately 80% of the emitted intensity to be reflected at the skin boundary (even with gel removing any air between the probe and the skin). Thus most of the sound energy would not enter the body. A returning echo would also have about 80% of its intensity reflected, so only a small portion would exit the tissue and enter the transducer. Therefore the received echo intensity for a perfect (100%) reflector would be only 4% ($0.2 \times 1.00 \times 0.2$) because only approximately 20% of the intensity enters and only about 20% of the echo intensity exits the body. To solve this problem, a **matching layer** is usually placed on the transducer face (see Fig. 3.3E). This material has an impedance that is an intermediate value between those of the transducer elements and the tissue. The material reduces the reflection of ultrasound at the transducer element surface, thereby improving sound transmission in both directions across it. This is analogous to the thin coating on eyeglasses or camera lenses that reduces light reflection at the air-glass boundary. Given the broad bandwidth of modern transducers, many frequencies (and therefore wavelengths) are present in the short ultrasound pulses transmitted. Hence, multiple matching layers will improve sound transmission across the element-tissue boundary better than a single layer. Typically, two layers are used, although in some cases, one or three layers are used. The lower impedance of piezocomposite elements assists in the impedance-matching process, allowing more of the ultrasound energy to exit the front of the element into the patient rather than being lost as heat in the damping material.

ADVANCED CONCEPT

For continuous-wave ultrasound, a single matching layer of quarter-wave thickness and an impedance that is the geometric mean of the two impedances at the boundary (i.e., of the transducer and the skin) provides the best match. The geometric mean is the square root of the product of the two impedances. Because ultrasound pulses are characterized by a bandwidth rather than a single frequency, multiple layers (usually two for practical purposes) of varying impedance values and thicknesses match the impedances better than a single matching layer would. Even so, the matching layers still act as a bandpass filter, limiting the bandwidth of the pulses transmitted from the elements to the tissues.

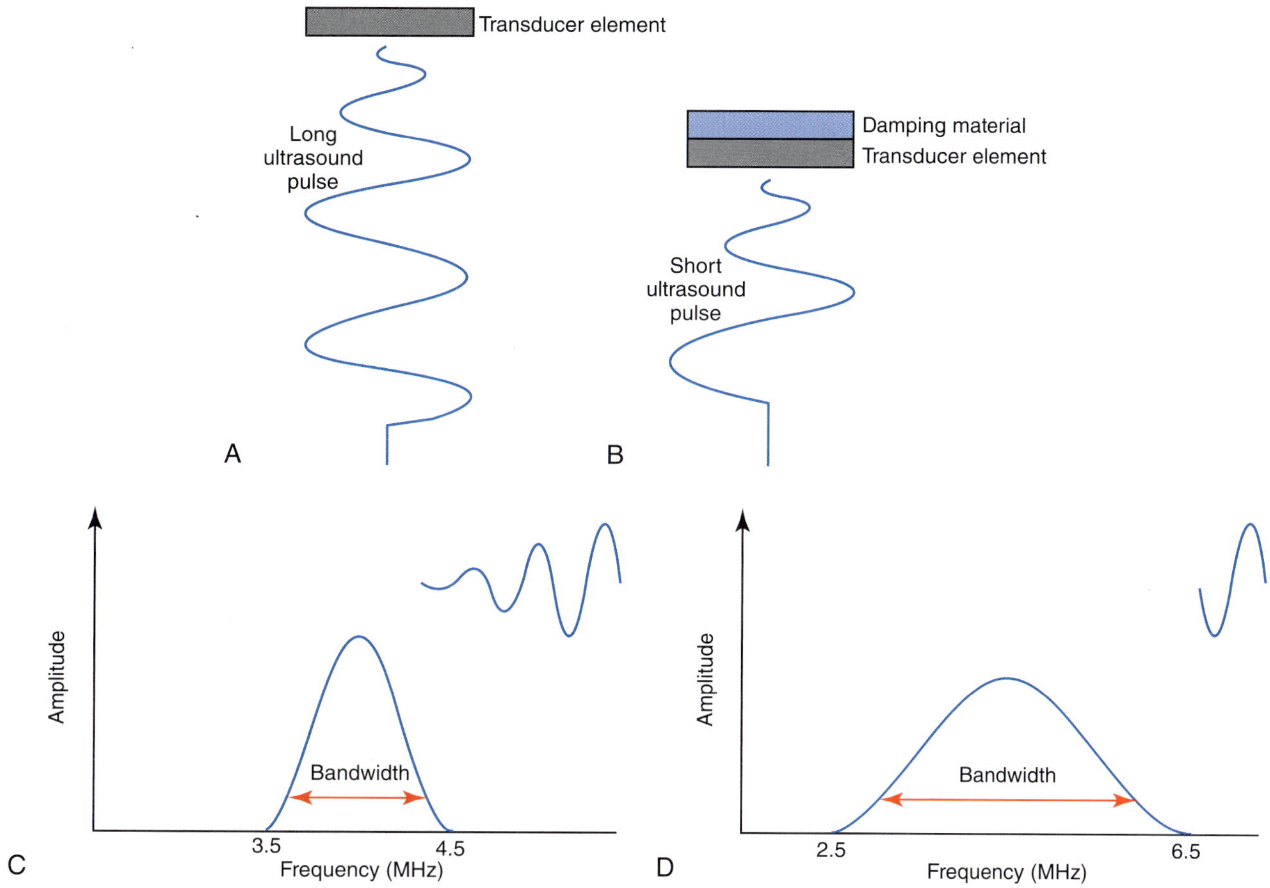

Fig. 3.7 **A,** Without damping, a transducer element produces a long ultrasound pulse of many cycles. **B,** With damping material on the rear face of the transducer element, a short ultrasound pulse of a few cycles is produced. This figure shows each pulse traveling (*down*) away from the transducer in space so that the bottom end is the beginning or leading edge of the pulse while it travels down. **C–D,** Plots of the frequencies present in the ultrasound pulses (from **A** and **B,** respectively). Component amplitude is the amplitude of each frequency component present. Bandwidth is the frequency range within which the amplitudes exceed a reference value. Compare the frequency spectrum for a narrowband, undamped pulse **(C)** with the frequency spectrum for a broadband, damped pulse **(D)**.

Coupling Medium

Because of its very low impedance, even a very thin layer of air between the transducer and the skin surface reflects virtually all the sound, preventing any penetration into the tissue. For this reason, a coupling medium, usually an aqueous gel, is applied to the skin before transducer contact. This eliminates the air layer and facilitates the passage of sound into and out of the tissue. Thus the combination of matching layers and the coupling medium enables the efficient passage of ultrasound into the body and the return of echoes from the body into the transducer.

> Matching layers and coupling media facilitate the passage of ultrasound in both directions across the transducer-skin boundary.

Invasive Transducers

Some transducers are designed to enter the body (Fig. 3.8) via the vagina, rectum, esophagus, or via a blood vessel (catheter-mounted transducer assemblies). These approaches allow the transducer to be placed closer to the anatomy of interest, which avoids echoes from intervening tissues (e.g., lung or gassy bowel) and reduces the sound transmission path length (i.e., depth). This reduction in the imaging depth yields lower attenuation and, therefore, allows higher frequencies to be used, which in turn improves detail resolution.

BEAMS AND FOCUSING

A continuous wave ultrasound beam contains ultrasound at all time points and locations within the beam similarly to how a flashlight beam is "filled" with light. A pulsed beam does not. What is then meant by "the beam" in the case of pulsed ultrasound? The term *beam* refers to the width of a pulse as it travels away from the transducer. Generally, the width in the scan plane is not the same as the width perpendicular to the scan plane. The width in the scan plane determines the **lateral resolution (LR)**, whereas the width perpendicular to the scan plane determines the extent of the section thickness artifact (discussed in Chapter 7).

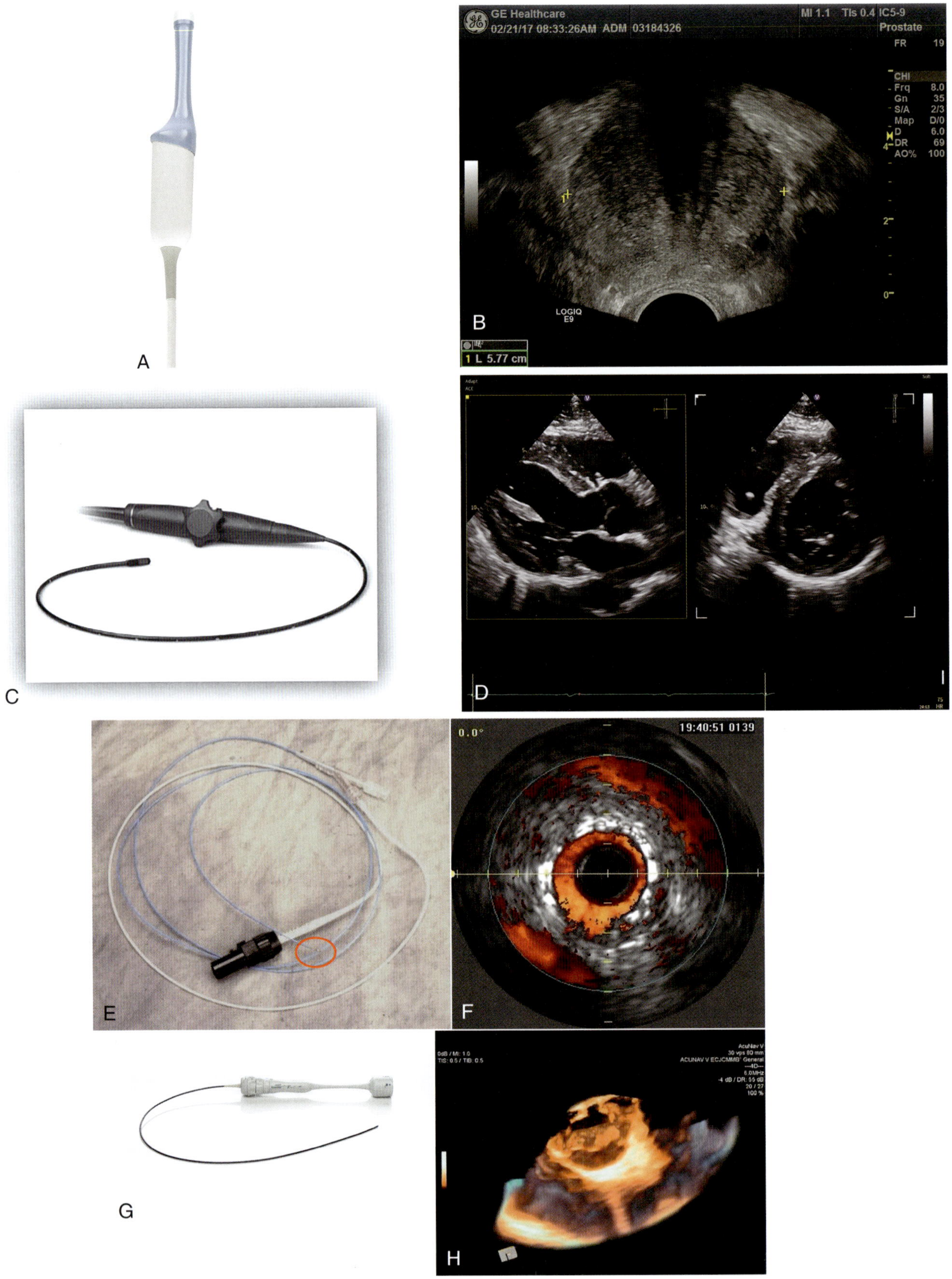

Fig. 3.8 **A,** Endocavitary transducer. **B,** Transrectal view of the prostate. **C,** Transesophageal probe for echocardiography. **D,** Transesophageal view of the adult heart showing real-time biplane imaging. **E,** Catheter-mounted transducer (*circle*) for viewing the interior of a blood vessel. **F,** Interior view of a blood vessel. **G,** Intracardiac catheter transducer. **H,** View of aortic valve with the intracardiac catheter transducer. (**A–F,** Courtesy GE HealthCare. **I and J**, Courtesy Siemens Healthineers.)

ADVANCED CONCEPT

The formation of a focused (narrow transmit) beam from an aperture of some size and shape is explained by Huygens principle and the concept of diffraction. Diffraction is the deviation of the direction of a wave that is *not* attributable to reflection, scattering, or refraction. Diffraction occurs when a wave passes an obstacle or a small (similar to the wavelength) aperture. Huygens principle states that all points on a wave front or at a source can be considered as point sources for the production of spherical (secondary) wavelets. As these wavelets propagate, the wave front location and orientation at later times can be constructed by the summation of these wavelets. This principle can be applied to the surface of a transducer to determine the beam profile of the wave that emanates from that surface.

The near-zone length is given by

$$NZL = \frac{(a_p)^2}{4\lambda} = \frac{(a_p)^2 f}{4c}$$

where a_p is the disk aperture, that is, diameter, and c is the propagation speed.

The beam width (w_b) at any location depends on wavelength (λ), aperture (a_p), and distance from the transducer (d).

In the approximation of Fig. 3.9, at the end of the near zone, the beam width is equal to one-half the transducer width (Fig. 3.10). At a distance of two times the near-zone length, the beam width is equal to the transducer diameter. Beyond this distance, the beam width increases in proportion to the distance. As a pulse travels through the near zone, its width decreases; as it travels through the far zone, its width increases. In the near zone,

$$W_b = a_p - \frac{2\lambda d}{a_p} = a_p - \frac{2cd}{fa_p}$$

where a_p is the diameter for a circular aperture. For a rectangular aperture, the expression is more complicated. In the far zone,

$$W_b = \frac{2(\lambda \times d)}{a_p} = \frac{2cd}{f \times a_p}$$

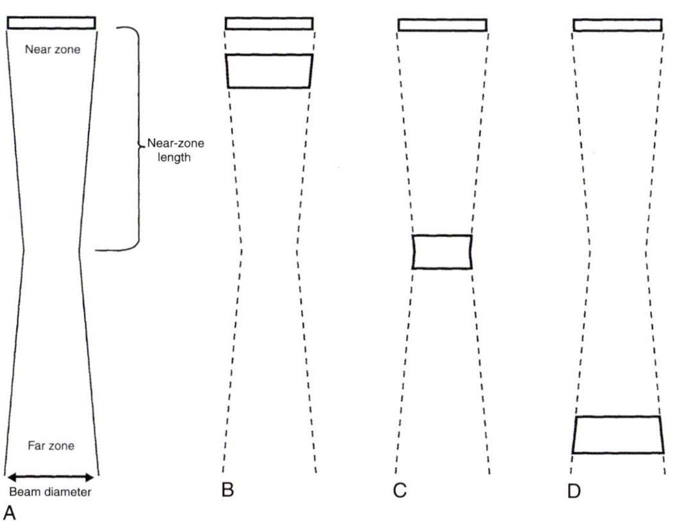

Fig. 3.9 **A,** Beam width for a single-element unfocused disk transducer operating in the continuous wave mode. The near zone is the region between the disk and the minimum beam width. The far zone is the region beyond the minimum beam width. Intensity varies within the beam, with intensity variations being greatest in the near zone. This beam approximates the changing pulse diameter as an ultrasound pulse travels away from a transducer. **B,** An ultrasound pulse shortly after leaving the transducer. **C,** Later, the ultrasound pulse is located at the end of the near-zone length, where its width is at a minimum. **D,** Still later, the pulse is in the far zone, where its width is increasing as it travels.

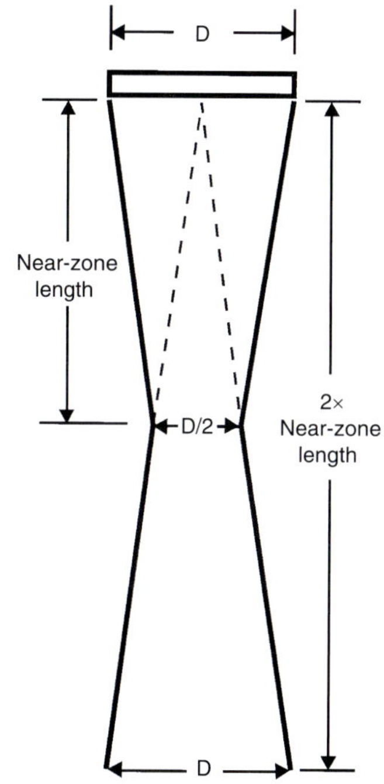

Fig. 3.10 Sound beam from a disk transducer. The beam width narrows to half the disk diameter *(D)* at the near-zone length and then widens to the disk diameter at twice the near-zone length.

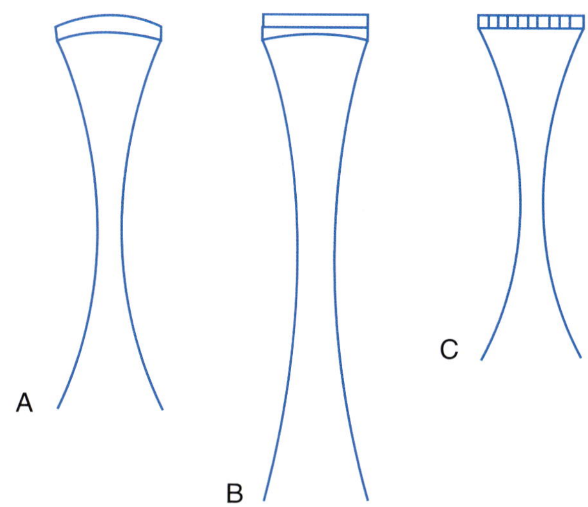

Fig. 3.11 Sound focusing by a curved transducer element, lens, or phased array. Lenses focus because the propagation speed through them is higher than through tissues. Refraction at the surface of the lens forms the beam so that a focal region occurs. The operation of phased arrays is described later in this chapter. **A,** Curved transducer element. **B,** Lens. **C,** Phased array.

Focusing

To improve resolution, diagnostic transducers and beams have traditionally been focused. Focusing sound in the same manner as focusing light reduces *beam* width. Sound may be focused (Fig. 3.11) by using curved (rather than flat) transducer elements, by using a **lens**, or by phasing (discussed later in this chapter). Focusing narrows the beam (hence the term *narrow transmit beam*). Beam width is decreased in the **focal region** (also called focal zone) and in the area between it and the transducer (termed the *near zone*), but it is widened in the region

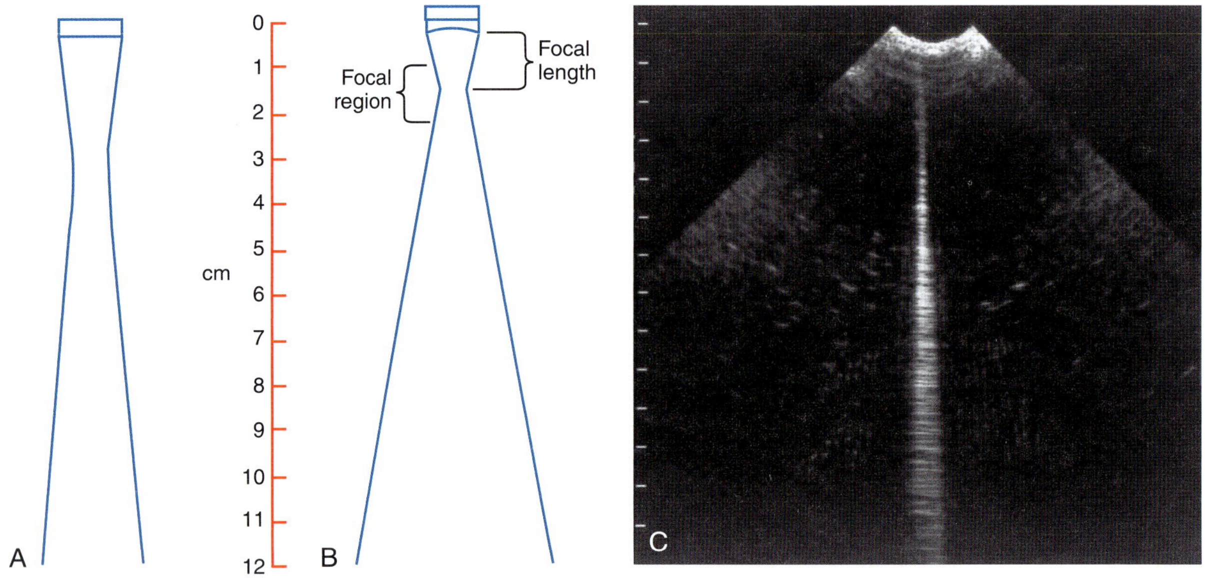

Fig. 3.12 Beam diameter for a 6-mm, 5-MHz transducer without **(A)** and with **(B)** focusing. Focusing reduces the minimum beam width compared with that produced without focusing. However, well beyond the focal region, the width of the focused beam is greater than that of the unfocused beam. **C,** A focused beam. This is an ultrasound image of a beam profile test object containing a thin vertical scattering layer down the center. Scanning this object generates a picture of the beam (the pulse width at all depths). In this case, the focus occurs at a depth of approximately 4 cm (this image has a total depth of 15 cm). Depth markers (in 1-cm increments) are indicated on the left edge of the figure.

beyond (termed the *far zone*) (Fig. 3.12). **Focal length** is the distance from the transducer to the center of the focal region. **Focal zone** length (called *depth of field* in photography) is the distance between equal beam widths that are some multiple (e.g., × 2) of the minimum value at the **focus**.

While the element or lens is increasingly curved (or phase-delay curvature in a **phased array** is increased), the focus moves closer to the transducer and becomes "tighter" (i.e., the beam width at the focus decreases). The limit to which a beam can be narrowed depends on wavelength, size of the source (the width of the element or group of elements and termed the **aperture**), and focal length.

It should be noted that diagnostic ultrasound imaging in general is transitioning toward employing broad (unfocused) transmit beam schemes instead of the traditional narrow (focused) transmit beams described above. Unfocused beams can now produce images that have excellent *focusing throughout the image* (through virtual beam forming) with significantly higher frame rates. The broad transmit beam schemes rely on virtual beam forming and will be described in more detail in Chapters 4 and 5.

Useful Frequency Range

To meet resolution and penetration requirements reasonably, the useful frequency range for most diagnostic applications is 1 to 35 MHz. The lower portion of the range is useful in cardiology or when increased depth (e.g., in an obese subject) or high attenuation (e.g., in transcranial studies) is encountered. The higher portion of the frequency range is useful when little penetration is required (e.g., in imaging breast, thyroid, or superficial vessels or in pediatric imaging) as well as in dermatological application. In most large patients, 3 to 6 MHz is a satisfactory frequency; however, in thin patients and in children, 7.5, 10, and 15 MHz can often be used. If frequencies less than 2 MHz are used, detail resolution is insufficient for anything except wall motion assessments in echocardiography. If frequencies from 20 to 35 MHz (<20 MHz in deeper applications) are used, the depth penetration is not sufficient in many applications except for ophthalmologic and dermatologic imaging. There are also catheter-mounted transducers operating at frequencies as high as 70 MHz for intravascular imaging, since penetration of only a few millimeters is sufficient. Table 3.2 lists values for typical imaging depths and axial resolution for various frequencies.

ADVANCED CONCEPT

For a rectangular aperture, the minimum beam width (at the focus)—that is, the focal beam diameter (d_f)—can be obtained by multiplying twice the wavelength by the f number (F), which is the focal length divided by the aperture.

$$d_f = 2 \times \lambda \times F = \frac{2(\lambda \times fl)}{a_p}$$

As the aperture is increased, the focus narrows, improving the resolution. Also, as frequency is increased, wavelength decreases, again narrowing the focus and improving resolution. Table 3.A shows f-number ranges in use. The best practical focus is with an f number of 2, yielding $d_f = 4\lambda$. Thus the best LR is about four times the best axial resolution (which is equal to wavelength for a two-cycle pulse).

These considerations only apply to narrow transmit beams and can be bypassed with virtual beam forming.

TABLE 3.A f-Number Ranges

Focus	f Number
Weak	>6
Moderate	2–6
Strong	<2

TABLE 3.2 Typical Imaging Depth and Axial Resolution (Two-Cycle Pulse and Traditional Narrow Transmit Beams) in Tissue

Frequency (MHz)	Imaging Depth (cm)	Axial Resolution (mm)
2.0	30	0.77
3.5	17	0.44
5.0	12	0.31
7.5	8	0.20
10.0	6	0.15
15.0	4	0.10

ARRAYS

Not only must the transducer emit ultrasound pulses and receive echoes, but it must also track the pulses through the many anatomic paths required to generate a two-dimensional (2D) image. This is sometimes called *scanning, sweeping*, or *steering* the beam through the tissue cross-sections to be imaged. Scanning is done rapidly and automatically so that many images, called *frames*, can be acquired and presented in rapid sequence within a second. Presenting 2D (grayscale) images in a rapid sequential format, similar to a movie or television, is called *real-time ultrasound imaging.*

Automatic steering of a sound beam is performed electronically with arrays, providing a means for sweeping the sound beam through the tissues rapidly and repeatedly to achieve real-time imaging (>10 frames per second). Transducer arrays, as the name implies, contain multiple transducer elements. These elements are rectangular and arranged in a straight line (a **linear array**; see Figs. 3.3E and 3.13A) or a curved line (a so-called **convex or curved array**; see Fig. 3.14B).

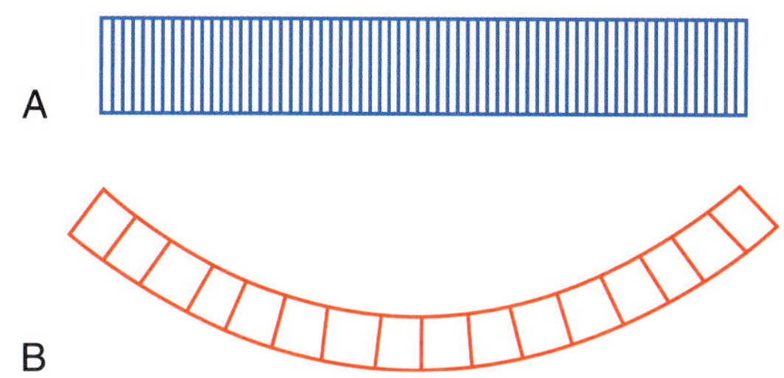

Fig. 3.13 A, Front view of a linear array with 64 rectangular elements. **B,** Side view of a convex array with 16 elements.

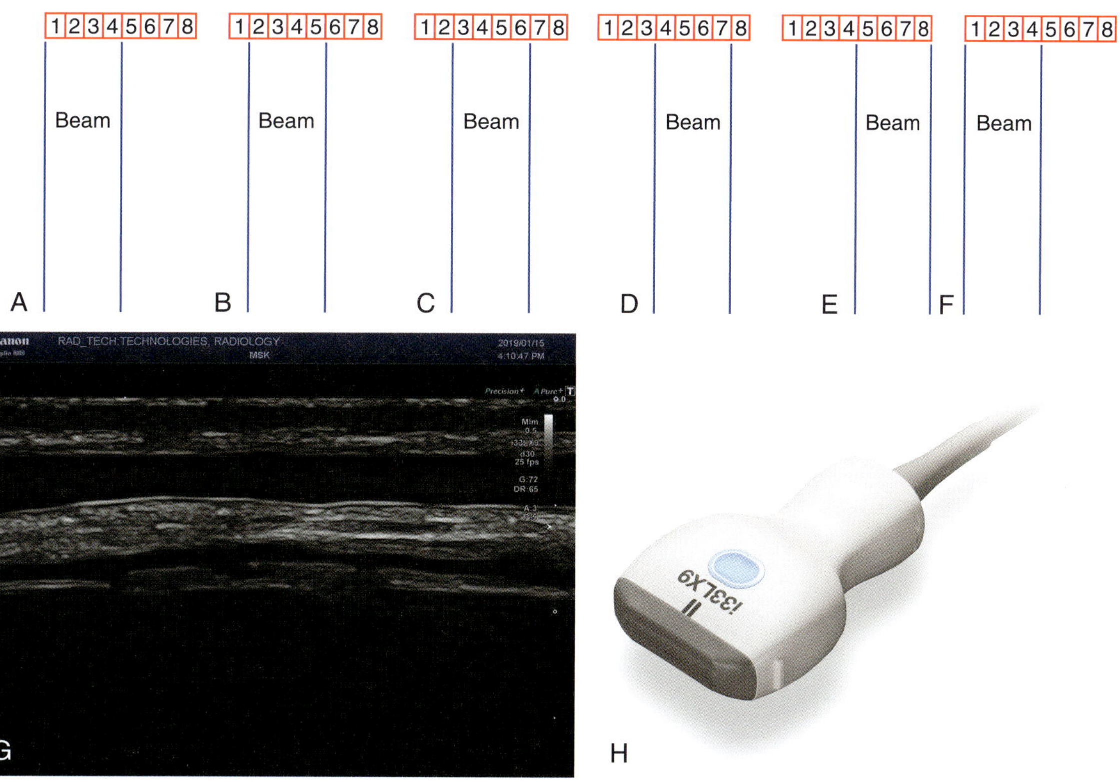

Fig. 3.14 A linear array (side view). A voltage pulse is applied simultaneously to all elements in a small group: first to elements 1–4 (for example) as a group **(A),** then to elements 2–5 (**B**), and so on across the transducer assembly **(C–E)**. The process is then repeated (**F**). **G,** An image generated from the linear array in **H**.

Linear Array

Arrays are operated in two ways, called *sequencing* and *phasing*. A more complete (but seldom used) name for what is commonly called a **linear array** is *linear sequenced array*. "Linear" describes construction, whereas "sequenced" describes operation. This array contains a straight line of rectangular elements, each approximately one wavelength wide, and is operated by applying voltage pulses to groups of elements in succession (Fig. 3.14). Each group of elements acts similarly to a larger transducer element, providing an aperture large enough to confine the ultrasound to a fine enough beam for satisfactory LR. As different groups are energized one by one (but with significant overlap between adjacent groups), the origin of the sound beam moves across the face of the transducer assembly from one end to the other. Thus the same effect as manual linear scanning with a single element the size (aperture) of each energized group is achieved. Such electronic scanning, however, can be done rapidly and consistently without involving any moving parts.

This electronic scanning is repeated rapidly enough that real-time (live) presentation (more than 10 images per second) of ultrasound echo information results. Real-time presentation requires scanning the beam across the transducer assembly many times per second. The aperture is the size of the group of elements activated to produce each pulse. The width of the entire image is approximately equal to the length of the array (Fig. 3.15). The linear image is a *rectangular image*, which consists of parallel scan lines produced by pulses originating at different points across the surface of the array (and across the top of the image) that all travel in the same vertical direction (parallel), as shown in Figs. 1.6, 3.14G and 3.15.

> A linear array produces rectangular images composed of many parallel, vertical scan lines.

The pulsing sequence described in Fig. 3.14 (eight elements, pulsed in groups of four) yields only five scan lines making up the image. This would certainly be a limited image. A 128 element array pulsed in groups of four would yield a 125 line display. Pulsing these elements individually (rather than in groups of four) would yield a 128 line display, but the small aperture (a single element is less than 1 mm in size) would cause excessive beam spreading and poor detail resolution. If the pulsing sequence alternated groups of three and four elements (e.g., elements 1 to 3, then 1 to 4, 2 to 4, 2 to 5, 3 to 5, 3 to 6, 4 to 6, 4 to 7, and on through the array), the number of scan lines would be doubled, to 250, thereby increasing line density and improving image quality but with reduced frame rates.

Curved Array

A curved array is constructed as a curved line of elements rather than a straight one. The operation of such an array is otherwise identical to that of the linear array (by sequencing groups of elements from one end of the array to the other), but because of the curved construction, the pulses travel out in different directions, producing a **sector**-type image (Fig. 3.16). The complete (but seldom used) name for this transducer is *convex sequenced array*, but *curved* or *curvi-linear array* is by far the most common terms.

> The curved array operates as a linear array but produces a sector image due to the different scan line orientations (i.e., the beams travel in different directions).

Phased Array

A **phased array** (also sometimes referred to as a *linear phased array*) contains a compact straight line of elements, each about one-quarter of a wavelength wide. The phased array is operated by applying voltage pulses to all (or most) elements (not a small group) in the assembly, but with small (<1 μs) time differences (called *phasing*) between them, so that the resulting sound pulse is sent out in a specific direction, as shown in Fig. 3.17. If the same time delays were used each time the process was repeated, the subsequent pulses would travel out in the same direction repeatedly producing a single line of sight (which can be used in Doppler mode, but obviously not for a complete anatomical image). However, the time delays are automatically changed

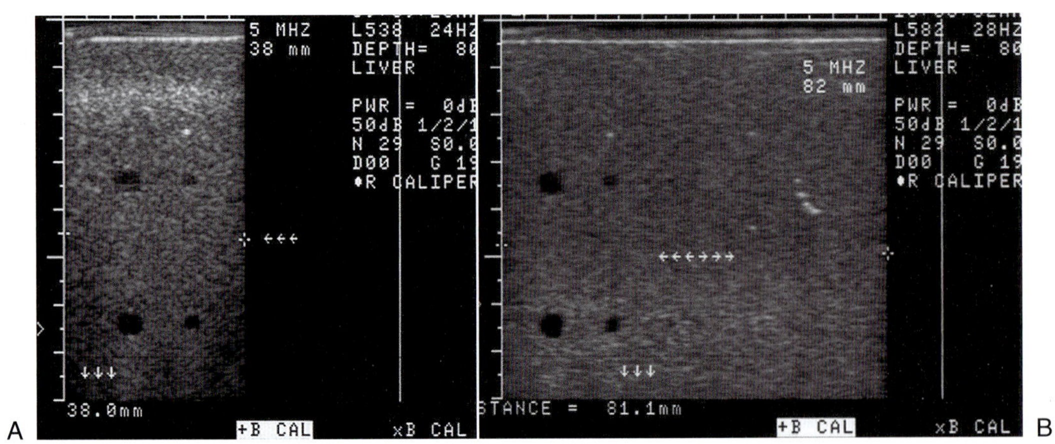

Fig. 3.15 The linear image width is determined by the length of the linear array used. **A,** In this example, a 5-MHz, 38-mm linear array (L538) produces an image that is 38 mm wide. **B,** A 5-MHz, 82-mm linear array (L582) produces an image that is 81 mm wide.

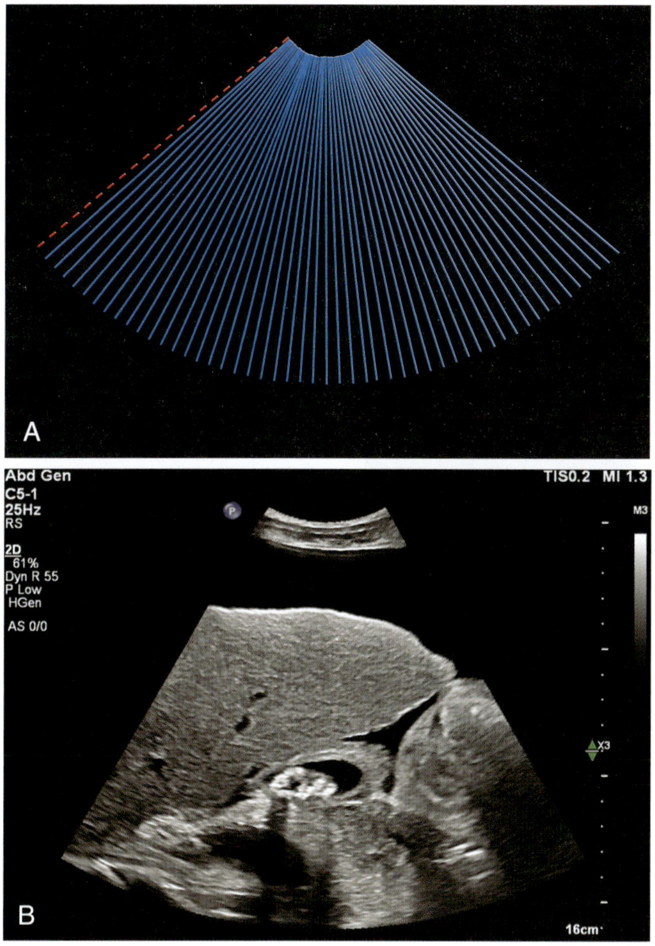

Fig. 3.16 A, Curved arrays send pulses out in different directions from different points across the curved array surface. **B,** A sector-type image with a curved top is produced by a convex array (here a liver with ascites).

slightly with each successive repetition so that subsequent pulses travel out in slightly different directions, and the beam direction continually changes (Fig. 3.18). This process results in the sweeping of the beam, with beam direction changing with each pulse, to produce a sector image (see Fig. 3.18F), the same effect as with manual rotation of a single element. Such electronic sector scanning, however, can be done rapidly and consistently without involving moving parts. The phased array is sometimes (but rarely) called an *electronic sector transducer*.

> A phased array scans the beam in sector format using short, incremental time delays between firings.

Phasing can also be applied to linear arrays to steer the beam from each element group in different directions by sending out pulses from each group with different phasing. Hence, rectangular images can be extended to sector images providing a wider field of view. A linear array with this capability is referred to as a *vector array*, which will be discussed in more detail later in this section. In addition, phasing can be used on both linear and curved/convex arrays to produce echoes from a specific anatomic location from several different viewing angles. The echo information from these multiple views is processed to present an image of improved quality (i.e., with reduced speckle). This is referred to as "spatial compounding" of an ultrasound image. This is discussed in more detail in the next chapter.

ADVANCED CONCEPT

As an example of the required delay to steer a beam (and scan line) in a specific direction, let us consider a 40 mm aperture containing 128 elements. We will calculate the case for a beam directed out at a 45° angle to the left of the transducer axis. The tangent of 45° is 1, which means that the opposite and adjacent sides in the equivalent triangle are equal (Fig. 3.19). In this equivalent triangle, the hypotenuse is the wavefront. The arrow shows the direction of travel that is always perpendicular to the orientation of the wavefront.

The length of the adjacent side of the triangle (also the length of the array aperture) is 40 mm. Thus the length of the opposite side is also 40 mm. The time required for that portion of the pulse to travel from the right-most element to a depth of 40 mm is $t = 40/1.54 = 26$ µs. At this instant in time, the left-most element has emitted its contribution to the pulse. Consequently, the total delay from right to left in energizing the elements is 26 µs. As the transducer has 128 elements in the 40-mm array, it has a 0.2 µs element-to-element delay (26/128) to achieve a pulse directed at 45° degrees off the array axis.

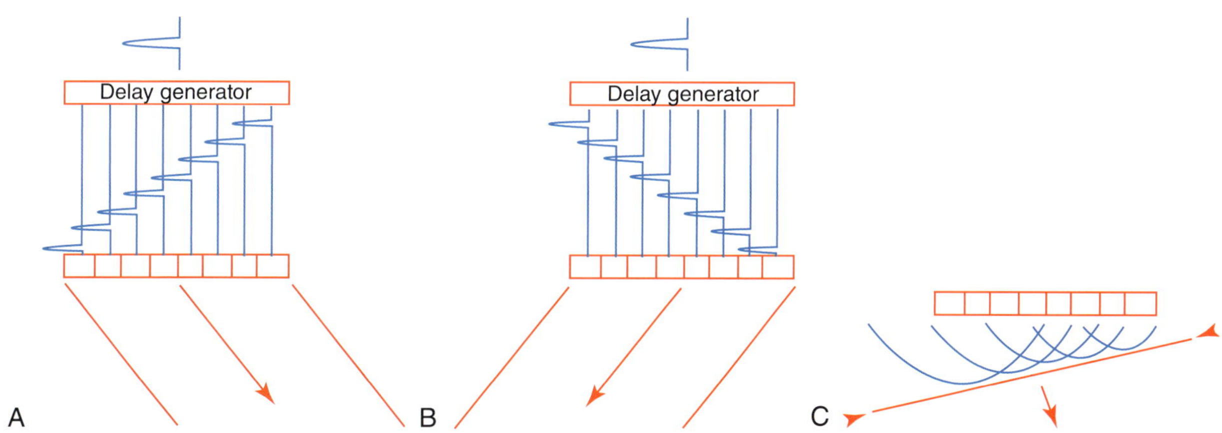

Fig. 3.17 A linear array (side view). **A,** When voltage pulses are applied in rapid progression from left to right, one ultrasound pulse is produced that is directed to the right. **B,** Similarly, when voltage pulses are applied in rapid progression from right to left, one ultrasound pulse is produced that is directed to the left. **C,** The delays in **A** produce a pulse, the combined pressure wavefront of which *arrowheads* is angled from lower left to upper right. A wave always travels perpendicular to its wavefront, as indicated by the *arrow.*

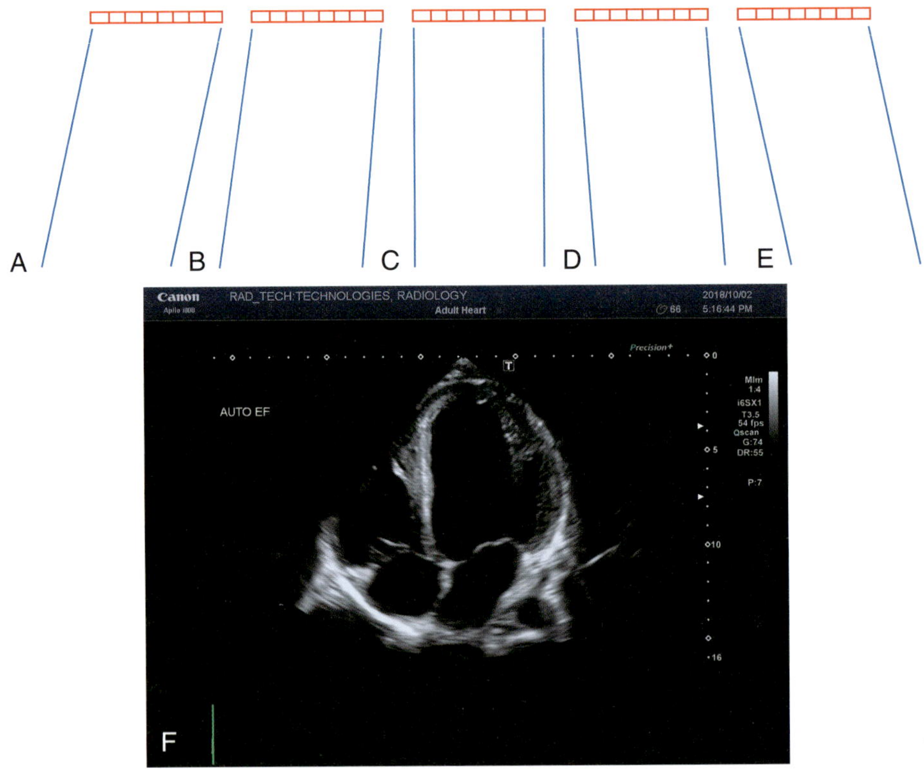

Fig. 3.18 A five-pulse sequence in which each pulse travels out in a different direction. **A,** The rapid voltage application progression is from right to left across the array. **B,** A right-to-left progression with slightly shorter time delays. **C,** No delays (all elements energize simultaneously). **D,** A left-to-right progression. **E,** A left-to-right progression with slightly longer delays. **F,** A4 chamber cardiac sector image produced by a phased array. The image comes to a point at the top.

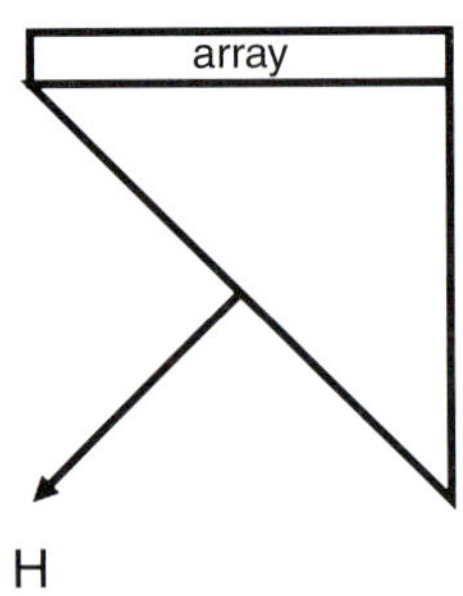

Fig. 3.19 Diagram for calculation of phase delay.

Electronic Focus

In addition to steering the beam, phased arrays can focus the beam as well (Fig. 3.20). An increase in the curved delay pattern (greater time delays between elements) moves the focus closer to the transducer, whereas a decrease (shorter delays) in curvature moves it deeper. Thus phasing provides electronic control of the location of the focus (Fig. 3.21).

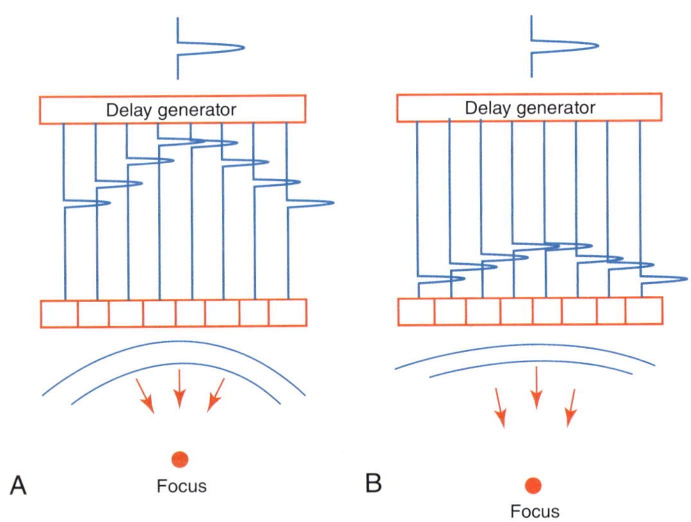

Fig. 3.20 By adding curvature to the phase delay pattern, a pulse is focused. **A,** Greater curvature places the focus closer to the transducer. **B,** Less curvature moves the focus deeper.

With narrow transmit beams, multiple foci can be used to achieve, in effect, a long focus (Fig. 3.22). In the simplest implementation, multiple foci require multiple pulses (per scan line), each focused at a different depth. Echoes from the focal region of each pulse are displayed, and the rest are discarded. The resulting image is a montage of the focal regions of the different pulses, which improves detail resolution by, in effect, yielding a longer focal region. However, the use of multiple pulses per scan line takes more time, and the frame rate is markedly reduced, which degrades temporal resolution (discussed later). Thus temporal resolution is sacrificed in this approach to improve detail resolution and it is therefore not used in modern scanners. Instead, one approach to bypass this dilemma is to create an amalgamated pulse that will be dynamically focused at multiple depths simultaneously (Fig. 3.22I)

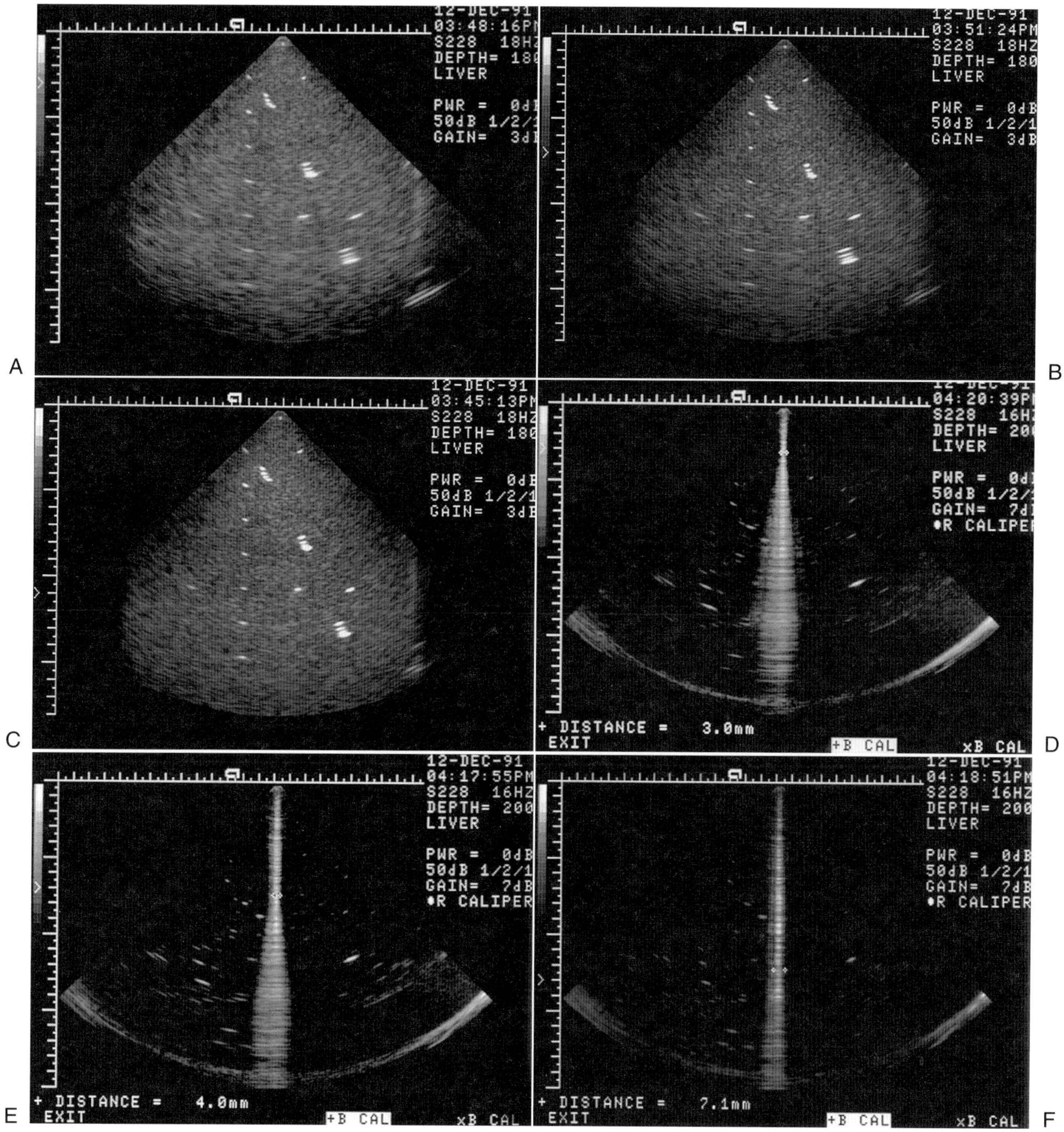

Fig. 3.21 Phase control of focal length. Focus located at 3 cm **(A)**, 7 cm **(B)**, and 11 cm **(C)**. Beam profiles show foci located at 3 cm **(D)**, 7 cm **(E)**, and 13 cm **(F)**.

> Electronic focusing is accomplished with a curved pattern of phased delays. An increase or decrease in the curvature of the delay pattern moves the focus shallower or deeper, respectively.

Phasing is also applied to linear arrays to provide electronic focal control (Fig. 3.23A–B). Rather than each group of elements being pulsed simultaneously, as in Fig. 3.15, the outer elements are pulsed slightly ahead of the inner ones (see Fig. 3.23C). This produces a curved pulse that is focused at a depth determined by the delay between the firing of the outer and inner elements. These pulses are focused, but not steered, by phasing. They still travel straight down to produce parallel vertical scan lines and a rectangular display. In a similar way, phased focusing is applied to curved arrays.

LR is improved by reducing the beam diameter, that is, by focusing (see Fig. 2.34). Fig. 3.24 shows a focused beam. The lateral smearing of a thin layer of scatterers indicates the beam width and LR at various depths. The best resolution is obtained

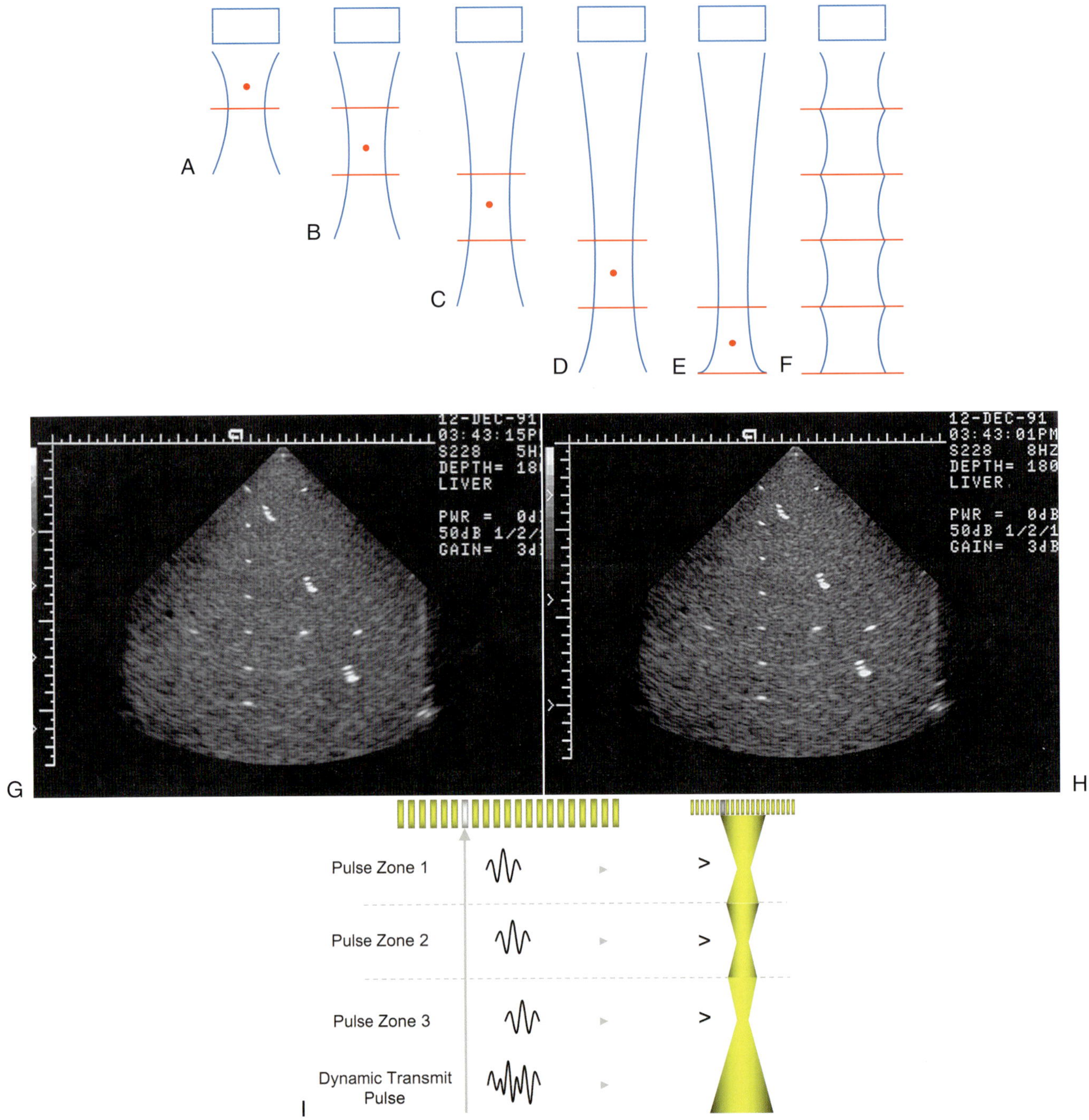

Fig. 3.22 Multiple-transmit focus uses a pulse for each focus. In this example, five pulses focused at different depths **(A–E)** are needed to produce a montage image **(F)** with an effectively long focus (narrow beam). Only the echoes from the focal region of each pulse are used to produce the image. The rest are discarded. **G,** Five foci at 2, 5, 8, 12, and 16 cm. **H,** Triple foci at 3, 9, and 15 cm. Note the reduced frame rates (5 and 8 Hz, compared with 18 and 16 Hz in Figure 3.21). **I,** Amalgamating 3 pulses focused at different depths into one dynamic transmit pulse produces a beam profile with a longer focus without the loss of frame rate.

at the focus (Figs. 3.23 and 3.24). Detail resolution is improved with increases in imaging frequency.

Variable Aperture

Recall that aperture, focal length, and wavelength determine the beam width at the focus when narrow transmit beams are employed. To maintain the same beam width at the focus for increasing focal lengths, the aperture must also be increased. This means that, in fact, not all elements of a phased array are used to generate all pulses. Smaller groups are used for short focal lengths, whereas larger groups are used for foci of increasing depth (see Fig. 3.23D–F).

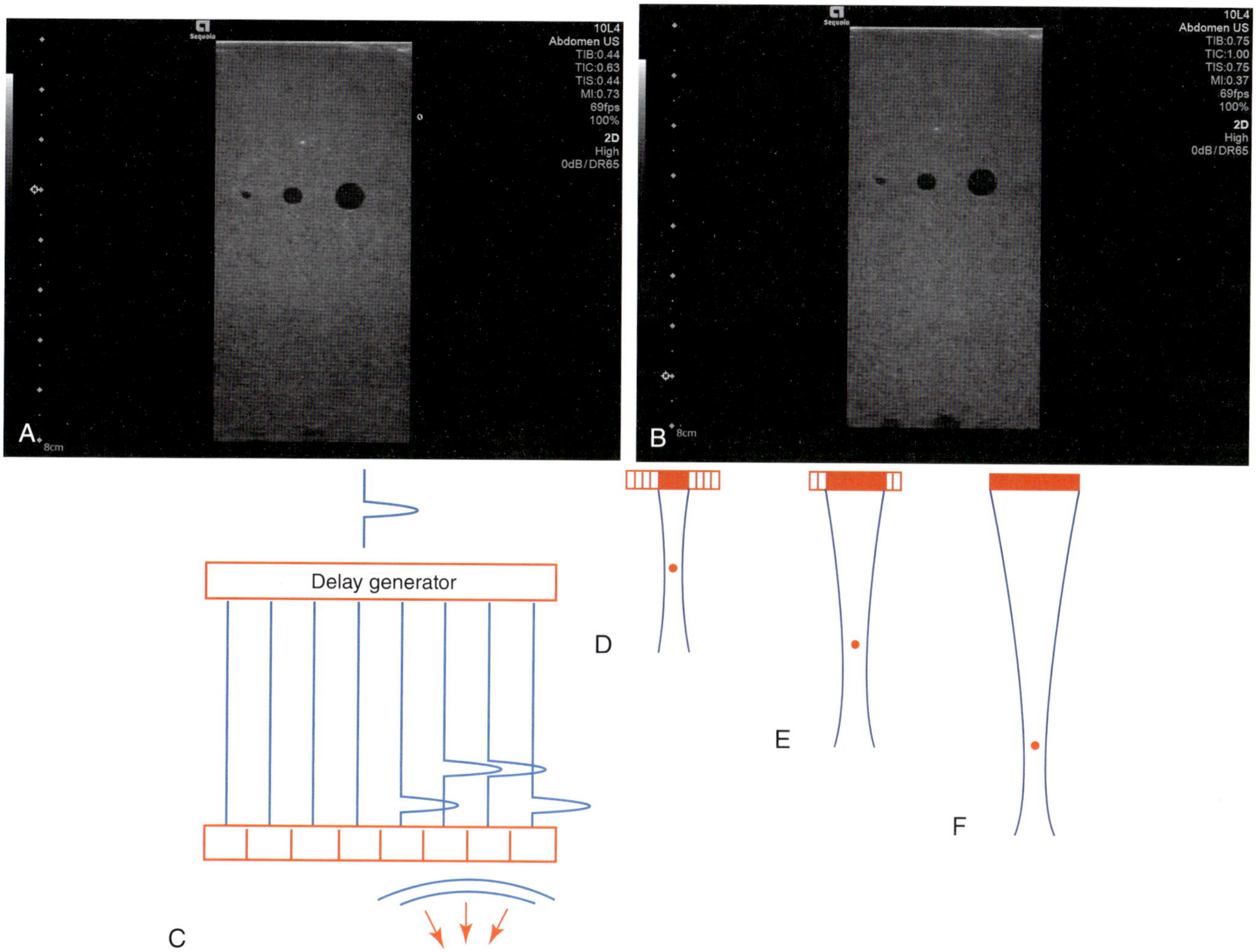

Fig. 3.23 **A,** A linear array with the focus located at 3.0 cm produces a clear image of the small cystic objects. **B,** When the focus is located at 7.0 cm (less phase delay curvature), a slight loss of image quality results for the simulated cysts. **C,** Phased delays are applied to each element group to focus the pulse. **D-F,** Variable aperture. To maintain comparable focal beam width at different depths, more array elements are used (increasing the aperture) while the focus is moved deeper. **D,** Four elements. **E,** Eight elements. **F,** Twelve elements.

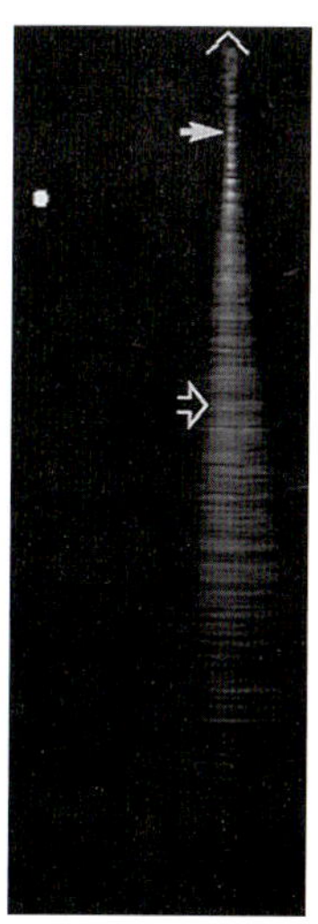

Fig. 3.24 Beam width is shown as lateral smearing of a thin vertical scattering layer in a test object. The beam indicates the lateral resolution at each depth. In this example, beam width is approximately 2 mm at the focus *(closed arrow)* and approximately 10 mm at a depth of 6 cm *(open arrow)*, well beyond the focus.

Two-Dimensional Arrays

A single line of elements can only be electronically focused or steered in the scan plane. Focus (fixed at one depth) can be achieved in the third dimension with a lens or with curved elements. With at least three rows of elements—that is, a 2D array—phasing can be applied to focus in the third dimension as well. Electronic focusing in the third dimension eliminates the need for a lens or curved elements and the focusing can be controlled over a much wider range of depths. This dimension, perpendicular to the scan plane, is called *slice thickness dimension* or *section thickness dimension*. Beam width in this dimension is important with regard to slice thickness artifacts, also called *partial-volume artifacts*. This third dimension and its associated slice thickness are shown in Figs. 1.7A and 1.9A.

Conventional arrays scan in rectangular or sector format in one dimension (Fig. 3.25A). 2D arrays with hundreds, thousands, or tens of thousands of elements have the ability to steer and focus in two dimensions rather than one. Biplane imaging (see Fig. 3.25B–D) and rapid electronic volume imaging (see Fig. 3.25E–F) are thus possible.

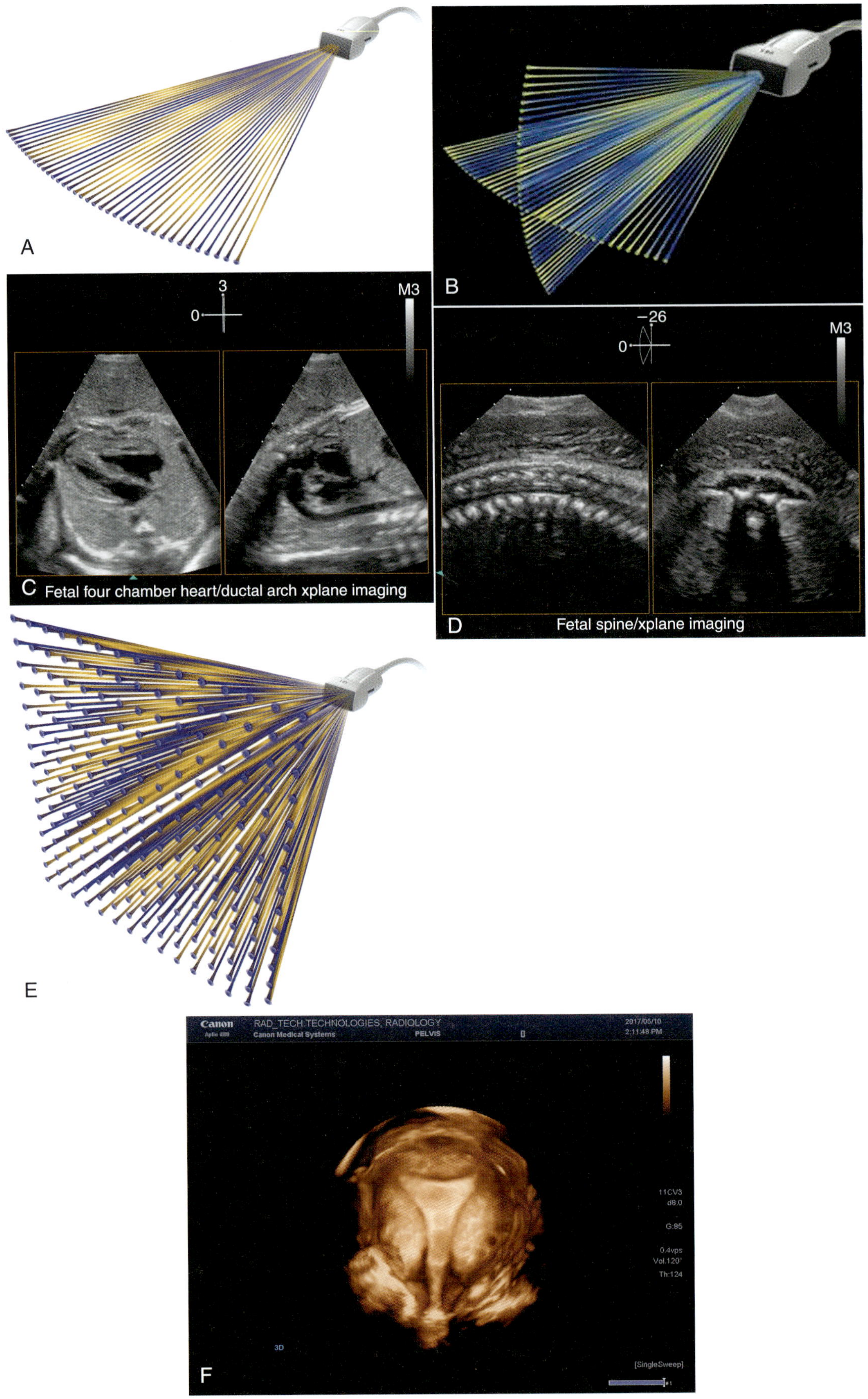

Fig. 3.25 A, Conventional two-dimensional scan. **B–D,** Biplane imaging. **E–F,** Rapid electronic volume (3D) imaging. (**A–E,** Courtesy Philips Medical Systems. **F,** Courtesy Canon Medical Systems USA)

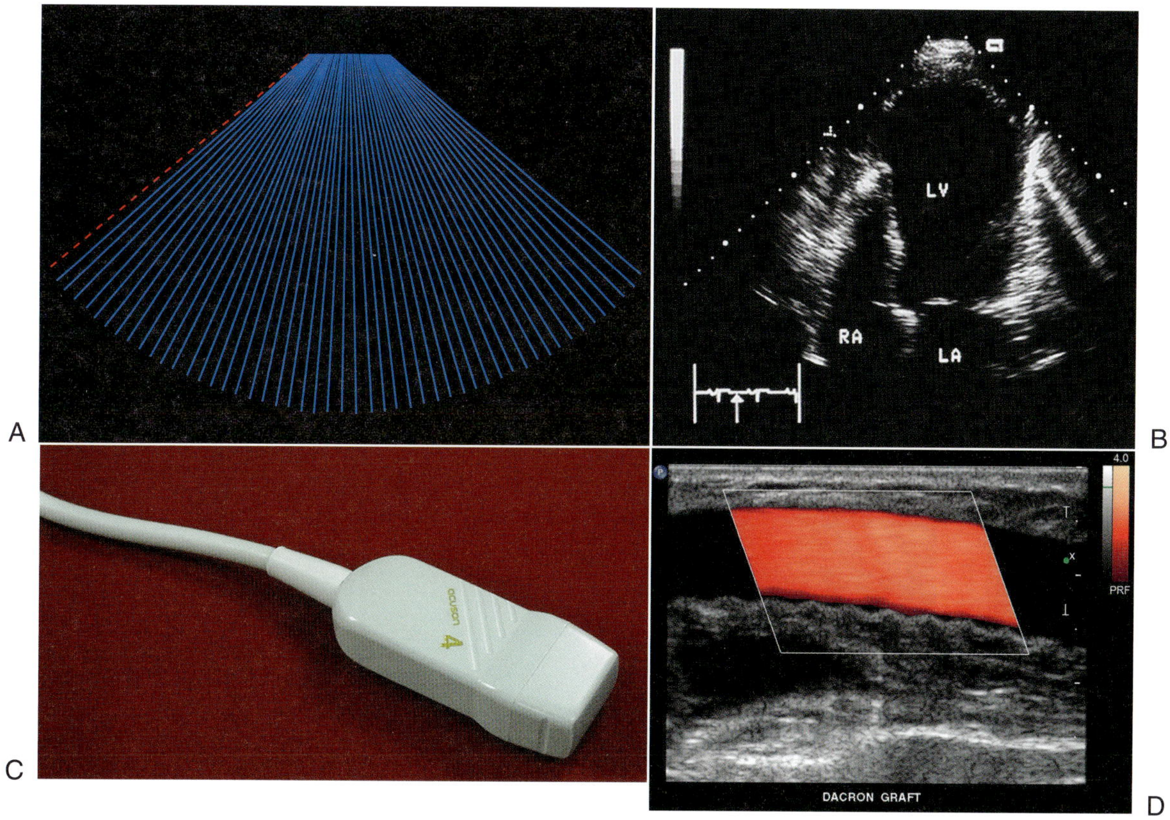

Fig. 3.26 **A,** A vector array sends pulses out in different directions from different starting points across the flat surface of the array. **B,** A cardiac scan produced by a vector array. **C,** A vector array transducer. **D,** A phased linear array producing a parallelogram-shaped color-Doppler display.

Grating Lobes

In addition to side lobes, a characteristic of single-element transducers, arrays have **grating lobes**, which are additional beams resulting from their multielement structure. Grating lobes can be reduced by driving the elements in a group nonuniformly (i.e., with different voltage amplitudes). Outer elements are driven at lower amplitudes than inner elements. Echo reception sensitivity is also less for outer elements. This is called **apodization**. Because optimal apodization changes continually with focusing and steering, it is called *dynamic apodization*. The downside of apodization is that some broadening of the main beam occurs with degradation of resolution. Subdicing of each element into a group of smaller elements is also done to weaken grating lobes and to reduce interelement interaction for improved electronic focusing. The subelements are tied together electrically so that they function as one element.

Alternatively, the use of 2D arrays provides control over the ultrasound beam in all three dimensions (i.e., axial, lateral, and elevational), which can be used to reduce or even eliminate grating lobes. In clinical practice, when using a modern scanner, no sonographer will encounter grating lobes that impact diagnostic evaluations.

Vector Array

Phasing can be applied to each element group in a **linear array** to steer pulses in various directions, in addition to initiating them at various starting points across the array. **Vector array** is the name applied to this type of transducer (Fig. 3.26). This transducer converts the image format of a linear array from rectangular to sector. Scan lines originate from different points across the top of the display and travel out in different directions. The image format is similar to that of a curved array except that the contact surface (footprint) is smaller and the top of the display is flat. More elements can be used at a time, allowing for larger apertures than can be achieved with curved arrays. Phasing can be applied to linear arrays as well in such a way that each pulse travels in the same direction (but not straight down). This converts a rectangular display to a parallelogram-shaped display useful in color-Doppler imaging (see Fig. 3.26D).

By now there are commercially available very high-frequency (30–33 MHz) vector arrays commercially available. These transducers are aimed at dermatology and ophthalmology applications, but they have also found use in more unusual clinical applications such as dental evaluations (Fig. 3.27).

> The vector array is a combination of linear and phased array operations. It presents a sector display that is flat across the top of the image.

Reception Steering, Focus, and Aperture

When an array is receiving echoes, the (electric) outputs of the elements can be timed or delayed so that the array is sensitive in a particular direction with a focus at a particular depth

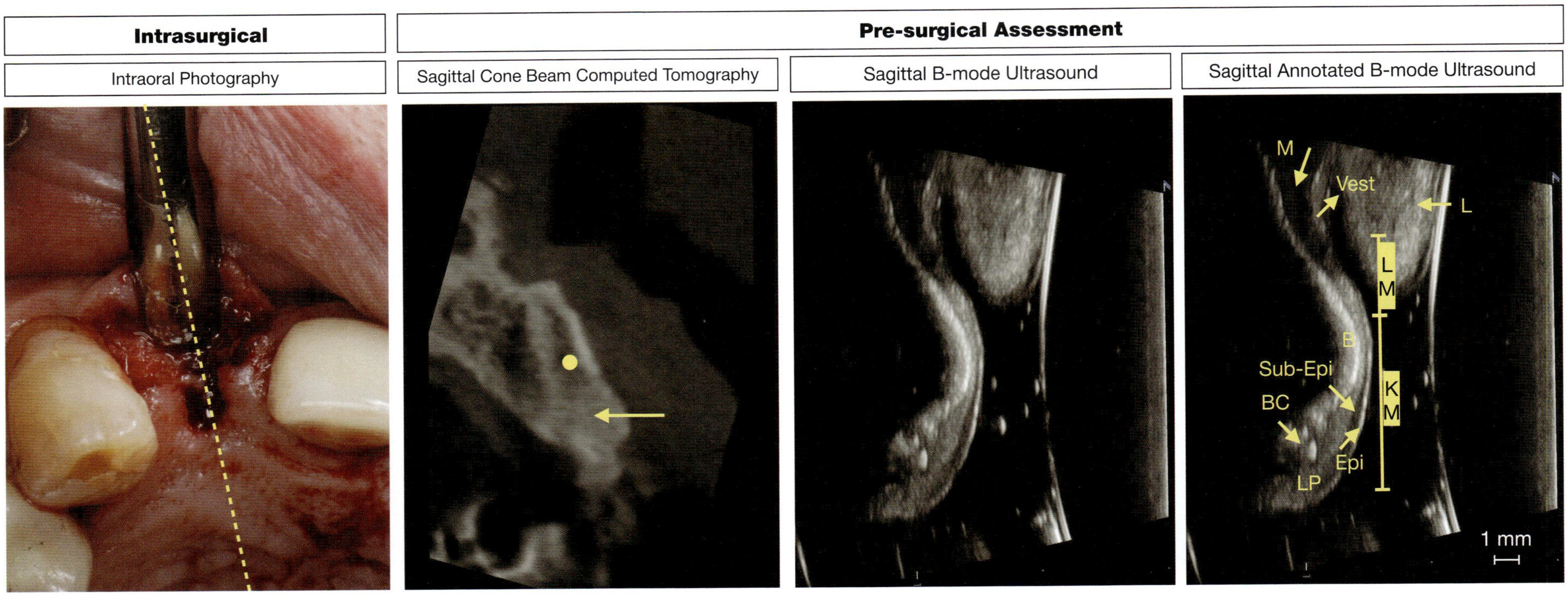

Fig. 3.27 Anatomical soft and hard tissue assessment of an edentulous crest for dental implant placement using a 33 MHz vector array. **Intrasurgical:** *Intraoral Photography* of the edentulous crest showing bone crest anatomy after flap opening. Note that the yellow dotted line represents the sagittal plane analyzed during pre-surgical assessment. **Presurgical assessment:** *Sagittal (view) Cone Beam Computed Tomography* of the edentulous crest. This image shows a hyperdense region (*yellow arrow*) of a placed bone graft and a yellow dot that marks a less dense region, here the native bone. *Sagittal B-mode Ultrasound image* of the facial (sagittal) mid-edentulous crest showing the bone, soft tissue, and lip. *Sagittal Annotated B-mode image of* hard tissues: bone crest (*BC*), bone (*B*), and soft tissue: muscle (*M*), lip (*L*), vestibule (*Vest*), keratinized mucosa (*KM*), lining mucosa (*LM*), epithelium (*Epi*), sub-epithelium (*Sub-Epi*), lamina propria (*LP*). Note: The muscle (S) is visible by its surface reflection only. (Courtesy Dr. Oliver Kripfgans, University of Michigan.)

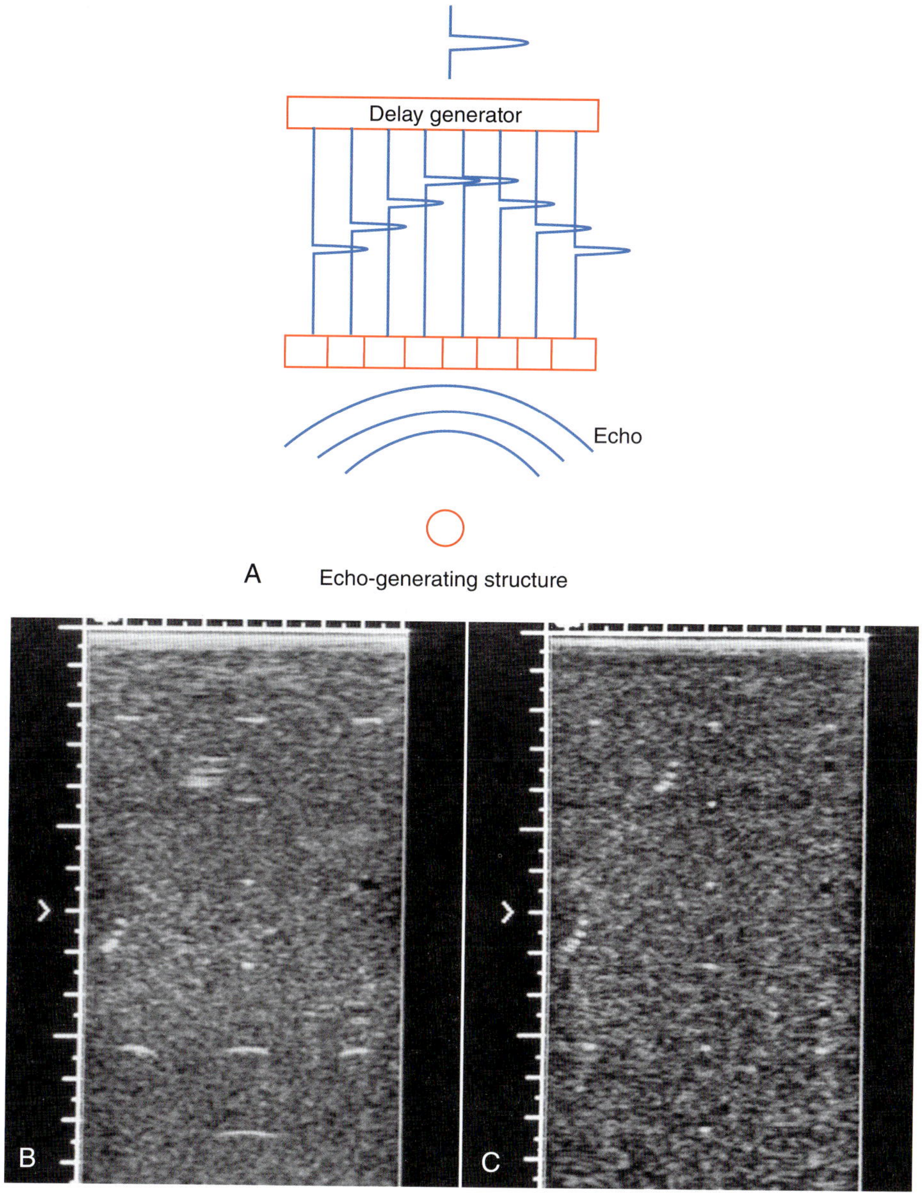

Fig. 3.28 **A,** A spherically shaped echo arrives at array elements at different times, producing noncoincident voltages in the various channels. If simply combined, a weak, long voltage (with poor resolution and sensitivity) would result. However, with proper delays, the voltages are made to coincide, producing a strong, short (good resolution and sensitivity) voltage. While echoes return from deeper and deeper locations, their curvature is reduced. Thus the delay correction must be reduced while echoes return. This is called dynamic focusing. **B,** Dynamic focus is off. **C,** When the dynamic focus is on, resolution improves.

(Fig. 3.28). This reception focus depth is increased continually as the transmitted pulse travels through tissues and the echoes arrive from deeper and deeper locations. This continually changing reception focus is called dynamic focusing. **Dynamic focusing** is similar to the continual change in focusing that occurs, for example, with a video camera when filming a child riding away on a bicycle. The combination of transmission focus and dynamic reception focus improves detail resolution over large depth ranges. As the focus continually changes during echo reception, the aperture increases to maintain a constant focal width. This is called **dynamic aperture**. The terms used to describe arrays relate to their construction and function as shown in Table 3.3. Box 3.1 and Tables 3.4 and 3.5 summarize transducer types, terminology, characteristics, and display formats.

With phasing, the reception "beam" is steered and dynamically focused.

TABLE 3.3 Terms Used to Describe Arrays

Term	Construction	Scanning	Focusing
Array	✓		
Linear	✓		
Sequenced		✓	
Convex/Curved	✓		
Phased		✓	✓

BOX 3.1 Common Transducer Types and Their Implied Array Terminology

- Linear array or (phased) linear (sequenced) array
- Curved array or (phased) convex/curved (sequenced) array
- Phased array or (linear) phased array
- Vector array or (phased and sequenced) (linear) vector array

The words in parentheses are implied in the abbreviated common terminology, which is used in day-to-day practice.

TABLE 3.4 Transducer Characteristics

Type	Beam Scanned by Sequencing	Beam Scanned by Phasing	Beam Focused by Phasing
Linear array	✓		✓
Curved array	✓		✓
Phased array		✓	✓
Vector array	✓	✓	✓

TABLE 3.5 Display Formats

Type	Rectangle or Parallelogram	Sector	Flat Top	Curved Top	Pointed Top
Linear array	✓		✓		
Curved array		✓		✓	
Phased array		✓			✓
Vector array		✓	✓		

REVIEW

The following key points are presented in this chapter:

- Transducers convert energy from one form to another.
- Ultrasound transducers convert electric energy to ultrasound energy, and vice versa.
- Transducers operate on the piezoelectric principle.
- Transducers are operated in pulse-echo mode.
- Operating frequency depends on element thickness.
- Pulsed transducers have damping material to shorten spatial pulse length for acceptable resolution.
- Transducers produce sound in the form of beams with near, focal, and far zones.
- Beam width can be reduced by focusing to improve LR.
- Detail resolution improves with increasing frequency.
- *Linear* and *curved* are types of array construction.
- *Sequenced*, *phased*, and *vector* are types of array scanning operations.
- Phasing also enables electronic control of focus.

EXERCISES

Answers appear in the Answers to Exercises section at the back of the book.

1. A transducer converts one form of __________ to another.
   a. energy
   b. force
   c. image
   d. scan
2. Ultrasound transducers convert __________ energy into __________ energy, and vice versa.
   a. electric, light
   b. heat, electric
   c. heat, light
   d. electric, ultrasound
3. Ultrasound transducers operate on the __________ principle.
   a. piezomagnetic
   b. piezoelectric
   c. electropiezo
   d. electromagnetic
4. Single-element transducers are in the form of __________.
   a. squares
   b. rectangles
   c. disks
   d. ovals
5. The __________ of a transducer element changes when voltage is applied to its faces.
   a. width
   b. height
   c. length
   d. thickness
6. The term *transducer* is used to refer to a transducer __________ or to a transducer __________.
   a. element, assembly
   b. matching, element
   c. backing, damping
   d. backing, assembly
7. A transducer __________ is part of a transducer __________.
   a. assembly, element
   b. element, assembly
   c. cable, matching
   d. backing, damping
8. An electric voltage pulse, when applied to a transducer, produces an ultrasound __________ of a(n) __________ that is equal to that of the voltage pulse.
   a. pulse, amplitude
   b. intensity, amplitude
   c. pulse, frequency
   d. pulse, duration

9. The resonance frequency of an element is determined by its ___________.
   a. width
   b. height
   c. length
   d. thickness
10. Operating frequency ___________ when transducer element thickness is increased.
   a. increases
   b. decreases
   c. is unchanged
   d. none of the above
11. The addition of damping material to a transducer reduces the number of ___________ in the pulse, thus improving ___________ ___________. It increases ___________.
   a. amplitudes, detail resolution, frequency
   b. amplitudes, lateral resolution, bandwidth
   c. cycles, lateral resolution, frequency
   d. cycles, axial resolution, bandwidth
12. Damping material reduces the ___________ of the transducer and ___________ of the diagnostic system.
   a. efficiency, sensitivity
   b. frequency, sensitivity
   c. frequency, efficiency
   d. frequency, penetration
13. Ultrasound transducers typically generate pulses of ___________ or ___________ cycles.
   a. five, ten
   b. five, six
   c. one, three
   d. two, three
14. For a particular transducer element material, if a thickness of 0.4 mm yields an operating frequency of 5 MHz, the thickness required for an operating frequency of 10 MHz is ___________ mm.
   a. 0.1
   b. 0.2
   c. 0.3
   d. 0.5
15. Which of the following transducer frequencies would have the thinnest elements?
   a. 2 MHz
   b. 3 MHz
   c. 5 MHz
   d. 7 MHz
   e. 10 MHz
16. The matching layer on the transducer surface reduces _______ caused by impedance differences.
   a. attenuation
   b. amplitude
   c. transmission
   d. reflection
17. A coupling medium on the skin surface eliminates reflection caused by ___________.
   a. air
   b. skin
   c. matching layer
   d. element
18. Damping lengthens the pulse. True or false?
19. Damping increases efficiency. True or false?
20. The damping layer is in front/back of the element.
21. The matching layer is in front/back of the element.
22. The matching layer has ___________ impedance.
   a. high
   b. low
   c. intermediate
   d. zero
23. Elements in linear arrays are in the form of ___________.
   a. rectangles
   b. squares
   c. rings
   d. disks
24. Transducer assemblies are also called ___________.
   a. transducers
   b. probes
   c. scanheads
   d. scan converters
   e. skinheads
   f. more than one of the above
25. Operating frequency is also called ___________ ___________.
   a. operating mode
   b. bandwidth mode
   c. operating bandwidth
   d. resonance frequency
26. Mixtures of a piezoelectric ceramic and a nonpiezoelectric polymer are called ___________.
   a. composites
   b. piezopolymers
   c. ceramopolymers
   d. piezocomposites
27. To operate a transducer at more than one frequency requires ___________.
   a. narrow bandwidth
   b. moderate bandwidth
   c. broad bandwidth
   d. no bandwidth
28. Is it practical to attempt to operate a 5-MHz transducer with a bandwidth of 1 MHz at 6 MHz?
29. Is it practical to attempt to operate a 5 MHz transducer with a bandwidth of 2.5 at 3 and 7 MHz?
30. A focused beam is divided into three regions, called the ___________ zone, the ___________ zone, and the ___________ zone.
   a. near, focal, far
   b. narrow, wide, extended
   c. forward, middle, reverse
   d. low, medium, high
31. The region between the transducer and the focal region is the ___________ length.
   a. narrow zone
   b. near zone
   c. wide zone
   d. far zone

32. Transducer size is also called ___________.
    a. aperture
    b. zone
    c. bandwidth
    d. width

Exercises 33–38 relate to Advanced Concept #3:

33. Near-zone length increases with increasing source ___________ and ___________.
    a. amplitude, intensity
    b. amplitude, frequency
    c. aperture, frequency
    d. aperture, amplitude
34. Which transducer element has the longest near zone?
    a. 6 mm, 5 MHz
    b. 6 mm, 7 MHz
    c. 8 mm, 7 MHz
35. A higher-frequency transducer produces a ___________ near-zone length.
    a. longer
    b. shorter
    c. unchanged
    d. none of the above
36. A smaller aperture produces a(n) ___________ near-zone length.
    a. longer
    b. shorter
    c. unchanged
    d. none of the above
37. A transducer with a near-zone length of 10 cm can be focused at 12 cm. True or false?
38. Which of the following transducer(s) can focus at 6 cm?
    a. 5 MHz, near-zone length of 5 cm
    b. 4 MHz, near-zone length of 6 cm
    c. 4 MHz, near-zone length of 10 cm
    d. b and c
    e. None of the above
39. Sound may be focused by using a ___________.
    a. curved element
    b. lens
    c. phased array
    d. more than one of the above
40. Focusing reduces the beam diameter at all distances from the transducer. True or false?
41. The distance from a transducer to the location of the narrowest beam width produced by a focused transducer is called focal ___________.
    a. length
    b. width
    c. depth
    d. height
42. Transducer arrays are transducer assemblies with several transducer ___________.
    a. elements
    b. layers
    c. cables
    d. backings
43. Linear arrays scan beams by ___________ element groups.
    a. phasing
    b. steering
    c. delaying
    d. sequencing
44. A phased linear array with a single line of elements can focus in ___________ dimension(s).
    a. one
    b. two
    c. three
    d. five
45. Focusing in section thickness can be accomplished with ___________ elements or a ___________.
    a. curved, sequencer
    b. round, sequencer
    c. curved, lens
    d. round, lens
46. Electronic focusing in section thickness requires multiple rows of ___________.
    a. lenses
    b. matchers
    c. dampers
    d. elements
47. Match the following (answers may be used more than once):
    a. Linear array _______.
    b. Phased array _______.
    a. Convex array _______.
    1. Voltage pulses are applied in succession to groups of elements across the face of a transducer.
    2. Voltage pulses are applied to most or all elements as a group, but with small time differences.
48. If the elements of a phased array are pulsed in rapid succession from right to left, the resulting beam is ___________.
    a. steered right
    b. steered left
    c. focused
49. If the elements of a phased array are pulsed in rapid succession from outside in, the resulting beam is ___________.
    a. steered right
    b. steered left
    c. focused
50. ___________ and ___________ describe how arrays are constructed (select two).
    a. linear
    b. phased
    c. sequenced
    d. vector
    e. convex
51. ___________, ___________, and ___________ describe how arrays are operated (select three).
    a. linear
    b. phased
    c. sequenced
    d. vector
    e. convex
52. Shorter time delays between elements fired from outside in result in ___________ curvature in the emitted pulse and a ___________ focus.

a. no, weak
b. less, shallower
c. less, deeper
d. greater, shallower
e. greater, deeper

53. A rectangular image is a result of linear scanning of the beam. This means that pulses travel in __________ __________ direction(s) from __________ starting point(s) across the transducer face.
a. two different, one
b. many different, many
c. the same, one
d. the same, different

54. A sector image is a result of sector steering of the beam. This means that pulses travel in __________ direction(s) from a common __________ at the transducer face.
a. two different, end
b. different, origin
c. the same, point
d. the same, end

55. In __________ and __________ arrays, pulses travel out in different directions from different starting points on the transducer face.
a. linear, convex
b. convex, phased
c. phased, vector
d. convex, vector

56. Match the following transducer assembly parts with their functions:
a. Cable ________
b. Damping material ______
c. Piezoelectric element ______
d. Matching layer ________
1. reduces reflection at transducer surface
2. converts voltage pulses to sound pulses
3. reduces pulse duration
4. conducts voltage pulses

57. Which of the following improve sound transmission from the transducer element into the tissue? (more than one correct answer)
a. matching layer
b. Doppler effect
c. damping material
d. coupling medium
e. refraction

58. A 5-MHz unfocused transducer with an element thickness of 0.4 mm, an element width of 13 mm, and a near-zone length of 14 cm produces two-cycle pulses. Determine the following:
a. Operating frequency if thickness is reduced to 0.2 mm: __________ MHz
b. Axial resolution in the case of (a): __________ mm at 5 MHz:
c. Depth at which lateral resolution is best: __________ cm
d. Lateral resolution at 14 cm: __________ mm
e. Lateral resolution at 28 cm: __________ mm
f. This transducer can be focused at depths less than __________ cm.

59. Lateral resolution is improved by __________.
a. damping
b. pulsing
c. focusing
d. matching
e. absorbing

60. For an unfocused transducer, the best lateral resolution (minimum beam width) is __________ the transducer width. This value of lateral resolution is found at a distance from the transducer face that is equal to the __________ __________ length.
a. equal to, near zone
b. half, near zone
c. equal to, far zone
d. half, far zone

61. For a focused transducer, the best lateral resolution (minimum beam width) is found in the __________ region.
a. near
b. far
c. local
d. focal

62. An unfocused 3.5-MHz, 13-mm transducer will yield a minimum beam width (best LR) of __________ mm.
a. 3.5
b. 13
c. 26
d. 6.5

63. An unfocused 3.5-MHz, 13-mm transducer produces three-cycle pulses. The axial resolution in soft tissue is __________ mm.
a. 0.7
b. 1.4
c. 13
d. 26

64. In Exercises 62 and 63, axial resolution is better than lateral resolution. True or false?

65. Axial resolution is often not as good as lateral resolution in diagnostic ultrasound. True or false?

66. The two resolutions may be comparable in the __________ region of a strongly focused beam.
a. near
b. far
c. local
d. focal

67. Beam diameter may be reduced in the near zone by focusing. True or false?

68. Beam diameter may be reduced in the far zone by focusing. True or false?

69. Match each transducer characteristic with the sound beam characteristic it determines (answers may be used more than once):
a. Element thickness: ________, ________, and ________
b. Element width: __________
c. Element shape (flat or curved): ________
d. Damping: ________

1. Axial resolution
2. Lateral resolution
3. Operating frequency

70. The principle on which ultrasound transducers operate is the ___________
- **a.** Doppler effect
- **b.** Acousto-optic effect
- **c.** Acoustoelectric effect
- **d.** Cause and effect
- **e.** Piezoelectric effect

71. Which of the following is not decreased by damping?
- **a.** Refraction
- **b.** Pulse duration
- **c.** Spatial pulse length
- **d.** Efficiency
- **e.** Sensitivity

72. Which three things determine beam diameter for a disk transducer?
- **a.** Pulse duration
- **b.** Frequency
- **c.** Aperture
- **d.** Distance from disk face
- **e.** Efficiency

73. The lower and upper limits of the frequency range useful in diagnostic ultrasound are determined by ___________ and ___________ requirements, respectively.
- **a.** penetration, attenuation
- **b.** penetration, resolution
- **c.** resolution, penetration
- **d.** attenuation, resolution

74. The range of frequencies useful for most applications of diagnostic ultrasound is ___________ to ___________ MHz.
- **a.** 0.1, 15
- **b.** 2, 35
- **c.** 1, 10
- **d.** 1, 5

75. At what depth is the best lateral resolution in Fig. 3.12C?
- **a.** 1 cm
- **b.** 2 cm
- **c.** 3 cm
- **d.** 4 cm

76. Match the transducer type with the display formats in Fig. 3.29.
- **a.** Linear array ___________
- **b.** Convex array ___________
- **c.** Phased array ___________
- **d.** Vector array ___________
- **e.** Phased linear array ___________

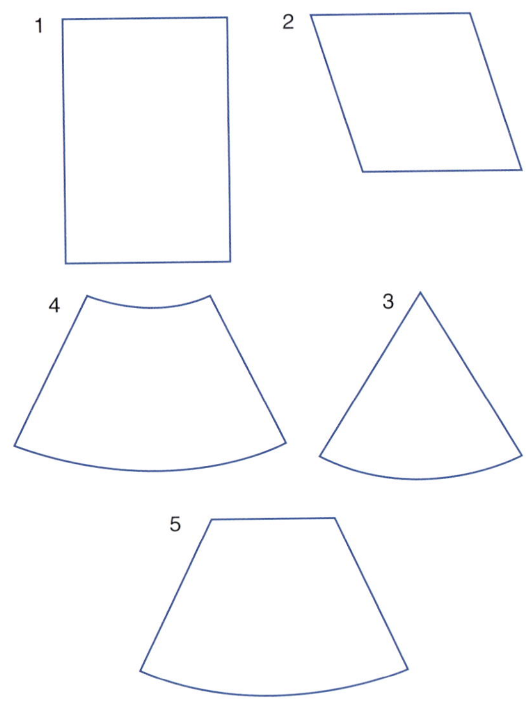

Fig. 3.29 Display formats. Illustration to accompany Exercise 100.

4

Instruments for Imaging Anatomy

LEARNING OBJECTIVES

After reading this chapter, the student should be able to do the following:

- Explain how ultrasound scanners work.
- Compare narrow and broad transmit beam operations.
- List the primary components of ultrasound imaging instruments.
- List the functions of each component including the beam former.
- Describe how images are stored electronically.
- Compare pre- and postprocessing.
- Compare signal processing and image processing.
- Explain the common displays and how they work.
- Define contrast resolution and list the factors that influence it.
- Define temporal resolution and list the factors that influence it.
- Explain how systems using broad transmit beams broad transmit beams work.
- List improvements in anatomical imaging with broad transmit beams.

CHAPTER OUTLINE

KEY TERMS

A mode
Amplification
Amplifier
Analog
Analog-to-digital converter
B color
B mode
B scan
Bandpass filter
Beam former
Bistable
Bit
Channel
Cine loop
Compression
Contrast resolution
Demodulation
Depth gain compensation
Detection
Digital
Digital-to-analog converter
Display
Dynamic range
Filtering
Flat-panel display
Frame
Frame rate
Freeze
Gain
Graphics processing unit (GPU)
Grayscale
Image memory
Image processor
Image former
Lateral gain control
M-mode
Persistence
Physical beam
Pixel
Postprocessing
Preprocessing
Pulse-echo principle
Pulse generator
Radio frequency
Real-time
Real-time display
Refresh rate
Scan line
Scanning
Signal
Signal processor
Spatial compounding
Temporal resolution
Time gain compensation
Virtual beam
Virtual beam forming
Volume imaging

In the preceding chapters, we discussed the means by which ultrasound is generated, how it interacts with tissues, and how echoes are received by the transducer. We now consider the scanners (instruments or systems) that receive echo voltages from the transducer and display them in the form of anatomical images. Diagnostic ultrasound systems are pulse-echo instruments. They determine echo strengths and locations of echo generation sites. The directions and arrival times of echoes returning from tissue structures determine the locations and depictions of these structures in the final display. This chapter describes how the scanner drives the transducer and how the returning echoes are processed and displayed by the ultrasound systems (Fig. 4.1) when using the traditional narrow transmit beams and when employing the more recent concept of unfocused broad transmit beams.

TWO MAIN PRINCIPLES OF SYSTEM OPERATION

For over 50 years, diagnostic ultrasound scanners have operated with narrow (focused) transmit beams and the pulse-echo principle as described in Chapters 1 and 3, where there is a one-to-one correspondence between the echoes received from

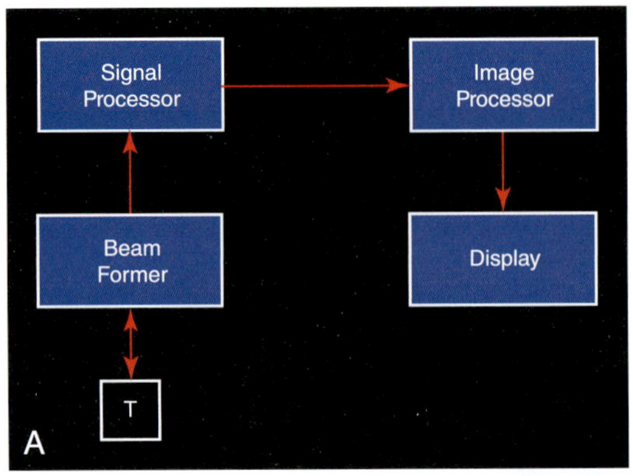

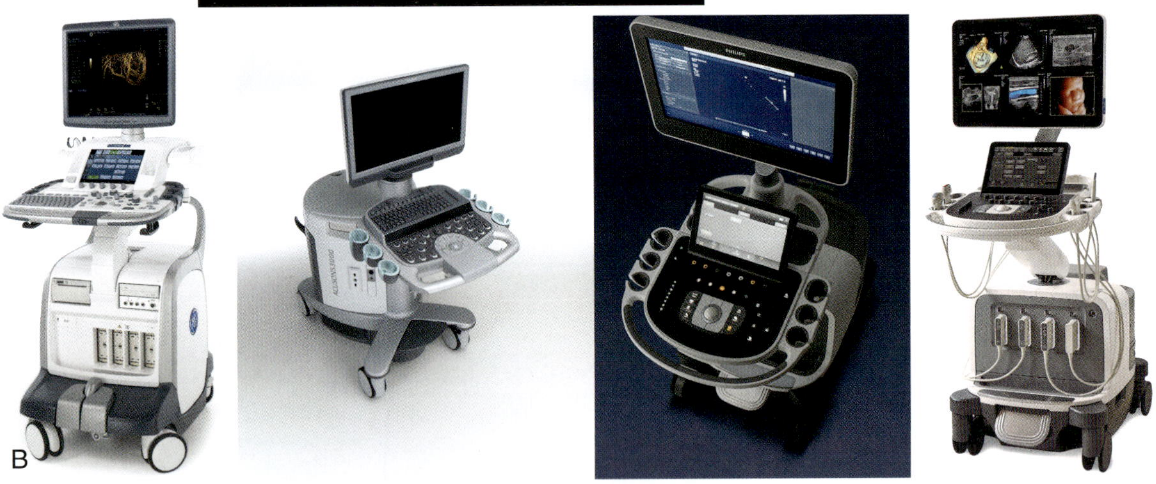

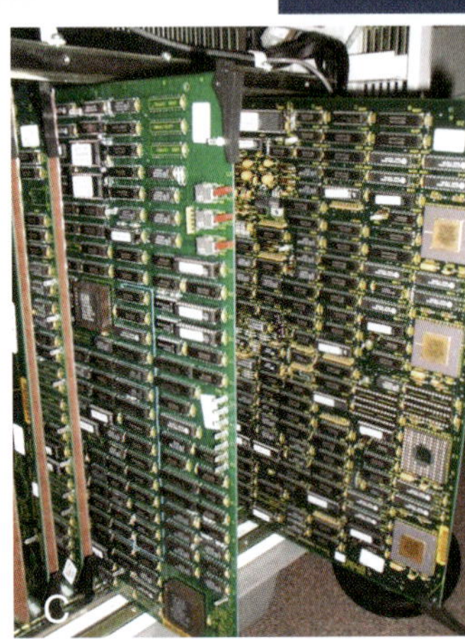

Fig. 4.1 **A,** The organization of a pulse-echo imaging system based on narrow transmit beams. The beam former produces electric pulses that drive the transducer and performs initial functions on the returning echo voltages from the transducer. The transducer produces an ultrasound pulse for each electric pulse applied to it. For each echo received from the tissues, an electric voltage is produced by the transducer. These voltages go through the beam former to the signal processor, where they are processed to a form suitable for input to the image processor. Electric information from the image processor drives the display, which produces the final displayed image of the cross-sectional anatomy interrogated by the system. **B,** Fully featured ultrasound scanners controlled through the control panel and/or touch-screens. **C,** Ultrasound scanners contain circuit boards, integrated circuits, and other electronic components.

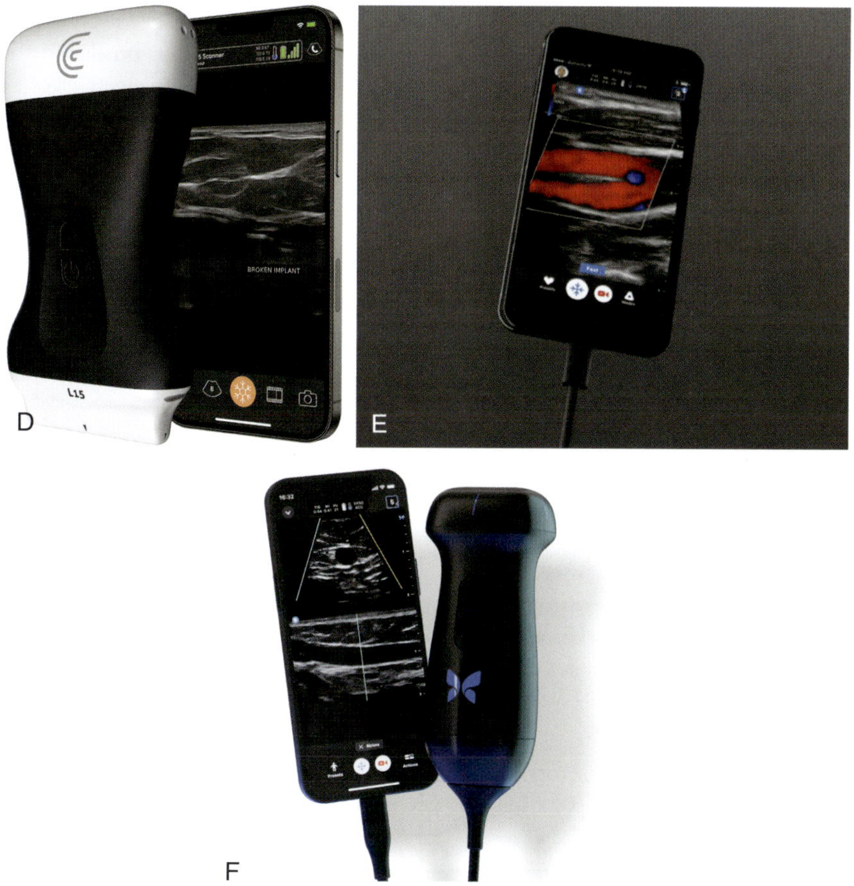

Fig. 4.1, cont'd D–F, Portable systems. (**B,** Courtesy GE HealthCare, Siemens Healthcare, and Philips Healthcare. **D,** Courtesy Clarius. **E,** Courtesy GE HealthCare. **F,** Courtesy Butterfly Networks.)

a transmitted ultrasound pulse and the displayed scan line (i.e., the final image). Recently, newer and more sophisticated ultrasound scanners (so-called high-end systems) have appeared that operate differently by using a broad transmit beam (one beam or a few; unfocussed or only weakly focused) and receiving echoes across the entire transducer aperture. Then virtual beam forming (described in more detail later in this chapter) is used to bring the entire image into focus providing excellent detail resolution throughout the final (displayed) image.

It should be noted that the "Sonography Principles and Instrumentation" examination administrated by the American Registry for Medical Diagnostic Sonography will mostly (entirely) concentrate on narrow transmit beam operation. However, most of tomorrow's sonographers will work and scan with scanners operating with broad transmit beams, which is why understanding this technology is important.

Comparing Narrow and Broad Transmit Beam Systems

As mentioned, narrow (focused) transmit beams have a one-to-one correspondence between the echoes received from a transmitted ultrasound pulse and the displayed scan line, that is, physical beam forming is directly coupled to the final displayed scan lines. The inherent time constraints associated with this serial line-by-line approach limit various characteristics of the image and force trade-offs such as between resolution and penetration (improving detail resolution by choosing a higher operating frequency will limit penetration). As another example, increasing the number of transmission focuses or increasing scan-line density (the number of lines per frame) aiming to improve detail resolution will also decrease frame rate (i.e., degrades temporal resolution). This interdependence can be avoided by taking a different approach to the pulse-echo principle.

Employing broad transmit beams may markedly reduce or even eliminate such limitations, enabling improvements in most (all) imaging characteristics. Fewer pulses (in the extreme a single pulse) are required with broad transmit beams, and transmission focusing, as described in Chapter 3, is no longer necessary. Nonetheless, the entire final image is going to be in focus, that is, with excellent detail resolution throughout. The dynamic-reception-focus principle, described in Chapter 3, is broadened to enable precise focusing at every pixel location in the image through virtual beam-forming. Given that fewer pulses are required to form the image, frame rates are much higher than in traditional scanners (as high as 5–6000 frames per second). Contrast resolution and penetration are also improved, while artifacts are reduced (as described in more detail later in this chapter). However, to achieve virtual beam forming at very high frame rates, significant computing power is required.

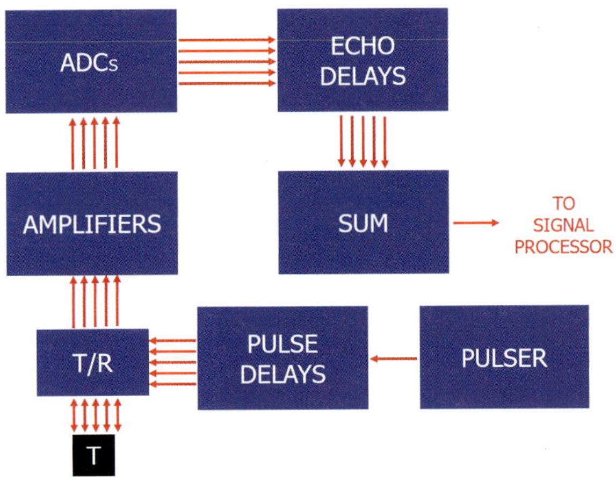

Fig. 4.2 The beam former consists of a pulser, delays, transmit/receive (*T/R*) switch, amplifiers, analog-to-digital converters (*ADCs*), and a summer (*SUM*). The beam former sends digitized echo-voltage streams to the signal processor. *T* is the transducer.

BOX 4.1 Functions of the Beam Former

- Generating the waveforms and voltages that drive the transducer.
- Determining pulse repetition frequency, coding, frequency, and intensity.
- Scanning, focusing, and apodizing the transmitted beam.
- Digitizing the echo voltage stream.
- Directing, focusing, and apodizing the received beam.
- Amplifying the returning echoes.
- Compensating for attenuation.

NARROW TRANSMIT BEAM INSTRUMENTS

Fig. 4.1, A presents a diagram of the organization of a diagnostic ultrasound imaging system utilizing narrow transmit beams. The scanner is composed of a **beam former**, a **signal processor**, an **image processor**, and a **display**.

BEAM FORMER

A simple diagram of the beam former, which is tasked with transmitting focused ultrasound pulses as well as receiving echoes and performing the initial focusing upon reception, is presented in Fig. 4.2. It consists of a **pulse generator**, pulse delays, **digital-to-analog converters** (DACs), transmit/receive (T/R) switch, **analog-to-digital converters** (ADCs), **amplifiers**, echo delays, and a summation component. It should be noted that in reality the pulse delays (on transmission) and the echo delays (on reception) are performed by the same set of digital switches, but they are shown separately to better illustrate the concept of a beam former. Box 4.1 lists the functions of a beam former.

Pulse Generator

The pulse generator produces the digital waveforms that the DACs transform into electric voltages (further on in the processing chain; Fig. 4.3) that drive the transducer. The driving voltages are typically in the form of a single cycle of voltage of the desired operating frequency and form the beam that sweeps through the tissue to be imaged. In response, the transducer converts electrical energy into mechanical energy and produces the ultrasound pulses that travel into the patient. The frequency of the voltage pulse determines the frequency of the resulting ultrasound pulse (see Fig. 4.3, B–E). Frequencies from 1 to 35 MHz clinical probes are available and will cover most applications.

> The pulse generator produces the digital waveforms that DACs transform into the voltages that drive the transducer.

Pulse-repetition frequency (*PRF*) is the number of voltage pulses sent to the transducer each second and thus the number of ultrasound pulses produced per second. The *PRF* ranges from 4 to 15 kHz (5–30 kHz for Doppler applications with the higher values associated with continuous wave [CW] Doppler modes). The ultrasound *PRF* is equal to the voltage *PRF*, because one ultrasound pulse is produced for each voltage pulse. Likewise, the ultrasound pulse repetition period is equal to the voltage pulse repetition period (the time from the beginning of one pulse to the beginning of the next).

The operator does not normally have direct control of the *PRF* in grayscale mode. Rather, the pulse generator adjusts it appropriately for the current imaging depth. To achieve a high frame rate (i.e., receive information for display at a rapid rate), a high *PRF* is desirable. However, all echoes from one pulse must be received before the next pulse is transmitted in order to properly display returning echoes, which limits how high the *PRF* can be. The timing sequence that is initiated by the pulse generator is shown in Fig. 4.4. For deeper imaging, echoes take longer time to return, thus forcing a reduction in *PRF* and the frame rate (i.e., number of images that are generated each second). Imaging depth—that is, penetration (*pen*) in centimeters—multiplied by *PRF* (in kHz) must not exceed 77 if echo misplacement is to be avoided (an artifact known as *range ambiguity*, which is discussed in Chapter 7). Hence:

$$pen(\text{cm}) \times PRF(\text{kHz}) \leq 77(\text{cm/ms})$$

The scanner automatically uses the highest *PRF* possible, while avoiding any range ambiguity. For a reduced operating frequency, penetration increases, and *PRF* is automatically reduced to avoid echo misplacement.

ADVANCED CONCEPTS

The 77 in the penetration-*PRF* limit equation (pen [cm] × PRF [kHz] ≤ 77 [cm/ms]) is derived as follows. The time required for the ultrasound pulse to travel to the maximum imaging depth (penetration) and return is

$$t(\mu\text{s}) = \frac{2 \times pen(\text{mm})}{c(\text{mm}/\mu\text{s})} = \frac{2 \times pen}{1.54} = \frac{pen}{0.77}$$

where *t* is time (in microseconds) and *c* is propagation speed (in millimeters per microsecond).

This is the minimum allowable time in microseconds between pulses (*PRP*). In milliseconds, $t = pen/770$. The reciprocal is the maximum allowable *PRF* (in kHz) to avoid echo misplacement, that is, $PRF_{max} = 1/PRP_{min} = 770/pen$.

ADVANCED CONCEPTS—cont'd

Thus, $pen \times PRF_{max} = 770$. Converting pen from millimeters to centimeters, $pen \times PRF_{max} = 77$. Thus pen (cm) $\times$ PRF (kHz) ≤ 77.

The greater the voltage amplitude produced by the pulse generator through the DAC, the greater the amplitude and intensity of the ultrasound pulse produced by the transducer. Transducer driving–voltage amplitudes reach approximately 100 V. Output level is sometimes shown on the display in terms of a percentage or decibels relative to maximum (100% or 0 dB) output (Fig. 4.5). Other output indicators account for relevant risk mechanisms. Reducing the acoustic output will also reduce received echo amplitudes (see Fig. 4.5, C). An increase in amplifier gain can compensate for this. A reduction in imaging depth also occurs, but this is surprisingly small. For example, a reduction of 50% in output from a 5 MHz transducer corresponds to only a 5% penetration reduction (from approximately 12.0 to 11.4 cm).

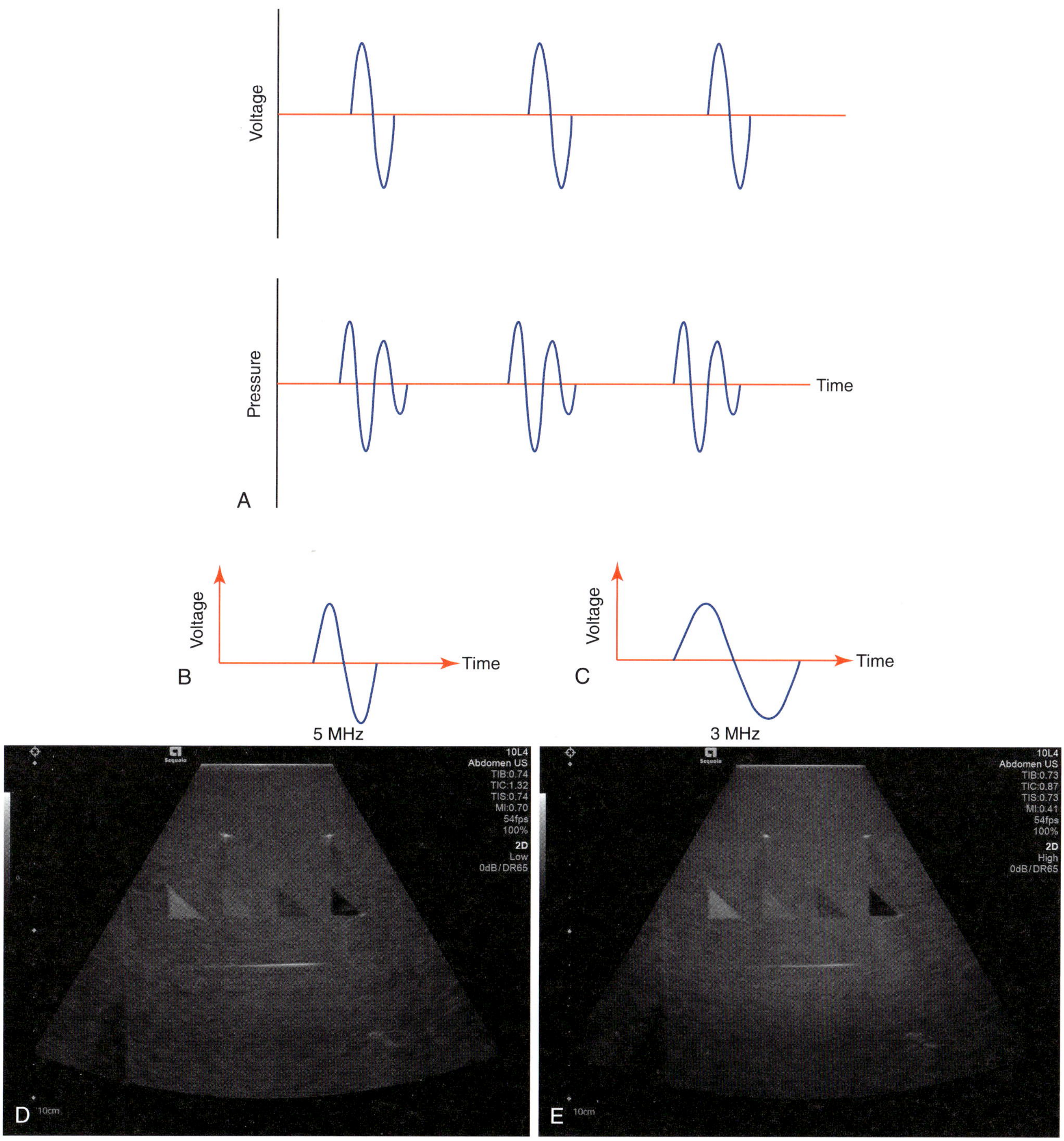

Fig. 4.3 With every voltage pulse applied **(A)**, an ultrasound pulse is produced by the transducer. Voltage pulses of different frequencies **(B–C)** produce ultrasound pulses of different frequencies. The operator can change the operating frequency without changing transducers. **D–E,** Images with 4–6 MHz and 8–10 MHz frequencies, respectively, with the same transducer.

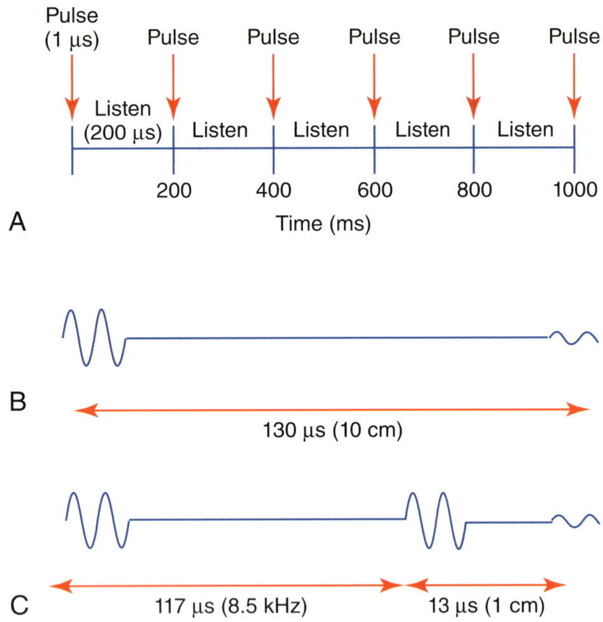

Fig. 4.4 A, Timing sequence for pulse-echo ultrasound imaging. The sequence is initiated by the production of a 1-μs pulse of ultrasound when the pulser sends a voltage pulse to the transducer. This is followed by a period of as long as 250 μs during which echoes are received from the tissue by the transducer. The length of this time is determined by the maximum depth from which the echoes return. For example, at a frequency of 5 MHz, echoes can return from as deep as 15 cm. The round-trip travel time (13 μs/cm × 15 cm) to this depth is 195 μs. This listening period is followed (5 μs later) by the next pulse. In this illustration, the listening period is 200 μs; that is, the pulse repetition period is 200 μs (the pulse-repetition frequency [*PRF*] is 5 kHz). If *PRF* was greater, the pulse repetition period would be decreased, resulting in emission of the next pulse before the reception of all the (deeper) echoes from the previous pulse. This would produce range-ambiguity artifact (see Chapter 7) and thus is avoided by the scanner. The *PRF* is automatically adjusted to avoid this problem: higher *PRF*s are used for superficial imaging, whereas lower *PRF*s are used for deep imaging (to allow for the longer time required for the arrival of deeper echoes). The latter causes a reduction in frame rate. **B,** An echo (from a 10 cm depth) arrives 130 μs after pulse emission. **C,** If the pulse repetition period were 117 μs (corresponding to a *PRF* of 8.5 kHz), the echo in B would arrive 13 μs after the next pulse was emitted. The instrument would place this echo at a 1-cm depth rather than the correct value. This is known as *range-ambiguity artifact*.

Delay Switches

Modern transducer arrays require complicated sequencing and phasing operations for transmission and reception performed in real time. Sequencing, phase delays, and variations in pulse amplitudes, which are necessary for the electronic control of beam **scanning**, steering, transmission focusing, aperture, and apodization, must be accomplished. The pulse generator produces the initial digital waveforms, which determine pulse amplitudes, while pulse delays (essentially digital switches) carry out all of the other tasks (as described in Chapter 3).

After ADCs and amplification, the echoes (represented by digital numbers) pass through digital delay lines (i.e., digital switches) to accomplish reception dynamic focus and steering functions (as discussed in Chapter 3).

Channels

The pulse delays have a single input from the pulse generator, but multiple outputs to the transducer elements; that is, there are actually many delay paths through the pulse delay switches. The reason for this is that each of the many elements in the array needs a different delay to form the ultrasound beam properly. Each independent delay and element combination constitutes a transmission **channel** (Fig. 4.6). An increased number of channels allows more precise control of beam characteristics. On reception, each independent element, ADC, amplifier, and delay path constitutes a reception channel. Typical numbers of channels in modern diagnostic ultrasound scanners range from 64 to 256 or at the most 512. Larger numbers are sometimes advertised, but a looser definition (than the one presented here) of the term *channel* is used in such advertisements. The number of channels does not exceed the number of elements in a transducer.

> A channel is an independent signal path consisting of a transducer element, delay switch, and possibly other components.

DACs and ADCs

In modern ultrasound scanners, the strategy is to digitize all **signals** as soon as possible (i.e., as close to the transducer as possible). On the transmission side, digital signals representing ultrasound pulses pass through DACs and are converted into analog voltages that are provided to the transducer elements. The term **analog** means "proportional," and the term **digital** means "in the form of discrete numbers." On the receive side, echo voltages are digitized; that is, they pass through ADCs (Fig. 4.7). An ADC (also called a *digitizer*) converts the voltage from analog to digital form and is the opposite of a DAC (i.e., it performs the reverse operation). After the ADC, echo voltages are replaced by a series of numbers, and further manipulation of the echoes is accomplished as digital signal processing (mathematical manipulation of numbers representing echoes).

The transition to all digital ultrasound imaging systems is similar to what has occurred in many aspects of consumer electronics, such as music players and mobile phones that handle, store, and process sound and pictures in digital form. The ADC interrogates (i.e., samples) the incoming voltage at regular intervals and determines its value at each interrogation instant. The interrogation rate must be twice the highest frequency involved in the interrogated voltage to preserve (in the subsequent digital number stream) all the harmonics contained in the voltage signal. For example, to digitize a 5 MHz CW voltage properly, the digitizing rate must be at least 10 MHz; that is, the voltage is interrogated 10 million times per second, yielding a stream of 10 million digitized values per second describing the original analog voltage.

> DACs convert digital waveforms to analog voltages for driving transducer elements, while ADCs convert the analog voltages representing echoes to numbers for digital signal processing and storage.

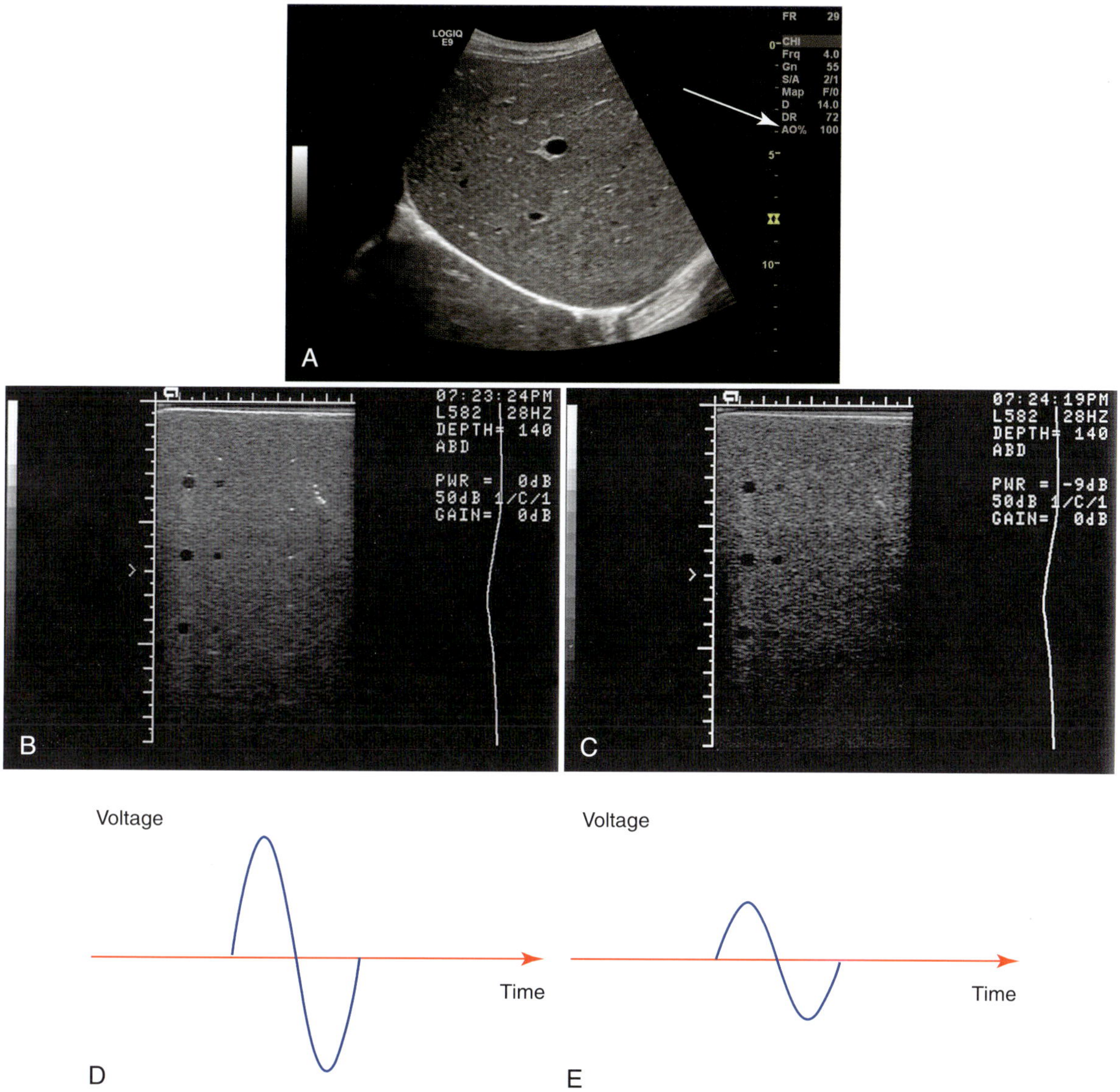

Fig. 4.5 **A,** The output indicator (*arrow*; acoustic output [*AO*]) shows a percentage relative to the maximum (100% in this example). **B–C,** The output indicator here shows decibels relative to the maximum. An output of 0 dB (100%) is compared with one of −9 dB (12.5%), in which the weaker echoes produce a darker image. **D–E,** Driving voltages from pulser to transducer for 0 and −6 dB, respectively. The voltage amplitude in **E** is half that in **D**, yielding one-fourth the power and intensity, thus −6 dB output compared with **D**.

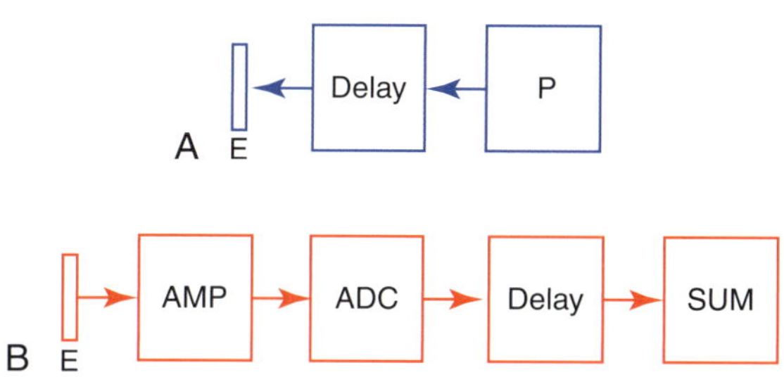

Fig. 4.6 **A,** A transmission channel consists of an independent delay and transducer element (*E*) combination. Several channels emanate from the pulser (*P*). **B,** A reception channel consists of an independent element (*E*), amplifier (*AMP*), analog-to-digital converter (*ADC*), and delay. The signals from many channels are combined in the summer (*SUM*).

ADVANCED CONCEPTS

The precision of the ADC digitization of the echo voltages depends on the number of bits available to the digitized binary number. For example, an 8-bit digitizer can yield any decimal number from 0 to 255 (2^8–1). If the maximum voltage being converted to a digital number is 10 V, the digitizer can determine its value at any interrogation to a precision of 10/255 or 0.039 V (0.4%). The temporal precision of the digitizer is determined by the digitizing frequency (i.e., the sampling frequency of the ADC). Each cycle of the voltage must be interrogated at least twice to determine its frequency. Thus changes in the voltage that occur at a faster rate than half the digitizing frequency cannot be followed by the digitizer and will be lost in the digitizing process. A 10-MHz digitizer interrogates 10 million times per second. Voltage frequencies of 5 MHz or less can be digitized properly in this ADC.

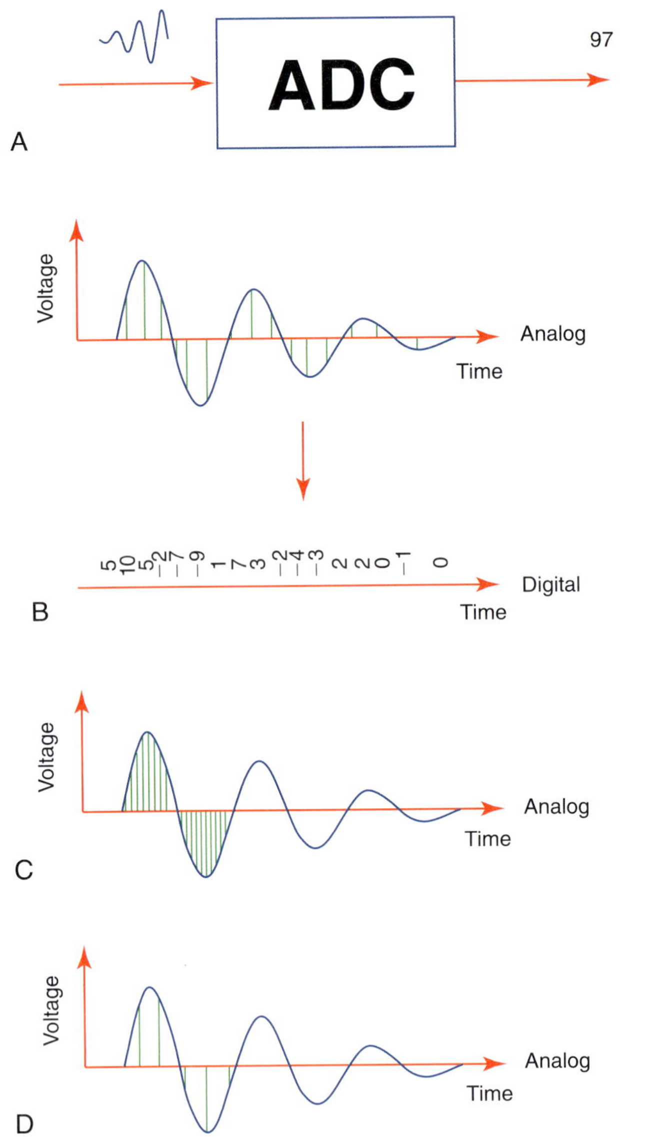

Fig. 4.7 **A,** The analog-to-digital converter (*ADC*) converts **(B)** the analog (proportional) echo voltage into a series of numbers representing the sampled voltage. The higher the sampling rate of the ADC, the better the temporal detail of the voltage is preserved. **C,** High sampling rate. **D,** Low sampling rate.

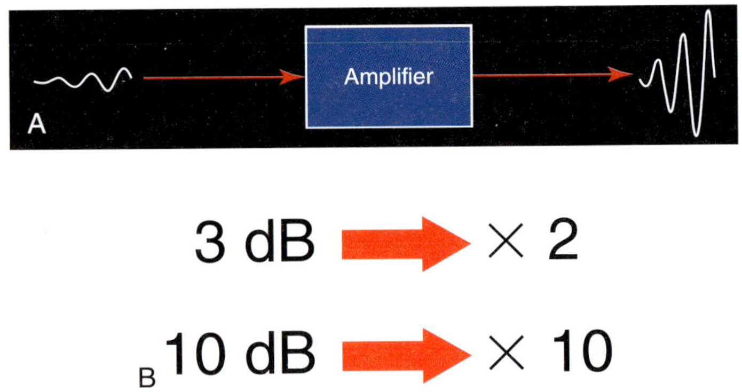

Fig. 4.8 **A,** Amplification (gain) increases signal amplitude, which is equivalent to voltage and, thus electric power. **B,** A gain of 3 dB corresponds to an output power equivalent to input power × 2; 10 dB corresponds to an input power × 10.

Transmit/Receive Switch

The T/R switch directs the driving voltages from the pulse generator and pulse delays via the DAC to the transducer during transmission and then directs the returning echo voltages from the transducer to ADC and onward to the amplifiers during reception. However, it is important to note that there are still plenty of ultrasound systems using analog beam formers with digitization taking place later in the processing chain. The T/R switch protects the sensitive input components of the beam former from the large driving voltages generated by the transmission components.

Conversely, in some scanners the DAC/ADC components are incorporated even closer to the transducer than indicated above and in Fig. 4.2—that is in the transducer handle itself. In this case, the T/R switch simply selects the transmission or reception pathway without shielding any beam former components (since that is not required when digital numbers are involved).

Amplifiers

Amplifiers increase signal amplitudes in each channel individually. **Amplification** is the conversion of the small signals received from the transducer elements (in analog beam formers/amplifiers voltages) to larger ones suitable for further processing and storage (Fig. 4.8). **Gain** is the ratio of amplifier output to signal or electric power input. The power ratio, which is expressed in decibels, is a parameter for analog amplifiers, and it is equal to the voltage ratio squared because electric power depends on voltage squared. For example, if the input voltage amplitude to an amplifier is 2 mV and the output voltage amplitude is 200 mV, the voltage ratio is 200/2, or 100. The power ratio is 100^2, or 10,000. As shown in Table 4.1, the gain is 40 dB. Beam former amplifiers typically have 60 to 100 dB of gain. Voltages from transducers to these analog amplifiers range from a few microvolts (μV; e.g., from blood) to a few hundred millivolts (mV; e.g., from bone or gas). For a 60 dB gain amplifier, the output power is 1 million times the power input, and the output voltage is 1000 times the input. For a 10 μV voltage input, the output voltage is 10 mV. If the gain of this amplifier is increased to 100 dB, the output voltage increases to 1 V.

> Amplifiers increase signal amplitudes. This increase is called *gain*.

Two useful decibel values to remember are 3 and 10 (see Fig. 4.8, B). Whereas 3 dB corresponds to a power gain of ×2, 10 dB corresponds to ×10. Values also can be combined; for example, 6 dB corresponds to two doublings (×4); 20 dB corresponds to ×10 ×10, or ×100; and 13 dB corresponds to ×10 ×2, or ×20.

Gain control (often a control panel button, but it varies from manufacturer to manufacturer and even from model to model) determines how much amplification is accomplished in the amplifier (Fig. 4.9). Gain control is similar in function to the level control

TABLE 4.1 Gain (Expressed in Decibels) and Corresponding Power and Amplitude Ratios

Gain (dB)	Power Ratio	Amplitude Ratio
0	1.0	1.0
1	1.3	1.1
2	1.6	1.3
3	2.0	1.4
4	2.5	1.6
5	3.2	1.8
6	4.0	2.0
7	5.0	2.2
8	6.3	2.5
9	7.9	2.8
10	10	3.2
15	32	5.6
20	100	10
25	320	18
30	1000	32
35	3200	56
40	10,000	100
45	32,000	180
50	100,000	320
60	1,000,000	1000
70	10,000,000	3200
80	100,000,000	10,000
90	1,000,000,000	32,000
100	10,000,000,000	100,000

The power (amplitude) ratio is output power (amplitude) divided by input power (amplitude).

on your sound system at home. With too little gain, weak echoes are not imaged. With too much gain, saturation occurs; that is, most echoes appear bright, and differences in echo strength are lost. More and more scanners have implemented automatic gain controls.

> Gain is set subjectively so that echoes appear with appropriate brightness, although more and more scanners do this automatically.

The amplifiers are also used to compensate for the effect of attenuation on the image. **Time gain compensation** (TGC; also occasionally called **depth gain compensation**) equalizes differences in received echo amplitudes caused by echoes originating at different depths. Reflectors with equal reflection coefficients will not result in echoes of equal amplitude arriving at the transducer (Fig. 4.10) if their travel distances are different (i.e., if the distances between the transducer and the reflectors are different), because sound is attenuated (or weakened) as it travels (on average by 0.5 dB/ [cm MHz]). Displaying echoes from similar reflectors in a similar way is obviously a requirement for any ultrasound imaging system. Longer path lengths result in greater attenuation and later arrival times. Therefore if echoes arriving later are amplified correctly (i.e., to a greater degree than earlier ones), attenuation compensation is accomplished. This is the goal of the TGC (Fig. 4.11). In other words, the later an echo arrives, the farther it has traveled and the weaker it will be. However, the later it arrives, the more it will be amplified. If this compensation is done properly, the resulting signal amplitude and thus displayed image will be the same as if there had been no attenuation.

The increase of gain with depth can be expressed in decibels of gain per centimeter of depth. When properly adjusted, it should correspond to the average attenuation in the tissue (i.e., in dB/cm of depth). Remember that each centimeter of depth corresponds to 2 cm of round-trip sound travel, so the resulting slope should be about 1 dB/(cm MHz), because the average attenuation in soft tissue is 0.5 dB/(cm MHz). The former refers to centimeters of depth, whereas the latter refers to centimeters of travel. The attenuation depends on depth (or rather travel distance), the attenuation of the tissues, and the frequency of the ultrasound beam, which requires the operator to subjectively adjust the TGC to compensate for these factors. TGC is set by the operator to achieve, on average, uniform brightness throughout the image. The average attenuation in the tissue cross-section at the operating frequency has been compensated when this is accomplished.

It is important to note that more and more scanners have incorporated "one button image optimization" algorithms, which typically adjust both overall gain and TGC settings automatically. Moreover, there are internal TGC curves that the operator will not have access to and which are varied depending on the system preset selected.

> Time gain compensates for the effect of attenuation on an image.

Typical TGC amplifiers compensate for approximately 60 dB of attenuation. At the depth at which maximum gain has been reached, the echo brightness begins to decrease, because the TGC can no longer compensate (the amplifier gain cannot be increased further). Hence, attenuation and maximum amplifier gain determine the maximum imaging depth. Maximum amplifier gain is reached when the amplifier noise and the weak echoes being amplified have comparable amplitude. Electronic noise (Fig. 4.12, A–B) exists in all electronic circuits and components. Any further increase in gain would only result in weaker echoes being lost in the noise and thus being unobservable.

Some instruments have **lateral gain control**, which allows adjustment of gain laterally across the image (see Fig. 4.12, C–D), typically in echocardiography. Regions with different attenuation values located laterally to each other can be compensated to yield consistent image brightness. For example, this is applied in echocardiography to provide consistent echo brightness laterally across the cardiac image.

The overall gain control is adjusted first to yield a perceptible image on the display. Then the TGC (and possibly the lateral gain) controls are adjusted to yield on-average uniform brightness over the image. Attenuation variations throughout

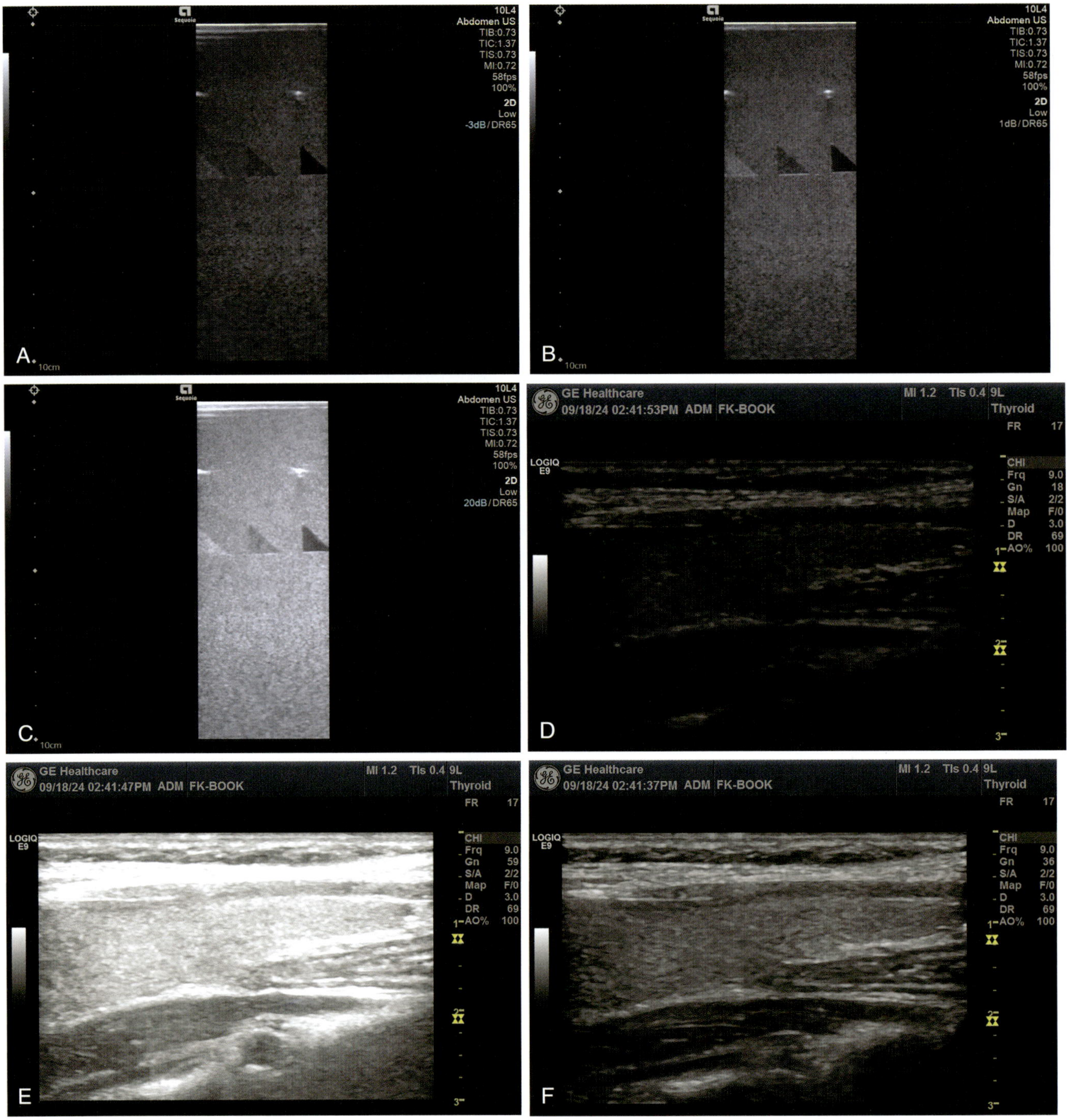

Fig. 4.9 **A,** Gain is too low (–3 dB). **B,** Proper gain (1 dB). **C,** Gain is too high (20 dB), causing saturation. Thyroid scans with low **(D),** high **(E),** and proper **(F)** gain.

the image are thus compensated for, yielding a good representation of the tissue cross-section (or plane) imaged. Again more and more scanners have implemented automatic gain controls (which can also include TGC and lateral gain settings).

Summer (Adder)

After all the channel signal components are delayed properly to accomplish the focus and steering functions, they are added together in the adder to produce the resulting scan line, which, along with all the others, will be displayed after signal processing and image processing. Reception apodization and dynamic aperture functions are also accomplished as part of this summation process.

> The beam former is responsible for electronic beam scanning, steering, focusing, apodization, and aperture functions.

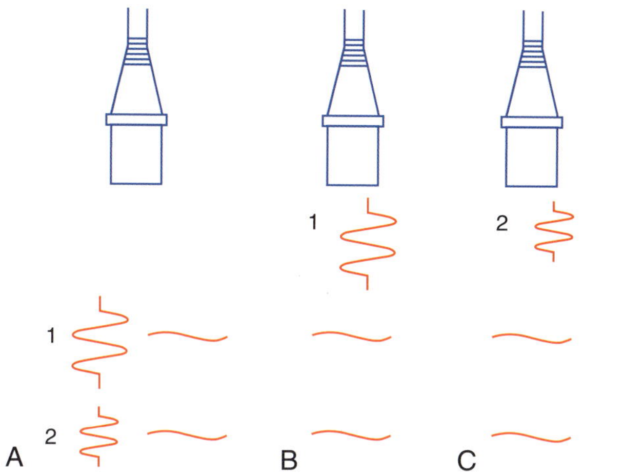

Fig. 4.10 Two identical reflectors are located at different distances from the transducer. **A,** The echo at the second reflector is weaker because the incident pulse had to travel farther to get there, thereby increasing attenuation. **B,** The echo from the first reflector arrives at the transducer. The echo is weaker than it was in **A** because of attenuation on the return trip. **C,** The echo from the second reflector arrives at the transducer later and in a weaker form than the first one did because of the longer path to the second reflector.

SIGNAL PROCESSOR

The receiving part of the beam former amplifies and combines the contributions from the individual elements and channels to form the stream of echoes returning from each transmitted pulse and sends them on to the signal processor. Operations carried out here include **filtering**, **detection**, and **compression**. A diagram of the signal processor is shown in Fig. 4.13. Box 4.2 lists the functions of the signal processor in its simplest form. These functions are commonly performed in this order although, in some cases, compression can precede detection and filtering can be associated with the amplifiers.

Filtering

Digital filters called *bandpass filters* operate at a specific frequency with a bandwidth that includes the frequencies in the returning echoes and eliminates signals (noise, etc.) outside that bandwidth. A **bandpass filter** is one that passes a range of frequencies (its bandwidth) and rejects those above and below the acceptance bandwidth (Fig. 4.14). Some bandpass filters dynamically move their frequency range to track the bandwidth of the returning echoes from a pulse. The echo bandwidth decreases as the echoes return, because the higher frequencies in the bandwidth are attenuated more than the lower ones.

Filtering eliminates frequencies outside the echo bandwidth, while retaining those that are most useful in a given type of operation.

Detection

Detection (also called **demodulation**) is the conversion of echo signals from **radio frequency** (RF) form to amplitude form (Fig. 4.15). This is done by detecting and connecting the maxima of the cyclic variations. This cyclic form is called

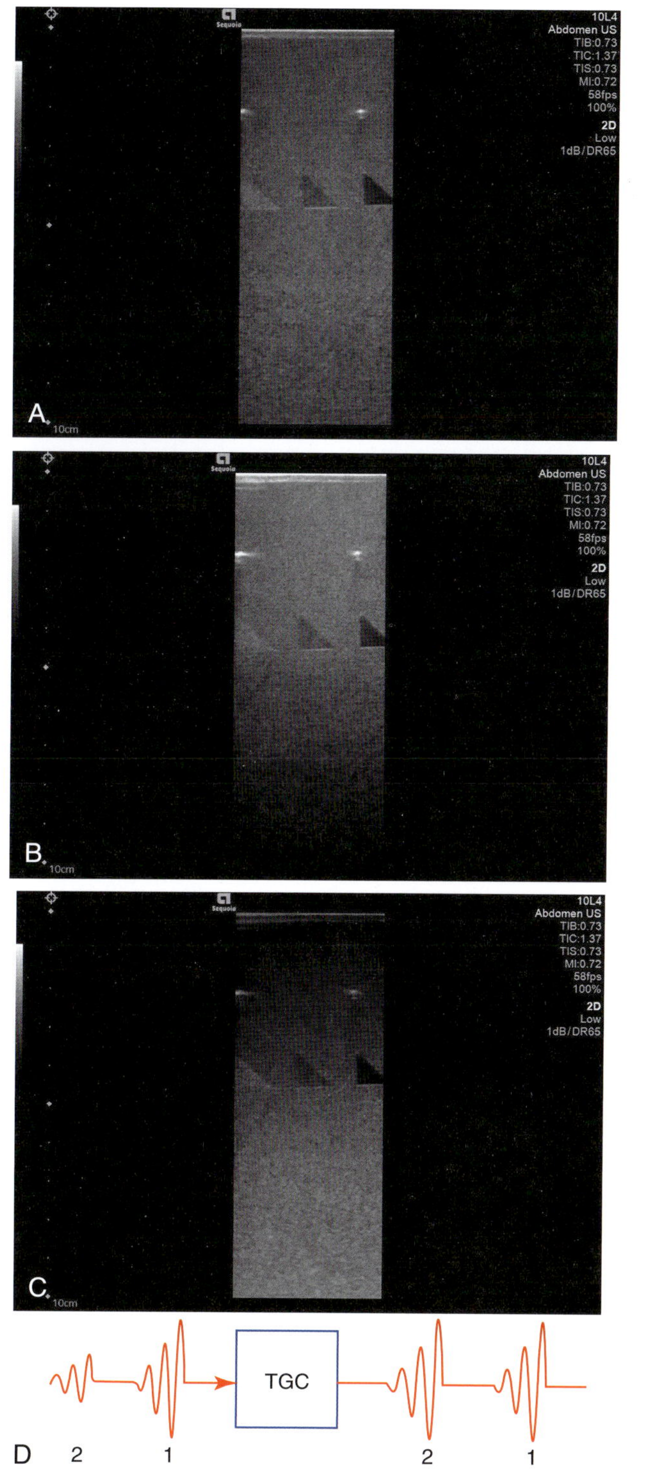

Fig. 4.11 Time gain compensation (*TGC*). Three scans of a tissue-equivalent phantom imaged at 4–6 MHz with correct TGC **(A)** and with the TGC set too high **(B)** or too low **(C)** in the near field. **D,** TGC controls (*arrow*) matching the image in **(C)**. Without TGC, the echo brightness (amplitude, intensity, strength) declines with depth (top to bottom). Average tissue attenuation is 0.5 dB/cm-MHz. This is calculated per centimeter of sound propagation. Average attenuation then is 1 dB/cm-MHz when the centimeter value is the distance from the transducer to the reflector. The sound must travel twice this distance (round trip), so the attenuation number doubles. Typical TGC slopes then will be about 1 dB/cm-MHz. **D,** Uncompensated echoes from identical structures at differing depths enter the TGC amplifier. The second (*2*) is weaker than the first (*1*) because it has come from a deeper site and has experienced more attenuation. After TGC, the amplitudes are identical.

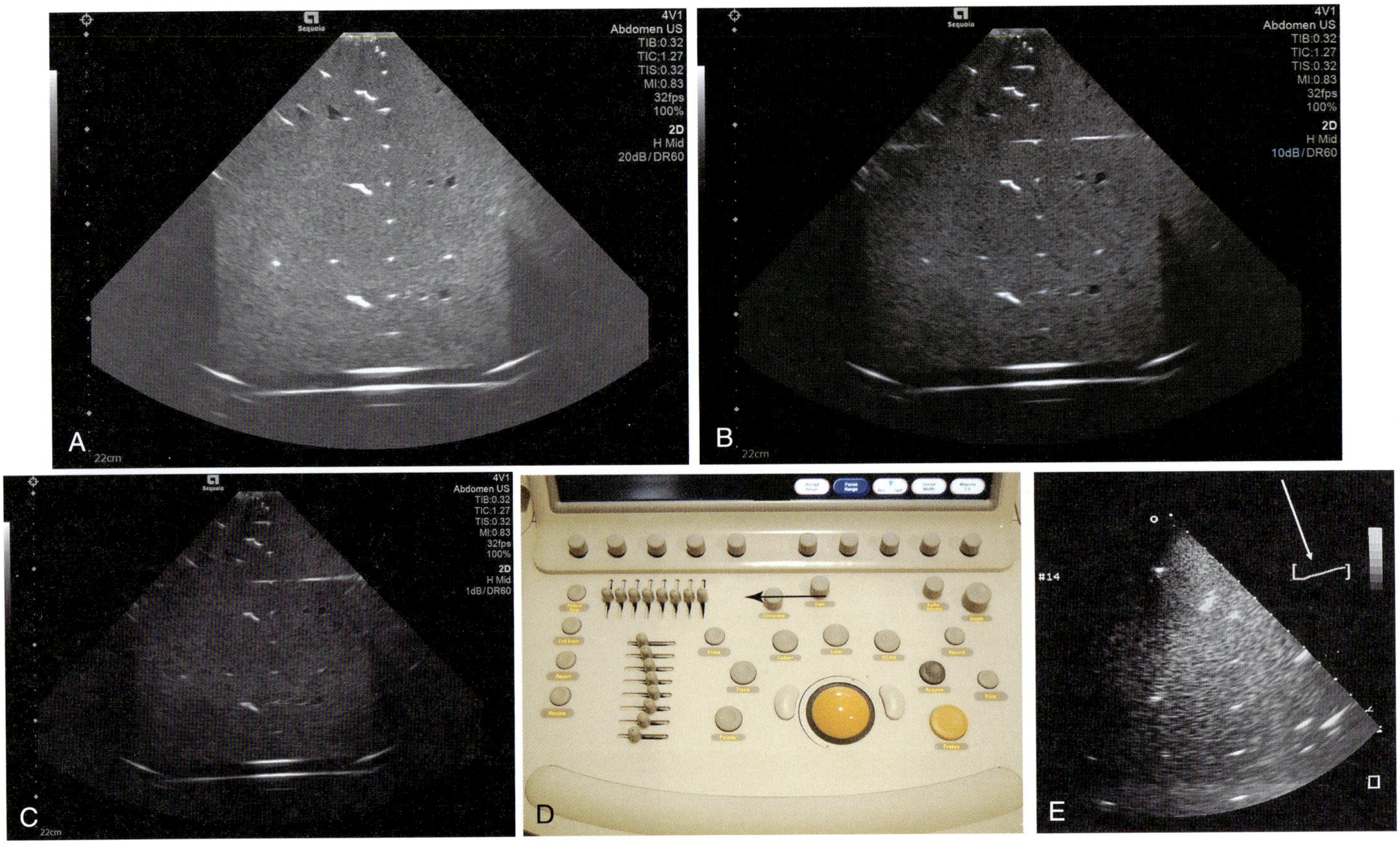

Fig. 4.12 **A,** Under conditions of high gain (20 dB), electronic noise (with its fuzzy appearance) can be seen on the edge of and beyond the phantom. **B,** With reduced gain (10 dB), these weak echoes are greatly reduced (but not eliminated). **C,** At a much lower gain (1 dB) these noise echoes are not amplified enough to be visualized. **D,** Lateral gain controls (*arrow*). **E,** Lateral gain adjusted to increase gain from left to right.

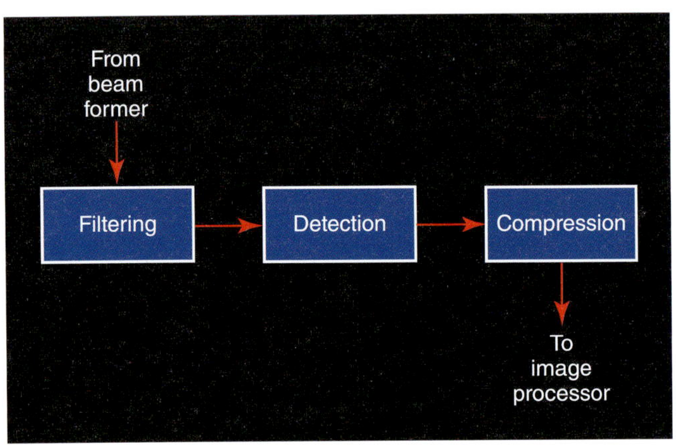

Fig. 4.13 The signal processor performs filtering, detection, and compression functions. The processor receives digital signals from the beam former and, after processing, sends them on to the image processor.

BOX 4.2 Functions of the Signal Processor

- Bandpass filtering
- Amplitude detection
- Compression (dynamic range reduction)

radio frequency, because it is similar to voltages found in a radio receiver. The detected form retains the amplitudes, but no phase information. Diagnostic ultrasound pulses do not have constant amplitude, and therefore when demodulated, they do not have the simplified blocked appearance shown in Fig. 4.15. Detection is not an operator-controllable function.

> Detection is the conversion of echoes from RF form to video form. The video form retains amplitudes of the echoes.

Compression

The ratio of the largest to the smallest amplitude (or power) that a system can handle is called the **dynamic range**. Dynamic range is expressed in decibels. For example, if an analog amplifier is insensitive to voltage amplitudes of less than 0.01 mV (because they are buried in electronic noise) and cannot properly handle voltage amplitudes of greater than 1000 mV, the ratio of usable voltage extremes is 1000/0.01 or 100,000. The power ratio of an analog amplifier is equal to the square of the voltage ratio: $100{,}000^2$ or 10,000,000,000. According to Table 4.1, the dynamic range of the amplifier is 100 dB. Amplifiers typically have dynamic ranges of 100 to 120 dB. System dynamic ranges

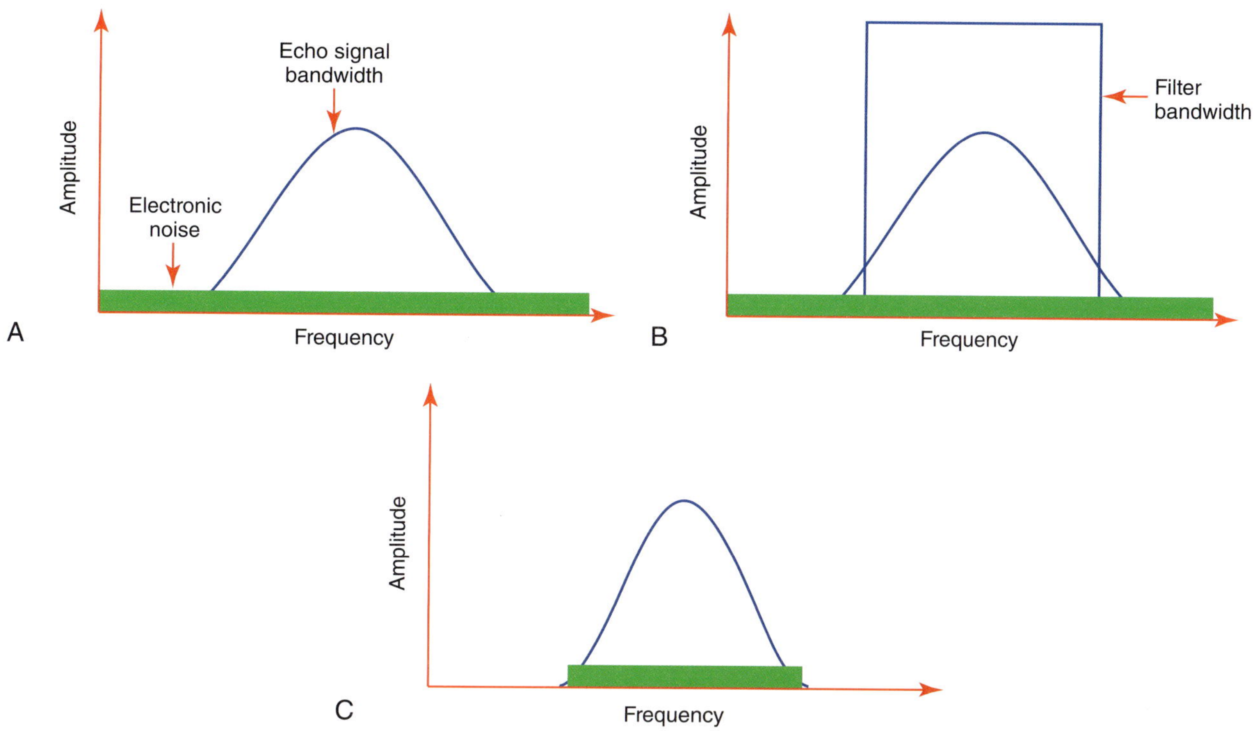

Fig. 4.14 **A,** Input to filter includes the echo signal bandwidth and the electronic noise with unlimited bandwidth. **B,** The filter bandwidth is designed to accommodate the signal bandwidth. **C,** The output from the filter has the frequencies above and below its bandwidth removed. Only the noise frequencies within the filter bandwidth remain.

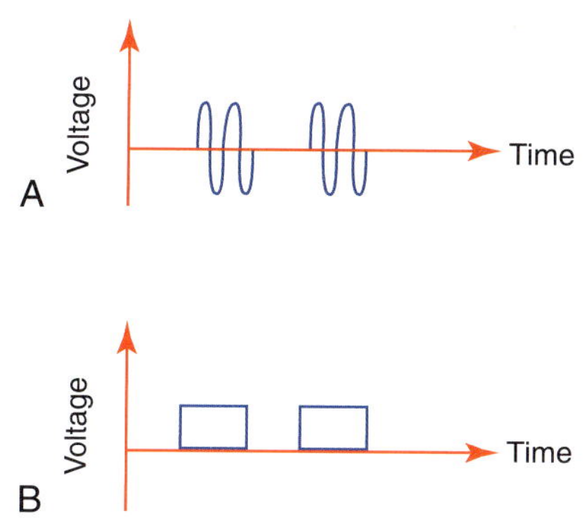

Fig. 4.15 Echo voltages are produced in a complicated cyclic form **(A)** called *radio frequency* (*RF*), which would be difficult to store and display. Furthermore, only the amplitude of each echo is needed for a gray-scale display of anatomy. Thus the RF form is converted to the simpler amplitude form **(B),** which retains the amplitude of each echo voltage.

are claimed to be as high as 170 dB. Greater values indicate the ability to detect weaker echoes, that is, greater sensitivity.

Other components of an ultrasound scanner have smaller dynamic range capabilities. Displays have dynamic ranges of 60 to 70 dB. Furthermore, human vision is limited to a dynamic range of approximately 100 dB, which means the largest display brightness can be approximately 100,000 times the smallest level (cf., Table 4.1). The echo dynamic range remaining after compensation is typically 50 to 100 dB. Compression is the process of decreasing the differences between the smallest and the largest echo amplitudes to a usable range for display (Fig. 4.16). The specific compression curve is almost always nonlinear with only a small range of brightness levels being linear.

> Compression reduces dynamic range—often nonlinearly—to a range suitable for display.

Compression is somewhat operator adjustable as a dynamic range control and by selecting a specific (nonlinear) compression curve (Fig. 4.17). These two elements reduce dynamic range by assigning some weak echo amplitude values to around zero and/or by assigning some of the strongest to maximum. Reassigned echoes may be at either end of the dynamic range or at both ends (see Fig. 4.17, J–L). A smaller dynamic range setting presents a higher contrast image, which is often desirable when evaluating endocardial border motion, but obviously not appropriate when searching for almost iso-echoic metastases in the liver. Gain control moves the dynamic range graph to the left or right (down or up the dynamic range) as gain is increased or decreased (see Fig. 4.17, M–N).

> Signal processing includes digital filtering, detection, and compression of echo data. The order in which these processes occur in the signal processor is usually filtering first, with detection and compression following in either order.

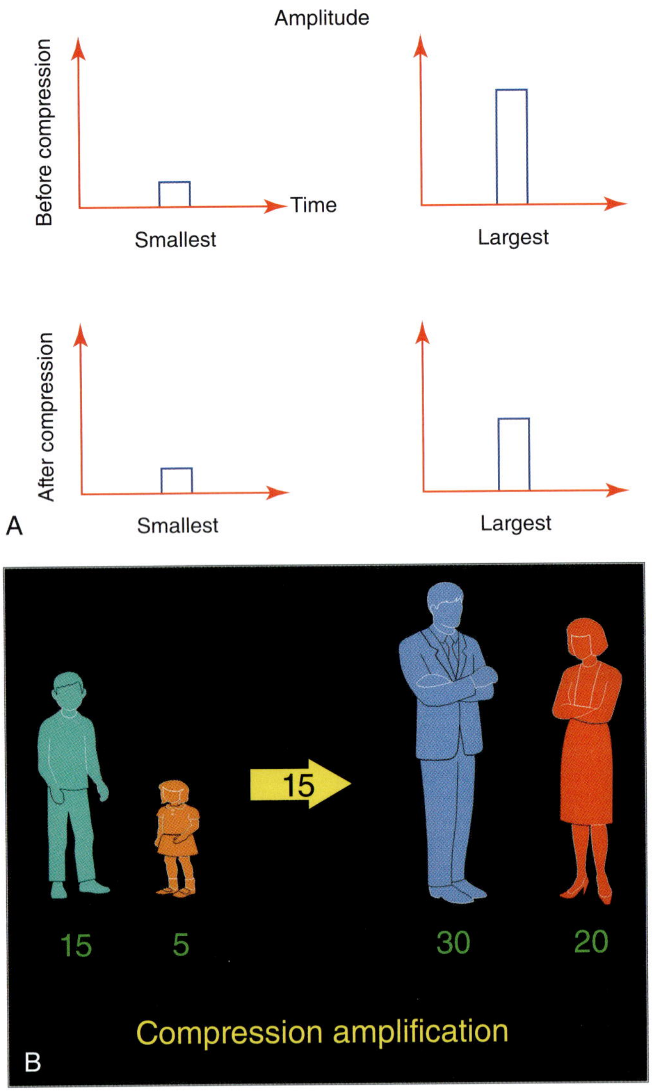

Fig. 4.16 Compression decreases the difference between the smallest and largest amplitudes passing through the system. **A,** In this example, the ratio of largest to smallest amplitudes before compression is 5. After compression, the ratio is 3. **B,** A family illustration of compression amplification. Big brother (age 15 years) is twice as tall (large dynamic range) as his little sister (age 5 years). Fifteen years later, the brother (age 30 years) is just slightly taller than the sister (age 20 years). Both have grown (amplification), but the shorter child grew more than the taller one, reducing the difference between them (compression).

IMAGE PROCESSOR

Until this point (through the beam former and signal processor), the echo data are traveling in scan-line form serially through the system, that is, one scan line at a time. No image has yet been formed. The image processor converts the digitized, filtered, detected, and compressed serial scan-line data into images that are stored in **image memory**, all in preparation for presentation on the scanner display. After detection of the echo amplitudes in the signal processor, the scan-line data enter the image processor, where they are preprocessed and stored in image form and then are processed in image form before finally being displayed on the system monitor (Fig. 4.18). Box 4.3 lists the functions of the image processor.

The image processor provides a means for correctly displaying the acquired echo information (i.e., in a linear or sector ultrasound image format). The direction of each scan line and the location of echoes in depth down each scan line are used to determine the proper location in the image memory (and thus on the display) for each echo. For example, a pulse transmitted from the transducer straight down into the body (so a linear array) will result in a series of echoes that are located in appropriate memory locations straight down a column in memory at various depths, that is, various row locations (Fig. 4.19, A). A pulse transmitted at an angle (an off-vertical direction) will result in a series of echoes that must be located in different rows and columns matching the scan-line orientation (see Fig. 4.19, B). The image processor properly locates each series of echoes corresponding to each scan line for each pulse transmitted from the transducer, which is the essence of ultrasound imaging with narrow transmit beams, and correctly fills up the image memory with echo information. This is accomplished in a fraction of a second, yielding one scan or **frame** of image information. This process is repeated many times per second to produce a rapid sequence of frames stored in the memory and presented on the display. This rapid-sequence presentation is called **real-time display** or real-time imaging for frame rates in excess of 10 frames per second (i.e., a frame rate of more than 10 Hz). The scanner depth control determines the depth being displayed and thus, the depth range covered by the image memory in the scan conversion process.

> The image processer formats digital echo data into image form for image processing, storage, and display.

Preprocessing

As part of the process of scan-line information going into the image memory, various processing functions may be performed on the image. This is called **preprocessing**, because it occurs before the echo data are stored in the image memory. Examples of preprocessing include edge enhancement (a function that sharpens boundaries to make them more detectable and measurements more precise), data (or **pixel**—meaning *picture element*) interpolation, persistence, and 3D volume data display formatting.

> Preprocessing is signal processing performed while echo data are being stored in the memory.

Pixel Interpolation

Image quality can be improved accomplished by filling in missing pixels. This occurs, for example, in sector scans where scan

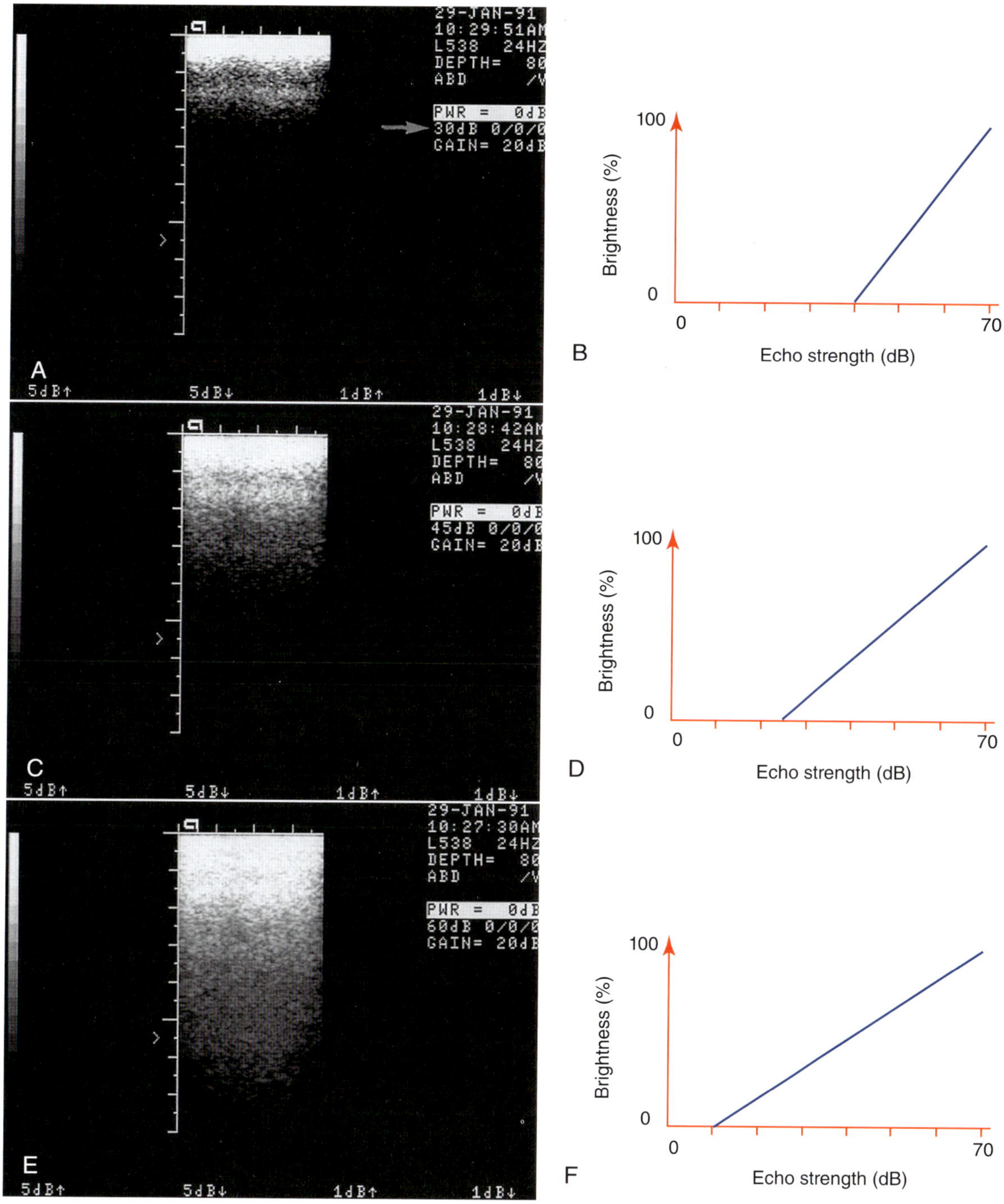

Fig. 4.17 **A,** The dynamic range setting (*arrow*) is 30 dB. The lower 40 dB of echoes returning from a tissue-equivalent phantom are set to 0 (*black portion*). The remainder show high contrast, with brightness progressing from black for 40-dB echoes to white for 70-dB echoes. **B,** A 30-dB dynamic range setting assigns the weakest 40 dB of echo dynamic range to zero (*black*) and the remaining 30 dB of dynamic range to linearly higher brightnesses. **C,** A display with a dynamic range of 45 dB. **D,** Brightness assignment for a 45-dB dynamic range. **E,** A display with a dynamic range of 60 dB. **F,** Brightness assignment for a 60-dB dynamic range.

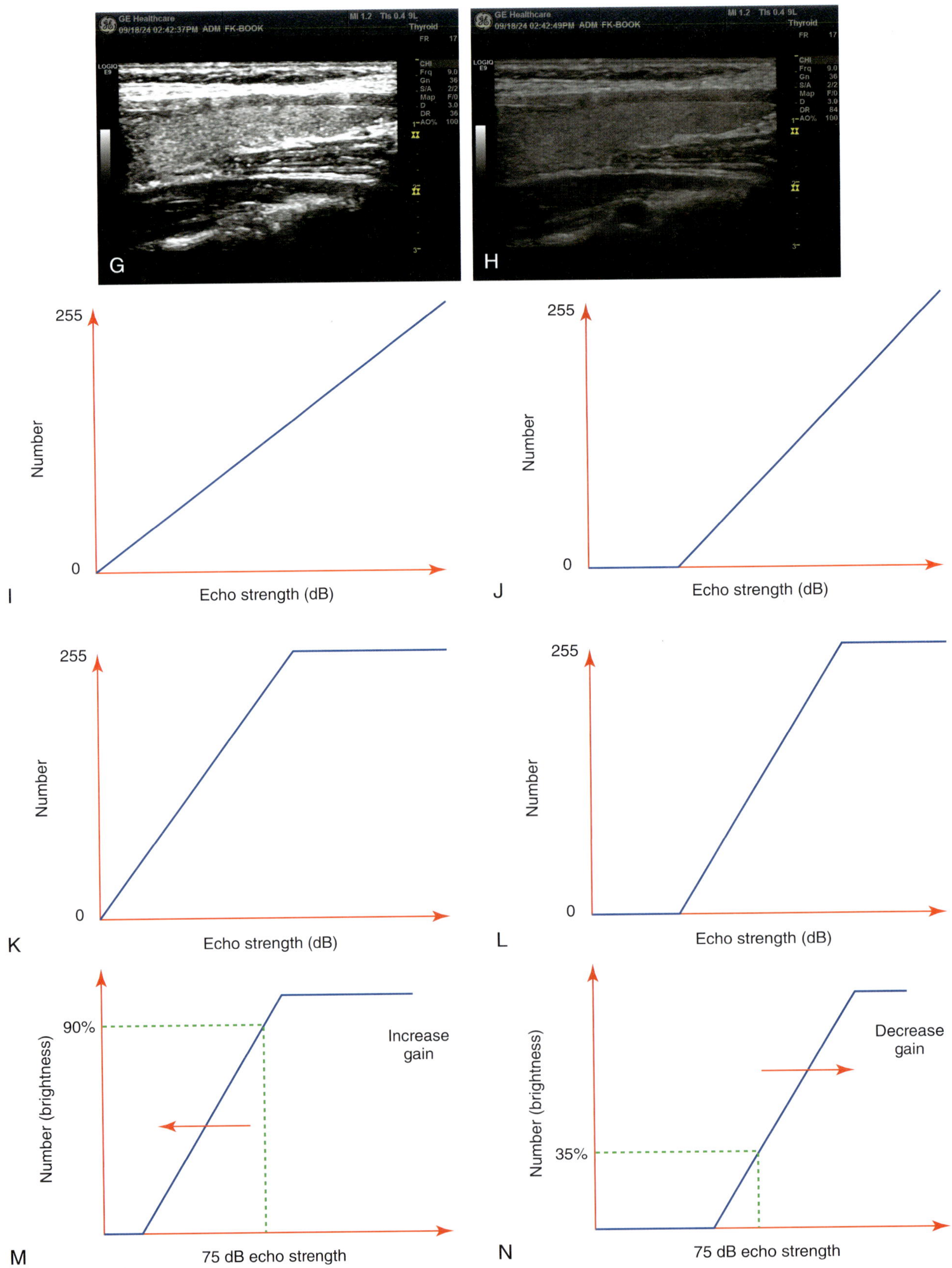

Fig. 4.17, cont'd G, Thyroid imaged with a dynamic range of 36 dB (notice how echoes tend to be either very white or very black) **(H)** and using a dynamic range of 84 dB, which produces a smoother image with more gray levels. **I,** Full system dynamic range displayed. **J,** Dynamic range reduced by setting a weaker portion to 0 (*black*). **K,** Dynamic range reduced by setting a stronger portion to maximum (*white*). **L,** Dynamic range reduced by setting weaker and stronger portions to black and white, respectively. **M,** This graph of brightness versus echo strength moves to the left as gain is increased. A midrange echo appears bright. **N,** The graph moves to the right for decreasing gain. The midrange echo appears dark.

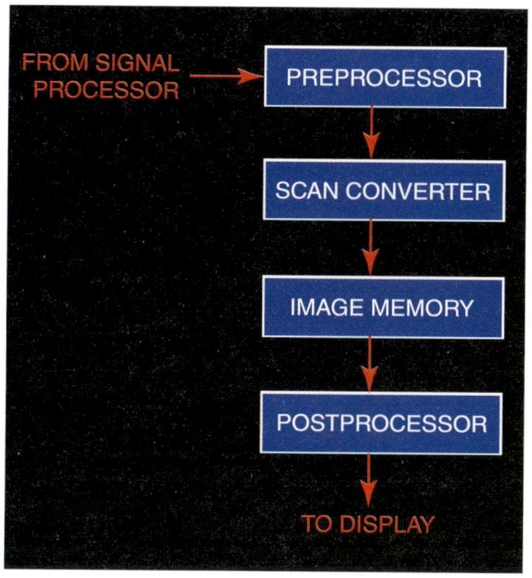

Fig. 4.18 The image processor converts scan-line data into images, processes the images before storing them in the image memory, processes them as they come out of the memory, and sends them on to the display.

lines diverge (i.e., have increasing separation) with distance from the transducer and intervening tissues are not interrogated meaning those pixels are left out. Interpolation assigns a brightness value to such a missed pixel, based on an average of the brightness of the adjacent pixels (see Fig. 4.19, C). Unlike sector scans, interpolation is not required with rectangular scans if there is a transmitted ultrasound pulse for each vertical

BOX 4.3 Functions of the Image Processor

- Preprocessing
- Persistence
- Storing image frames
- Cine loop
- Postprocessing
- Grayscale
- Color scale
- Three-dimensional data display

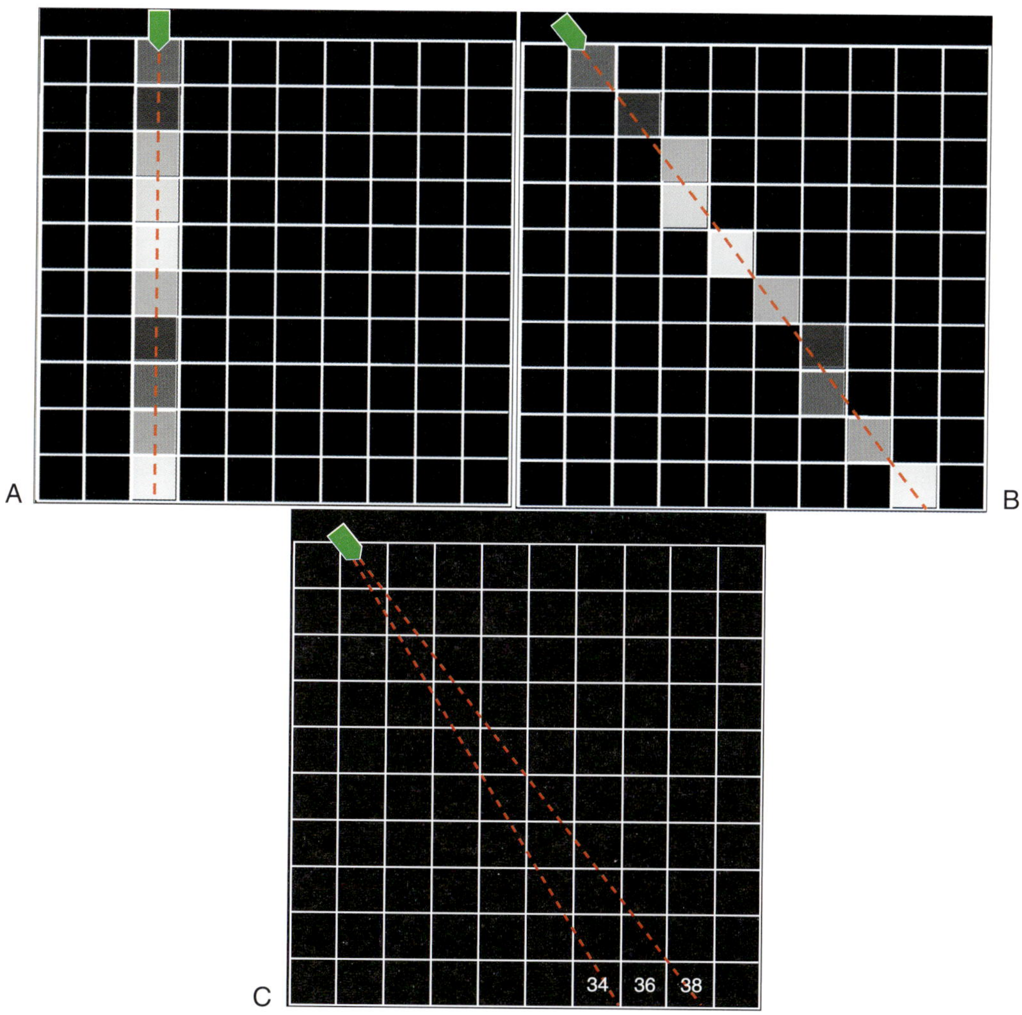

Fig. 4.19 **A,** A pulse emitted straight down into the body (*arrowhead and dashed line*) results in echoes located in a column of memory locations. **B,** A pulse emitted in another direction results in echoes located in various rows and columns. **C,** Pixel interpolation. Part of the image memory pixel grid is shown along with the paths of two pulses. At the bottom of the grid, the paths have separated sufficiently so that the pixel between them is missed. The interpolation calculation determines the mean value of the two adjacent pixels (34 and 38), which is 36. That value then is entered in the intervening pixel.

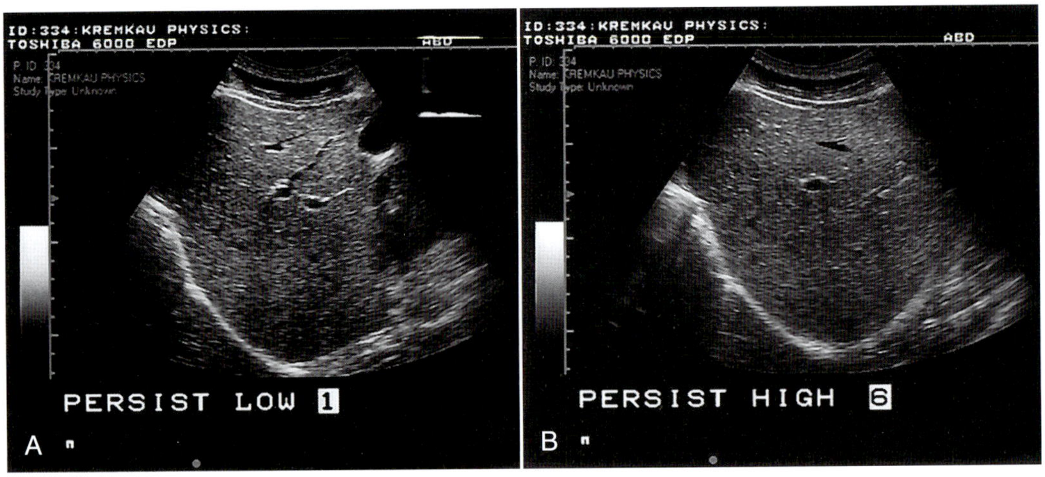

Fig. 4.20 **A,** Persistence off. **B,** Persistence on.

scan line displayed, although it may still be performed in order to improve overall image quality.

Persistence

Persistence is the averaging of sequential frames to provide a smoother image appearance and to reduce noise (Fig. 4.20). Noise, primarily speckle, is reduced because it can be considered as a random process. When several frames containing random content are averaged, the random content is reduced. Speckle reduction improves dynamic range and contrast resolution. However, frame averaging, in effect, reduces true FR, because averaged frames are no longer independent, although from the perspective of the observer if appears as if the frame rate is unchanged after the initial start of the averaging process. Operator control permits averaging of a selectable number of sequential frames from zero up to some maximum. Lower levels of persistence, or none at all, are appropriate for following rapidly moving structures. Higher levels are appropriate for slower moving structures.

> Persistence reduces noise and smooths the image by frame averaging.

Volume Imaging and Presentation

Three-dimensional imaging (3D, volume imaging) can be accomplished by acquiring many parallel two-dimensional (2D) scans (Fig. 4.21, A) and then processing this 3D volume of echo information in appropriate ways for presentation on 2D displays. The multiple 2D frames can be obtained by electronic scanning using 2D array transducers or by mechanically sweeping a regular transducer within one housing across a given arc. Common ways of presenting the 3D echo data include surface renderings, 2D slices through the 3D volume, and transparent views (see Fig. 4.21, B–G). The advantage of 2D slice presentation is that it is possible to present image-plane orientations that are impossible to obtain with conventional 2D scanning (e.g., the coronal plane at 90 degrees to the direction of pulse travel). Serial slice presentations similar to those in other imaging modes (magnetic resonance imaging and computed tomography) can be presented. Surface renderings are popular in obstetric imaging and echocardiography. Transparent views allow "see-through" imaging of the anatomy, as with plain-film radiographs. These presentation forms are postprocessing choices that present the stored 3D volume of echo information in different ways on the display.

A 3D volume image that can be acquired at rates sufficient for "live" or real-time presentations is often called *4D imaging*, in which the fourth dimension is time.

> A 3D volume of echo data can be displayed in several ways, including 2D slices, surface renderings, and transparent views.

Image Memory

After echo data are preprocessed, the image frames are stored in the image memory. Storing each image in the memory while the sound beam is scanned through the anatomy permits display of a single image (frame) out of the rapid sequence of frames acquired each second in real-time ultrasound scanners. Holding and displaying one frame out of the sequence is known as freeze. Instruments typically store a few to several hundreds of the last frames acquired before freezing (i.e., pushing the freeze button). This is called cine loop, cine review, or image review feature.

Pixels and Bits

Image memories used in ultrasound scanners are digital; that is, they are computer memories that store numbers (digits) just as digital cameras on your phone do (Fig. 4.22, A). Digital memories are discrete rather than continuous, which means that they can store only whole numbers in each pixel location. The 2D image plane is divided, similar to a checkerboard (see Fig. 4.22, B), into squares called *pixels* (picture elements), in a rectangular matrix, for example, 1024 × 768, 1920 × 1200 or 3840 × 2160. The pixels number hundreds of thousands to millions (786,432, 2,304,000, and 8,294,400 in the previous examples), so they are tiny and not noticeable unless magnified sufficiently. A number that corresponds to the echo strength received from the location

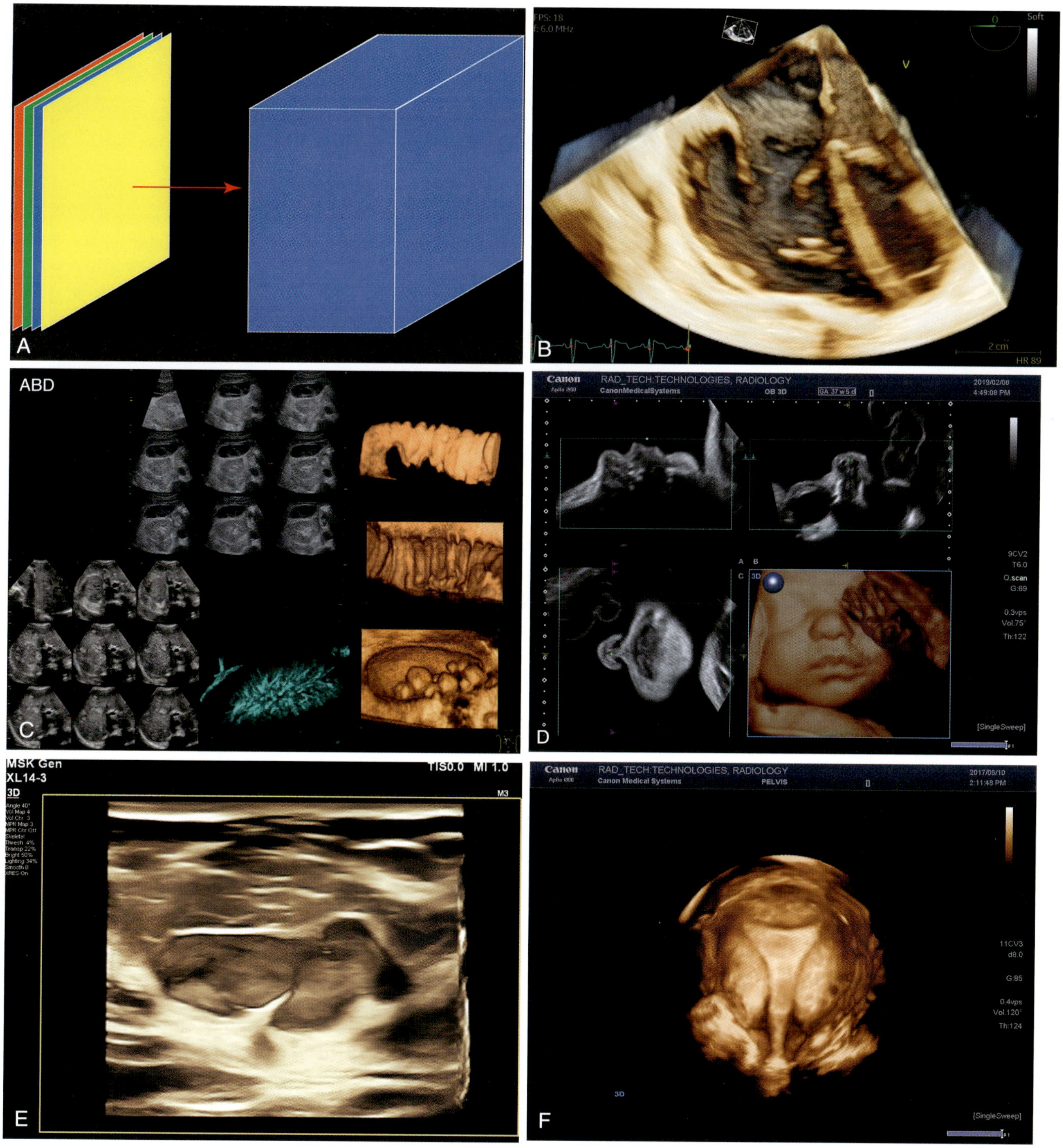

Fig. 4.21 Various presentations of three-dimensional images. **A,** Three-dimensional echo data are acquired by obtaining many parallel two-dimensional sections of echo information from the imaged anatomy yielding various postprocessing choices for presenting three-dimensional images. **B,** Cardiac image. **C,** Volume imaging of the abdomen. **D,** Fetal imaging. **E,** A breast cyst. **F,** pelvic 3D.

within the anatomy corresponding to that memory position (see Fig. 4.22, C) is stored in each of the pixel locations in the memory. The more pixels there are, the finer the spatial detail in the stored image (see Fig. 4.22, D–G).

If the digital memory were composed of a single-layer matrix checkerboard, each pixel location could store only one of two numbers: a zero or a one. The reason is that the memory element assigned to each pixel is binary, similar to an on-off switch, and thus can operate only in two conditions corresponding to one or zero. This would allow only **bistable** (black-and-white) imaging (see Fig. 4.23, A–B). To produce a **grayscale** image (hundreds of shades of gray or brightness, in addition to black and white),

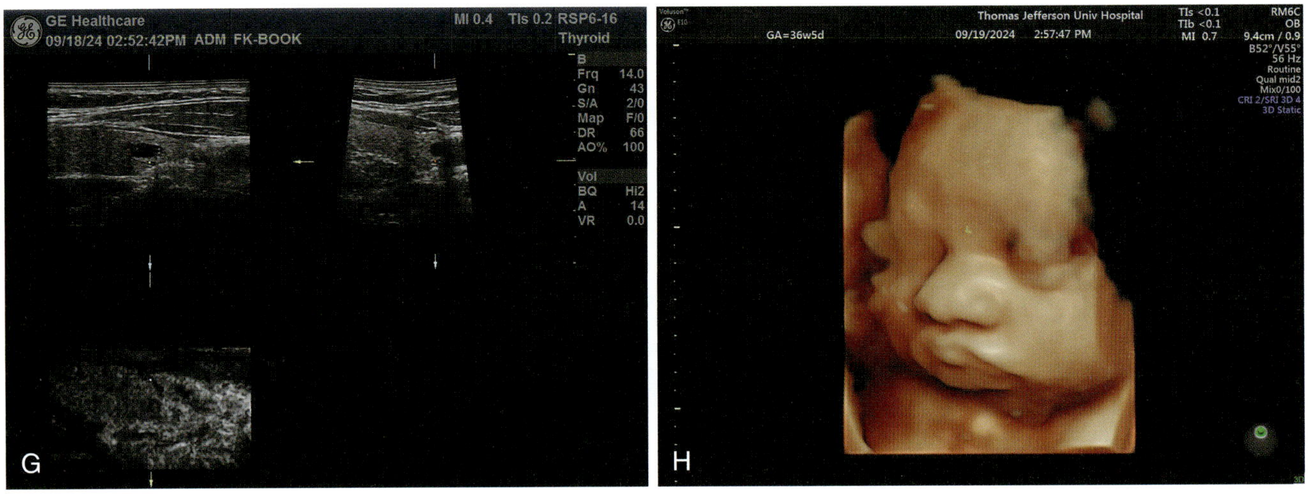

Fig. 4.21, cont'd **G,** Cyst in the thyroid. **H,** Fetal head. (**B,** Courtesy GE HealthCare. **D and F,** Courtesy Canon Medical Systems USA. **E,** Courtesy Philips Medical Systems. **H,** Courtesy Corinne DeStefano and Vincenzo Berghella, Thomas Jefferson University Hospital.)

storage of one of a multitude of possible numbers in each memory location is necessary. This requires the memory to have more than one matrix. These "checkerboards" can be thought of as being layered back to back. In a four-binary-digit memory, there are four checkerboards back to back (see Fig. 4.23, C) so that each pixel has 4 **bits** (binary digits) associated with it. In the binary numbering system, this allows numbers from 0 to 15 to be stored (a 16 shade system). Thus a 4 bit memory is a 16 shade memory. A 4 bit memory has four binary digits assigned to each pixel, that is, four layers of memory.

> The memory divides the image into pixels, such as a matrix of 1920 × 1200.

Binary Numbers

Because the memory elements are binary, digital memories use the binary numbering system to store echo information in the image memory. Computer memories and processors use binary numbers to carry out their functions, because they contain electronic components (switches) that operate in only two states, representing the numbers 0 and 1.

Binary digits (bits) consist of only zeros and ones, represented by their respective numeric symbols, 0 and 1. Other values must be represented by moving these symbols to different positions (columns). In the decimal system, in which there are 10 different symbols, 0 through 9, there is no single symbol for the number 10 (9 is the largest number for which there is a single symbol). To represent 10 in symbolic form, the symbol for 1 is used, but it is moved to the left, to the second column. A 0 is placed in the right column to clarify this, resulting in the symbol 10. The same symbol used to represent 1 is used, but in such a way that it no longer represents one, but rather 10 (i.e., the second column represents 10 to the power of 1 which is 10, and the third column will represent 10 to the second power or 100).

A similar procedure is used in the binary numbering system. The symbol 1 represents the largest number (1) for which there is a symbol in this system. To represent the next number (2), the same thing is done as in the decimal system; that is, the symbol 1 is placed in the next column to represent the 2 to the power of 1 which is 2. In this case, a 1 in the second column represents a value of 2 rather than 10, as in the decimal system. Columns in the two systems represent values as shown in Fig. 4.23, B–D. In the decimal system, each column represents 10 times the column to its right (10^0, 10^1, 10^2, 10^3, … or 1, 10, 100, 1000, …). In the binary system, each column represents 2 times the column to its right (so 2^0, 2^1, 2^2, 2^3, … or 1, 2, 4, 8 …).

Table 4.2 lists the binary forms of the decimal numbers 0 to 63. Numbers 64 to 127 would have one additional digit (representing the "sixty-fours" column or 2^6) and so forth with higher multiples of 2.

> Binary numbers use only the digits 0 and 1. Each column of a binary number represents double the column to its right.

Table 4.3 provides several examples of digital memories, where the discrete numbers that can be stored in the memory range from zero to the maximum determined by the number of bits per pixel. Fig. 4.23, C shows a 4 bit (per pixel) memory. Table 4.4 gives the total number of memory elements in various digital memories. A group of 8 bits is called a *byte*, and 1024 bytes (8192 bits) are called a *kilobyte*. In today's ultrasound instruments, 8, 12, and (at most) 16 bit memories are present.

Postprocessing

Signal processing and image processing performed before storage of the echo information in the image memory are called *preprocessing*. In general, preprocessing includes all that is done to echoes before they are stored in the memory (Fig. 4.24). Image processing that is accomplished after the echoes are stored in the memory is called *postprocessing*. In general, postprocessing includes all of the procedures performed with echoes while they

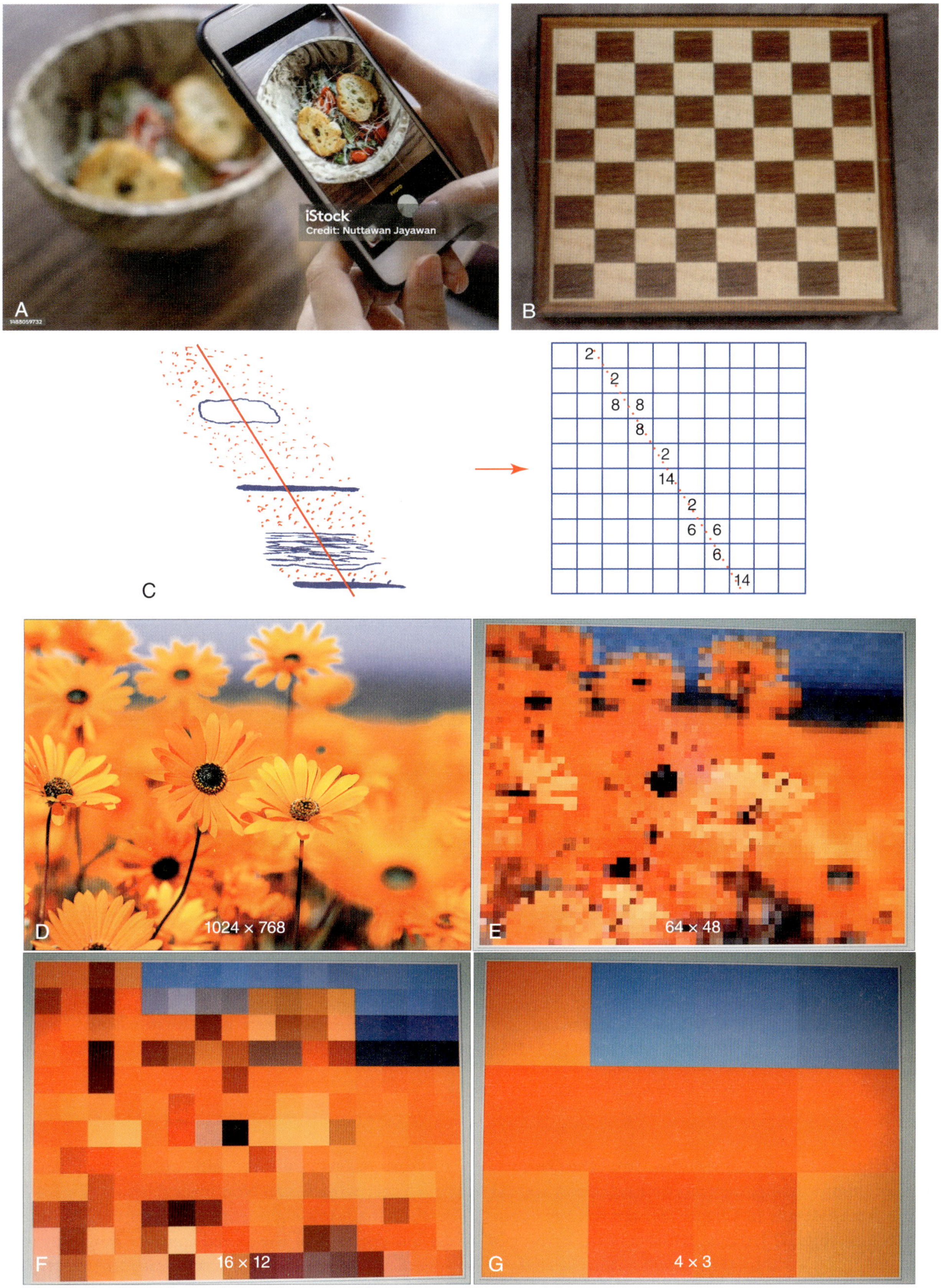

Fig. 4.22 **A,** Digital camera in a phone. **B,** A chessboard or checkerboard is divided into eight rows and eight columns of squares, for a total of 64 "pixels." **C,** Anatomic cross-section to be scanned, and the front view of a portion of the image memory. Numbers are stored in the memory elements according to the intensity of the echoes received from corresponding anatomic locations as an ultrasound pulse passes through them. **D–G,** Digital photos at pixel resolutions of 1024 × 768, 64 × 48, 16 × 12, and 4 × 3, respectively.

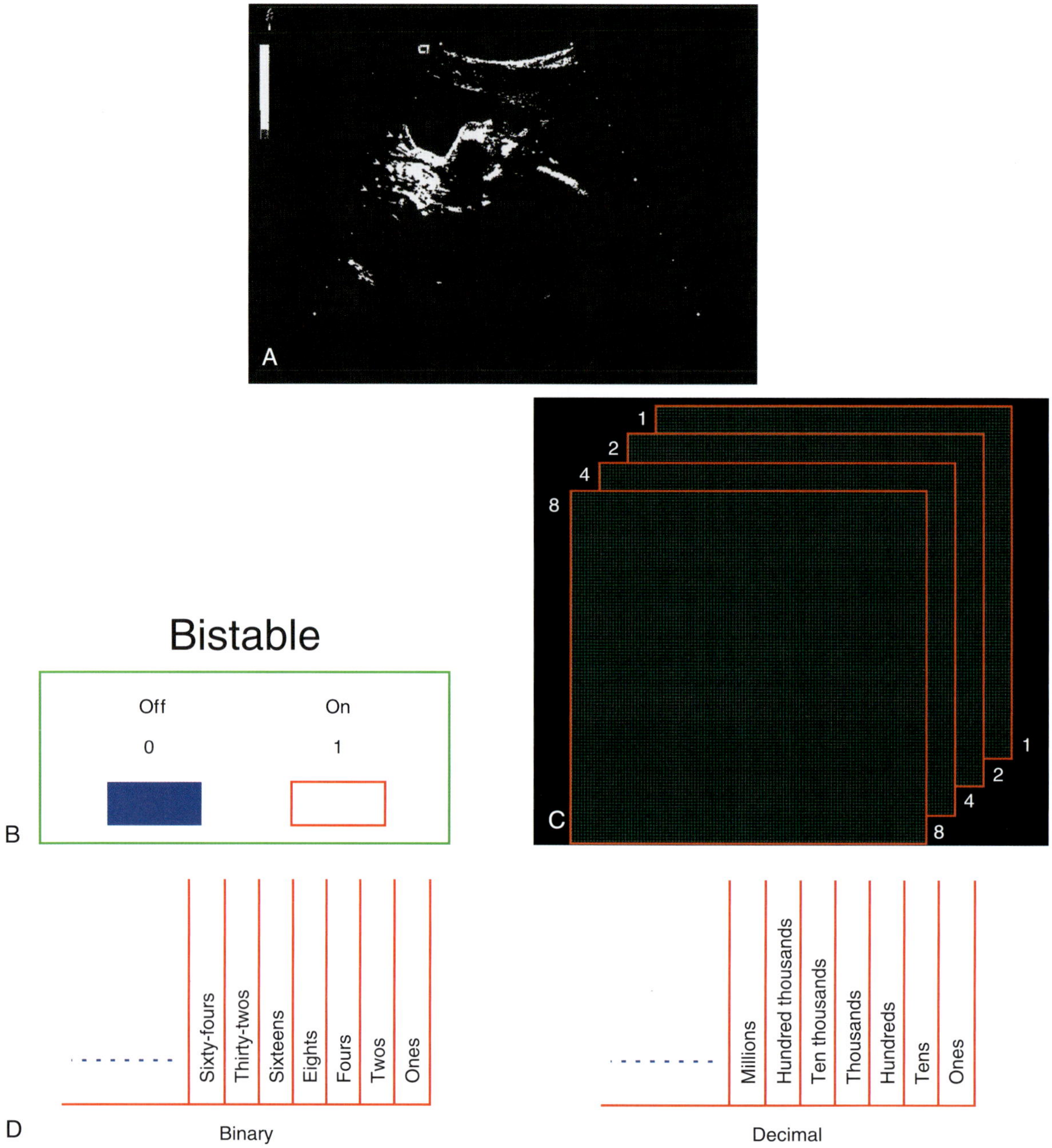

Fig. 4.23 **A,** Bistable image of fetal head and neck. **B,** In bistable imaging, only two values are used: memory element off represents 0 and is presented as black; memory element on represents 1 and is presented as white. **C,** A 10 × 10-pixel, 4-bit-deep (4 bits per pixel) digital memory. **D,** Columns in decimal numbers represent multiples of 10, whereas those in binary numbers represent multiples of 2.

are brought out of the memory to be displayed. Read magnification is an example. **Postprocessing** is the assignment of specific display brightness to numbers retrieved from the memory. Some aspects of preprocessing, such as persistence and **spatial compounding** (more details in Chapter 6), are operator controllable. Postprocessing is partially an operator-controllable process.

> Postprocessing is image processing performed on image data retrieved from the memory. Postprocessing determines how echo data stored in the memory will appear on the display.

Preprogrammed postprocessing brightness assignment schemes are typically selectable by the operator. The specific curve is always nonlinear with only a small range of brightness levels being linear. Nonlinear schemes (Figs. 4.25 and 4.26, A–B) that allow assignment of more of the brightness range to certain portions of the stored number range capability of the system are always used in clinical practice. This can improve the presentation and perception of small echo strength differences stored in the memory (improved contrast resolution, discussed later).

Many ultrasound instruments have the postprocessing ability to present echo intensities in different colors rather than in

TABLE 4.2 Binary and Decimal Number Equivalents

Decimal	Binary	Decimal	Binary
0	000000	32	100000
1	000001	33	100001
2	000010	34	100010
3	000011	35	100011
4	000100	36	100100
5	000101	37	100101
6	000110	38	100110
7	000111	39	100111
8	001000	40	101000
9	001001	41	101001
10	001010	42	101010
11	001011	43	101011
12	001100	44	101100
13	001101	45	101101
14	001110	46	101110
15	001111	47	101111
16	010000	48	110000
17	010001	49	110001
18	010010	50	110010
19	010011	51	110011
20	010100	52	110100
21	010101	53	110101
22	010110	54	110110
23	010111	55	110111
24	011000	56	111000
25	011001	57	111001
26	011010	58	111010
27	011011	59	111011
28	011100	60	111100
29	011101	61	111101
30	011110	62	111110
31	011111	63	111111

gray levels, that is, the ability to colorize echoes. In theory, the eye can differentiate more color tints than gray shades, which should mean color displays offer improved contrast resolution capability (discussed later). This process is called **B color** or *colorscale* (compared with grayscale). A color bar is included in such displays to show how colors are assigned to various echo levels. Fig. 4.26, C–E provides some examples. In practice, this is not an option that is used very often.

B color is a form of postprocessing that assigns colors, rather than gray level, to different echo strengths.

In summary, the procedure for moving the echo information required for display of the 2D cross-sectional image into a digital memory is as follows:

- The beam is scanned through the patient in such a way that it illuminates (or rather when it is a sound wave *insonifies*) the tissue cross-section being imaged.
- Echoes received from all points on this cross-section are converted to numbers (digitized) that are stored at corresponding pixel locations in the digital memory.
- All the information necessary for displaying this cross-sectional image now is stored in the memory.
- The information then can be taken out of the memory and presented on a 2D display in such a way that the numbers coming out of the memory are displayed as corresponding pixel brightness on the face of the display (Fig. 4.27).

Fig. 4.28 shows examples of such presentations. To enlarge the pixels, read magnification (sometimes called *zoom*) is used. In this presentation, rather than showing all the pixels in the memory, the display shows a smaller group of pixels in expanded (magnified) fashion. This increases pixel size, making the pixel composition of the image more obvious. Read zoom is a postprocessing function. Write magnification is also available on some systems. This allows a smaller anatomic field of view to be written into the entire memory, thereby enlarging the image without enlarging the pixel size (Fig. 4.29). Write zoom is a preprocessing function.

TABLE 4.3 Characteristics of Digital Memories

	LOWEST NUMBER STORED		HIGHEST NUMBER STORED		
Bits per Pixel	Decimal	Binary	Decimal	Binary	Number of Shades
8	0	00000000	255	11111111	256
12	0	000000000000	4095	111111111111	4096
16	0	0000000000000000	65,535	1111111111111111	65,536

TABLE 4.4 Bits (Binary Digits or Memory Elements) in Digital Memories With 1920 × 1200 (2,304,000) Pixels

Bits per Pixel	Total Bits	Total Kilobytes[a]
8	18,432,000	2250
12	27,648,000	3375
16	36,864,000	4500

[a]1 byte = 8 bits; 1 kilobyte = 1024 bytes, or 8192 bits.

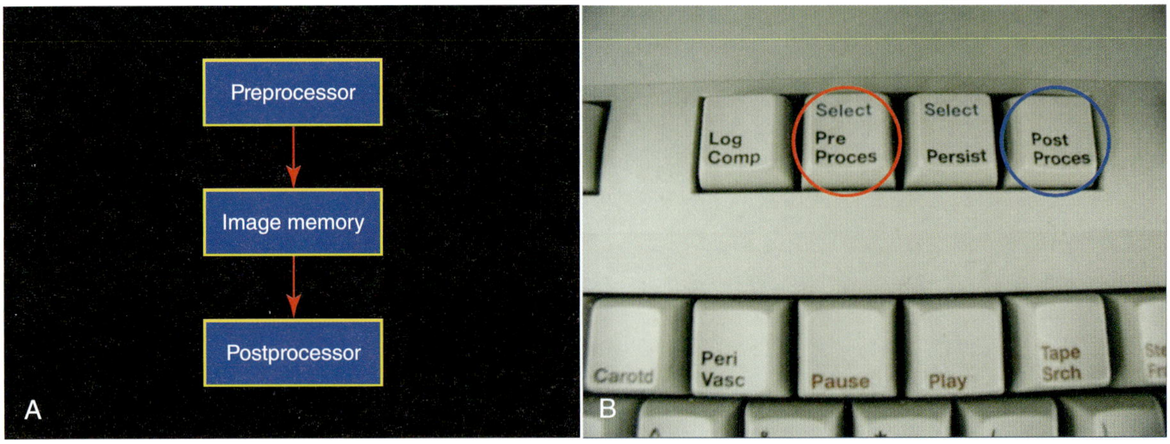

Fig. 4.24 **A,** Preprocessing (*red circle* in **B**) includes operations performed on echoes before storage in memory. **B,** Postprocessing (*blue circle*) includes operations performed after information is stored in memory.

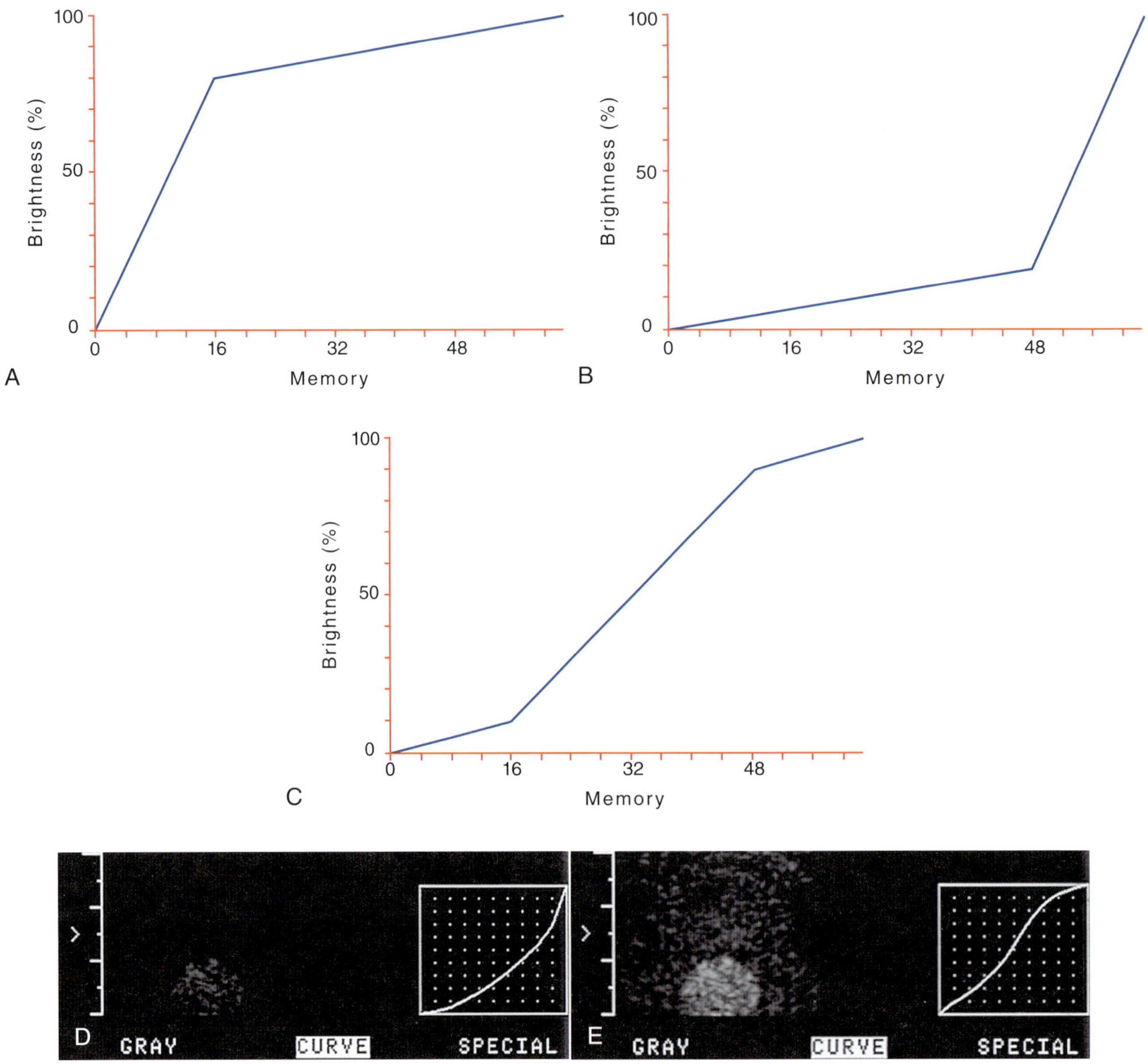

Fig. 4.25 Nonlinear postprocessing assignment schemes. A large brightness range is reserved for weak **(A),** strong **(B),** and intermediate-strength **(C)** echoes. Each area has improved contrast resolution (discussed later) at the expense of poorer contrast resolution in the remainder of the dynamic range. **D,** A display using a postprocessing curve similar to that in **B**. **E,** A display using a postprocessing curve similar to that in **C**.

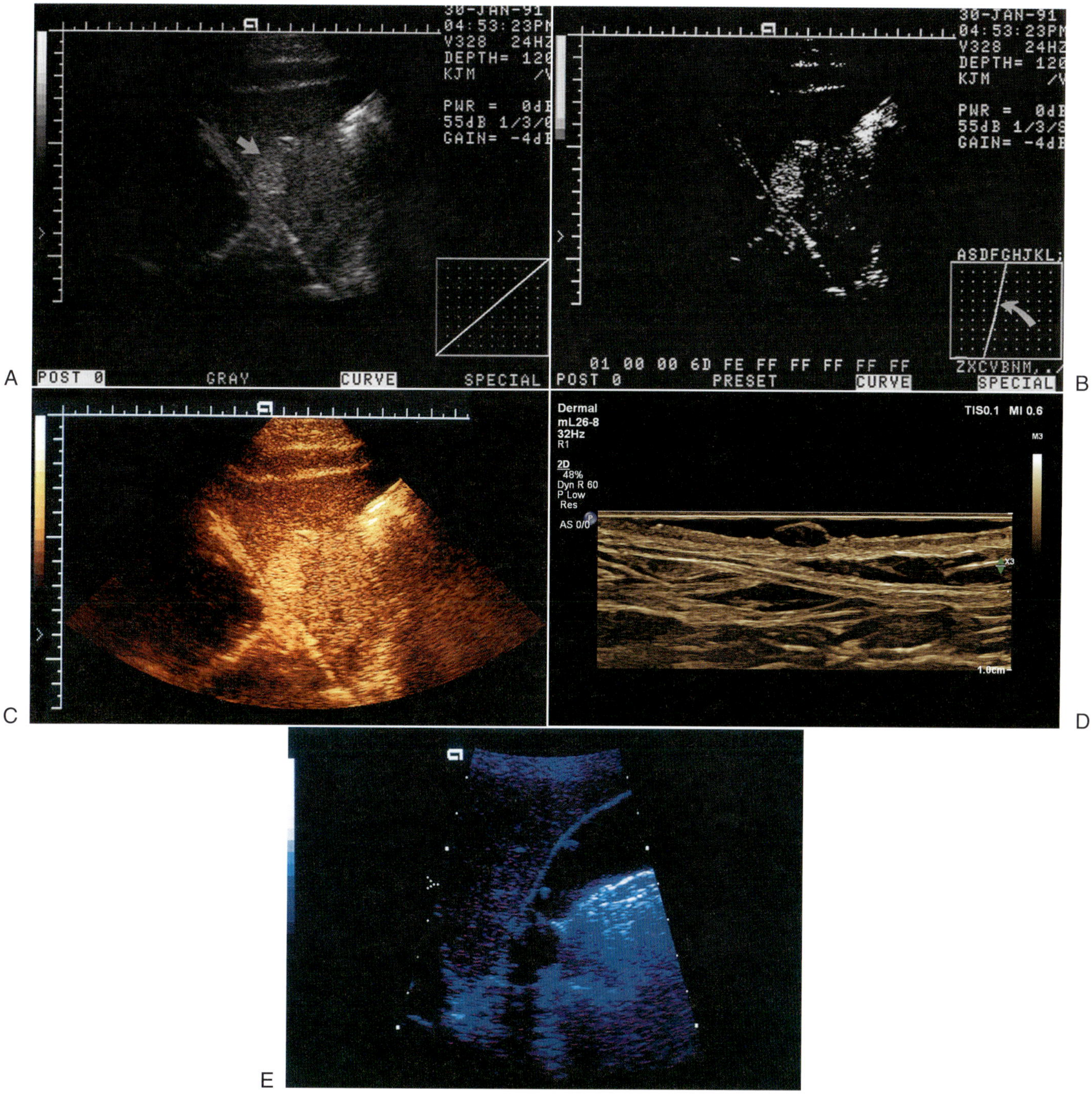

Fig. 4.26 **A,** An image of a hemangioma (*arrow*) obtained by using linear postprocessing. **B,** An image of a hemangioma with a steep postprocessing assignment (*curved arrow*) designed to produce a great contrast between these normal and abnormal tissue echoes. **C,** Color display of a hemangioma (compare with **A** and **B**), dermal lesion **(D)**, and gallbladder **(E)**. Color assignments are shown in the color bars on the side.

For a 1024 × 2048 matrix in which the represented anatomic width and depth are 10 and 20 cm, respectively, each pixel represents an anatomic dimension of 0.1 mm. This represents the spatial (detail) resolution of the memory matrix. If the width and depth are 5 and 10 cm, then the memory spatial resolution is 0.05 mm. However, the actual detail resolution of an ultrasound image is limited by spatial pulse length and beam width rather than by pixel density in the memory.

Finally, although in this overview, we have recognized memory only as image memory in the image processor, different ultrasound scanners may store echo information at various points along the processing chain, including storing RF echo data before amplitude detection. We have simplified the discussion by dealing with memory only as image memory in the image processor.

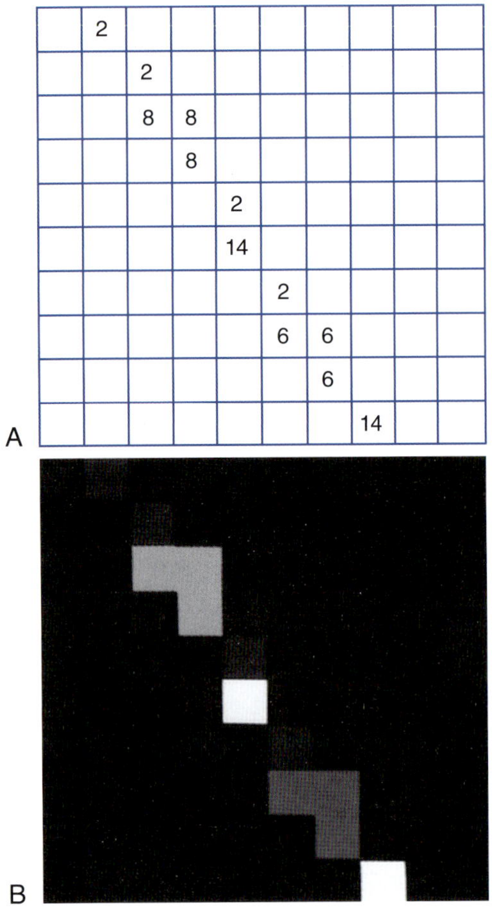

Fig. 4.27 For display of scanned anatomic structures, numbers are read out of pixel locations in digital memory **(A)** and applied to the display in such a way that pixel brightness corresponds to those stored numbers **(B)**. The display for the scan line acquired in Fig. 4.22, C is shown.

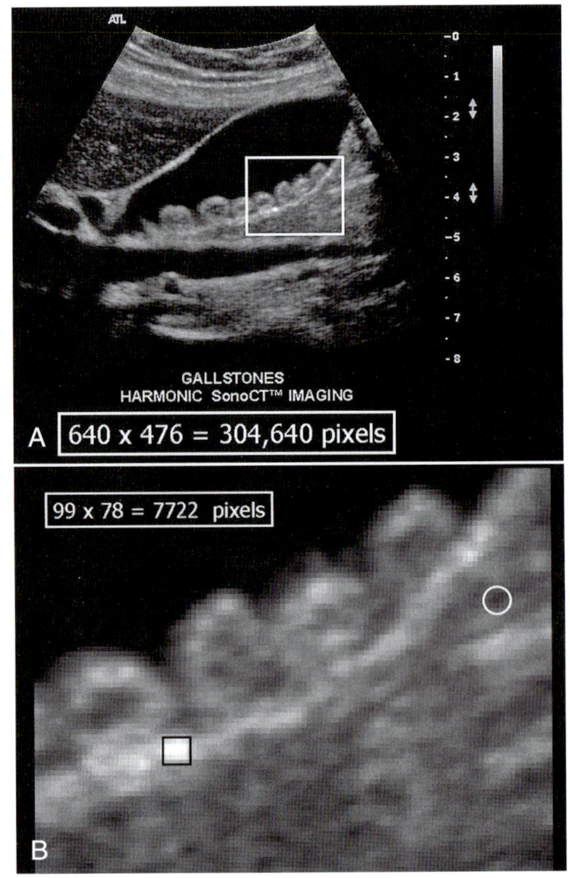

Fig. 4.28 Displays of pixels of various brightnesses representing various numbers in the corresponding memory locations. The display is magnified (*zoom*) here to make the square pixels more easily discernible. Normally, the pixels are too small and numerous to be seen individually. **A,** Unmagnified abdominal image containing 304,640 unresolved pixels. The box encloses the region magnified in **B.** Magnification reveals the 7722 pixels included within the box in **A.** The circle and the box enclose regions of small and large numbers (weak and strong echoes, respectively) in the image memory, respectively.

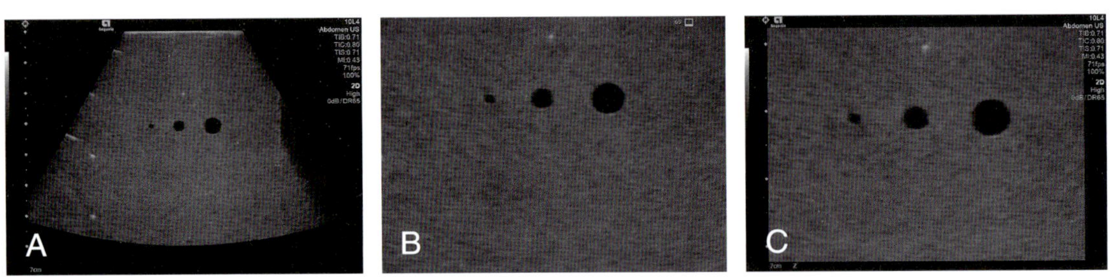

Fig. 4.29 Write and read zoom or magnification. **A,** A scan of a phantom without write magnification. **B,** A scan using write magnification. Included are 2, 4, and 6 mm simulated cysts. **C,** Read magnification, or zoom, magnifies the stored pixels; albeit mot nearly to the degree encountered a decade or more ago.

DISPLAY

The image memory is filled with echoes from many pulses as the beam is scanned through the anatomy to be imaged. The brightness (grayscale) displayed is proportional to the echo strength. The 2D grayscale scan is a brightness image that represents an anatomical cross-section in the scan plane. Each individual image is called a *frame.* Acquiring and presenting many frames (from tens to hundreds of frames) every second is called *real-time display.* A group of 2D scans can also be acquired to form a 3D volume of stored echo information.

Frame rate is the number of 2D ultrasound images (or 3D volumes) entered into the image memory per second, whereas **refresh rate** is the number of times per second that images are retrieved from the memory and presented on the display. These two rates can be but are not necessarily, equal.

The information delivered to the display can be presented in several ways. Common to all clinical applications is the brightness mode, also called **B mode**, **B scan**, or *grayscale imaging.* Grayscale anatomical displays can be in 2D or 3D forms. In echocardiography, motion mode (**M mode**) is also

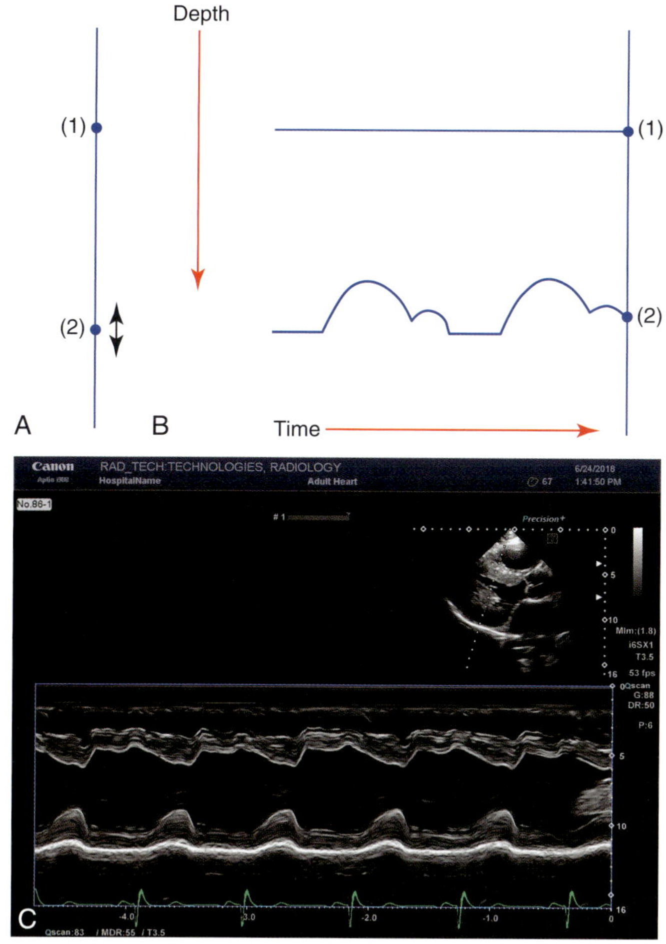

Fig. 4.30 **A,** B mode presentation of echo depth with echoes from both a stationary structure (*1*) and a moving one (*2*). **B,** If pulses are sent down the same path repeatedly, and vertical scan lines are placed next to each other, a display of depth versus time results. The pattern of motion of moving structures (*2*) is traced out on the display for evaluation. This is called *M mode display*. **C,** M mode presentation of moving cardiac structures. Depth is the vertical axis while, time increases to the right. The two-dimensional real-time anatomic cross-sectional image also is shown (*upper right*). The *dotted line* in the anatomical image indicates the repeating path of the ultrasound pulses used to generate the M mode display.

used (Fig. 4.30). M mode is a display form that presents depth (vertical axis) versus time (horizontal). An uncommon display (except in ophthalmology) shows the amplitudes of echoes and is called the **A mode** (Fig. 4.31). A mode is a depth versus amplitude display. The sound beam is stationary in both these presentations. Ultrasound pulses travel down the same path over and over. In the M mode display, the vertical scan lines are written next to each other across the horizontal time axis.

Flat-Panel Display

Ultrasound images are presented on computer displays because they represent the digital information stored in the image (computer) memory. Computer displays present image information in the form of horizontal lines (Fig. 4.32, A). Each horizontal display scan line corresponds to a row of digital data in the image memory. The information is read out of the memory, row by row (much as we read a page of text), and is written on the display, line by line, similar to writing on a lined sheet of paper. Because the display includes more than the actual image (such as alphanumeric data, icons, or a Doppler spectral display), the data in the memory vary. Nonetheless, whatever is stored in a given pixel in the memory (whether it is part of a grayscale image, part of a letter, or anything else) will appear at the corresponding pixel location on the display with the appropriate brightness and color (to allow for color Doppler images, etc.). Color displays are the *de facto* standard for ultrasound scanners.

> The display is a flat-panel display that presents an image in horizontal lines from top to bottom.

Flat-panel displays are used on computers, television sets, and ultrasound systems (see Fig. 4.32, B–C). A computer monitor is a digital display that presents data retrieved from the memory in a 2D pixel matrix according to some audio/video standard (typically using high-definition multimedia interface) and refreshing the display often (e.g., 60 times per second). A **flat-panel display** is a backlighted liquid crystal display (LCD) or a matrix of light-emitting diodes (LEDs). Such a display is composed of a rectangular matrix of thousands of digital LCD or LED elements (e.g., a 1920 × 1200 matrix contains 2,304,000 elements). These elements can be turned on or off individually and act as tiny light valves for blocking or passing the light from the light source behind the matrix. More specifically, the elements can be turned on partially to allow a measured amount of light through, usually in 256 steps of luminance, that is, 256 displayed gray levels from black to white.

Groups of red, green, and blue (RGB) elements allow what is called *24 bit color* (8 bits or 256 luminance values for each primary color element) yielding 16,777,216 possible colors presented at each pixel location. RGB are known as *primary additive colors*, because various combinations can produce nearly any color desired. For example, red and green, mixed equally, produce yellow. Green and blue produce *cyan*, the technical term for aqua. Red and blue produce magenta. RGB, equally mixed, produce white (or gray, depending on brightness).

CONTRAST AND TEMPORAL RESOLUTIONS

Contrast Resolution

For linear assignment of echo intensities to numbers in the memory, the echo dynamic range is equally divided throughout the gray levels of the system. Table 4.5 gives, for 4 to 8 bit systems, the number of decibels of dynamic range covered by each shade (for two different echo dynamic range values, 40 and 60 dB, after attenuation compensation) and the average intensity difference between two echoes required for assignment to different numbers (different shades) in the memory. This relates to contrast resolution, which is the ability to visualize subtle echo strength differences between adjacent tissues. An increase in the number of bits per pixel (more grayscale levels) improves contrast resolution. For a 4 bit, 40 dB dynamic range system, an echo must have nearly twice the intensity of another for it to be assigned a different level of gray. With a 60 dB dynamic range, more than twice the intensity would be required. For an 8 bit, 40 dB system, only a 3.8% difference is required, while a 12 bit, 60 dB system, a 0.2% difference is sufficient. Table 4.5 and Fig. 4.33 show how a greater number of shades or a reduced dynamic range improve contrast resolution.

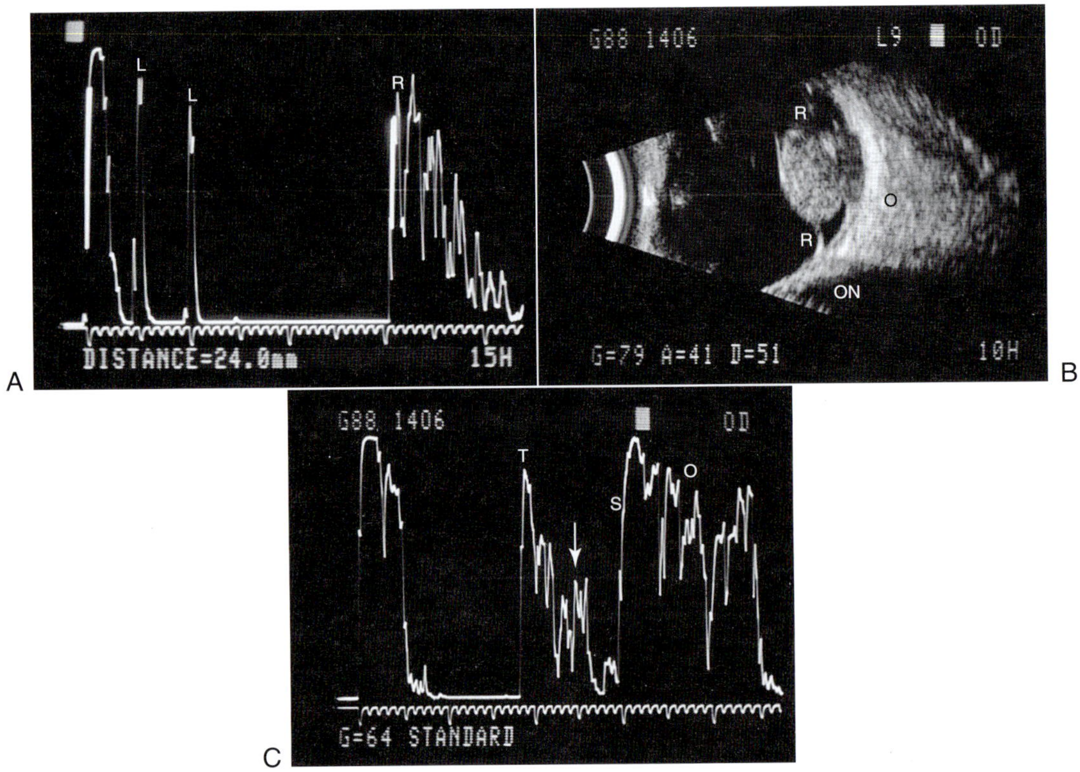

Fig. 4.31 A, A normal ophthalmologic A mode presentation, where *L* represents lens echoes and *R* represents the retina. A longitudinal B scan **(B)** and standardized A mode presentation **(C)** demonstrate the typical acoustic appearance of a choroidal melanoma. The B scan shows a mushroom-shaped mass with exudative retinal detachment (*R*) at the tumor margins. The A mode scan demonstrates a high spike from the tumor surface (*T*) and low to medium echogenicity within the lesion (*arrow*). In this figure, the horizontal axis represents depth. *O*, Orbital fat; *ON*, optic nerve; *S*, sclera.

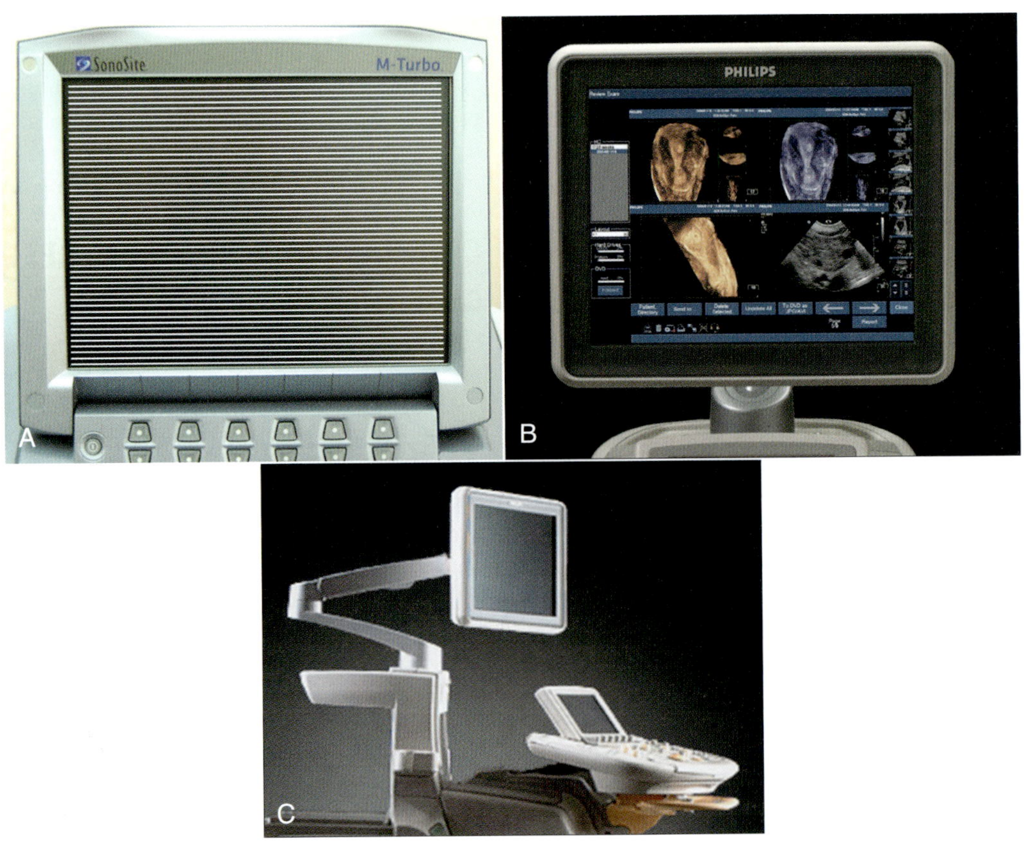

Fig. 4.32 A, An image on a display is scanned from left to right, top to bottom in horizontal lines, each corresponding to a row of echo-amplitude numbers in image memory. **B–C,** Flat-panel displays.

TABLE 4.5 Contrast Resolution of Digital Memories

	40 dB DYNAMIC RANGE		60 dB DYNAMIC RANGE	
Bits per Pixel	**Decibels per Shade[a]**	**Intensity Difference (%)[b]**	**Decibels per Shade[a]**	**Intensity Difference (%)[b]**
4	2.50	77.8	3.75	137.1
8	0.16	3.8	0.23	5.4
12	0.01	0.2	0.01	0.2

[a]Contrast resolution (dB per shade) = dynamic range/number of shades (e.g., 16 shades for 4 bits/pixel).
[b]The average difference required between two echoes for the echoes to be assigned different shades.

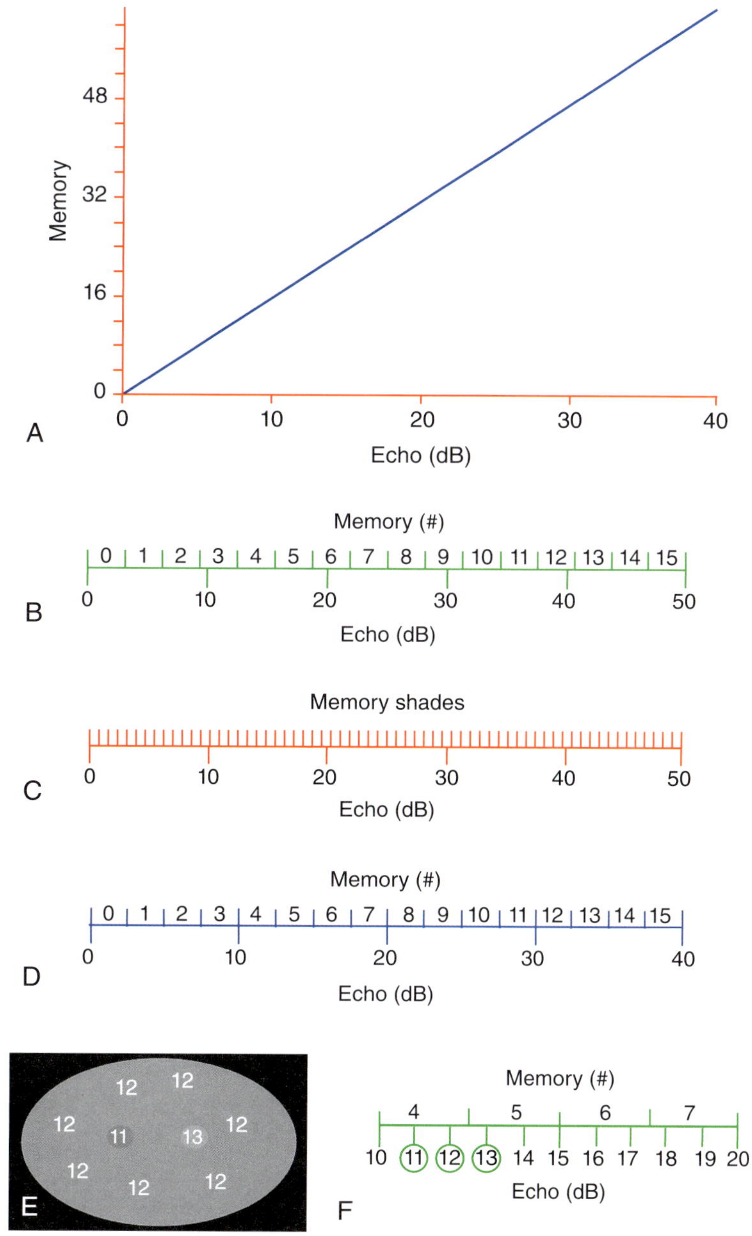

Fig. 4.33 **A,** Assignment of numbers (to be stored in the memory) to echo intensities. Echo intensity is expressed in decibels in the form of a straight-line assignment (relative to the weakest echo, which is represented as 0 dB; the strongest echo is 40 dB, which is 10,000 times the intensity of the weakest). An instrument dynamic range of 40 dB and a 6-bit (64-shade) memory are assumed. **B,** With a 4 bit memory, a 50 dB dynamic range is divided into 16 regions (shades). **C,** With a 6 bit memory, a 50 dB dynamic range is divided into 64 regions, which are numbered 0–63. **D,** With a 4 bit memory, a 40 dB dynamic range is divided into 16 regions. **E,** Liver echoes are 12 dB in strength on the dynamic range scale, whereas two metastatic regions have strengths 11 and 13 dB, respectively. These regions should be displayed slightly darker and lighter as shown. **F,** The 10 to 20 dB dynamic range portion of **D** is expanded. If normal liver echoes were 12 dB (assigned 4 in the memory) and metastases were 13 dB (slightly hyperechoic; assigned 5), the normal and abnormal would be different in the memory and would appear with different brightnesses on the display. If the metastases were 11 dB (slightly hypoechoic), they would be assigned 4 in the memory, just as would the normal echoes, and the difference would be lost (identical displayed brightnesses).

Continued

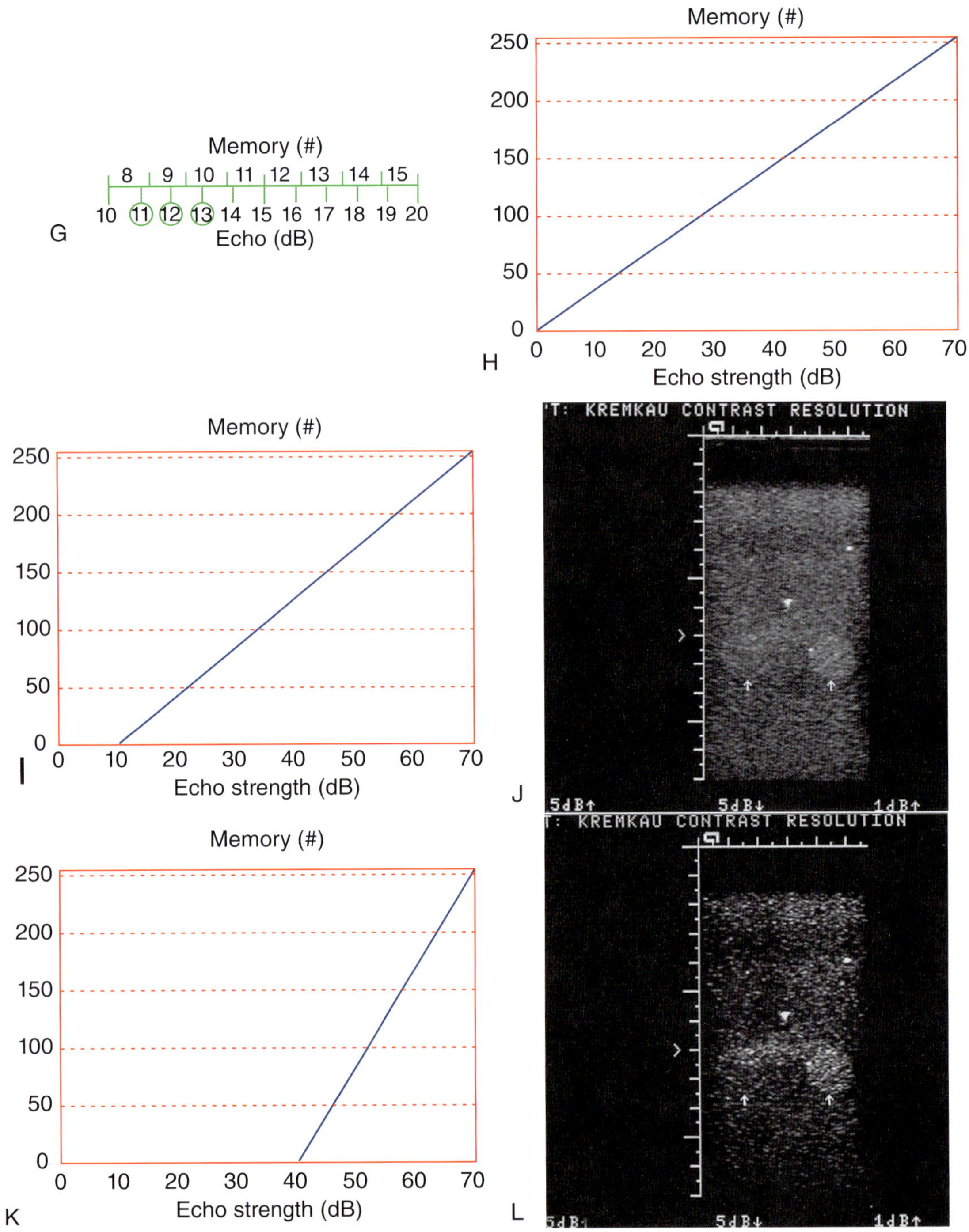

Fig. 4.33, cont'd G, With a 5 bit (32 shade) memory, both metastatic regions in **E** would be assigned numbers different from those for normal liver and different from each other; that is, contrast resolution would be maintained for both. A dynamic range or compression (preprocessing) control reassigns echo intensities in memory, with the weaker portion as zeros and the remainder in linear fashion. With an 8-bit memory, the compression control is set at maximum (70 dB; **H**), 60 dB **(I–J),** and 30 dB **(K–L)**. With decreasing dynamic range, more of the weaker portion is assigned to zero in memory (black on the display), and the contrast of the remainder (displayed) is enhanced with improved contrast resolution.

> Contrast resolution is the ability of a grayscale display to distinguish between echoes of slightly different intensities. Contrast resolution depends on the number of bits per pixel in the image memory and the dynamic range selected for the monitor.

The importance of contrast resolution is demonstrated in Fig. 4.34 showing examples of HCC in the liver, which can be slightly more or less echogenic (i.e., hyperechoic or hypoechoic) than the surrounding (normal) liver tissue. The smaller the difference in echogenicity, the more difficult it is to visualize the masses. One way to improve contrast resolution would be to scan with an ultrasound system with more bits per pixel (i.e., more shades of gray), since this increases the possibility that the echoes from the metastases would populate the image memory with different numbers than those for the surrounding liver. This is, obviously, not a very practical strategy to employ in clinical practice.

However, if a linear postprocessing assignment is used, small number differences in the memory may not be observable in the display. For example, in Fig. 4.34, D, if normal and abnormal tissue echoes differed by one digit in the memory (e.g., normal = 40 and abnormal = 41), there would only be a 0.4% difference in brightness. Alternatively, the postprocessing compression curve shown in Fig. 4.34, E, in which more grayscale values are assigned to the weaker echoes, would create a 1.2% difference in grayscale brightness between the two tissues. This improvement in contrast resolution for weaker echoes (because

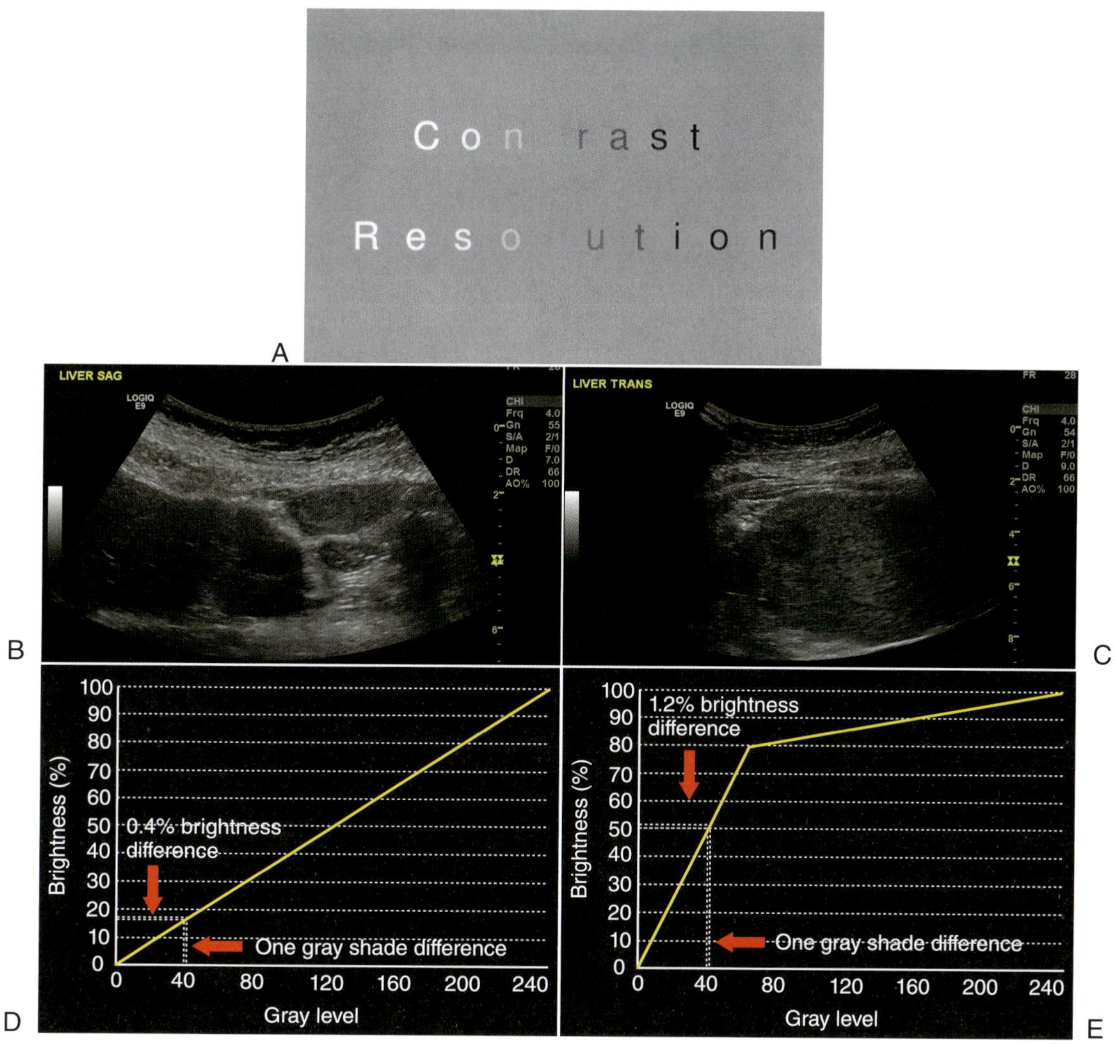

Fig. 4.34 A, Contrast resolution is the ability of a gray scale display to distinguish between echoes of slightly different amplitudes or intensities. **B,** Hepatocellular carcinoma (HCC) in a liver that is less echogenic (and therefore darker) than the surrounding liver tissue. **C,** HCC in a liver that is not as easily visualized as in **B,** because it is only slightly hypoechoic compared to the normal liver. Two tissue regions with slightly different echogenicities require good contrast resolution to be observed with different brightnesses. This requires enough gray levels so that echoes from the two regions are stored in the memory with different numbers to indicate their different strengths (echogenicities). Even then, the differences may not be observed on the display if they are minimal. **D,** In this example, one tissue region has echoes stored as gray level 40, whereas an adjacent region has echoes stored at gray level 41. These two regions would differ in brightness by 0.4% using a linear postprocessing assignment. This difference would not be seen by a human observer. **E,** With a different postprocessing choice, the brightness difference is 1.2%, which could be observed.

of the steeper slope for echoes assigned values 0–64 in the memory) is accomplished at the cost of degraded contrast resolution for the remainder of the dynamic range (a more shallow slope for echoes that are assigned values 65–255 in the memory). Fig. 4.26, A–B shows a hemangioma depicted using a specially crafted, steep postprocessing assignment for the echo levels that correspond to the echogenicity of the hemangioma. The contrast between abnormal and normal tissues is greatly increased.

Temporal Resolution

Ultrasound scanners store many frames of echo information in the image memory per second. This *frame rate* corresponds to the rate at which the sound beam is steered through the imaging plane (i.e., tissue cross-section) by the transducer. The effective FR observed on the display is limited by the monitor refresh rate. For example, the echo information may be entering the image memory at a FR of 100 Hz, but if the refresh rate is 75 Hz, echo information is retrieved from the memory 75 times per second, and only 75 images per second are then viewed on the display. However, there is an advantage to storing at an FR that is higher than the refresh rate. When the freeze mode is activated, the individual frames within the cine loop retain the temporal relationship achieved with the data acquisition FR.

Temporal resolution is the ability of a display to distinguish closely spaced events in time and to present rapidly moving structures correctly. Temporal resolution is expressed in milliseconds (ms), which is the time from the beginning of one frame to the beginning of the next one. This is also the time required to generate one complete frame. Temporal resolution improves while the FR increases (Fig. 4.35) because less time elapses from one frame to the next.

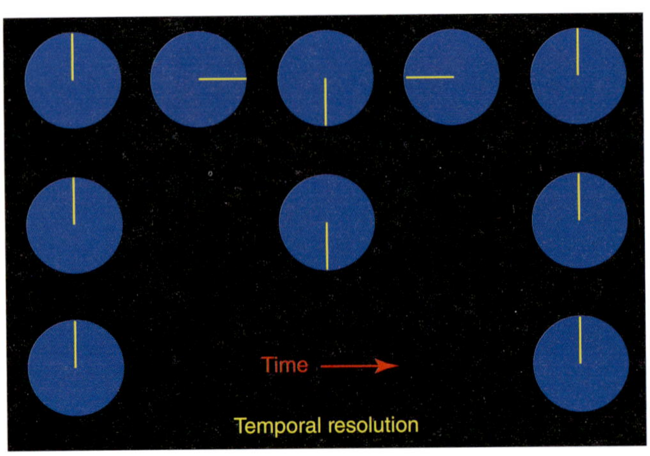

Fig. 4.35 Temporal resolution improves with frame rate. *Top row,* A wheel is rotated in a clockwise direction. Four images are taken during one revolution; thus the frame rate is four per revolution. *Middle row,* With a frame rate of two per revolution, it can be seen that the wheel is rotating, but the direction is ambiguous: it could be clockwise or counterclockwise. *Bottom row,* The frame rate is one per revolution. The motion of the wheel is not observed; indeed, it appears to be stationary. A similar result would occur in echocardiography if one frame per cardiac cycle was acquired at the same instant in each cycle. The heart would appear to be inactive.

Each frame in a narrow transmit beam system will be composed of many scan lines, most likely with more than one focus per line. In the simplest operating mode, each focus on each scan line in each frame, requires a transmit pulse. The required *PRF,* in this scheme, is determined by the chosen number of foci (*n*), lines per frame (*LPF*), and the *FR* in *Hz*. Indeed, the required *PRF* is equal to these three quantities multiplied together. However, most modern ultrasound scanners employ an amalgamated pulse that will be dynamically focused at multiple depths simultaneously, as described in Chapter 3, specifically (Fig. 3.23, I), or the broad transmit beam strategy (described later in this chapter). Both of these approaches will bypass the *PRF* limitations outlined above.

> Traditionally, each focus on each scan line in each frame requires transmission of a pulse. Hence, the following relationship applies:
>
> $$PRF\,(\mathrm{Hz}) = n \times \mathrm{LPF} \times \mathrm{FR}\,(\mathrm{Hz})$$
>
> However, most modern ultrasound scanners use either an amalgamated pulse (dynamically focused at multiple depths simultaneously) or a broad transmit beam with virtual beamforming to bypass this *PRF* limitation.

> In a narrow transmit beam system:
> To increase the number of lines per frame, the *PRF* must increase.
> To increase the FR, the *PRF* must increase.

However, time is required for echoes to return as a pulse travels into the tissue. The greater the penetration (pen), the longer it takes for all of the echoes to return (remember the "13 μs/cm rule"). To avoid confusing late arriving echoes from an earlier pulse with shallow echoes from a later pulse (leading to misplacement of echoes on the display; the range-ambiguity artifact), all echoes from one pulse must be received before the next pulse is transmitted. To accomplish this, *PRF* must decrease while penetration increases.

Hence, if a lower operating frequency is used, penetration is increased, and the *PRF* must decrease to avoid echo misplacement. This will occur as a FR reduction (Fig. 4.36) for lower operating frequencies. The FR decreases when displayed depth is increased (see Fig. 4.36, C–D). Likewise, more scan lines and multiple foci also reduce the FR (Fig. 4.37) because more time may be required to generate each frame. The (simplistic) relationship between these competing variables is as follows:

$$pen\,(\mathrm{cm}) \times n \times \mathrm{LPF} \times \mathrm{FR}\,(\mathrm{Hz}) \leq 77{,}000\ \mathrm{cm/s}$$

> If penetration increases, the *PRF* must decrease.
> If penetration increases, the FR decreases.
> If the lines per frame increases, the FR decreases.
> And to a lesser degree:
> If the number of foci increases, the FR decreases.

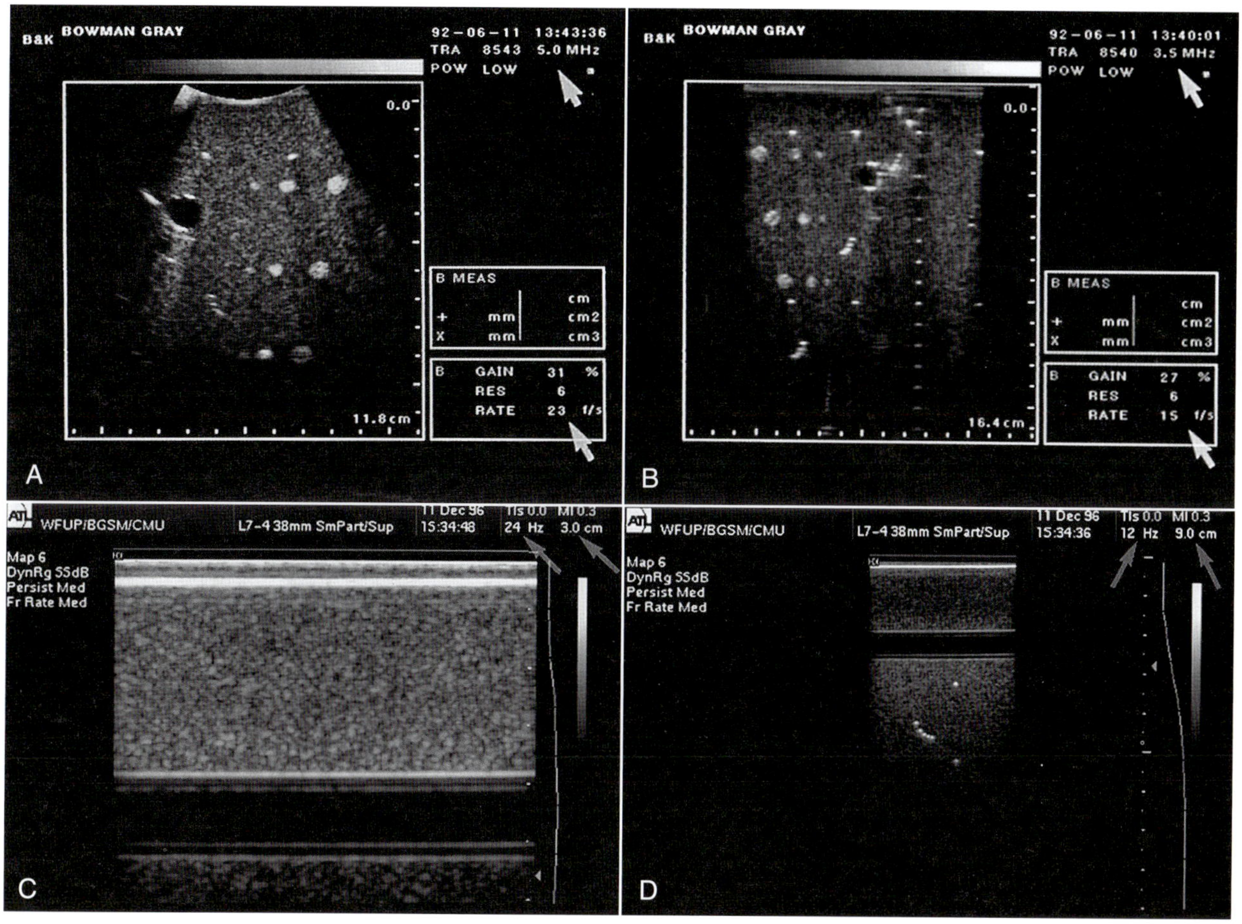

Fig. 4.36 A lower operating frequency allows greater penetration, thereby necessitating longer echo arrival time, which slows down the frame rate. **A,** 5 MHz, penetration of 9 cm, 23 frames per second. **B,** 3.5 MHz, penetration of 13 cm, 15 frames per second. **C,** With a displayed depth of 3 cm, the frame rate is 24 frames per second (Hz; *arrow*). **D,** A displayed depth increase to 9 cm reduces the frame rate to 12 Hz. At first this seems surprising because the operating frequency (5.5 MHz) and therefore the penetration are the same in both cases. However, the effective penetration is reduced with the reduced displayed depth in **C** by increasing pulse repetition frequency. The echoes from beyond the displayed depth are weaker because of attenuation. When the next pulse is sent, the amplifier gain drops with the restarting of the time gain control. Thus the deeper echoes are not amplified enough to be seen (in incorrect locations, i.e., range ambiguity artifact).

ADVANCED CONCEPTS

Above, we saw that

$$pen(\text{cm}) \times PRF(\text{kHz}) \leq 77(\text{cm/ms})$$

This equation is equivalent to

$$pen(\text{cm}) \times PRF(\text{Hz}) \leq 77{,}000(\text{cm/s})$$

and because

$$PRF = n \times LPF \times FR$$

we have

$$pen(\text{cm}) \times n \times LPF \times FR(\text{Hz}) \leq 77{,}000(\text{cm/s})$$

The number 77,000 is one-half the average speed of ultrasound in tissues (154,000 cm/s or 1540 m/s). The one-half results because the penetration (expressed in centimeters) is only half the round-trip distance the sound must travel for the deepest echoes.

Table 4.6 lists the allowable *PRF*s and FRs for various penetration and lines-per-frame values. Multiple foci reduce permitted FRs inversely (e.g., two foci with a penetration of 20 cm and 100 lines per frame are equivalent to one-half × 38, or 19 frames per second). It is important to note that Table 4.6 is ONLY valid for narrow transmit beam systems with a one-to-one correspondence between transmitted beams and displayed scan lines.

Temporal resolution in M and A modes is equal to pulse the repetition period because each pulse produces a new line of echo information on these displays.

> Temporal resolution is the ability to follow moving structures in detail over time. Temporal resolution depends on FR, which depends on depth, lines per frame, and to a lesser degree number of foci.

BROAD TRANSMIT BEAM INSTRUMENTS

It is important to emphasize that the discussion above on beam forming and temporal resolution applies to conventional, pulse-echo, narrow transmit beam ultrasound systems, which forces interdependence between detail and

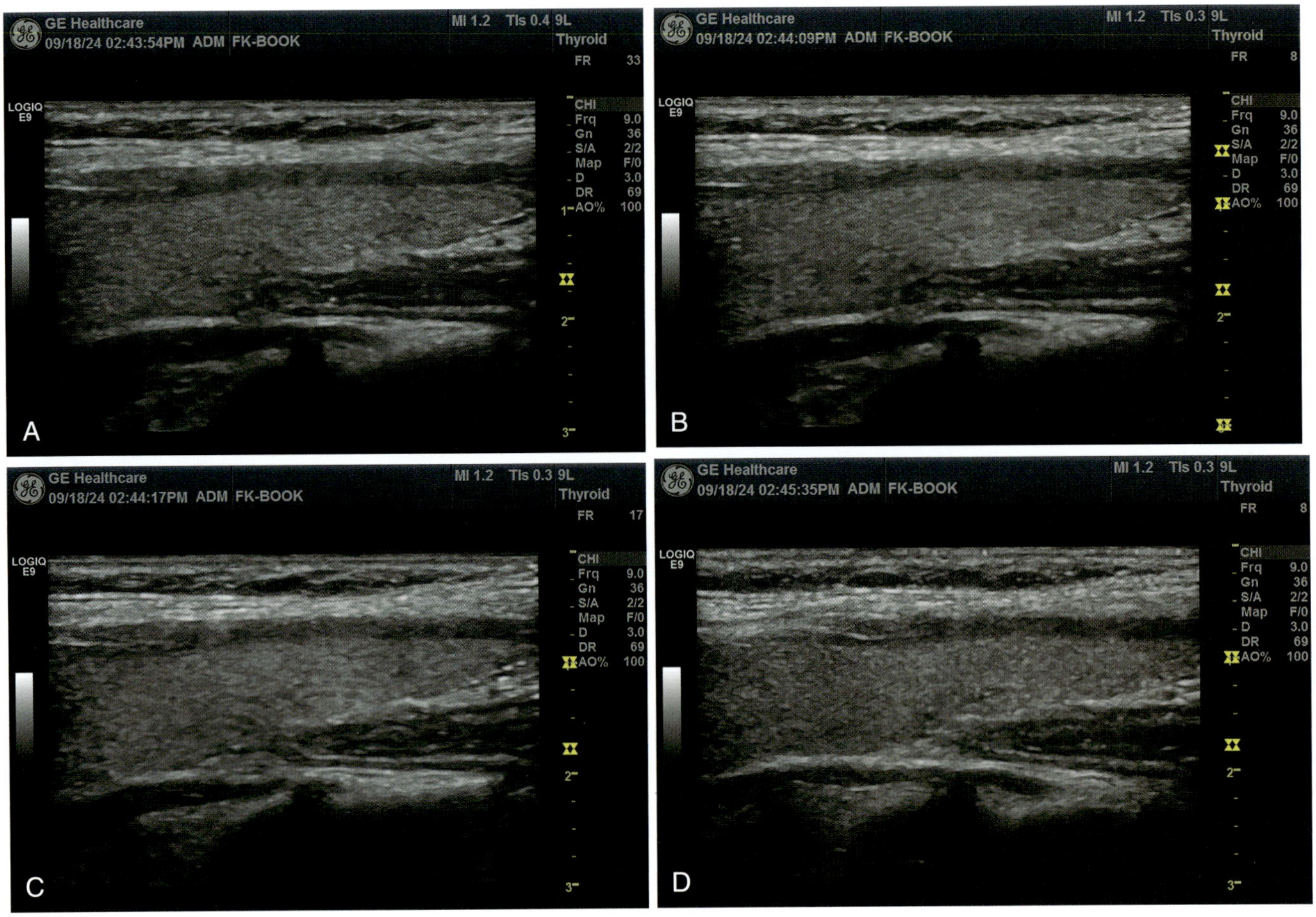

Fig. 4.37 **A,** One focus; frame rate of 33. **B,** Multiple foci (3) reduce the frame rate to 8. **C,** Frame rate of 17. **D,** An increased line density (doubling the number of scan lines) reduces the frame rate to 8.

TABLE 4.6 Pulse Repetition Frequency and Frame Rate Permitted for Various Single-Focus Imaging Depths (Penetration) and 100 or 200 Scan Lines per Frame

		FR	
Penetration (cm)	***PRF* (Hz)**	**100 Lines**	**200 Lines**
20	3850	38	19
15	5133	51	25
10	7700	77	38
5	15,400	154	77

FR, Frame rate; *PRF*, pulse repetition frequency.

temporal resolutions. As mentioned, using weakly focused or unfocused, broad transmit beams markedly reduce or even eliminate such limitations, enabling improvements in most (all) imaging characteristics.

Fig. 4.38 presents a diagram of the organization of an ultrasound imaging system operating with broad transmit beams. As with traditional scanners (cf., Fig. 4.1), these ultrasound systems are composed of a beam former, a signal processor, and a flat-panel display. However, the image processor is performing fundamentally different functions, which is why it is replaced by an **image former** in Fig. 4.38. While this naming convention

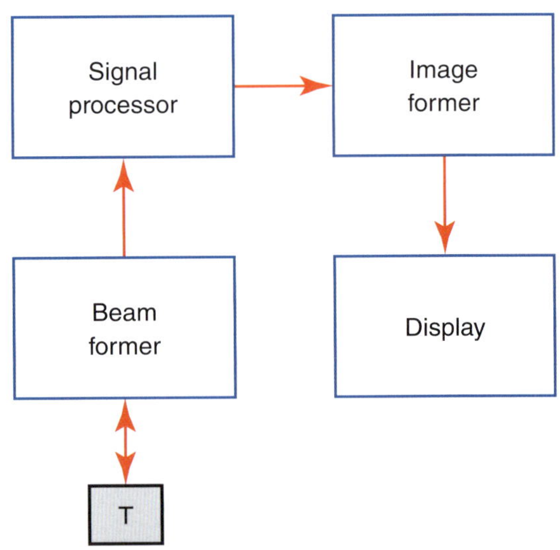

Fig. 4.38 The organization of a pulse-echo imaging system using broad transmit beams. The beam former produces the pulses that drive the transducer (T) and performs initial functions on the returning echo voltages from the transducer. Echoes received from the tissues are converted by the transducer into electric voltages or digital numbers. These echo values go through the beam former to the signal processor, where they are processed to a form suitable for input to the image former. Information from the image former drives the display, which produces the final image of the cross-sectional anatomy and/or motion or flow information.

BOX 4.4 Functions of the Beam Former

- Generating voltages that drive the transducer.
- Determining pulse-repetition frequency, coding, frequency, and intensity.
- Scanning the transmitted beam.
- Amplifying the returning echo voltages.
- Compensating for attenuation.
- Digitizing the echo voltage stream.

BOX 4.5 Functions of the Signal Processor

- Bandpass filtering
- Amplitude detection
- Compression (dynamic range reduction)

is more of a semantic concept, it helps illustrate the difference between narrow and broad transmit beam scanners.

In broad transmit beam instruments, the image processor is replaced by the image former.

Beam Former and Signal Processor

In principle, the beam former in scanners using broad transmit beam performs similar functions as those in traditional ultrasound imaging systems. However, many (sometimes all) elements in the transducer are employed to transmit a few (1–4, typically) of broad, unfocused or weakly focused, pulses into the anatomy, although some focusing is needed in certain applications such as contrast-enhanced ultrasound imaging or *CEUS* using contrast specific imaging modes (discussed in Chapter 6). Consequently, the entire field of view for the image is insonified in a few pulses (i.e., beams) resulting in much higher frame rates and improved temporal resolution.

The beam former sends the transmitted ultrasound pulses through the tissue cross-section in rectangular or sector format and determines the *PRF*, operating frequency, and output intensity as described previously in this chapter. The beam former carries out the functions of pulse transmission, forming and scanning a few broader transmit beams. It performs these functions as previously described for traditional, narrow transmit beam instruments except for the last item—directing, focusing, and apodizing the received beam (Box 4.4). Those functions are now performed by the image former in a much more processing intensive way that is termed *virtual beam forming*. The functions of the signal processor (Box 4.5) and display are not markedly changed compared to traditional imaging systems (i.e., operating with narrow transmit beams).

Image Former

Because the beam former is transmitting weakly focused or unfocused pulses, echoes from all portions of the insonified region from a given pulse arrive at different times at all the elements when in receive mode. In other words, the echoes arrive

BOX 4.6 Functions of the Image Former

- Store echo information received from the signal processor for each emitted pulse
- Sort out the combined echo information to determine the precise echo from each pixel location and store (virtual beam forming)
- Send the stored echo information to the display

at all the transducer elements completely mixed up and must be sorted out to determine the echo information for each location in the image. Massive, high-speed, parallel processing (across all receive channels simultaneously), which is now feasible, sorts out the echoes from all of this combined echo information, placing them in image memory in their proper locations. This process is referred to as virtual beam forming and can be considered a form of retrospective beam forming, which will be discussed in more detail in the next section. Because each transmitted pulse provides much of the echo information for the image, rather than that for just one scan line, the frame rate is increased dramatically so that frame rates in the high hundreds or even several thousands per second can be achieved, improving temporal resolution significantly.

Box 4.6 lists the functions of the image former.

In the **image former**, massive parallel processing enables rapid image acquisition with exquisite detail resolution, contrast resolution, and very high frame rates enabling excellent temporal resolution.

Virtual Beam Forming

Retrospective or virtual beam forming is a complicated, computational process that we will not describe in mathematical detail here. Virtual beam forming is accomplished by massive, parallel, high-speed, computational postprocessing using **graphics processing units** (GPUs), which include 1000 to 10,000 processing cores running in parallel in order to reach 10 to 100 trillion operations per second. However, we can think of it conceptually as follows: An echo from a given location arrives at the elements of a transducer in a specific pattern or sequence depending on its originating location (Fig. 4.39). Echoes from different origination locations arrive at the elements across the transducer aperture in different sequences depending on the distance and direction of travel (i.e., the angle that a given element has to the location where the echoes was created). This information varies with transmission and reception, but once determined (i.e., calculated) it can be used to sort out what arrived from each pixel location. This computational, retrospective beam forming can be thought of as producing a **virtual receiving beam** and as an extension of the dynamic focusing on receive principle described in Chapter 3. There is no physical echo scan line (i.e., receive beam) associated with a given direction of travel. Instead, the broad transmit beam can be thought of as going out to a specific pixel location, determining what is there (echo amplitude and, in some cases, Doppler shift) and bringing a set of echoes back to the transducer and, ultimately, to the image former.

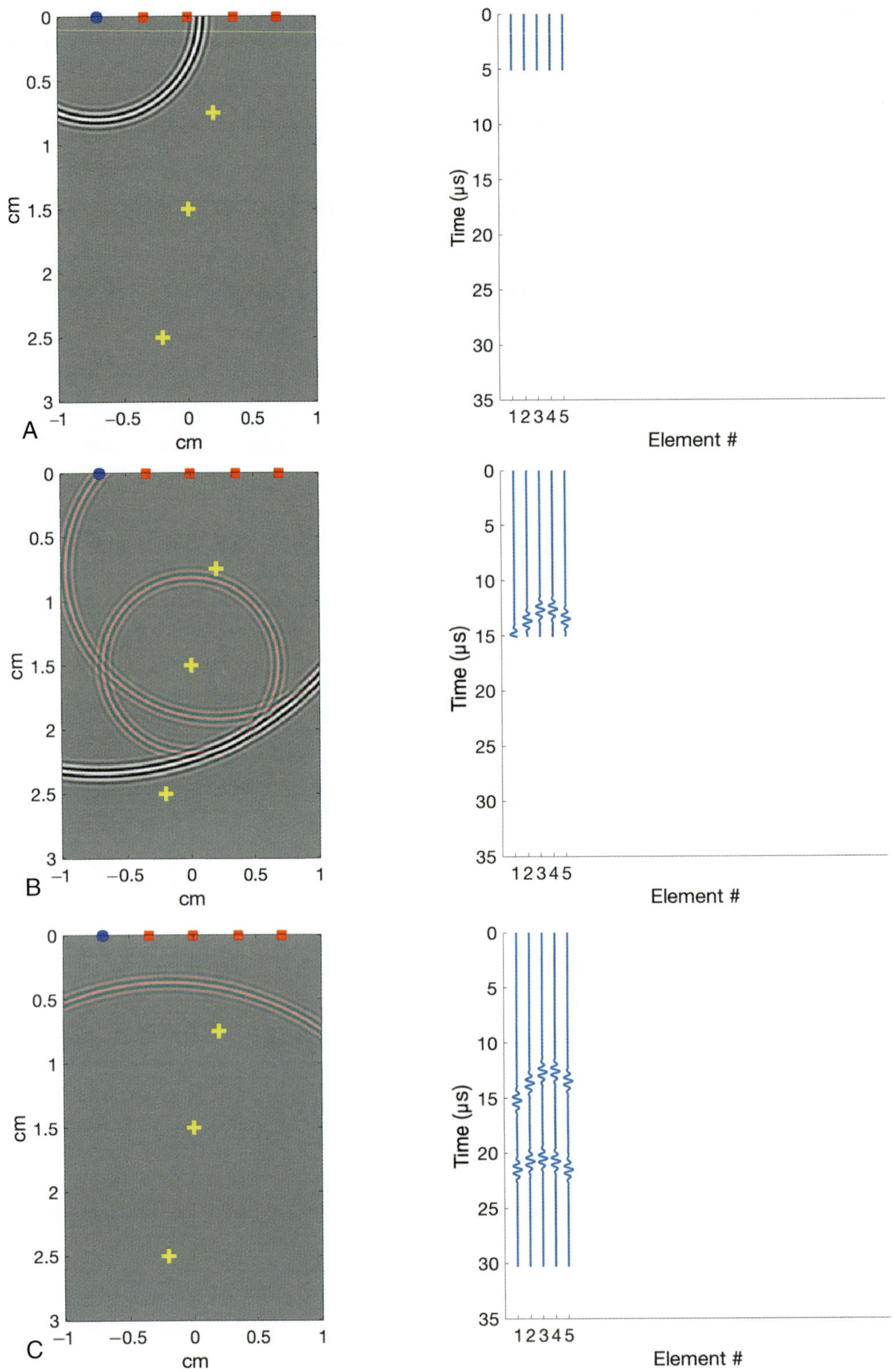

Fig. 4.39 A transducer employs five elements to transmit broad unfocused beams into a phantom with three scatterers (*yellow crosses*) **A,** A beam travelling from the left-most element (*in blue*) along with the corresponding time traces of received echoes from all five elements (*panel on the right*). **B–C,** Echoes from the scattering structures (*in red*) arrive at the transducer elements as can be seen in the time traces, while the transmitted pulse (*in white*) travels deeper.

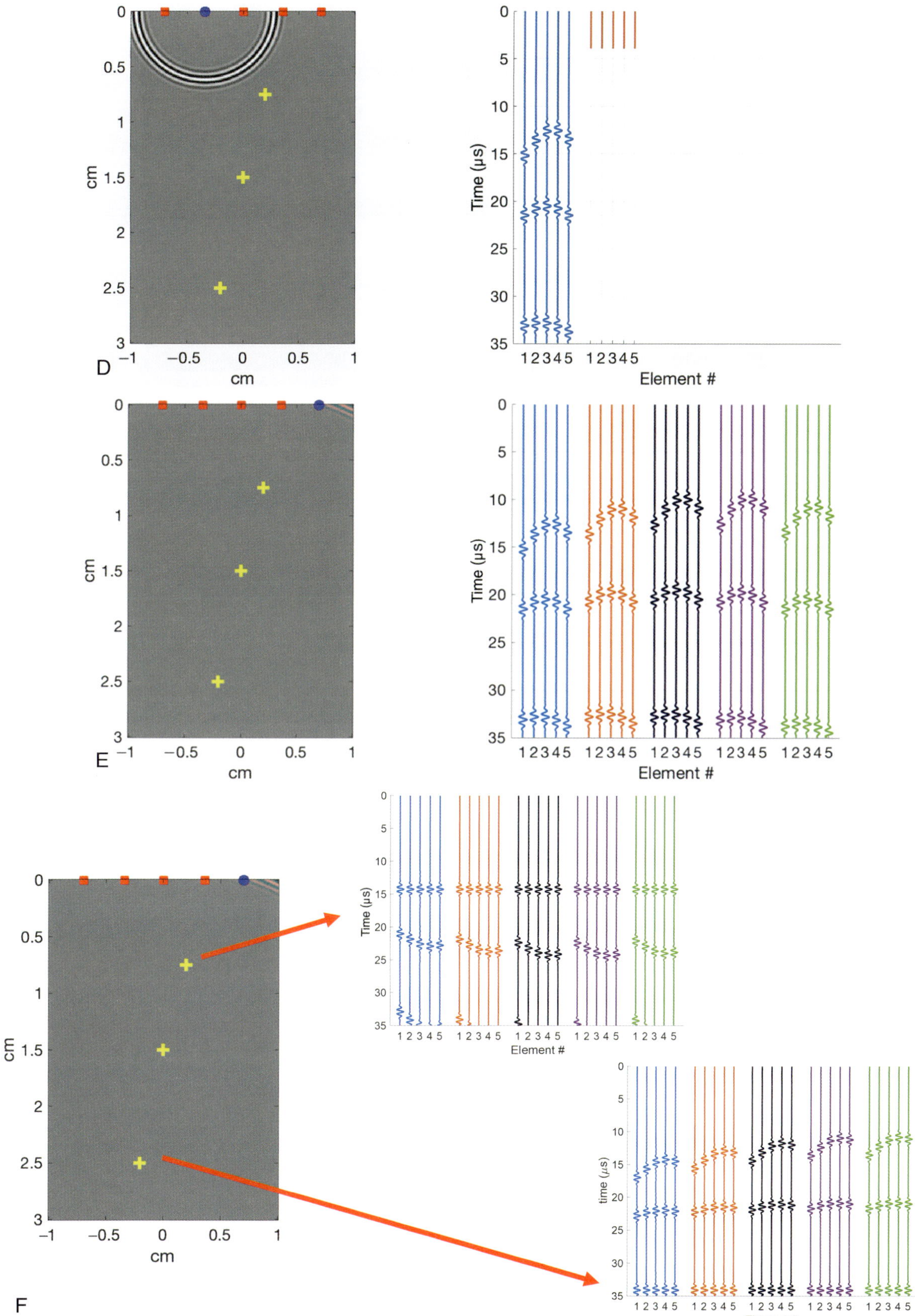

Fig. 4.39, cont'd D, Then the next element (*in blue*) transmits another broad unfocused beam and the process repeats, **(E)** until all elements have transmitted beams and received echoes. Notice how all the echoes are located at slightly different times due to the different travel paths of the pulses and their generated echoes. **F,** In virtual beamforming, the echoes associated with each pixel location are aligned (by compensating for the travel distances and therefore echo arrival times) in real time as shown for two of the scatterers (*red arrows*).

Continued

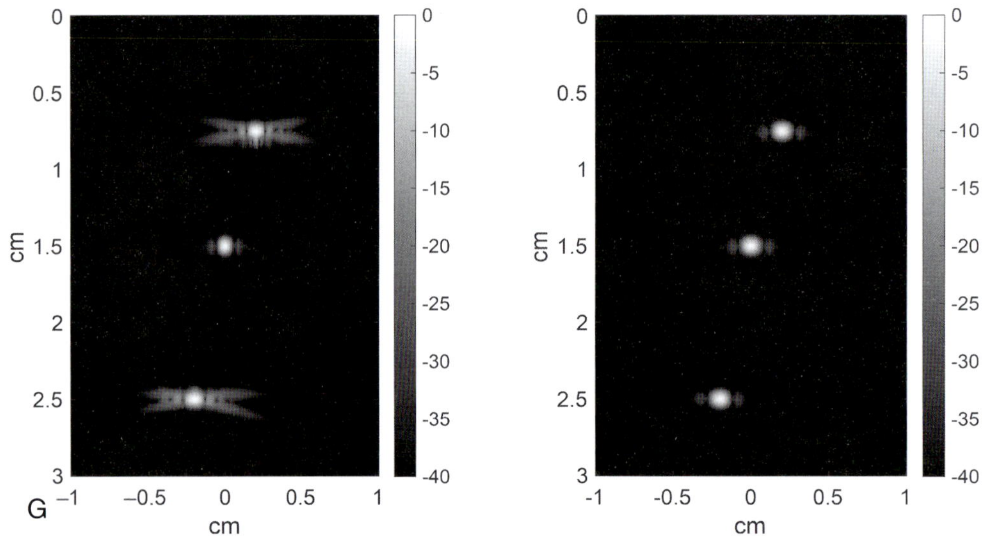

Fig. 4.39, cont'd G, This allows each pixel in the final image to be in focus at all times and transforms a traditional narrow transmit beam image of the 3 scatterers (*left panel*) into the optimally focused broad transmit beam image of the *right panel*. (Courtesy Stephen McAleavey, University of Rochester.)

This retrospective, computed beam forming process can be described as a computed time-reversal approach that mimics backward propagation of the transmitted pulse, revealing, in focus, all the structures that produced all the echoes received. This signal processing technique effectively achieves the excellent detail resolution that a laser-thin transmission beam, essentially a **virtual transmission beam**, would achieve through all portions of the image. The virtual beam forming approach yields images that are in focus throughout the image at all depths simultaneously. The axial resolution is determined by pulse length as described previously in Chapter 3, but the lateral and elevational resolution are markedly improved. Images appear as if a laser-thin ultrasound beam (which is not physically feasible at frequencies necessary for imaging depths appropriate for human anatomical imaging) had been transmitted. Virtual beam forming enhances the focus on reception as well as on transmission so that, in effect retrospectively, each echo of the image is precisely located and optimally imaged. Effectively, there is a transmit and receive focus at each pixel location (cf., Fig. 4.39). Section thickness is also reduced with this approach, improving elevational resolution.

Frame rates in scanners utilizing broad transmit beams in order to operate in virtual beam forming mode cannot be calculated as described in this chapter for narrow transmit beams with a one-to-one correspondence between echoes received from a transmitted ultrasound pulse and the displayed scan lines. Instead, frame rates are determined by how many (or rather how few) transmit beams are used, the computational methods used for virtual beam forming, and the speed of the processing (i.e., the speed of the GPU).

Detail, Contrast, and Temporal Resolutions

Detail resolution is determined by pulse length (axial resolution), which is improved by increasing operating frequency, and pulse width (lateral resolution), which is improved by focusing (see Chapter 3). The best detail resolution in the image occurs in the focal region of the transmitted **physical beam**—assuming a narrow transmit beam system. To achieve a more consistent focus over a greater depth, multiple foci per scan line can be implemented, but with a corresponding reduction in frame rate and, therefore, degradation of temporal resolution.

With broad transmit beams and virtual beam forming, there is no direct relationship between the number of scan lines and the number of pulses required to produce the image. The number of virtual beams is greater than the number of physical beams used to acquire the image. The number of virtual beams and the time to produce them is determined by the computational, retrospective, beam forming approach used in the image former and the speed of the GPUs. Straightforward calculation of frame rate (as described previously in this chapter) is not possible when employing broad transmit beams. Detail resolution and frame rate are determined by the computational processes used and the speed of the processors (i.e., the GPU). For example, an examination question could be as follows:

If the initial frame rate is 30 Hz and the number of foci is increased from 1 to 3, the frame rate is

a. unchanged
b. increased to 60 Hz
c. increased to 90 Hz
d. decreased to 15 Hz
e. decreased to 10 Hz

The straightforward answer for narrow transmit beam operations is that the frame rate is decreased to 10 Hz (30/3 or answer e). However, traditional calculations of detail and temporal resolutions are not even relevant for broad transmit beam operations. Conventional focusing is not used, let alone the concept of multiple transmit foci. Frame rates with virtual beam forming depend first and foremost on the GPU processing speed.

> Virtual beam forming improves detail, contrast and temporal resolutions, sensitivity, and penetration.

Anatomical Imaging

Using broad transmit beans and virtual beam forming significantly improves nearly every aspect of anatomical (i.e., grayscale) ultrasound imaging as well as Doppler motion detection and presentation (as color images or spectral displays; more detail in Chapter 5). As mentioned, the resulting images are similar to what extremely thin, laser-like ultrasound beams would produce, and while such beams cannot be produced physically, virtual beam forming computationally yields comparable results. Physical ultrasound beam forming is still necessary (pulses have to be transmitted in order to create echoes), but it is no longer coupled directly to displayed scan lines. Rather, computed and displayed scan lines can be thought of as produced by virtual beams. After the entire echo content of the image is acquired, electronic focus is applied to each pixel, as illustrated in Fig. 4.39, thus, the concept of the virtual receive beam.

Broad transmit beams yield improvement in nearly every aspect of diagnostic, grayscale (i.e., anatomical) ultrasound imaging (Box 4.7 and Figs. 4.40 and 4.41).

BOX 4.7 Improvements in Anatomical Imaging With Broad Transmit Beams

- Detail resolution improved dramatically
  - Laser-thin virtual beam
  - Entire image in focus
- Contrast resolution improved
  - Section thickness reduced
- Temporal resolution improved significantly
  - Broad transmit beam (fewer pulses required)
  - No multiple focus needed
  - Frame rates of 200–5000 Hz

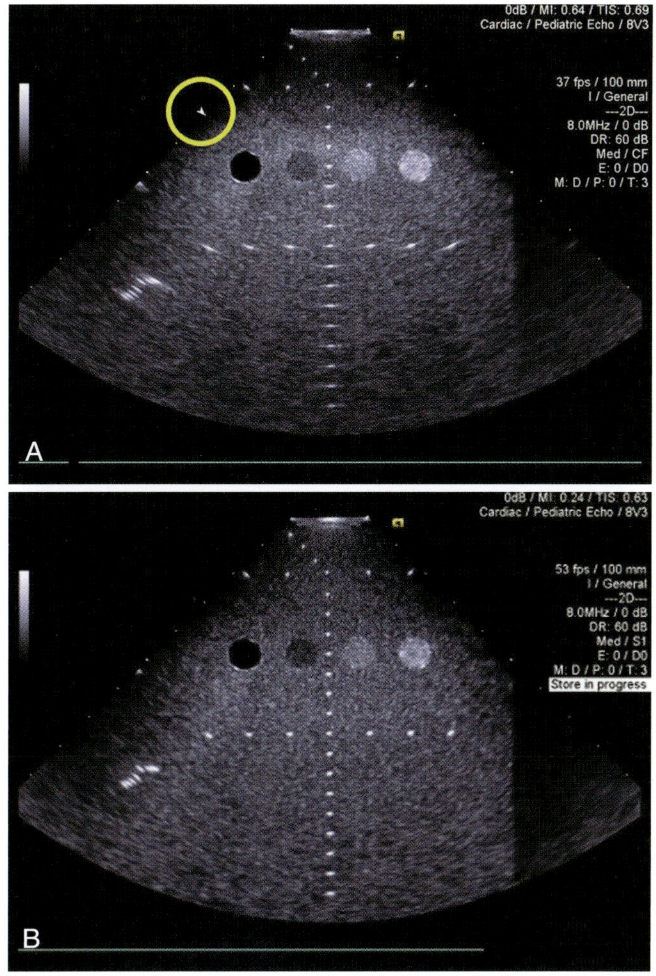

Fig. 4.40 **A,** Detail-resolution phantom with a focused narrow transmit beam (*arrowhead in circle* indicates focus). The nylon lines in cross-section are tiny dots in the focal region but are laterally smeared beyond the focus. **B,** Detail resolution phantom with an unfocused broad transmit beam (note there is no arrowhead). The entire image is in focus as indicated by the lack of lateral smearing of the nylon lines that all appear as tiny dots. (Courtesy © Siemens Healthineers 2019.)

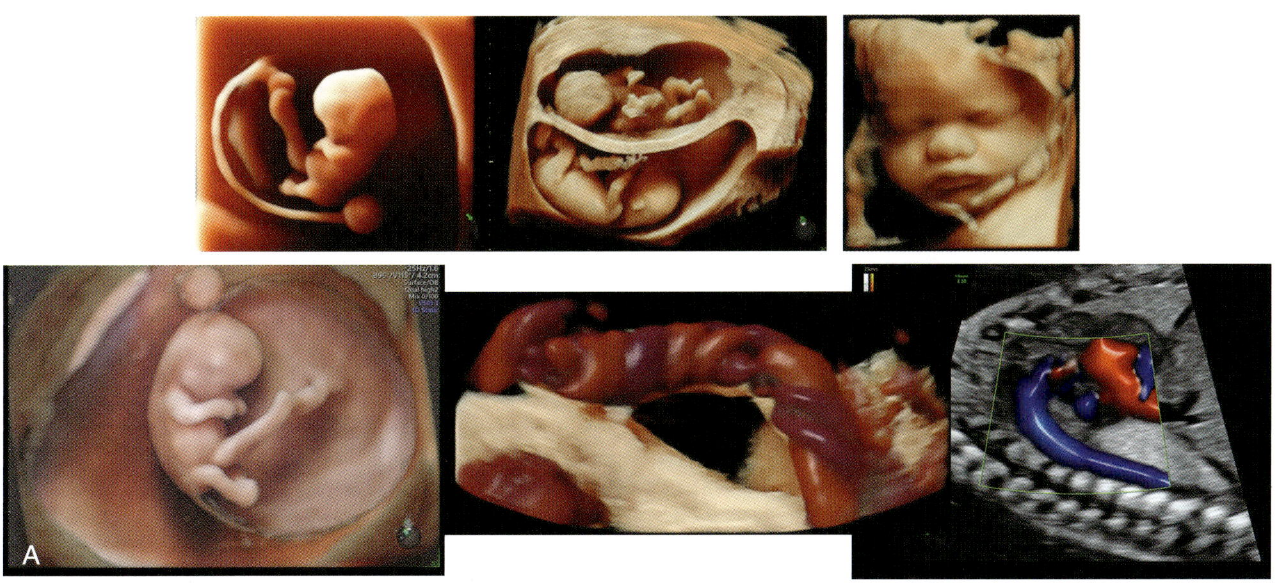

Fig. 4.41 Examples of the superb detail resolution achievable with broad transmit beams and virtual beamforming **A,** Obstetrical images.

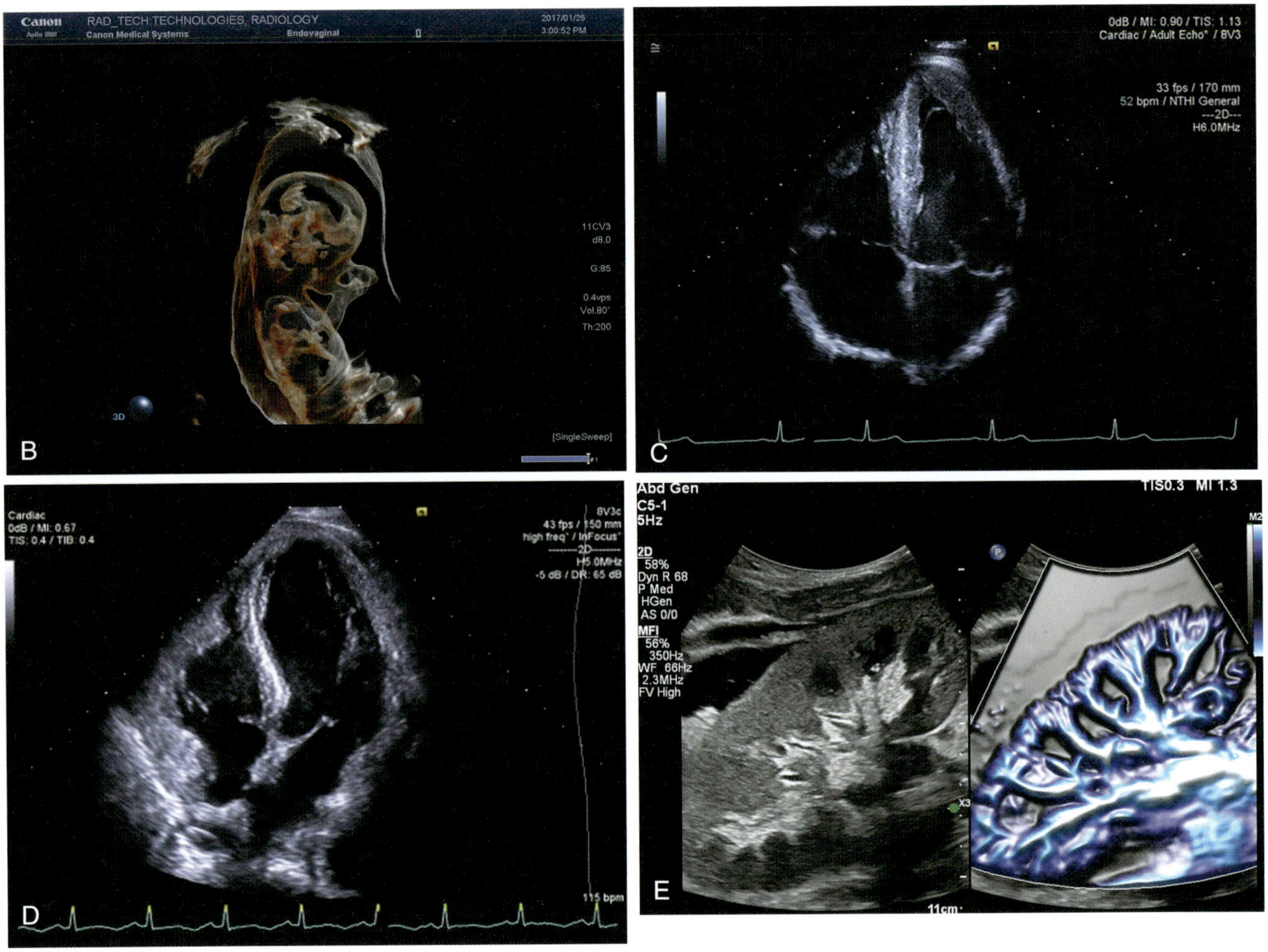

Fig. 4.41, cont'd **B,** 3D fetal rendering. **C–D,** Cardiac examples. **E,** Abdominal and vascular example. (**A,** Courtesy GE Healthcare. **B,** Courtesy Canon Medical Systems USA. **C and D,** Courtesy Siemens Healthineers. **E,** Courtesy Philips Medical Systems.)

REVIEW

The following key points are presented in this chapter:

- There are two operating principles in current commercially available ultrasound imaging systems using narrow and broad transmit beams.
- Ultrasound scanners are of the pulse-echo type.
- Scanners use the strength, direction, and arrival time of received echoes to generate A, B, and M mode displays.
- Ultrasound imaging systems include the beam former, signal processor, image processor, and display, and often these are attached to peripheral recording and display devices.
- The beam former is responsible for directing, focusing, and apodizing the ultrasound beam on transmission and reception. The beam former also amplifies the echo voltages, compensates for attenuation using TGC, and digitizes the voltages.
- The signal processor filters, detects, and compresses the echo signal.
- The image processer converts the echo data in scan-line format to image format for storage and display.
- A mode presents depth versus echo amplitude.
- B and M modes use a display of echo strength as brightness.
- M mode shows reflector motion in time. M mode is a presentation of echo depth versus time.
- B mode scans show anatomical cross-sections through the scan plane.
- Image memories store echo intensity information as binary numbers in memory elements.
- Contrast resolution improves with increasing bits per pixel.
- Real-time imaging is the rapid sequential display of ultrasound images (frames).
- Real-time imaging requires rapid, repeatable, sequential scanning of the sound beam through the tissue. This is accomplished with electronic transducer arrays.
- Increasing FR improves temporal resolution.
- With broad transmit beams operations, the image processor is replaced by the image former.
- In the image former, massive parallel processing with GPUs enables rapid image acquisition with exquisite detail resolution, contrast resolution, and very high frame rates, enabling excellent temporal resolution.
- Virtual beam forming improves detail, contrast and temporal resolutions, sensitivity, and penetration.

EXERCISES

Answers appear in the Answers to Exercises section at the back of the book.

1. The ultrasound *PRF* is equal to the voltage ___________ repetition frequency of the pulser.
   a. amplitude
   b. pulse
   c. period
   d. duration
2. Increased voltage amplitude produced by the pulser increases the ___________ and ___________ of ultrasound pulses produced by the transducer.
   a. amplitude, intensity
   b. amplitude, frequency
   c. frequency, period
   d. frequency, intensity
3. If a 6 MHz transducer images to a depth of 10 cm, to avoid range ambiguity, the maximum *PRF* permitted is ___________.
   a. 7.7 kHz
   b. 6.0 kHz
   c. 10.0 kHz
   d. 1.54 MHz
4. Functions performed by the signal processor include ___________, ___________, and ___________.
   a. amplification, digitizing, filtering
   b. amplification, filtering, digital-to-analog conversion
   c. amplification, filtering, compression
   d. filtering, detection, compression
5. Match the following functions with what they accomplish.
   a. Amplification
   b. Compensation
   c. Filtering
   d. Detection
   a. Compression
      1. converts pulses from radio frequency to amplitude form.
      2. increases all amplitudes.
      3. decreases dynamic range.
      4. corrects for tissue attenuation.
      5. reduces noise.
6. If the input voltage to an amplifier is 1 mV and the output voltage is 10 mV, the voltage amplification ratio is ___________. The power ratio is ___________. The gain is ___________ dB.
   a. 10, 20, 30
   b. 10, 100, 100
   c. 10, 100, 20
   d. 10, 10, 10
7. An amplifier with a gain of 60 dB has 1 mW of power applied to the input. The output power is ___________ W.
   a. 60
   b. 1
   c. 10
   d. 1000
8. An amplifier with a gain of 60 dB has 10 mV of voltage applied to the input. The output voltage is ___________ mV.
   a. 10
   b. 100
   c. 1000
   d. 60
9. Time gain compensation is accomplished in the ___________.
   a. pulser
   b. beam former
   c. signal processor
   d. postprocessor
   e. image processor
10. Compensation takes into account reflector ___________.
    a. impedance
    b. size
    c. amplitude
    d. depth
11. Compensation amplifies echoes differently, according to their arrival ___________.
    a. times
    b. positions
    c. directions
    d. strengths
12. Compression decreases the ___________ range to a range that the ___________ and human ___________ can handle.
    a. frequency, instrument, intelligence
    b. dynamic, display, vision
    c. amplitude, display, hearing
    d. dynamic, pulser, vision
13. If a display has a dynamic range of 20 dB and the smallest voltage it can handle is 200 mV, then the largest voltage it can handle is ___________ V.
    a. 20
    b. 2.0
    c. 0.2
    d. 0.02
14. Detection converts voltage pulses from ___________ form to ___________ form.
    a. ultrasound, infrasound
    b. infrasound, ultrasound
    c. radio frequency, amplitude
    d. ultrasound, radio frequency
15. Filtering widens bandwidth. True or false?
16. Filtering is accomplished in the ___________.
    a. pulser
    b. beam former
    c. signal processor
    d. postprocessor
    e. image processor
17. The compression or dynamic range control reduces the range of echo amplitudes displayed by reducing the weakest to ___________ and/or the strongest ones to the

__________ value and assigning the others to increasing values. This produces a(n) __________ contrast image with elimination of weakest and maximizing of strongest echoes.

a. minimum, maximum, higher
b. zero, 100, zero
c. zero, maximum, higher
d. 10, 100, optimum

18. An amplifier has a power output of 100 mW when the input power is 0.1 mW. The amplifier gain is __________ dB.
a. 10
b. 20
c. 30
d. 40

19. If the beam-former output to the transducer is reduced by 3, 6, or 9 dB, the ultrasound pulse output intensity is reduced by __________%, __________%, or __________%, respectively.
a. 50, 75, 87.5
b. 50, 25, 12.5
c. 6, 12, 18
d. 33, 66, 99

20. One watt is __________ dB below 100 W.
a. 1
b. 2
c. 10
d. 20

21. One watt is __________ dB above 100 mW.
a. 1
b. 2
c. 10
d. 20

22. If the input power is 1 mW and the output is 10,000 mW, the gain is __________ dB.
a. 10
b. 20
c. 30
d. 40

23. If an amplifier has a gain of 15 dB, the ratio of output power to input power is __________. (Refer to Table 4.1.)
a. 15
b. 22
c. 30
d. 32

24. If the output of a 22 dB gain amplifier is connected to the input of a 23 dB gain amplifier, the total gain is __________ dB. The overall power ratio is __________. (Refer to Table 4.1.)
a. 22, 45
b. 45, 23
c. 45, 32,000
d. 32,000, 45,000

25. If a 17-dB electric attenuator is connected to a 15-dB amplifier, the net gain is __________ dB. The net attenuation is __________ dB. For a 1-W input, the output is __________ W. (Refer to Table 2.3.)
a. 2, 2, 2
b. 2, −2, −2
c. −2, 2, 6.3
d. −2, 2, 0.63

26. For the digital memory shown in Fig. 4.42, enter the number stored in each pixel location.
a. Lower right: __________
b. Middle right: __________
c. Upper right: __________
d. Upper middle: __________
e. Upper left: __________

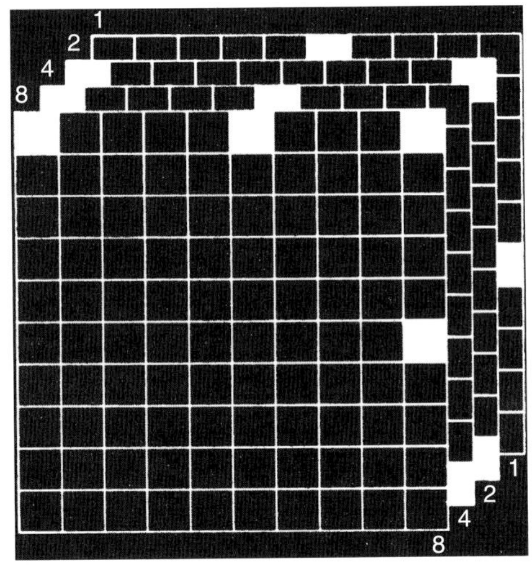

Fig. 4.42 Digital memory description. Illustration to accompany Exercise 26. The white color indicates that the memory device is on.

27. The contrast resolution for an instrument that has an echo dynamic range of 43 dB and 32 shades is __________ dB per shade.
a. 1.3
b. 3.2
c. 4.3
d. 32
e. 43

28. The contrast resolution for an instrument that has a 6-bit memory and a 45-dB echo dynamic range is __________ dB per shade.
a. 0.3
b. 0.5
c. 0.7
d. 0.9
e. 6

29. Match the following:
a. Analog:
b. Digital:
c. Preprocessing:
d. Postprocessing:
e. Pixel:
a. Bit:
1. picture element
2. assignment of stored numbers
3. discrete

4. binary digit
5. proportional
6. assignment of displayed brightness

30. Typical image pixel dimensions are at least ___________.
a. 640 × 1080
b. 4096 × 64,000
c. 100 × 100
d. 512 × 1540
e. 1024 × 768

31. How many bits per pixel are required for each number of shades?
a. 16: ___________
b. 32: ___________
c. 64: ___________
d. 128: ___________
e. 256: ___________

32. ___________ total memory elements are required for a 100 × 100 pixel, 5 bit digital memory.
a. 500
b. 1000
c. 5000
d. 10,000
e. 50,000

33. Memories of ___________ bits per pixel are common in ultrasound today.
a. 4–12
b. 4–6
c. 8–16
d. 5–9
e. 10–11

34. Digital memories store ___________.
a. logarithms
b. electric magnetism
c. electric current
d. electric charge
e. numbers

35. ___________ is commonly controllable by the operator.
a. Postprocessing
b. Pixel matrix
c. Bits per pixel
d. Digitization
e. All of the above

36. In binary numbers, how many symbols are used?
a. 0
b. 1
c. 2
d. 4

37. The term binary digit is commonly shortened into the single word ___________.
a. bigit
b. binit
c. bidig
d. bit

38. Each binary digit in a binary number is represented in the memory by a memory element, which, at any time, is in one of ___________ states that are ___________ or ___________.
a. 2, on, off
b. many, odd, even
c. 4, high, low
d. 10, odd, even

39. Match the following (see Fig. 4.23, D)

Column in an 8-bit binary number hgfedcba:	Decimal number represented by a 1 in the column:
a. ___________	1. 64
b. ___________	2. 32
c. ___________	3. 1
d. ___________	4. 16
e. ___________	5. 8
f. ___________	6. 128
g. ___________	7. 2
h. ___________	8. 4

40. The binary number 10110 represents zero 1, one 2, one 4, zero 8, and one 16; that is, the decimal number 0 + 2 + 4 + 0 + 16 = 22. What decimal number does the binary number 11001 represent?
a. 15
b. 20
c. 25
d. 35

41. The decimal number 13 is made up of one 1, zero 2, one 4, and one 8 (8 + 4 + 0 + 1 = 13). The number therefore is represented by the binary number ___________.
a. 1011
b. 1101
c. 1110
d. 0111

42. Match the following:

Decimal Number	Binary Number
a. 1 ___________	1. 0001111
b. 5 ___________	2. 0011001
c. 10 ___________	3. 0001010
d. 15 ___________	4. 0110010
e. 20 ___________	5. 0000001
f. 25 ___________	6. 1100100
g. 30 ___________	7. 0101000
h. 40 ___________	8. 0011110
i. 50 ___________	9. 0010100
j. 100 ___________	10. 0000101

43. How many binary digits are required in the binary numbers representing the following decimal numbers?
a. 0 ___________
b. 1 ___________
c. 5 ___________
d. 10 ___________
e. 25 ___________
f. 30 ___________
g. 63 ___________
h. 64 ___________
i. 75 ___________
j. 100 ___________

44. How many bits are required to represent each decimal number in binary form?
   a. 7 ___________
   b. 15 ___________
   c. 3 ___________
   d. 511 ___________
   e. 1023 ___________
   f. 63 ___________
   g. 255 ___________
   h. 1 ___________
   i. 127 ___________
   j. 31 ___________
45. How many bits are required to store numbers representing each number of different gray shades?
   a. 2 ___________
   b. 4 ___________
   c. 8 ___________
   d. 15 ___________
   e. 16 ___________
   f. 25 ___________
   g. 32 ___________
   h. 64 ___________
   i. 65 ___________
   j. 128 ___________
46. The primary formats of image presentation are called ___________ *mode*, ___________ *mode*, and ___________ *mode*. They are used in ___________, ___________, and ___________ types of clinical imaging, respectively.
   a. B (brightness), M (motion), A (amplitude), all, cardiac, ophthalmic
   b. A (amplitude), B (brightness), M (motion), all, cardiac, ophthalmic
   c. B (brightness), M (motion), A (amplitude), cardiac, all, ophthalmic
   d. B (brightness), M (motion), A (amplitude), ophthalmic, all, cardiac
47. ___________ mode is used for studying the motion of a structure such as a heart valve.
   a. A
   b. B
   c. M
   d. all of the above
48. B scan presents a cross-section through the ___________ plane.
   a. longitudinal
   b. transverse
   c. elevational
   d. scan
49. A display that shows various echo strengths as different brightnesses is called a ___________-___________ or ___________ ___________ *display*.
   a. grayscale, B mode
   b. cross-sectional, anatomic mode
   c. sono-scan, sectional mode
   d. gray-mode, square pixel
50. The ___________ ___________ stores the gray-scale image and allows it to be displayed on a computer monitor.
   a. signal processor
   b. preprocessor
   c. postprocessor
   d. image memory
51. Match the following (use answers more than once):
   a. linear array ___________ 1. rectangular image
   b. convex array ___________ 2. sector image
   c. phased array ___________
   d. vector array ___________
52. If the *PRF* of an instrument is 1 kHz and it displays (single focus) 25 frames per second, there are ___________ lines per frame.
   a. 20
   b. 40
   c. 60
   d. 100
53. The *PRF* is ___________ Hz if 30 frames (40 lines each) are displayed per second (single focus).
   a. 600
   b. 1200
   c. 30
   d. 40
54. Imaging involving 10 cm depth penetration, a single focus, 100 scan lines per frame, and 30 frames per second can be accomplished without range ambiguity. True or false?
55. The maximum frame rate permitted for 15 cm penetration, 3 foci, and 200 scan lines per frame is ___________.
   a. 3.0
   b. 5.5
   c. 8.5
   d. 15
   e. 30
56. The primary components of a diagnostic ultrasound imaging system are the ___________, ___________, ___________, ___________, and ___________.
   a. transducer, beam former, signal processor, image processor, display
   b. transducer, image former, echo processor, scan convertor, output
   c. pulser, pulser delay, T/R switch, echo delays, summer
   d. amplifier, digital convertor, analog convertor, scan convertor, display
57. The information that can be obtained from an M mode display includes ___________.
   a. distance and motion pattern
   b. transducer frequency, reflection coefficient, and distance
   c. acoustic impedances, attenuation, and motion pattern
   d. none of the above
58. The TGC control compensates for ___________.
   a. machine instability in the warmup time
   b. attenuation
   c. transducer aging
   d. the ambient light in the examining area
   e. patient examination time
59. A grayscale display shows ___________.
   a. gray color on a white background
   b. echoes with one brightness level

c. white color on a gray background
d. a range of echo amplitudes

60. The dynamic range of an ultrasound system is ___________.
a. the speed with which ultrasound examination can be performed
b. the range over which the transducer can be manipulated while an examination is performed
c. the ratio of the maximum amplitude to the minimum echo strength that can be displayed
d. the range of voltages applied to the transducer

61. A ______________ formats scan line data to image form.
a. beam former
b. scan convertor
c. signal processor
d. image formatter

62. Which of the following is not performed by a signal processor?
a. detection
b. filtering
c. digital-to-analog conversion
d. radio frequency–to–amplitude conversion
e. compression

63. In a digital memory, echo intensity is represented by ___________.
a. positive charge distribution
b. a number stored in the memory
c. electron density of the display writing beam
d. a and c
e. all of the above

64. If there were no attenuation in tissue, ___________ would not be needed.
a. filtering
b. compression
c. detection
d. TGC

65. Echo imaging includes ultrasound generation, propagation and reflection in tissues, and reception of returning ___________.
a. echoes
b. impedances
c. propagations
d. transmissions

66. The diagnostic ultrasound systems in common clinical use today are of the ___________-___________ type.
a. transmit-receive
b. pulse-echo
c. through-transmission
d. A-mode

67. Grayscale instruments show echo amplitude as ___________ on the display.
a. numbers
b. color
c. spikes
d. brightness

68. Pulse-echo instruments look for three things: the ___________, ___________, and arrival ___________ of echoes returning from tissues.
a. amplitude, frequency, location
b. strength, direction, time
c. focus, delay, direction
d. frequency, duration, delay

69. An image memory stores image information in the form of ___________ numbers.
a. electric charge
b. binary
c. decimal
d. impedance
e. none of the above

70. Imaging systems produce a visual ___________ from the electric ___________ received from the transducer.
a. display, voltages
b. map, numbers
c. presentation, amplifiers
d. display, numbers

71. The transducer is connected to the signal processor through the ___________ ___________.
a. pulser delay
b. image processor
c. scan convertor
d. beam former

72. The transducer receives voltages from the ___________ in pulse-echo systems.
a. pulser delay
b. image processor
c. scan convertor
d. beam former

73. The ___________ receives digitized echo voltages from the beam former.
a. signal processor
b. image processor
c. scan convertor
d. beam former

74. Increasing gain generally produces the same effect as ___________.
a. decreasing attenuation
b. increasing attenuation
c. increasing compression
d. increasing rectification
e. b and c

75. The ADC is part of the ___________.
a. beam former
b. signal processor
c. image processor
d. display
e. a and b
f. c and e

76. Voltage pulses from the pulser are applied through delays to the ___________.
a. digitizer
b. transducer
c. ADCs
d. preprocessor

77. Detection is a function of the ___________.
a. beam former

b. signal processor
c. image processor
d. display
e. a and b

78. If gain is reduced by one-half, with input power unchanged, the output power is ____________ what it was before.
a. equal to
b. twice
c. one-half
d. none of the above

79. If gain is 30 dB and output power is reduced by one-half, the new gain is ____________ dB.
a. 15
b. 60
c. 33
d. 27
e. none of the above

80. If four shades of gray are shown on a display, each twice the brightness of the preceding one, the brightest shade is ____________ times the brightness of the dimmest shade.
a. 2
b. 4
c. 8
d. 16
e. 32

81. The dynamic range displayed in Exercise 80 is ________ dB.
a. 10
b. 9
c. 5
d. 2
e. 0

82. In which units are gain and attenuation usually expressed?
a. dB
b. dB/cm
c. cm
d. cm/3 dB
e. None of the above

83. Time gain compensation makes up for the fact that reflections from deeper reflectors arrive at the transducer with greater amplitude. True or false?

84. The modes that show one-dimensional (depth) real-time images are ____________ and ____________ modes.
a. A, B
b. A, C
c. B, M
d. A, M

85. The mode that shows two-dimensional real-time images is the ____________ mode.
a. A
b. B
c. C
d. M

86. A real-time B mode display may be produced by rapid ____________ scanning of a transducer array.
a. electronic
b. manual
c. visual
d. reverse

87. Each complete scan of the sound beam produces an image on the display that is called a ____________.
a. picture
b. frame
c. window
d. movie

88. For a single focus, the number of lines in each frame is equal to the number of times the transducer is ____________ while the frame is produced; that is, while the sound beam is scanned.
a. quiet
b. focused
c. pulsed
d. delayed

89. In real-time scanning, the required *PRF* depends on the number of ____________ per frame and ____________ rate.
a. lines, frame
b. scans, scan
c. echoes, pulsing
d. focuses, propagation

90. Increasing the number of foci may reduce ____________ ____________.
a. detail resolution
b. contrast resolution
c. pulse repetition
d. frame rate

91. To correct for attenuation, TGC must ____________ the gain for increasing depth.
a. increase
b. decrease
c. correct
d. decelerate

92. If a higher frequency is used, resolution is ____________, imaging depth ____________, and the TGC slope must be ____________.
a. improved, decreases, increased
b. degraded, increases, decreased
c. unchanged, increases, eliminated
d. improved, increased, increased

93. For pixel dimensions 512 × 512 and 1920 × 1200, calculate the number of image pixels.
a. 262,144; 2,304,000
b. 262,144; 786,432
c. 786,432; 1,524,288
d. 324,288; 3,262,144

94. Which type of array gives a wide view close to the transducer? ____________ Which of the following produce(s) a sector format image? ____________ (Choose from the list below for both answers.)
a. vector
b. linear
c. phased
d. convex
e. more than one of the above

95. In Fig. 4.43, if two foci were used, the frame rate would be ___________.
 a. 33
 b. 22
 c. 11
 d. 6
 e. 1

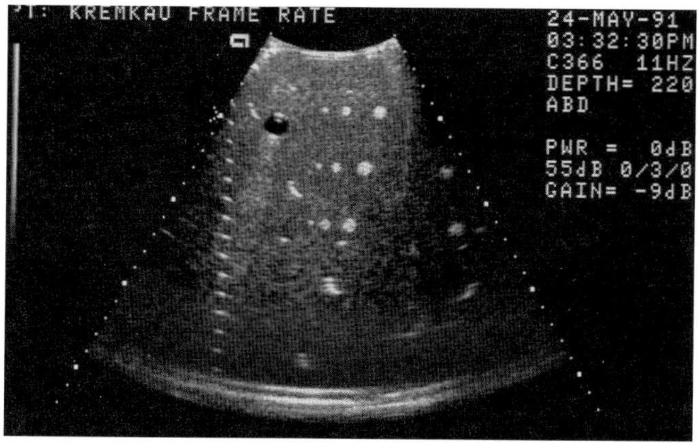

Fig. 4.43 Illustration to accompany Exercise 95.

96. What is adjusted improperly in Fig. 4.44?
 a. gain
 b. time gain compensation
 c. compression
 d. frame rate
 e. rejection

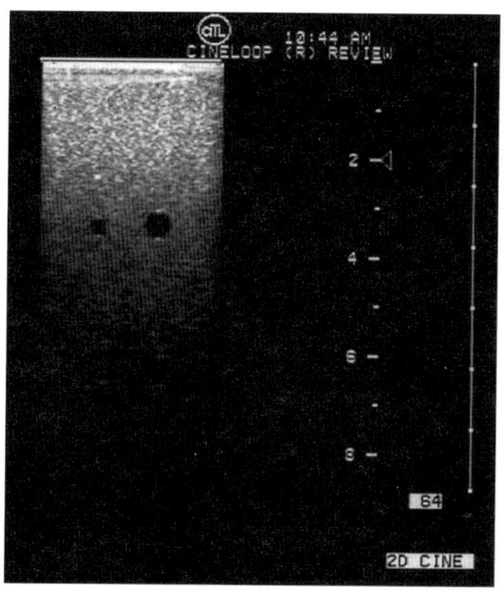

Fig. 4.44 Illustration to accompany Exercise 96.

97. The decreasing gain of the time gain compensation curve (*arrows*) in Fig. 4.45 is caused by ___________.
 a. weak attenuation
 b. refraction
 c. strong attenuation
 d. beam broadening
 e. beam narrowing

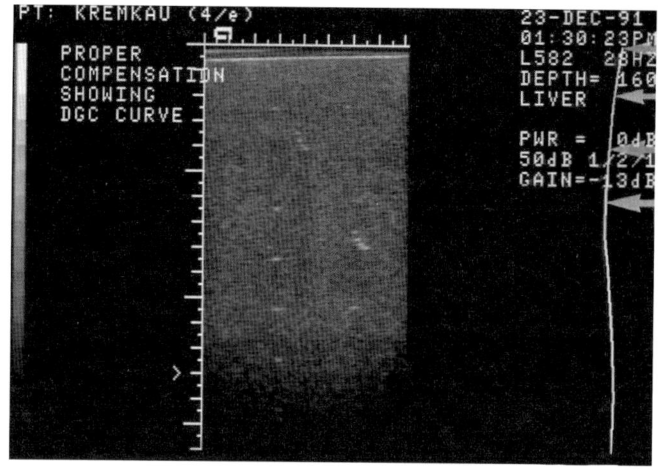

Fig. 4.45 Illustration to accompany Exercise 97.

98. In the linear amplifier of Fig. 4.46, the gain is ___________ dB.
 a. 1000
 b. 300
 c. 100
 d. 60
 e. 10

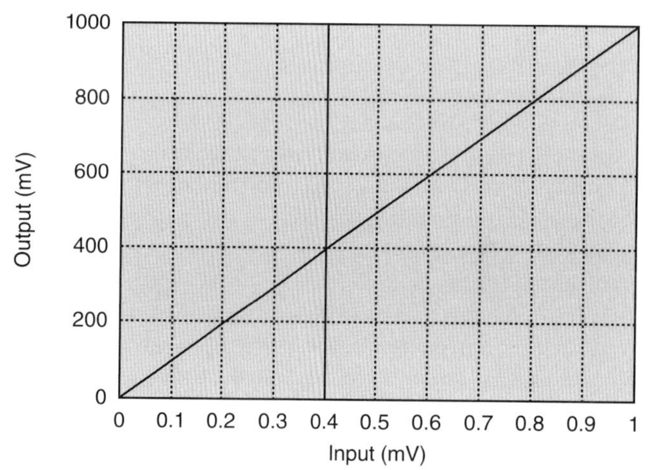

Fig. 4.46 Illustration to accompany Exercise 98.

99. Compression is a function of the ___________.
 a. beam former
 b. signal processor
 c. image processor
 d. postprocessor

100. The underlying principle upon which broad transmit beam systems operates is
 a. the Doppler principle
 b. the compressional wave principal
 c. the virtual beam principle
 d. the pulse-echo principle

101. With an unfocused transmit beam in virtual-beam ultrasound imaging, which zone(s) is/are in focus?
 a. near zone
 b. far zone

c. no zones
d. all zones

102. Which is not needed with broad transmit beam instruments?
a. transmitted beam
b. multiple-transmit focus
c. reception focus
d. TGC

103. Which is not a reason for improvement of detail resolution with broad transmit beam systems?
a. shorter transmit pulses
b. reception focus at each pixel location
c. massive postprocessing with GPU(s)
d. retrospective beam forming

104. Which is not a reason for improvement of temporal resolution with broad transmit beams?
a. shorter transmit pulses
b. fewer transmit pulses
c. no multiple focusing
d. speed of GPU(s)

105. Which is not significantly improved with broad transmit beam instruments?
a. axial resolution
b. lateral resolution
c. temporal resolution
d. contrast resolution

106. Physical beam forming applies to ______________ imaging.
a. narrow transmit beam
b. broad transmit beam
c. both narrow and broad transmit beams
d. neither narrow nor broad transmit beams

107. Virtual beam forming applies to
a. narrow transmit beam
b. broad transmit beam
c. both narrow and broad transmit beams
d. neither narrow nor broad transmit beams

108. Multiple transmission focus control applies to
a. narrow transmit beam
b. broad transmit beam
c. both narrow and broad transmit beams
d. neither narrow nor broad transmit beams

109. Retrospective beam forming applies to
a. narrow transmit beam
b. broad transmit beam
c. both narrow and broad transmit beams
d. neither narrow nor broad transmit beams

110. Improving detail resolution sacrifices temporal resolution is true for
a. narrow transmit beam
b. broad transmit beam
c. both narrow and broad transmit beams
d. neither narrow nor broad transmit beams

111. Simultaneous grayscale, color-Doppler, and spectral-Doppler applies to
a. narrow transmit beam
b. broad transmit beam
c. both narrow and broad transmit beams
d. neither narrow nor broad transmit beams

112. Narrow transmit beam instruments yield higher frame rates than broad transmit beam instruments. True or false?
a. true
b. false

113. Broad transmit beams enable the entire image to be in focus. True or false?
a. true
b. false

114. Broad transmit beam instruments produce laser-thin ultrasound beams. True or false?
a. true
b. false

115. Multiple transmit focuses degrade temporal resolution with
a. narrow transmit beam
b. broad transmit beam
c. both narrow and broad transmit beams
d. neither narrow nor broad transmit beams

116. Reception focus applies to
a. narrow transmit beam
b. broad transmit beam
c. both narrow and broad transmit beams
d. neither narrow nor broad transmit beams

5

Instruments for Imaging Motion and Flow

LEARNING OBJECTIVES

After reading this chapter, the student should be able to do the following:

- List and compare the various kinds of flow encountered in blood circulation.
- Explain how a stenosis affects flow.
- Define and discuss the Doppler effect, the Doppler shift, and the Doppler angle.
- Explain how flow detection is localized to a specific site in tissue by using pulsed Doppler techniques.
- Describe spectral analysis.
- Discuss examples of how spectral analysis is applied to evaluate flow conditions at the site of measurement and proximal and distal to it.
- Explain how two-dimensional flow information is color-encoded on a grayscale image.
- Compare Doppler-velocity with power Doppler color flow displays.
- List improvements in motion and flow imaging with broad transmit beams.

CHAPTER OUTLINE

Flow
Doppler Effect
Spectral Doppler Displays
Color Doppler Displays
Motion and Flow Imaging With Broad Transmit Beams

KEY TERMS

Autocorrelation
Baseline shift
Bernoulli effect
Clutter
Color Doppler display
Compliance
Continuous wave Doppler
Cosine
Disturbed flow
Doppler angle
Doppler effect
Doppler equation
Doppler shift
Doppler spectrum
Duplex mode
Eddies
Ensemble length
Fast Fourier transform
Filter
Flow
Fluid
Frequency spectrum
Gate
Hue
Inertia
Laminar flow
Luminance
M-mode
Parabolic flow
Phase quadrature
Plug flow
Poise
Poiseuille equation
Power Doppler display
Priority
Pulsatile flow
Pulsed Doppler
Range gating
Resistance
Sample volume
Saturation
Scan line
Spectral analysis
Spectral broadening
Spectral Doppler display
Spectrum analyzer
Stenosis
Streamlines
Tissue Doppler imaging
Turbulence
Variance
Virtual beamforming
Viscosity
Volumetric flow rate
Wall filter
Window

In addition to anatomical imaging, ultrasound can also detect and display information about motion. Motions of interest diagnostically include (cardiac) tissue motion of the beating heart and the motion of the resulting blood **flow** within the circulation. Tissue motion can be detected directly in **M-mode** or by using the **Doppler effect**, which is also how blood flow is detected with ultrasound. In this chapter, we first consider characteristics of blood flow in the human circulatory system, the flow that will be detected, quantified, and evaluated with Doppler ultrasound. Next, we discuss details of the Doppler effect and how the motion information is presented in audible and visual such as *spectral Doppler* and *color Doppler*.

FLOW

The circulatory system consists of the heart, arteries, arterioles, capillaries, venules, and veins, altogether containing approximately 5 L of blood. The heart is the pump that produces blood flow through the circulatory system. It is a contracting and relaxing muscle (the myocardium) with four chambers: two atria and two ventricles. Blood flows from the superior and inferior vena cava and pulmonary veins into the right and left atria, respectively, and from there into the ventricles. From the left and right ventricles, blood flows into the aorta and pulmonary artery, respectively. When the heart contracts, the result (under normal conditions) is forward flow into the aorta and pulmonary artery. Valves are present in the heart to permit forward flow and prevent reverse flow. Malfunctioning valves can restrict forward flow by not opening sufficiently (**stenosis**) or allow reverse flow by not closing completely (insufficiency or regurgitation). Doppler ultrasound is useful to detect both of these conditions.

Flow in the heart, arteries, and veins can be detected with Doppler ultrasound. The capillaries are the tiniest vessels, measuring 5 to 10 μm in diameter or 0.005 to 0.010 mm. The human body contains approximately 1 billion capillaries. Across the capillary walls, the exchange of gases, nutrients, and waste products within the cells takes place, sustaining their life. This is the role of the circulatory system.

Fluid

Matter generally is classified into three categories: gas, liquid, and solid. Gases and liquids are **fluids**; that is, they are substances that flow and conform to the shape of their containers. To flow is to move in a stream, continually changing position and, possibly, direction. Water can flow downstream in a river or through a garden hose. Air can flow through a fan. Similarly, blood flows through the heart, arteries, capillaries, and veins.

> Gases and liquids are fluids, materials that flow.

Viscosity is the **resistance** to flow offered by a fluid in motion. Viscosity is given in units of kilogram per meter-second (kg/m-s) or in **poise**. One poise is 1 g/cm-s or 0.1 kg/m-s. Water has a relatively low viscosity compared with molasses, for example, which has a high viscosity. The viscosity of blood plasma is approximately 50% greater than that of water. The viscosity of normal blood ranges from 0.0035 kg/m-s (or 0.035 poise) to 0.0050 kg/m-s (or 0.050 poise) at 37°C, approximately five times that of water. Blood viscosity can vary from approximately 0.002 kg/m-s (or 0.02 poise; with anemia) to approximately 0.010 kg/m-s (or 0.02 poise; with polycythemia). Blood viscosity also varies with flow speed.

> Viscosity is the resistance of a fluid to flow.

Pressure, Resistance, and Volumetric Flow

Pressure is the force driving fluid flow. Pressure is force per unit area expressed as N/m^2 or Pascal (Pa). Pressure is equally distributed throughout a static fluid and exerts its force in all directions. Hydrostatic pressure is a term that describes the force of gravity on a volume of static fluid. A pressure difference is required for flow to occur. If the pressure is greater at one end than of a liquid-filled tube at the other, the liquid will flow from the higher pressure end to the lower pressure end (while equal pressure applied at both ends will result in no flow). A pressure difference can be generated by a pump (e.g., the heart in the circulatory system) or by the force of gravity (e.g., by raising one end of a tube higher than the other). This is the situation in the lower extremity veins in a standing person, and therefore these vessels have valves to prevent reverse flow. The greater the pressure difference, the greater the flow rate. This pressure difference is often referred to as the *pressure gradient* (although, strictly defined, pressure gradient is the pressure difference *divided by the distance between the two pressure locations*). While the pressure decreases from one end of the tube to the other, this decrease can be thought of as a slope (i.e., the pressure difference divided by the distance over which the pressure drop occurs; Fig. 5.1). A constant driving pressure produces steady flow (i.e., the flow doesn't change over time). The driving pressure produced by the heart varies with time (as in the cardiac cycle). This concept will be considered in more detail later in this section.

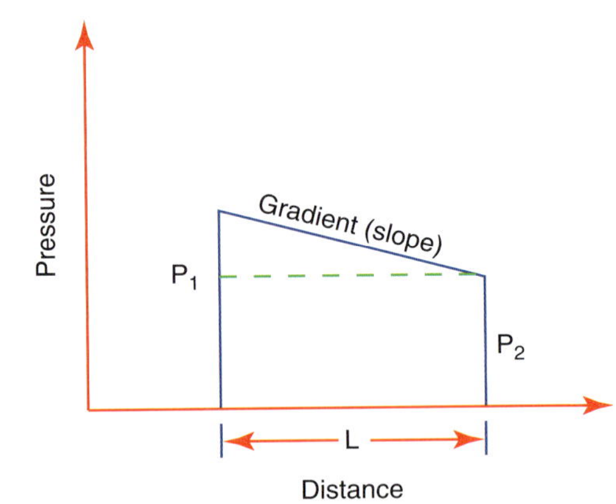

Fig. 5.1 The pressure gradient or slope is the pressure difference ($P_1 - P_2$) divided by the separation (L) between the two pressure locations.

> Fluid flow in a tube is a response to a pressure difference between the ends of the tube.

Volumetric flow rate (Q) (commonly called *flow*) refers to the volume of blood passing a point per unit of time. Volumetric flow rate is usually expressed in milliliters per minute or per second. The total adult blood flow rate (cardiac output) is approximately 5000 mL/min (i.e., the total blood volume circulates through the body in approximately 1 minute). The volumetric flow rate in a long straight tube is determined not only by the pressure difference (ΔP measured in Pa) but also by the resistance (R measured in kg/m-s) to flow.

$$Q(mL/s) = \frac{\Delta P(Pa)}{R(kg/m-s)}$$

> If the pressure difference increases, then the volumetric flow rate also increases.

> If the resistance to flow increases, then the volumetric flow rate decreases.

The flow resistance in the human circulation cannot be expressed in a simple equation. However, the specific situation of a long, straight tube is much simpler and here resistance depends on the fluid viscosity (v) and the tube length (L) and radius (r), as follows:

$$R(g/cm^4 - s) = 8 \times L(cm) \times \frac{v(kg/m-s)}{\pi \times r^4 (cm^4)}$$

From this equation, we can see that an increase in viscosity or tube length increases resistance, whereas an increase in the radius or diameter of the tube decreases resistance. The latter effect is particularly strong, with resistance depending on radius to the fourth power (r^4). Thus doubling the radius of a tube decreases its resistance to one-sixteenth its original value. From experience, we know that a longer or smaller (in radius) garden hose reduces water flow. Likewise, if we tried to force a higher viscosity fluid, such as molasses, through a hose, we would not get nearly the flow rate that we would with water.

Poiseuille Equation

If we combine the flow resistance equation and the flow rate equation above, while replacing radius with tube diameter (d), we get the **Poiseuille equation** for volumetric flow rate:

$$Q(mL/s) = \frac{\Delta P(Pa) \times \pi \times d^4 (cm^4)}{128 \times L(cm) \times v\ (kg/m-s)}$$

It is important to remember that this equation is **only** valid for steady flow in long, straight tubes. Thus it provides only a rough approximation to the conditions encountered in human blood circulation. The equation is useful, however, in making qualitative conclusions and predictions, and the relationships that it describes are referred to as **Poiseuille's law**.

> If pressure difference increases, flow rate increases.

> If diameter increases, flow rate increases.

> If length increases, flow rate decreases.

> If viscosity increases, flow rate decreases.

The resistance of the arterioles accounts for approximately half of the total resistance in the systemic circulation. The muscular walls of arterioles can constrict or relax, producing dramatic changes in flow resistance. This is how the vessel walls control blood flow to specific tissues and organs in response to their needs.

> **Poiseuille's law** states that the volumetric flow rate in a tube depends on the pressure difference, the length and diameter of the tube, and the viscosity of the fluid.

Types of Flow

Flow can be divided into five categories: (1) plug, (2) laminar, (3) parabolic, (4) disturbed, and (5) turbulent depending on its spatial distribution. At the entrance to a tube, the speed of the fluid is essentially constant across the tube (Fig. 5.2). This is called **plug flow** because it is similar to the motion of a solid object (such as a plug) that does not flow but moves as a unit. Plug flow is a special form of **laminar flow**. Laminar flow (meaning flow in layers) is a flow condition in which **streamlines** (which describe the motion paths of fluid particles) are straight and parallel. While the fluid flows down the tube, **parabolic flow** develops (Fig. 5.3). Flow speed is maximum at the center of the tube and minimum (including zero) at the tube walls. A decreasing profile of flow speeds from the center to the wall is present. Successive layers of fluid slide over each other with relative motion. The pressure

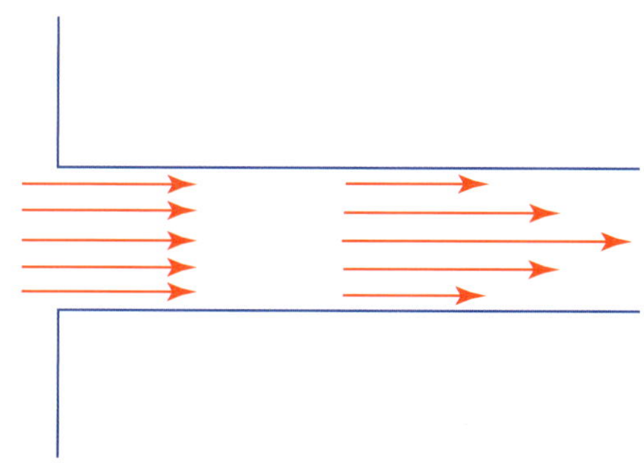

Fig. 5.2 At the entrance to a tube or vessel, plug flow exists. After some distance, laminar flow is achieved.

difference between each end of the tube overcomes the viscous resistance of the layers sliding over each other, maintaining the laminar flow throughout the tube. Steady flow in a long, straight tube results in a parabolic flow profile. Parabolic flow is a particular pattern of laminar flow in which varying flow speeds across the tube are described by a parabola (see the curved dashed line in Fig. 5.3). In the case of parabolic flow, the average flow speed across the vessel is equal to one-half of the maximum flow speed (i.e., at the center). Parabolic flow is not commonly seen in blood circulation, because blood vessels generally are not long and straight. However, nonparabolic laminar flow is commonly seen; indeed, its absence is often an indicator of abnormal flow conditions at a site where there is vascular or cardiac-valvular disease.

> Laminar flow is flow in which layers of fluid slide over each other in straight lines.

Disturbed flow occurs when the parallel streamlines describing the flow (see Fig. 5.2) are altered from their straight form (Fig. 5.4). This occurs, for example, in the region of a stenosis or at a bifurcation where a vessel splits into two. In disturbed flow, particles of fluid still flow in the forward direction. Parabolic and disturbed flows are both forms of laminar flow.

In the final category, turbulent flow, or **turbulence**, the flow pattern is random and chaotic, with particles moving at different speeds in many directions, even in circles called **eddies**, with forward net flow still maintained. While flow speed increases in a tube, turbulent flow eventually will occur (Fig. 5.5). Turbulence may also occur in the transition from high flow speed in a narrow tube to slower flow in a broad tube, such as when the flow from the common carotid artery enters the carotid bulb (Fig. 5.6).

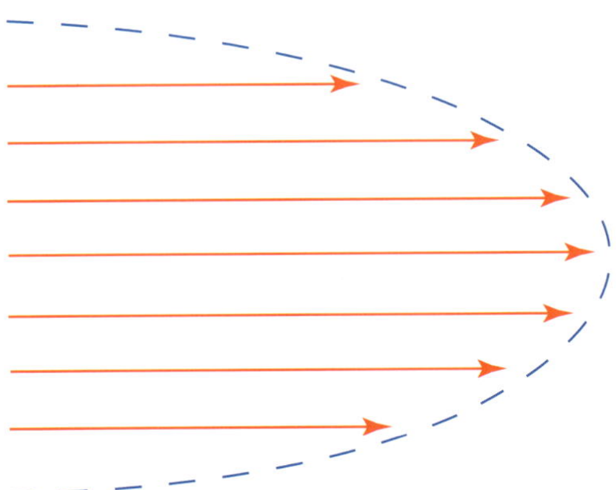

Fig. 5.3 Parabolic flow profile. The *dashed line* is a parabola.

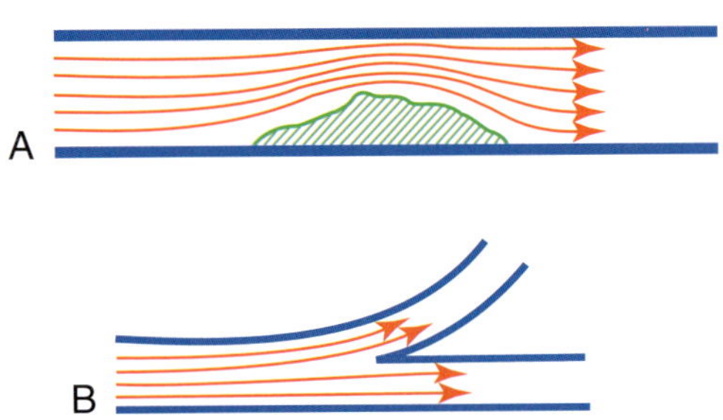

Fig. 5.4 Disturbed flow at a stenosis **(A)** and at a bifurcation **(B)**.

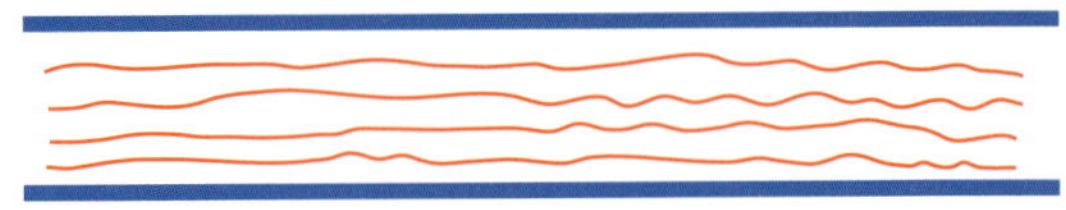

Fig. 5.5 Turbulent flow in a vessel may result from too great a flow speed.

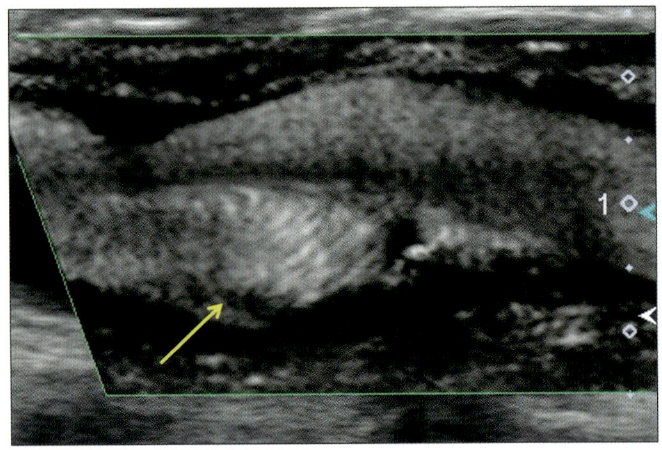

Fig. 5.6 As the flow from the common carotid artery enters the carotid bulb a distal area of flow reversal and turbulence can be seen (*yellow arrow*).

> **Disturbed flow** is a form of laminar flow in which streamlines are not straight. Turbulent flow is nonlaminar flow with random and chaotic speeds and directions.

Pulsatile Flow

Thus far, we have considered steady flow in which pressures, flow speeds, and flow patterns do not change over time. This is generally the situation on the venous side of the circulatory system, although cardiac pulsations or respiratory cycles can influence venous flow in some locations, such as the inferior venae cava or IVC. However, in the heart and the arterial circulation, flow is pulsatile, being controlled by the beating heart with pulsatile variations of increasing and decreasing pressure and flow speed. For steady flow, volumetric flow rate is simply related to pressure difference and flow resistance. With **pulsatile flow**, the relationship between the varying pressure and flow rate depends on flow impedance, which includes resistance, as discussed earlier; the **inertia** of the fluid as it accelerates and decelerates; and the **compliance** (expansion and contraction) of the nonrigid vessel walls. The mathematical analysis is complex and will not be presented here.

Instead, we will focus on two dominant characteristics of interest in pulsatile flow, which are the Windkessel effect and flow reversal. When the pressure pulse forces a fluid into a compliant vessel, such as the aorta, the vessel expands and increases the volume within. (This is why it is easy to feel the pulse on the wrist or neck.) Later in the cycle, when the driving pressure is reduced, the compliant vessel is able to contract, producing extended flow later in the pressure cycle. This process is known as the *Windkessel effect*. In the aorta, the Windkessel effect results in continued

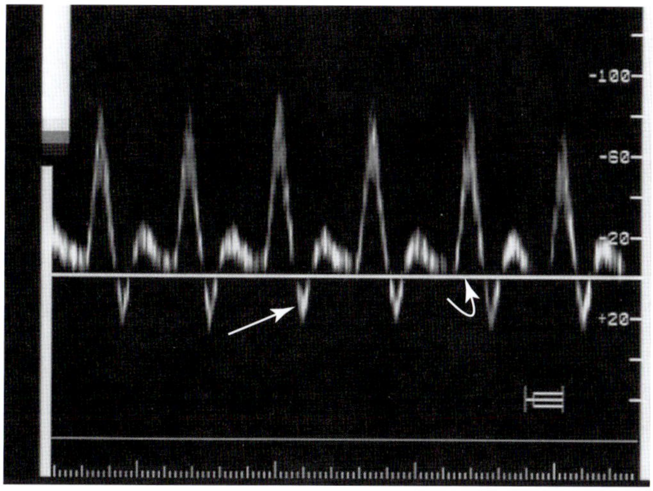

Fig. 5.7 Flow reversal (*straight arrow*) below the baseline (*curved arrow*) is seen in the superficial femoral artery in diastole.

flow in the forward direction because aortic valve closure prevents backward flow into the heart. In the distal circulation, the expansion of distensible vessels results in the reversal of flow in diastole, while the pressure decreases and the distended vessels contract. Flow reversal is a normal occurrence where there are no valves to prevent it (Fig. 5.7). Pulsatile flow in compliant vessels thus, includes added forward flow and/or flow reversal in diastole, depending on the location within the arterial circulation. Arterial diastolic flow (absence, presence, direction, quantity) reveals much information concerning the state of downstream arterioles, where flow cannot be measured directly with ultrasound.

> Pulsatile flow is nonsteady flow, with acceleration and deceleration over the cardiac cycle.

> Pulsatile flow in distensible vessels includes added forward flow and/or flow reversal over the cardiac cycle in some locations within the circulation.

Continuity Rule

A narrowing of the lumen of a vessel, or a stenosis, produces disturbed (see Fig. 5.4) and possibly turbulent flow (see Fig. 5.6). The average flow speed in the stenosis must be greater than the average flow speed proximal and distal to the stenosis so that the volumetric flow rate is constant throughout the vessel. Volumetric flow rate must be constant in all three regions—proximal to the stenosis, at the stenosis, and distal to the stenosis—because blood is neither created nor destroyed while it flows through a vessel. This concept is called the continuity rule.

> Flow speed increases at a stenosis, and turbulence can occur distal to it.

The volumetric flow rate is equal to the average flow speed across the vessel multiplied by the cross-sectional area of the vessel. Therefore, if a stenosis has an area measuring one-half of the area of the proximal and distal vessel, the average flow speed within the stenosis is twice the average flow speed proximal and distal to the stenosis. If a stenosis has a diameter that is one-half the diameter of the adjacent area, the area at the stenosis is one-fourth that of the adjacent area, so the average flow speed in the stenosis must increase by a factor of 4 (i.e., quadruple).

The apparent contradiction of Poiseuille's law and the continuity rule for a stenosis is sometimes puzzling to students. Poiseuille's law states that flow speed decreases with smaller diameters, whereas the continuity rule says that flow speed increases with smaller diameters. How can this be so? The answer is that the two situations are different. Poiseuille's law deals with a long, straight vessel with no stenosis. The diameter in Poiseuille's law refers to the diameter of the *entire vessel*. By contrast, the diameter in the continuity rule refers to the diameter of a short portion of a vessel (i.e., the stenosis). If the diameter of the entire vessel is reduced (as in vasoconstriction), flow speed is reduced. If the diameter of only a short segment of a vessel is reduced (stenosis), the flow speed in the vessel is unaffected, except at the stenosis, where it is increased. Flow speed increases because the stenosis has little effect on the overall flow resistance of the entire vessel if the stenosis length is small compared with the vessel length and if the lumen in the stenosis is not too small (does not approach complete occlusion). Fig. 5.8 illustrates these dependencies of volumetric flow rate and flow speed at the stenosis with increasing stenosis. The maximum normal flow speed in the circulation is approximately 100 cm/s. However, in stenotic regions, flow speeds can increase to a few meters per second. Doppler ultrasound is useful for detecting flow speed increases that are associated with vascular disease.

The increased flow speed within a stenosis can cause turbulence distal to the stenosis. Sounds produced by turbulence, which can be heard with a stethoscope, are called bruits. The ultimate stenosis is called an *occlusion*, in which the vessel is blocked and there is no flow. Using our garden hose analogy again, we can compress the hose (not near the nozzle) and see little effect on the flow at the nozzle until the hose is compressed to near occlusion. At that point, turbulence may occur, and vibration can be felt on the surface of the hose.

Bernoulli Effect

At a stenosis, the pressure is less than it is proximal and distal to the stenotic area (Fig. 5.9). This pressure difference (i.e., decrease within a stenosis) is necessary to allow the fluid to accelerate into the stenosis and decelerate out of it and also to maintain volumetric flow rate continuity. This difference in pressure across regions of high flow speed is known as the **Bernoulli effect** and is described by the Bernoulli equation (ignoring viscous losses and height differences). The difference in pressure (ΔP) that results a region with two different flow speeds (v_1 and v_2) is

$$\Delta P = \tfrac{1}{2}\rho(v_2^2 - v_1^2)$$

where ρ is the density of blood (about 1060 kg/m^3). In an even more simplified form of the equation, specifically describing a stenosis, the flow speed proximal to the stenosis is assumed to be small enough, compared with the flow speed in the stenosis,

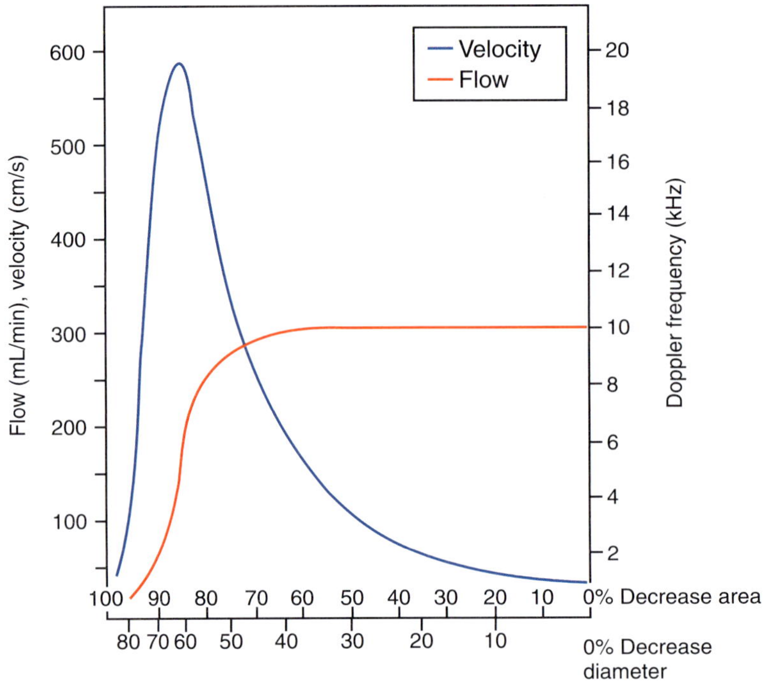

Fig. 5.8 As the diameter of the stenosis is reduced (moving to the left on the horizontal axis; tighter stenosis), volumetric flow rate (Q) is unaffected initially because the stenosis does not contribute substantially to the total vessel resistance. While the diameter continues to decrease, however, the vessel resistance increases, reducing the volumetric flow rate (eventually to zero at occlusion). Flow rate and, thus, distal pressure begin to drop significantly beyond a diameter reduction of approximately 50% (area reduction of 75%). While the diameter of the stenosis decreases, the flow speed increases (because of the flow continuity requirement), reaches a maximum, and then decreases to zero as the increasing flow resistance effect dominates. (Modified from Spencer MP, Reid JM: Quantitation of carotid stenosis with continuous-wave (C-W) Doppler ultrasound, *Stroke* 10:326–330, 1979.)

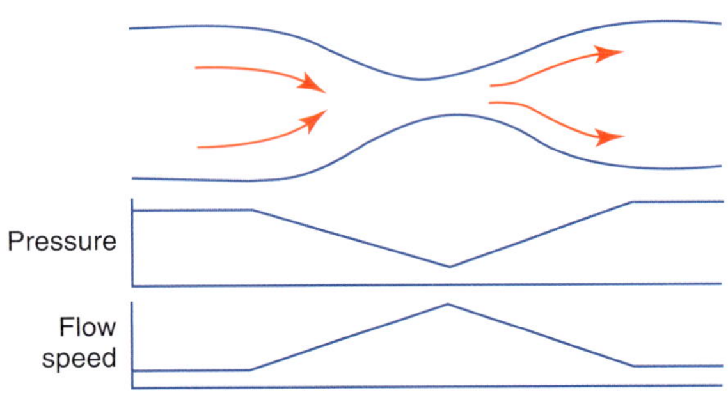

Fig. 5.9 To maintain flow continuity, flow speed must increase through a stenosis. In conjunction with this, the pressure drops (the Bernoulli effect) in the stenosis. (From Kremkau FW: Fluid flow III, *J Vasc Technol* 17:153–154, 1993.)

to be ignored. Hence, calculating pressure drop across a stenosis or a stenotic valve uses the following form of the equation:

$$\Delta P \sim 4(v_2)^2$$

where v_2 is the flow speed (meters/second) in the jet and ΔP (millimeters of mercury or mmHg) is the pressure drop across the valve. For example, if the flow speed in the jet is 5 m/s, the pressure drop is 100 mmHg. Thus pressure drop can be calculated from a measurement of flow speed at the stenotic valve by using Doppler ultrasound.

> If flow speed increases, the magnitude of the pressure drop increases.

> The Bernoulli effect is a reduction in pressure associated with high flow speed at a stenosis.

DOPPLER EFFECT

The Doppler effect is a change in frequency (and wavelength) caused by the relative motion of a sound source, receiver, or reflector. If a reflector is moving toward the source and receiver, the received echo has a higher frequency that would occur without the motion. Conversely, if the motion is away (receding) from the source and receiver, the received echo has a lower frequency. The amount of increase or decrease in frequency depends on the relative speed of the reflector, the angle between the wave propagation direction and the direction of motion, and the frequency of the wave emitted by the source.

A quantitative description of the Doppler effect is provided by the **Doppler equation**. A moving reflector (Fig. 5.10) or scatterer of a wave is a combination of a receiver and a source moving relative to each other. In diagnostic ultrasound, the most common scenario is a moving reflector approaching a stationary source, which means more cycles of a wave are encountered in 1 second than if the reflector were stationary.

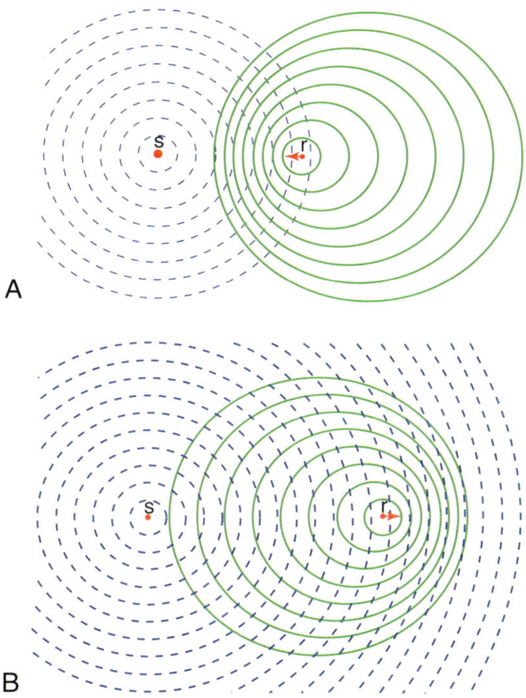

Fig. 5.10 A moving reflector (*r*) returns a higher frequency echo if it is approaching the source and receiver (*s*) **(A)** and a lower frequency echo if it is moving away from the source and receiver **(B)**.

This is because the reflected cycles are compressed in front of the reflector, while it moves into its own reflected wave. This reduction in wavelength increases the frequency of the reflected wave (echo).

Doppler Shift

The change in frequency caused by motion is called the Doppler-shift frequency or, more commonly, the **Doppler shift** (f_D). The Doppler shift is equal to the received frequency (fR) minus the frequency transmitted by the source (f_T). For an approaching reflector (scatterer), the Doppler shift is positive; that is, the received frequency is greater than the source frequency. For a receding reflector moving away from the source, the Doppler shift is negative; that is, the received frequency is smaller than the source frequency. The relationship between the Doppler shift and the reflector speed (v) is expressed by the simplified Doppler equation (which only considers motion directly toward or away from the source):

$$f_D(\text{kHz}) = f_R(\text{kHz}) - f_T(\text{kHz}) = f_T(\text{kHz}) \times \frac{2 \times v(\text{cm/s})}{c(\text{cm/s})}$$

> If the scatterer speed increases, the Doppler shift increases. If source frequency increases, the Doppler shift increases.

> The Doppler shift is the difference between the transmitted and the received frequency (i.e., the echo frequency returning from moving scatterers).

TABLE 5.1 Doppler Frequency Shifts for Various Scatterer Speeds Toward[a] the Sound Source at a Zero Doppler Angle

Incident Frequency (MHz)	Scatterer Speed (cm/s)	Reflected Frequency (MHz)	Doppler Shift (kHz)
2	50	2.0013	1.3
5	50	5.0032	3.2
10	50	10.0065	6.5
2	200	2.0052	5.2
5	200	5.013	13.0
10	200	10.026	26.0

[a]Motion away from the source would yield negative Doppler shifts.

Take, for example, a source frequency of 5 MHz, and a scatterer speed of 50 cm/s (0.5 m/s) relative to a propagation (sound) speed of 1540 m/s. When the scatterer is approaching the source, the received frequency is greater than the source frequency, producing a positive Doppler shift of 0.0032 MHz or 3.2 kHz. For a scatterer moving away from a receiver, the Doppler shift is −3.2 kHz. Other examples that use various source frequencies and scatterer speeds are given in Table 5.1.

ADVANCED CONCEPTS

The Doppler effect occurs for a moving source (Fig. 5.11) or receiver (detector) (Fig. 5.12) and for relative motion between them. The Doppler equation for a source moving at speed v_s is

$$f_D = f_T\left(\frac{v_s}{c - v_s}\right)$$

And the equation for a receiver moving at speed v_r is

$$f_D = f_T\left(\frac{v_r}{c}\right)$$

A moving reflector (Fig. 5.10) is a combined moving receiver and source. For a reflector moving at speed v, the Doppler equation is

$$f_D = f_T\left(\frac{2v}{c - v}\right)$$

For example, if $f_T = 5$ MHz, $v = 5$ m/s (500 cm/s), and $c = 1540$ m/s. The Doppler shift f_D is then 0.032 MHz (or 32 kHz).

Physiologic blood flow speeds, even in extreme cases, are less than 1% of the speed of sound in tissues. Because blood flow speed is small compared with sound speed, it may be ignored in the denominator of the foregoing Doppler equation, yielding the commonly used simplified form of the Doppler equation for a moving reflector given above. Using the same values as in the previous example yields $f_D = 32$ kHz again.

The factor of two in the Doppler equation (for a moving reflector or scatterer) is the result of two Doppler shifts: (1) the Doppler shift that occurs when a moving receiver (the scatterer) encounters the wave, and (2) the Doppler shift that occurs when the moving emitter (the scatterer again) reradiates the wave. Another way to view the factor of two is to consider the transducer to be the source and receiver of sound separated by the round-trip sound path distance, which is twice the distance from the transducer to the reflector. As the reflector approaches or recedes from the transducer, this round-trip distance is reduced at a rate that is double the speed of the reflector.

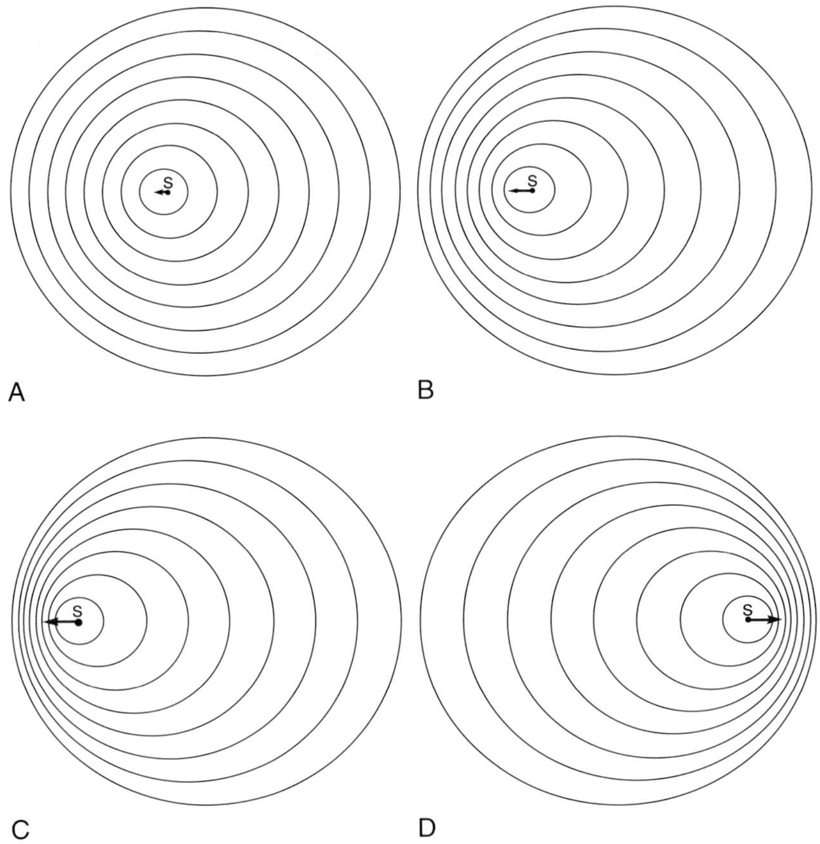

Fig. 5.11 A moving source of sound *(s)* produces a shorter wavelength (higher frequency) ahead of it and a longer wavelength (lower frequency) behind it compared with the wavelengths at the sides, which are the same as for a stationary source. **A,** Slow speed. **B,** Medium speed. **C,** High speed. **D,** High-speed movement in the opposite direction.

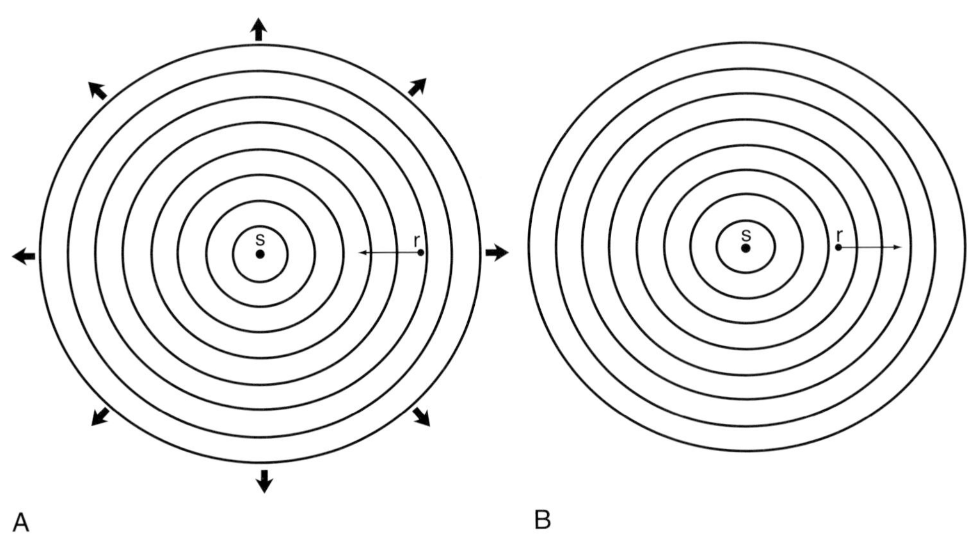

Fig. 5.12 **A,** A receiver (*r*) moving toward the source (*s*) experiences a higher frequency (more cycles per second) than a stationary one would because it is moving against the sound propagation direction. **B,** A receiver moving away from the source experiences a lower frequency than a stationary one would because it is moving along with the sound propagation direction.

However, in diagnostic ultrasound—specifically Doppler ultrasound—we are interested in the speed of the blood flow or (less often) tissue motion, not the Doppler shift itself. To facilitate this, the Doppler equation is rearranged to place the velocity alone on the left side of the equation. Substituting the speed of sound in tissues (154,000 cm/s) and by using units as indicated for the various quantities, the equation becomes:

$$v(\text{cm/s}) = \frac{77(\text{cm/ms}) \times f_D(\text{kHz})}{f_T(\text{MHz})}$$

ADVANCED CONCEPTS

The speed of sound used in the Doppler equation is the average speed of sound in soft tissues: 1540 m/s or 1.54 mm/μs. Using the speed of sound in blood (1570–1575 m/s) is tempting. Strictly speaking, however, this is not appropriate because the scatterers (blood cells) are not moving through their medium (blood plasma) but along with it; that is, there is no relative motion between the cells and their suspending medium to produce a Doppler shift. Where then does the Doppler shift occur? Doppler shift occurs where the relative motion exists, that is, at the blood-intima boundary for plug flow, in which case the tissue sound speed is relevant. For other types of flow (laminar, disturbed, and turbulent), relative motion occurs between flow layers (laminae), and some (unknown) combination of sound speeds for tissue and blood would be appropriate. Fortunately, this level of accuracy is not required for Doppler techniques to be useful.

The Doppler equation relates the flow speed to Doppler shift and transmit frequency.

The fact that the Doppler shift is proportional to the blood flow speed explains why the Doppler effect is so useful in medical diagnosis. Blood flow is what interests us and the Doppler shift is measured in a Doppler mode and the Doppler equation is solved to yield the flow speed information.

Doppler Ultrasound

With diagnostic medical ultrasound, stationary transducers are used to transmit and receive the ultrasound. The Doppler effect is a result of the motion of blood, the flow of which we wish to measure, or the motion of tissue that we wish to evaluate. Physiologic flow speeds, even in highly stenotic jets, do not exceed a few meters per second and the corresponding Doppler shifts are shown in Table 5.1. Detectable blood flow speed with Doppler ultrasound ranges from a few millimeters per second to a few meters per second, depending on the measurement parameters.

The Doppler shift is proportional to flow speed.

Operating Frequency

For a given flow in a vessel, the Doppler shift measured is proportional to the operating frequency of the instrument (Fig. 5.13; also see Table 5.1). Thus measuring the same flow in the same vessel using two transducers operating at 2 and 4

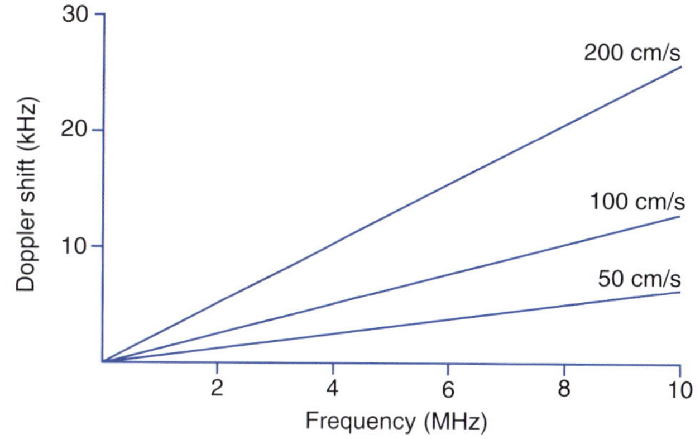

Fig. 5.13 The Doppler shift as a function of operating frequency, as determined by the Doppler equation for various flow speeds (at a zero Doppler angle).

MHz will yield two different Doppler shifts. The higher frequency transducer will have a Doppler shift that is twice that of the lower frequency transducer. Therefore when comparing Doppler shifts, one must consider the transmit frequency of the transducer employed. The operating frequency is incorporated into the calculation of flow speed through the Doppler equation. Thus comparisons of flow speeds between different instruments and transducers have taken this variable into account.

The Doppler shift is proportional to the operating frequency.

Doppler frequencies used in vascular studies are lower than those used for anatomical imaging (i.e., B-mode), because echoes from blood are a lot weaker than echoes from soft tissues (by 40–100 dB).

Doppler Angle

If the direction of sound propagation is exactly opposite the flow direction, the maximum positive Doppler shift is obtained, as described in the simplified Doppler equation. Likewise, if the flow speed and propagation speed directions are the same (parallel), the maximum negative Doppler shift is obtained. However, if the angle between these two directions (Fig. 5.14) is nonzero (nonparallel), lesser Doppler shifts will occur. The Doppler shift depends on the cosine of the Doppler angle (θ) and the Doppler Equation becomes:

$$f_D(\text{kHz}) = \frac{f_T(\text{kHz}) \times 2 \times v(\text{cm/s}) \times \cos\theta}{c(\text{cm/s})}$$

$$v(\text{cm/s}) = \frac{77(\text{cm/ms}) \times f_D(\text{kHz})}{f_T(\text{MHz}) \times \cos\theta}$$

Table 5.2 gives cosine values for various angles. Only the portion of the motion direction that is parallel to the sound beam contributes to the Doppler effect. The cosine gives the component of the flow velocity vector that is parallel to the sound beam (Fig. 5.15). For a given flow, the larger the Doppler angle, the less the Doppler shift (see Fig. 5.14, B–C). Table 5.3 lists examples of Doppler shifts for various angles.

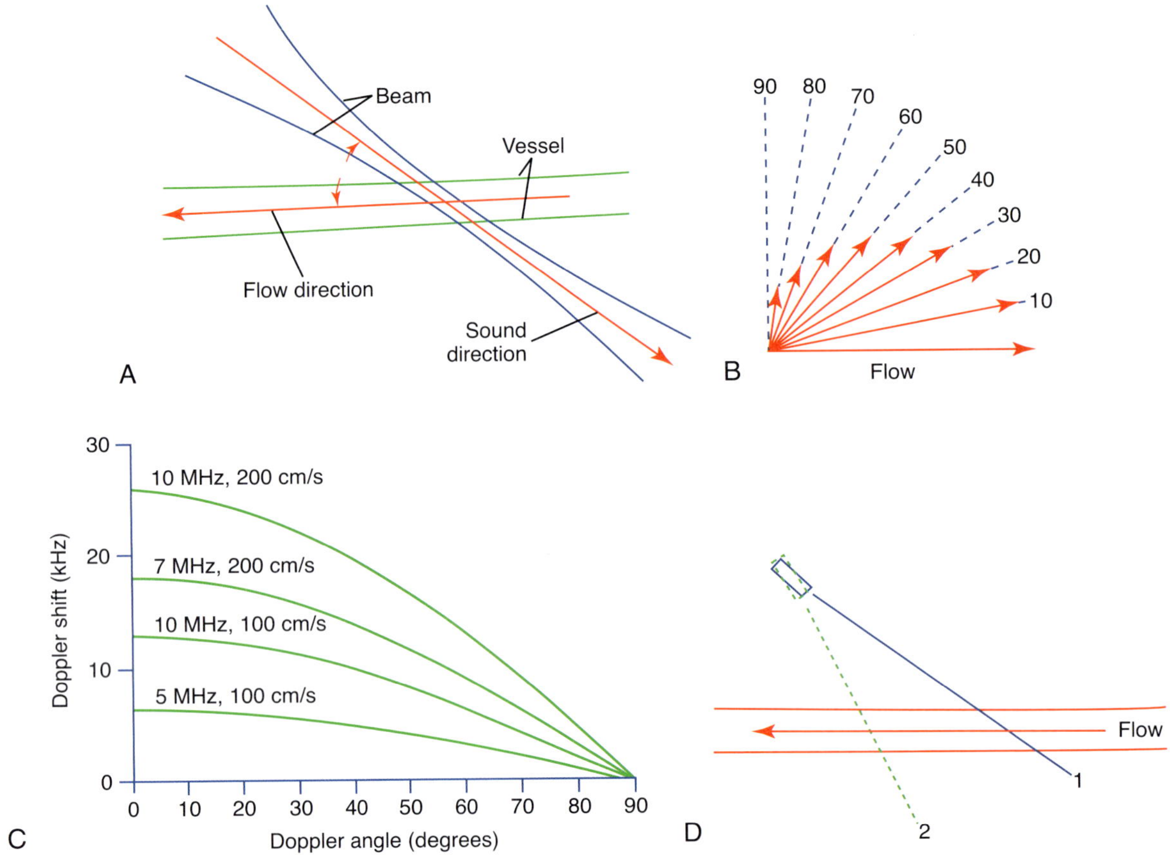

Fig. 5.14 **A,** The Doppler angle θ is the angle between the direction of flow and the sound propagation direction. **B,** With constant flow, while the Doppler angle increases, echo Doppler-shift frequency decreases. The length of the *arrows* indicates the magnitude of the Doppler shift as the Doppler angle increases. **C,** The Doppler shifts as a function of angle, as determined by the Doppler equation for various incident frequencies and scatterer speeds. **D,** The same flow in a vessel, viewed at different angles, yields different Doppler shifts.

TABLE 5.2 Cosines for Various Angles

Angle A (Degrees)	Cosine A
0	1.000
5	0.996
10	0.98
15	0.97
20	0.94
25	0.91
30	0.87
35	0.82
40	0.77
45	0.71
50	0.64
55	0.57
60	0.50
65	0.42
70	0.34
75	0.26
80	0.17
85	0.09
90	0.00

Notice that for a 90-degree Doppler angle, the Doppler shift is zero (as cos 90 = 0), irrespective of the blood flow velocity being interrogated.

> If the cosine increases, the calculated scatterer speed decreases.

> If the Doppler angle increases, the calculated scatterer speed increases.

Doppler displays present information on the presence, direction, speed, and character of blood flow (Box 5.1) and on the presence, direction, and speed of tissue motion. This information is presented in audible, color Doppler, and/or spectral Doppler forms (Box 5.2).

SPECTRAL DOPPLER DISPLAYS

Initial instrumentation for Doppler measurements of flow in the heart and in blood vessels used spectral Doppler operating in either continuous wave (CW) or pulsed wave (PW) mode. CW operation is based on two separate transducers (or groups of transducer elements) and detects Doppler-shifted echoes in

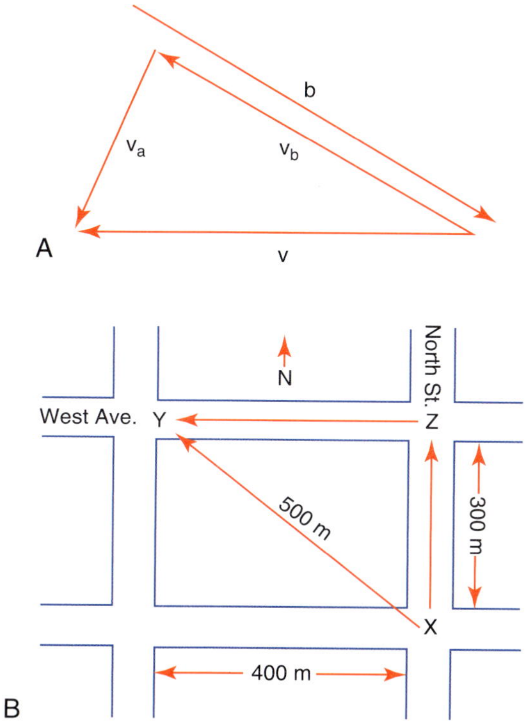

Fig. 5.15 A, The flow velocity vector (*v*) can be broken into two components: one (v_b) that is parallel to the sound beam (*b*) direction and one (v_a) that is perpendicular to the sound beam direction. Only the component parallel to the beam contributes to the Doppler effect. **B,** A city block can be used as an analogy to the vector components in A. To get from point X to point Y, one could walk diagonally across the block, a distance of 500 m. However, if buildings blocked that path, an alternative route would be 300 m north on North Street and then 400 m west on West Avenue. The 500-m northwest vector from X to Y is equivalent to a 300-m north vector plus a 400-m west vector (i.e., the result is the same: depart from X and arrive at Y). In this example, the component of the XY vector parallel to North Street is the XZ vector, and the component parallel to West Avenue is the ZY vector.

TABLE 5.3 Doppler Frequency Shifts for Various Angles and Scatterer Speeds Toward the Sound Source of Frequency 5 MHz

Scatterer Speed (cm/s)	Angle (Degrees)	Doppler Shift (kHz)
100	0	6.5
100	30	5.6
100	60	3.2
100	90	0.0
300	0	19.0
300	30	17.0
300	60	9.7
300	0	0.0

the region of overlap between the beams of the transmitting and receiving transducer elements. In PW mode, ultrasound pulses are transmitted and received using a single group of transducer elements (i.e., parts of an array) or even a single-element transducer (in the 1960s and 1970s). The pulses in PW Doppler are longer than those used in imaging to improve the signal-to-noise ratio (SNR) and enable Doppler frequency shift detection. Through **range gating**, PW Doppler has the ability to select information from a particular depth along the beam. To use PW Doppler effectively, it commonly utilized in combination with grayscale ultrasound. Such operation is called *duplex scanning* because of the dual functions (anatomic imaging and flow measurement). CW and PW operations present Doppler-shift information in an audible form and as a visual display.

BOX 5.1 Types of Flow Information Provided by Doppler Ultrasound

- Presence of flow
- Yes
- No
- Direction of flow
  - Forward (toward the transducer)
  - Reverse (away from the transducer)
- Speed of flow
  - Slow
  - Fast
  - Quantitative velocities (cm/s)
- Character of flow
  - Laminar (plug and parabolic)
  - Turbulent

BOX 5.2 Various Forms of Presenting Doppler Information

- Audible sounds
- Spectral display
- Color Doppler display
- Power Doppler display

Continuous Wave Doppler Systems

CW Doppler instruments include a CW oscillator and a Doppler detector that detects the changes in frequency (Doppler shifts) resulting from scatterer motion and presents them as audible sounds and as a visual display corresponding to the motion. A diagram of the components of a CW Doppler system is presented in Fig. 5.16, A. The oscillator produces a continuously alternating voltage typically at a frequency of 2 to 10 MHz, which is applied to the source transducer element. The ultrasound frequency is determined by the oscillator and is set to equal the operating frequency of the transducer. In the transducer assembly, there is a separate receiving transducer element that produces voltages with frequencies equal to the frequencies of the returning echoes. If there is scatterer motion, the reflected ultrasound frequencies and the ultrasound produced by the source transducer will be different. The difference between these two frequencies, which is the Doppler shift, is identified by the Doppler detector and then drives a set of loudspeakers (one for positive and one for negative Doppler shifts or forward and reverse flew) at this frequency. Doppler shifts are typically one-thousandth of the operating frequency,

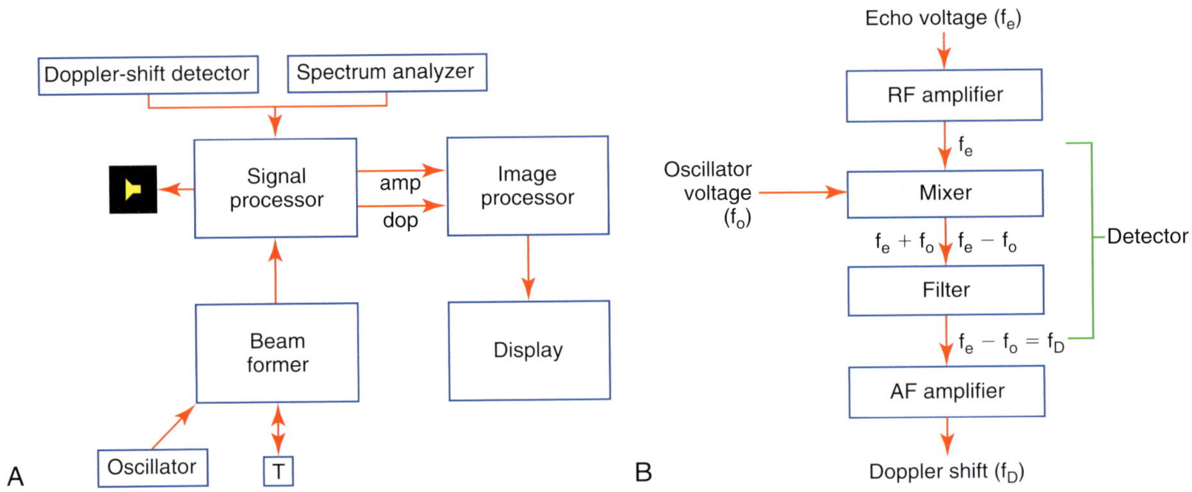

Fig. 5.16 **A,** Block diagram of a sonographic instrument functioning in continuous-wave Doppler mode. The oscillator (part of the beam former) produces a continuously alternating voltage that drives the source transducer element (*T*). The receiving transducer element (*T*) produces a continuous voltage in response to echoes it is continuously receiving. The signal processor includes a Doppler-shift detector that detects differences in frequency between the voltages produced by the oscillator and by the receiving element. The Doppler shifts produce voltages that drive the loudspeakers and a visual display. The frequency of the audible sound is equal to the Doppler shift and is proportional to the reflector speed and to the cosine of the angle between the sound propagation direction and the boundary motion. **B,** Block diagram of a continuous-wave Doppler detector. The radio frequency (*RF*) amplifier increases the echo voltage amplitude. The frequency of the echo voltage is fe. In the mixer, this frequency is combined with the oscillator voltage, the frequency of which is fo. The mixer yields the sum and difference of these two frequency inputs ($f_e + f_o$ and $f_e - f_o$). The low-pass (high-frequency rejection) filter removes $f_e + f_o$, leaving $f_e - f_o$, which is the Doppler-shift frequency (f_D). This frequency then is strengthened in the audio frequency (*AF*) amplifier. The mixer and filter together constitute the Doppler detector.

which puts them in the audible range. Doppler shifts also are commonly sent through a **spectrum analyzer** to a **spectral Doppler display** for visualization and evaluation.

The detector (see Fig. 5.16, B) amplifies the echo voltages it receives from the receiving element, detects the Doppler-shift information in the returning echoes, and determines the motion direction from the sign of the Doppler shift. Doppler shifts are determined by mixing the returning voltages with the CW voltage from the oscillator. This produces the sum and difference of the oscillator and echo frequencies (see Fig. 5.16, B). The difference is the desired Doppler shift. The sum is a much higher frequency (approximately double the operating frequency) and is filtered out. The difference is zero for echoes returning from stationary structures. In the case of echoes from moving structures (e.g., vessel walls) or flowing blood, this difference is the Doppler shift, which provides information about motion and flow (positive or negative).

> The Doppler detector detects Doppler shifts and determines their sign (positive or negative), that is, the direction of the flow.

Positive and negative shifts indicate motion toward and away from the transducer, respectively. The detector shown in Fig. 5.16, B does not provide this directional information. Determining direction and separating Doppler-shift voltages into separate forward and reverse channels is accomplished by the **phase quadrature** detector.

ADVANCED CONCEPTS

In the phase quadrature detector, two voltages from the oscillator (one leading by one-quarter of a cycle [Fig. 5.17], i.e., "quad") are mixed with the returning echo voltages to yield the difference, which is the Doppler shift. The echo voltages contain the Doppler shifts representing flow toward (ft) and away from (fa) the transducer. The filter outputs of the direct channel and the delayed (quadrature) channel are the Doppler shifts from the echo voltage input. If the Doppler shift is positive, the shift in the direct channel lags behind that in the quadrature channel by one-quarter of a cycle (90 degrees). If the Doppler shift is negative, the shift in the quadrature channel lags behind that in the direct channel by one-quarter of a cycle. The Doppler shifts in both of these channels are next shifted by a quarter cycle. A negative Doppler shift in the direct channel at that point leads the one in the quadrature channel (before the additional 90-degree shift) by half a cycle. When added, these two voltages cancel (Fig. 5.18), yielding no output. Positive Doppler shifts in these two channels are in phase (no lead or lag), yielding output from the direct channel adder. Positive shifts in the quadrature channel lead those in the direct channel by half a cycle, whereas negative shifts in the two channels are in phase. Thus the negative shifts are the output of the quadrature channel adder. The outputs of the two adders are sent to separate loudspeakers so that forward and reverse Doppler shifts can be heard separately. The outputs are also sent to a spectral display to show positive and negative Doppler shifts above and below the display baseline, which represents zero Doppler shift.

The forward and reverse channel signals are sent to separate loudspeakers so that forward and reverse Doppler shifts can be heard separately. The signals also are sent to a spectral display to show positive and negative Doppler shifts above and below the display baseline, which represents zero Doppler shift (Fig. 5.19).

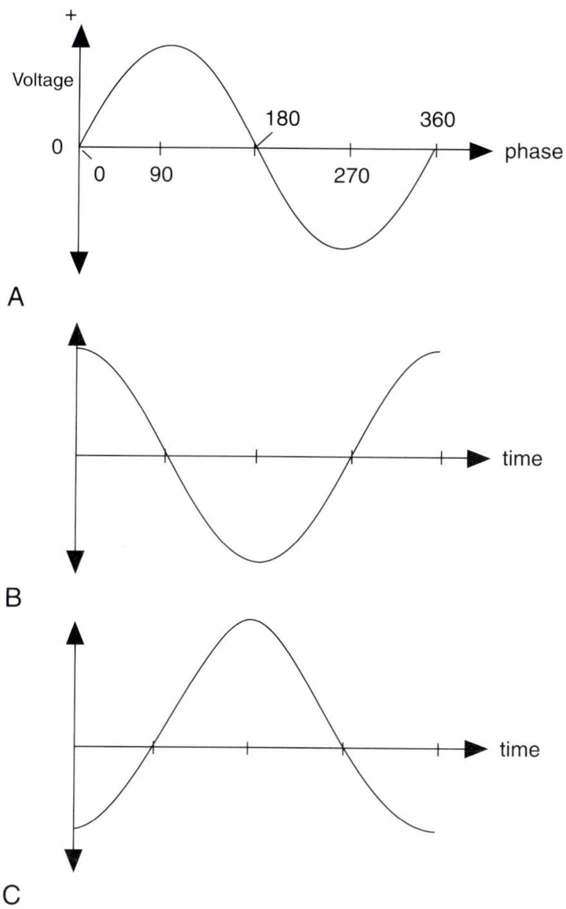

Fig. 5.17 Phase. **A,** One complete variation (cycle) of alternating voltage may be thought of as traveling around a 360-degree circle. One-quarter of a cycle is 90 degrees of phase angle. Phase is a description of progression through a cycle (analogous to the phase of the moon). One-quarter of a cycle is 90 degrees, and one-half of a cycle is 180 degrees. The completion of a cycle occurs at 360 degrees, but this is also the 0-degree phase of the next cycle. **B,** This voltage leads that in A by 90 degrees (one-quarter cycle). **C,** This voltage lags that in A by 90 degrees and lags that in B by 180 degrees. If the voltages in B and C are added together, a zero voltage results. (The two voltages are equal and opposite, so they cancel each other when summed.)

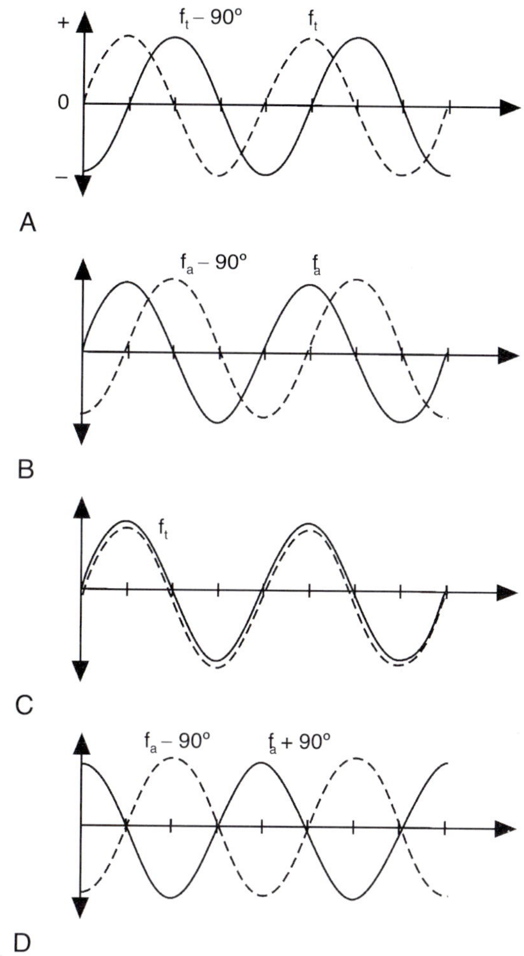

Fig. 5.18 The *solid curves* refer to the direct channel, whereas the *dashed curves* refer to quadrature. The vertical axis represents voltage, and the horizontal one represents time. **A,** Positive Doppler shifts (f_t) at the output of the direct channel filter lag those in the quadrature channel by 90 degrees. **B,** Negative Doppler shifts (f_a) at the output of the quadrature channel lag those in the direct channel by 90 degrees. **C,** Positive Doppler shifts at the input to the direct channel adder are in phase (0-degree phase difference), yielding an f_t output. **D,** Negative Doppler shifts at the input to the direct channel adder are 180 degrees out of phase, yielding a zero f_a output.

Continuous Wave Sample Volume

CW operation detects flow that occurs anywhere within the intersection of the transmitting and receiving beams of the dual-transducer assembly (Fig. 5.20). The sample volume is the region from which Doppler-shifted echoes return, in other words the overlapping region of the transmitting and receiving beams. Because the sample volume is large, CW Doppler systems often produce complex and confusing presentations if two or more different motions or flows are included in the sample volume (e.g., two blood vessels viewed simultaneously). However, the large sample volume of a CW system is helpful when searching for a Doppler maximum associated with a vascular or valvular stenosis (the latter is really the only clinical use outside of OB).

> The Doppler sample volume of a CW Doppler instrument is relatively large, being the overlapping region of the transmission and reception beams.

Because a distribution of flow velocities is encountered by the beam as it traverses a vessel, a distribution of many Doppler-shifted frequencies returns to the transducer and, thus, the Doppler scanner. In the arterial circulation or the heart, these Doppler shifts are changing continually over the cardiac cycle and are displayed as a function of time with appropriate real-time frequency spectrum processing (Fig. 5.21). These displays provide quantitative data for evaluating Doppler-shifted echoes. The displayed Doppler information is stored in the digital memory before it is displayed so that it can be frozen and backed through the last few seconds of preceding information.

Wall Filter

In Doppler studies, a wall filter that rejects frequencies below an adjustable value is used to eliminate high-intensity, low-frequency Doppler shifted echoes, so-called clutter, caused by the heart or any moving tissues or vessel walls or cardiac valve

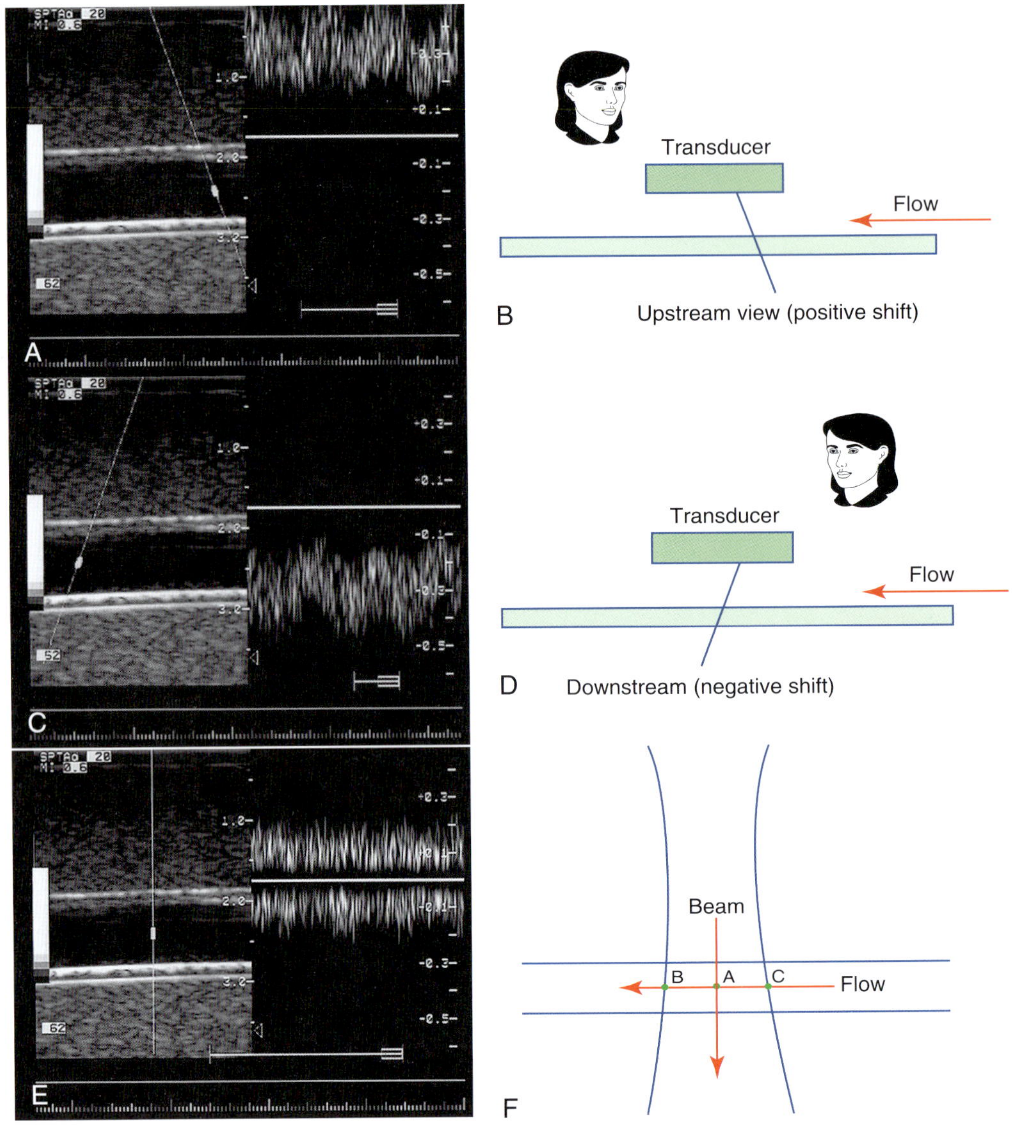

Fig. 5.19 The beam is steered to the right, and positive Doppler shifts are received **(A).** Thus this is an upstream view **(B),** and flow is from right to left. Therefore steering the beam to the left **(C)** would provide a downstream view **(D)** with negative Doppler shifts. With the beam perpendicular to the flow **(E),** Doppler shifts are received, both positive and negative, because of beam width **(F);** that is, a portion of the beam views upstream while a portion views downstream. The beam axis portion (90-degree angle) yields a zero Doppler shift (baseline).

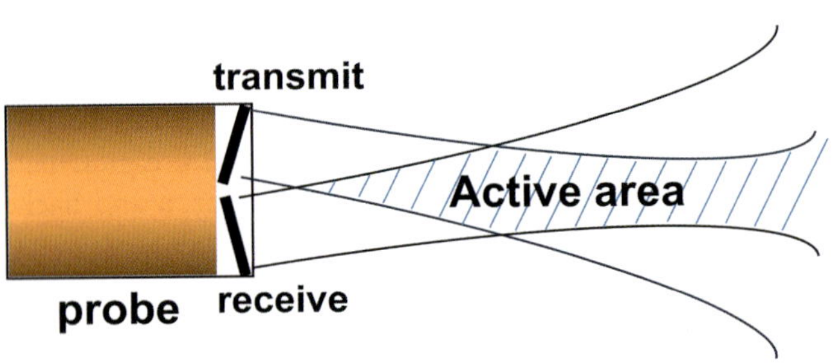

Fig. 5.20 Continuous wave Doppler systems have dual-element transducer assemblies, one for transmitting and one for receiving. The region over which Doppler information can be acquired (the active area or rather the Doppler sample volume) is the region of overlap between the transmitting and receiving beams (*blue region*).

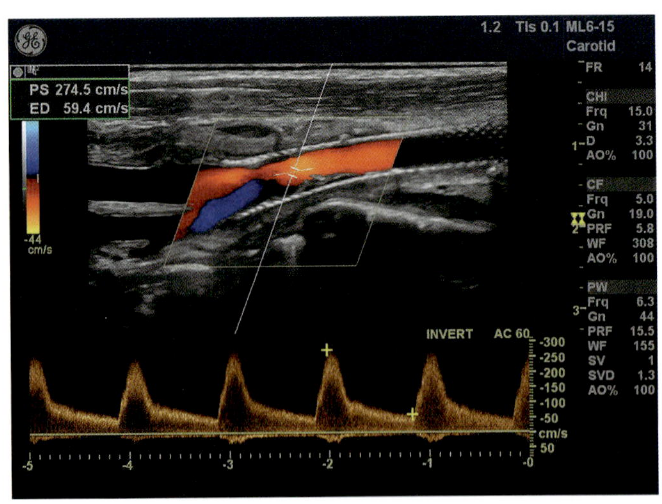

Fig. 5.21 A spectral display of vascular pulsed wave Doppler-shift frequencies (or rather velocities—the conversion from frequency shifts to velocities will be covered later in this chapter) in a carotid artery as a function of time. (Courtesy GE HealthCare.)

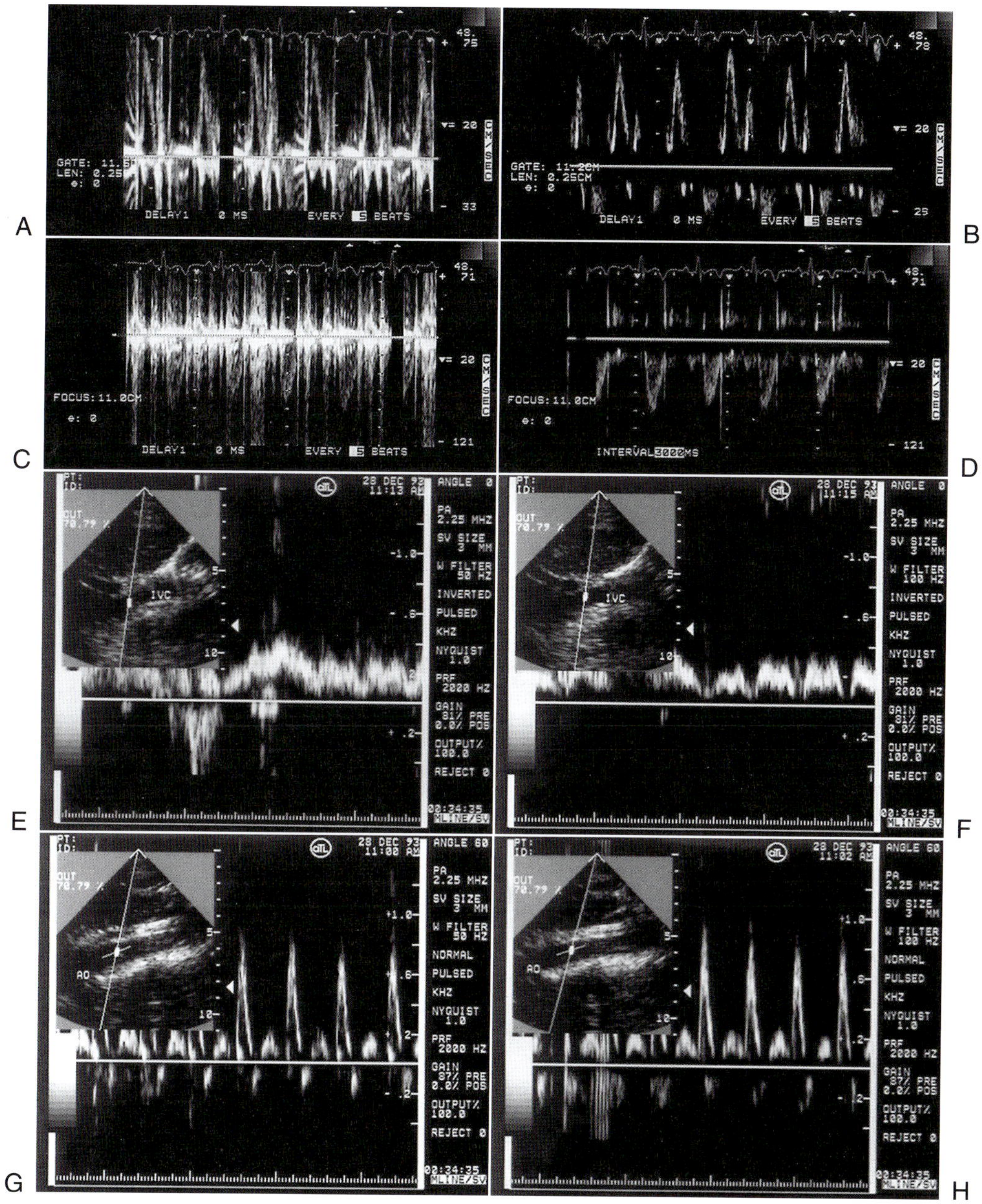

Fig. 5.22 **A,** Clutter in the spectrum of inflow at the mitral valve is shown. **B,** The clutter in A is removed by increasing the wall filter setting. **C,** Clutter in the spectrum of the left ventricular outflow tract. **D,** The clutter in C is removed with an increase in the wall filter setting. **E,** Clutter in the display of inferior vena caval flow. **F,** The clutter shown in E is removed by adjusting the wall filter from 50 to 100 Hz. **G,** Clutter in the display of aortic flow. **H,** The clutter shown in G is removed by adjusting the wall filter.

motion (Fig. 5.22). Sometimes called a *wall-thump filter*, the filter rejects these strong echoes that otherwise would overwhelm the weaker echoes from blood. These strong echoes have low Doppler-shift frequencies, because the tissue structures do not move as fast as blood does. The upper limit of the filter is sometimes (but not always) adjustable by the user over a range of approximately 25 to 3200 Hz. However, the filter, if not properly used, can erroneously alter conclusions with regard to diastolic flow and distal flow resistance by eliminating legitimate lower frequency Doppler shifts (Fig. 5.23).

> Wall filters remove clutter (low-frequency Doppler shifts from moving tissue).

Pulsed Wave Doppler Systems

A diagram of the components of a PW Doppler system is given in Fig. 5.24, A. The pulser (in the beam former) functions as it does in grayscale imaging, except that it generates longer pulses consisting of several voltage cycles that in turn drive the transducer generating Doppler ultrasound pulses. While imaging pulses are two or three cycles long, pulses used in Doppler instruments, however, have pulse lengths of approximately 4 to 48 cycles. This is necessary to overcome the abysmal SNR associated with Doppler shifts (up to 100 dB below clutter echoes). Echo voltages from the transducer are processed in the detector. In the detector, echo voltages are amplified, their frequency

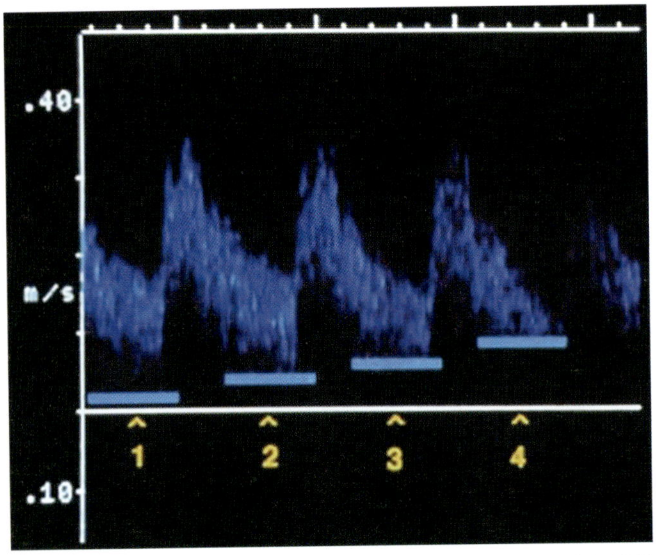

Fig. 5.23 Four different wall filter settings (125, 250, 500, and 1000 Hz) eliminate frequencies as shown until erroneously only the peak systolic part of the spectrum is left.

is compared with the pulser frequency, and Doppler shifts are determined. Doppler shifts are sent to loudspeakers for audible output and to the display for visual observation.

However, even with a longer pulse, a PW Doppler system cannot overcome the poor SNR of Doppler ultrasound with a single firing. Instead, PW Doppler systems transmit a train of pulses—typically 32 to 512 pulses. The frequency of pulse transmission within such a pulse train is known as the pulse repetition frequency (*PRF*). Each pulse yields a single sample of the Doppler signal. In other words, a PW Doppler system samples the Doppler signal at a rate equal to *PRF* (i.e., the sampling frequency is the *PRF*). Each of the returning Doppler shifted echoes yields a sample of the Doppler shift from the Doppler detector. These samples are connected and smoothed (filtered) to yield the sampled waveform (see Fig. 5.24, B–E).

> A PW Doppler system samples the Doppler signal.

Range Gate

While CW Doppler systems have no range (i.e., depth) selection, Pulsed-Doppler systems solve this problem by detecting motion or flow at a selected depth with a relatively small sample volume or range gate. Based on their arrival time (remember the 13 μs/cm rule), motion information may be obtained from a specific by selecting an appropriate delay time for opening up (or gating) the signal processor (see Fig. 5.24, A). This is called range gating. The operator controls the gate length and location.

> Range gating controls depth selection and the Doppler sample volume size.

The gate indicates the sample volume location from which returning Doppler-shifted echoes are accepted, while echoes from outside this location are rejected (i.e., the sample volume gate is closed; Table 5.4 and Figs. 5.25–5.27). The width of the sample volume is equal to the beam width. The gate has some length (i.e., time) over which it permits reception (Table 5.5). For example (applying the 13 μs/cm rule), a gate that passes echoes arriving from 13 to 15 μs after pulse generation is listening over a depth range of 10.0 to 11.5 mm. Hence, the gate is located at a depth of 10.8 mm with a length (depth range) of ±0.8 mm. Longer gate lengths are used when searching for the desired vessel and flow location, and shorter gate lengths are used for spectral analysis and evaluation. The shorter gate length improves the quality of the spectral display.

The Doppler sample volume is determined by beam width, gate length, and emitted pulse length. One-half of the pulse length (i.e., the axial resolution inherent in the transmitted pulse) is added to gate length to yield the effective sample volume length (Table 5.6). Thus the pulse length must shorten as the gate length is reduced. The sample volume width is equal to the beam width at the sample volume depth.

Duplex Mode

Including PW Doppler capabilities in a grayscale ultrasound scanner allows what is commonly referred to as **duplex mode**, which has the capacity to image anatomic structures and analyze flow at a given location in the imaging plane more or less at the same time (i.e., within the same image). Imaging enables the user to position the sample volume and perform angle correction in a PW Doppler system (Fig. 5.28).

When using narrow transmit beams, duplex systems must be time-shared; that is, imaging and Doppler flow measurements cannot be done simultaneously. Electronic scanning with arrays permits rapid switching between imaging and Doppler functions (reaching frame rates of 25 Hz and above), allowing what can appear to be simultaneous acquisition of real-time image and Doppler flow information. Duplex imaging frame rates are slower than in imaging-only modes to allow for the acquisition of Doppler information between frames. Similarly, a time-out from the spectral display is taken to acquire and present a grayscale image frame (but this gap in the spectral display is filled in with artificial system-generated signals for esthetical reasons).

> Duplex instruments enable the operator to place the Doppler sample volume by showing its location in the grayscale (i.e., anatomical) image.

Angle Adjustment or Correction

To convert a display correctly from Doppler shift (in Hz) versus time to flow velocity (in cm/s; cf., Fig. 5.28) versus time, the Doppler angle (i.e., the beam-to-vessel angle) must be incorporated accurately into the calculation process. This adjustment is commonly called angle correction and is essential for comparisons across patients (since blood velocity is a physiological parameter unlike Doppler shifts). A lack of angle adjustment leaves the scanner to assume that the Doppler angle is zero, which is incorrect unless the angle is, in

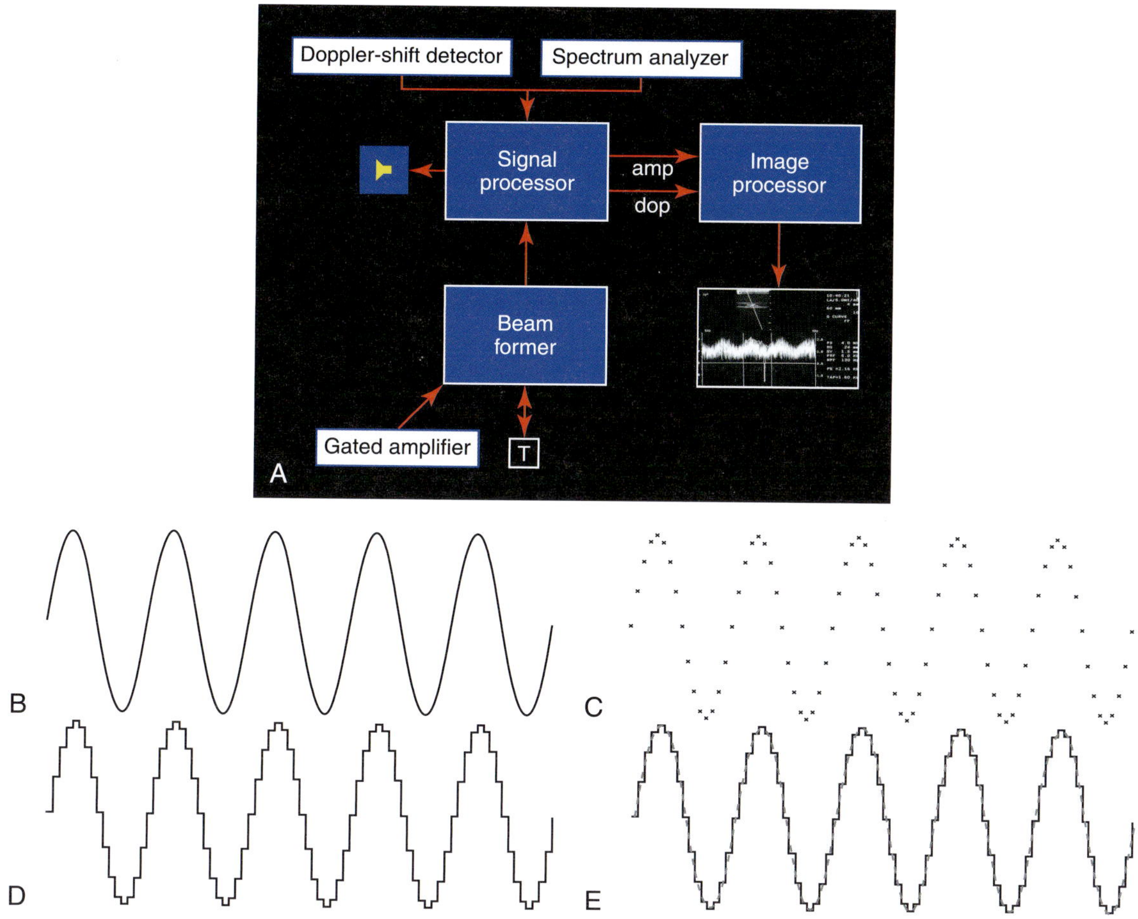

Fig. 5.24 A, Block diagram of a sonographic instrument functioning in pulsed wave (PW) Doppler mode. The beam former produces voltage pulses of several cycles each, which drive the transducer (*T*). The signal processor includes a Doppler-shift detector, where shift frequencies are compared with the frequency of the outgoing pulses. The difference (the Doppler shift) is sent to the loudspeakers and, through the spectrum analyzer and image processor, to the display. The beam former also contains a gate that selects echoes from a given depth according to arrival time and thus gives motion information from a selected depth. **B,** Five cycles of a 500-Hz Doppler-shift frequency occurring in 10 ms of time. **C,** In a PW Doppler instrument, each pulse yields echoes from the sample volume. These echoes, after Doppler detection, yield samples (x) of the Doppler shift from the sample volume. In this example, 80 samples are determined in a 10 ms time period. Therefore the pulse-repetition frequency of the instrument is 8 kHz (with each pulse yielding one sample of the Doppler shift). **D,** The PW Doppler gate is also called a *sample-and-hold amplifier*. It samples the returning stream of echoes (resulting from one emitted pulse of ultrasound) at the appropriate time for the desired depth (see Table 5.7) and holds the value until the next pulse and sample are accomplished. **E,** Low-pass filtering (which removes higher frequencies) smooths the sampled result (*solid line*), yielding the desired Doppler-shift waveform (*dashed line*) comparable with that shown in **B**.

fact, zero. The beam-to-vessel angle estimation is achieved by placing a cursor on the anatomical display (i.e., the gray-scale image) that it is parallel to the posterior vessel wall (this assumes the direction of flow is parallel to the vessel wall, which is valid only for a straight vessel with no flow obstruction). This is a subjective operation performed by the operator of the ultrasound scanner (typically the sonographer), although there are now automatic adjustment algorithms available on high-end scanners (so-called single button optimization functions).

As angle increases, the cosine decreases, increasing the calculated flow velocity. Thus when the angle indicator on the Duplex image is set at 60 degrees, the scanner responds by doubling the calculated flow speed from what it would have been at a Doppler angle of zero, since the cosine in the denominator of the Doppler equation is set at 0.5. This compensates for the reduction in the Doppler shift caused by the Doppler angle actually involved in the ultrasound beam and flow intersection by doubling the measured flow velocity to the correct value. Without doing that, the calculated flow speed would be half the correct value.

In principle, if the angle is incorporated correctly, the calculated flow speed in the vessel should be the same, regardless of the Doppler angle; that is, the actual flow speed is certainly not altered by the Doppler angle used in detecting it (Table 5.7). Not surprisingly, however, inaccuracies in angle estimation do

TABLE 5.4 Echo Arrival Time for Various Reflector Depths (Gate Locations)

Depth (mm)	Time (μs)
10	13
20	26
30	39
40	52
50	65
60	78
70	91
80	104
90	117
100	130
150	195
200	260

occur. Errors in the estimation of the Doppler angle are more critical at large angles than at small ones, because the cosine changes rapidly at large angles. Table 5.8 gives error values for various angles. For example, if the correct Doppler angle is 60 degrees but the estimation is 5 degrees in error (the angle estimate is 55 or 65 degrees), the error in the cosine value is approximately 15%, yielding a calculated velocity that is incorrect by approximately 18%. Fig. 5.29 shows how the error in the calculated flow speed increases with angle. For this reason, and because Doppler-shift frequencies become very small at large angles, thereby reducing the system sensitivity, Doppler measurements (and particularly the calculated flow velocities) are not reliably achieved at Doppler angles greater than approximately 60 degrees.

Moreover, we generally do not go below about 30 degrees, because it is not anatomically accessible. One generally achieves success, then, at angles greater than this. However, in Doppler

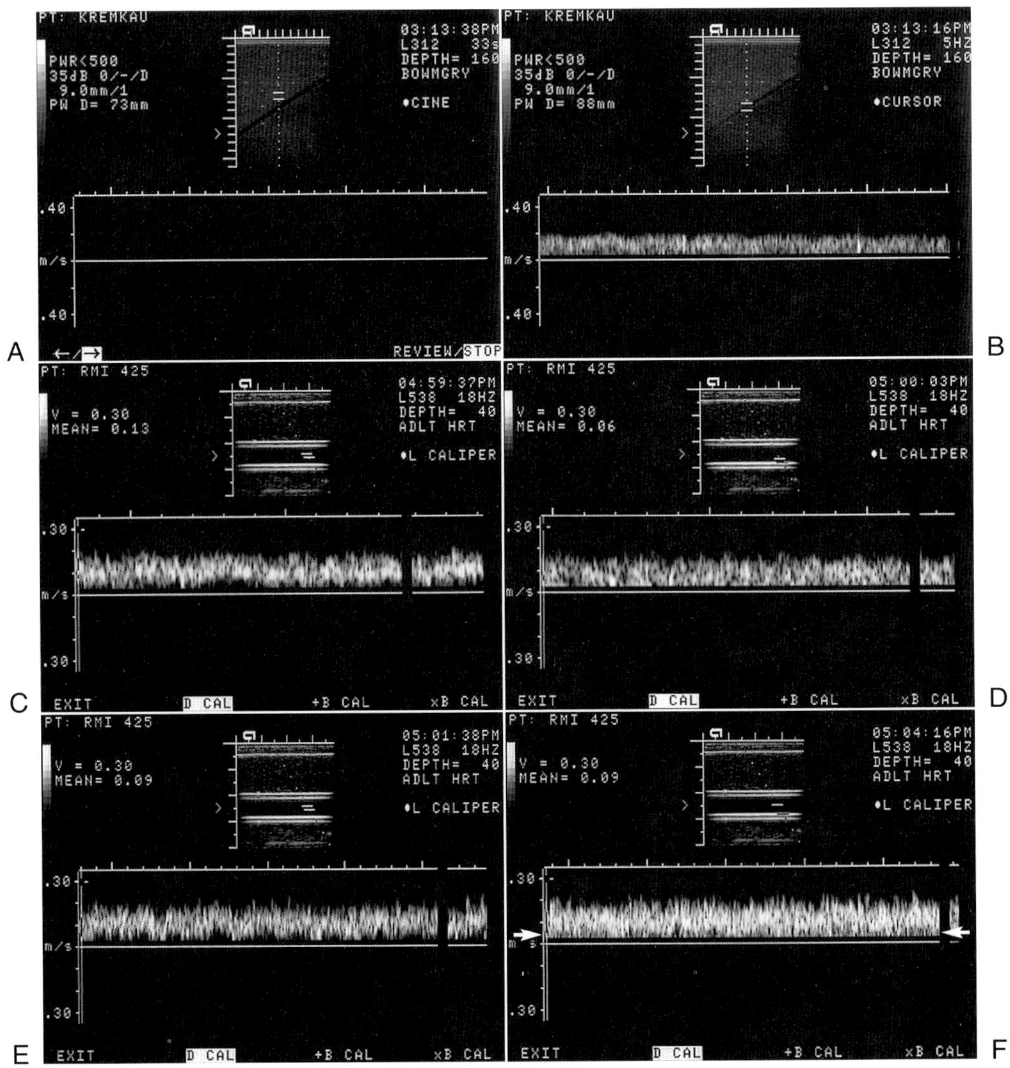

Fig. 5.25 A, The pulsed wave Doppler sample volume is located at 73 mm of depth (95 μs arrival time). No Doppler shift is seen on the lower display because Doppler-shifted echoes from within the tube arrive at about 114 μs. **B,** When the gate is open later (corresponding to a depth of 88 mm), Doppler shifts are received and displayed (indicating a constant flow rate in the tube). **C,** The gate is located in the center of the tube. **D,** The gate is located near the tube wall. Mean flow speed is 6 cm/s compared with 13 cm/s in C. This is the expected result with laminar flow. **E,** The gate is again located at the center of the tube. **F,** The gate length is extended to include the flow from the center, out to the tube wall. Note the strengthening of the lower flow speeds (Doppler shifts) (*arrows*) compared with **E**, where the slower flow is not included in the sample volume.

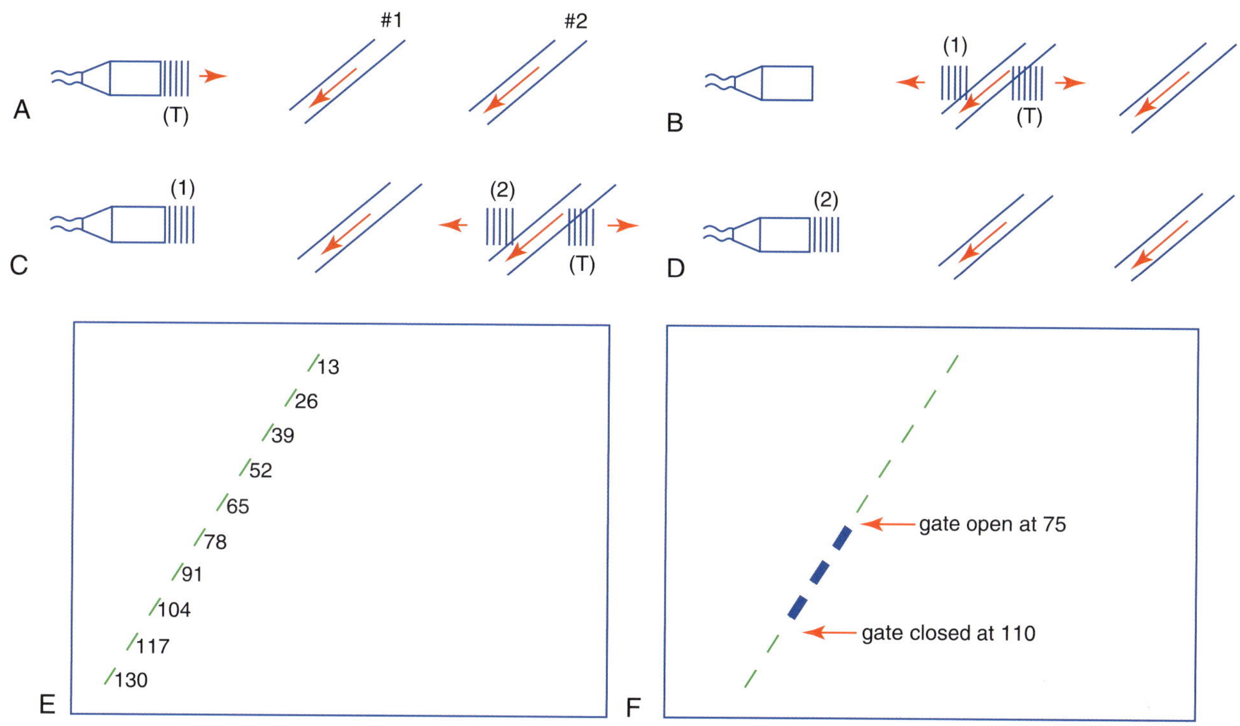

Fig. 5.26 **A,** A pulse (*T*) leaves the transducer. **B,** An echo (*1*) is generated in vessel number *1*. **C,** Echo *1* arrives at the transducer. At the same time, another echo (*2*) is generated at vessel number *2*. **D,** Echo *2* arrives at the transducer after echo *1*. These echoes will be processed by the instrument if the gate is open when they arrive. **E,** Echoes from 1, 2, 3, 4, 5, 6, 7, 8, 9, and 10 cm depths arrive at the times (microseconds) indicated. **F,** If the gate is open from 75 to 110 μs after pulse emission, only the echoes in **E,** arriving at 78, 91, and 104 μs, will be accepted. The others will be rejected.

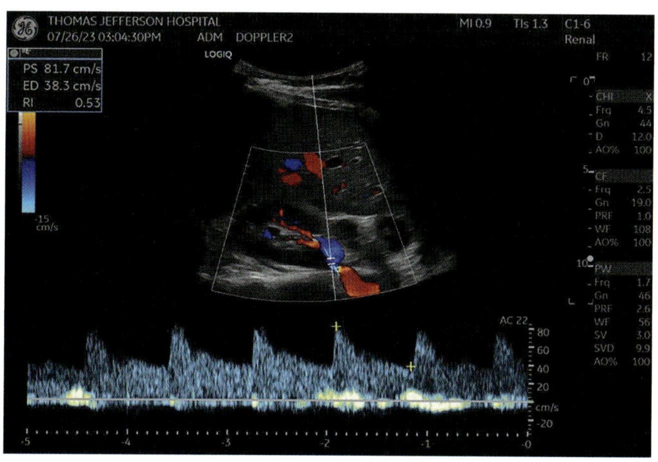

Fig. 5.27 Example of pulsed wave Doppler with the sample volume (i.e., the Doppler gate) placed in the renal artery.

echocardiography, Doppler angles of near zero are useful, and zero is commonly assumed (i.e., angle correction is not used in this application unlike in vascular applications). The angle between the beam and the heart wall is large, and obtaining a zero-degree beam to flow angle is relatively straightforward, which avoids any problem.

In the discussion above, we have considered the flow to be parallel to vessel walls, which is often not the case even in unobstructed vessels. Off-axis flow will impact the accuracy of the angle correction and, thus, the accuracy of the estimated flow velocities. As shown in Fig. 5.30 even for a relatively small 20

TABLE 5.5 Spatial Gate Length for Various Temporal Gate Lengths

Length (mm)	Time (μs)
1	1.3
2	2.6
3	3.9
4	5.2
5	6.5
10	13.0
15	19.5
20	26.0

TABLE 5.6 Amount Added to Effective Gate Length by Pulse Length for Various Cycles per Pulse and Frequencies

Amount Added (mm)	Cycles	f (MHz)
1.9	5	2
3.8	10	2
7.7	20	2
0.8	5	5
1.5	10	5
3.1	20	5
0.4	5	10
0.8	10	10
1.5	20	10

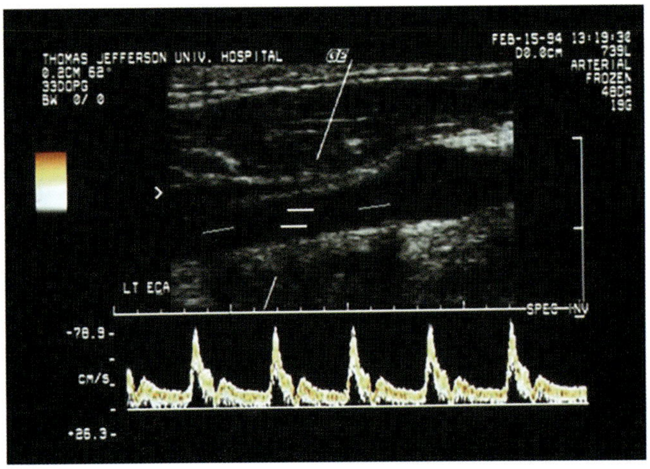

Fig. 5.28 Duplex Doppler of the external carotid artery demonstrating how grayscale ultrasound imaging is being used to guide the Doppler sample volume placement. Notice that the Doppler shifts are expressed as velocities (in cm/s) rather than in Hz.

TABLE 5.7 Doppler Shifts (for 4 MHz) at Various Doppler Angles for the Same Flow Yielding a Consistent Calculated Flow Speed

Calculated Flow Doppler Shift (kHz)	Angle (Degrees)	Speed (cm/s)
2.25	30	50
1.99	40	50
1.84	45	50
1.67	50	50
1.30	60	50

TABLE 5.8 Cosine and Calculated-Speed Errors for Angle Errors of 2 and 5 Degrees

True Angle (Degrees)	COSINE ERROR (%) +2 Degrees	COSINE ERROR (%) +5 Degrees	SPEED ERROR (%) +2 Degrees	SPEED ERROR (%) +5 Degrees
0	-0.1	-0.4	+0.1	+0.4
10	-0.7	-1.9	+0.7	+2.0
20	-1.3	-3.6	+1.3	+3.7
30	-2.1	-5.4	+2.1	+5.7
40	-3.0	-7.7	+3.1	+8.3
50	-4.2	-10.8	+4.4	+12.1
60	-6.1	-15.5	+6.5	+18.3
70	-9.6	-24.3	+10.7	+32.1
80	-19.9	-49.8	+24.8	+99.2

degrees of off-axis flow, errors of 20% to 55% will occur with increasing errors for increasing Doppler angles. Moreover, angle adjustment also assumes that the flow (and thus the Doppler angle) is completely within the scan plane. However, you should remember that the flow may not be parallel to the imaging scan plane, which includes the Doppler beam; thus, there may be a component of Doppler angle between the flow direction and the scan plane. It is important to keep in mind the

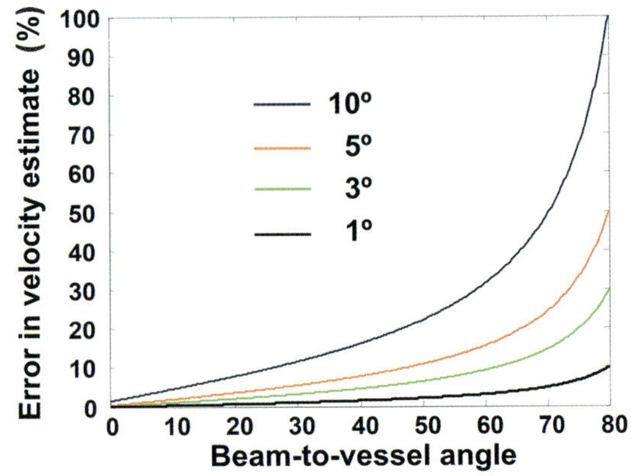

Fig. 5.29 A, Error in the velocity estimate (in %) as a function of beam-to-vessel angle for 1-, 3-, 5-, and 10-degree angle errors.

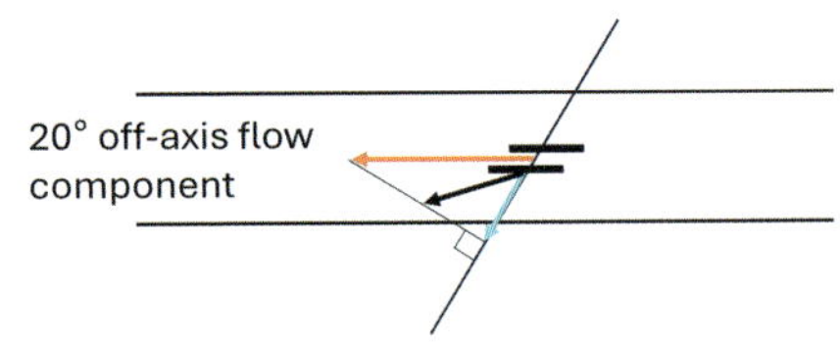

Beam-to-vessel angle	Actual velocity	Measured velocity	Error
60°	100 cm/s	153 cm/s	53%
50°	100 cm/s	135 cm/s	35%
40°	100 cm/s	123 cm/s	23%

Fig. 5.30 Schematic of off-axis flow demonstrating how the measured Doppler shift in kHz (*blue arrow*) gets adjusted to the blood flow velocity (in cm/s; *red arrow*) even though off-axis flow (in this example at a 20-degree angle; *black arrow*) would produce the same measure Doppler shift (in kHz). The error this would induce in the final velocities is indicated below and ranges from 23% to 53% for an actual velocity of 100 cm/s.

three-dimensional character of the components involved in the angle correction (really velocity estimation) process (e.g., vessel anatomy, flow direction, and ultrasound image scan plane).

Finally, there is an argument to be made for consistency in Doppler angle selections and that since the commonly acceptable range of 30 to 60 degrees, errors are inevitable and will increase with increasing Doppler angles. Hence, selecting a Doppler angle and sticking to it across all patients (or at the very least for a given individual patient) will tend to produce similar errors making changes of time more reliable (generally speaking at least). So, in summary, a consistent angle between 30 and 60 degrees is best, and picking an angle on the lower side is probably preferable to reduce errors, while maintaining an angle that can be achieved consistently in most vascular applications.

Spectral Analysis and the Frequency Spectrum

The Doppler-shifts extracted from the signal processor do not get displayed directly; otherwise, it would resemble Fig. 5.31, A, which is the visual picture of what a listener hears from the system loudspeakers. Instead, the signal undergoes further processing. Spectral analysis (see Fig. 5.31, A–C) provides a more meaningful way to visualize the Doppler information. The presentation is in the form of a Doppler **frequency spectrum**.

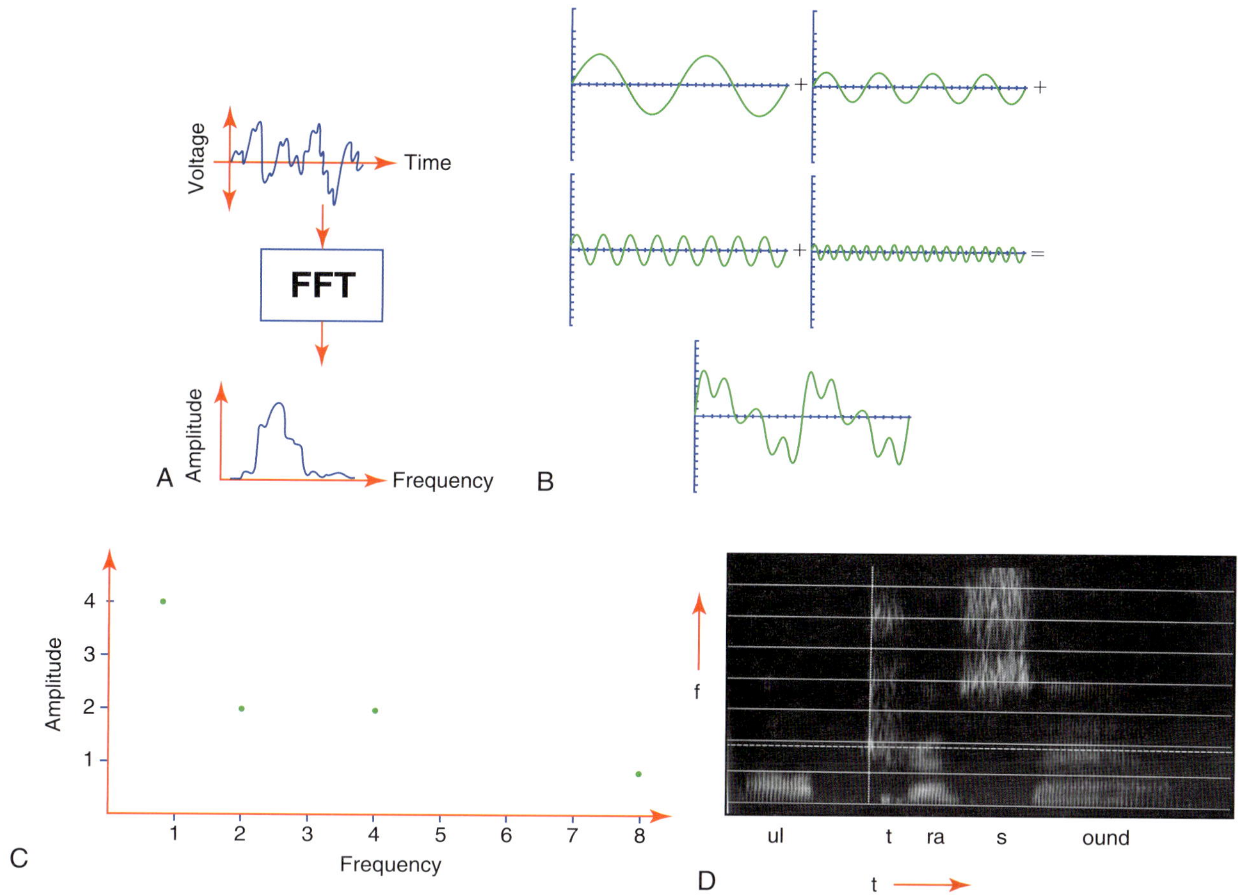

Fig. 5.31 Fast Fourier transform (*FFT*). **A,** The Doppler-shift signal (containing many frequencies) is transformed by the FFT into a spectrum. (See Fig. 5.49 for an example of the Doppler signal before [A] and after [B] FFT processing.) **B,** Four voltages of different frequencies are combined to give the complex result. **C,** The FFT analysis of this combined voltage yields this spectrum of four frequency components (a frequency of 1 with amplitude 4, two frequencies [2 and 4] with amplitude 2, and one frequency of 8 with amplitude of 1). **D,** Spectral analysis of the word *ultrasound*. Time progresses to the right while the word is uttered, and approximately 100 FFTs are performed. The vertical axis represents frequency. The low frequencies of the *ul, ra,* and *ound* syllables are seen, along with the high frequencies of the *t* and *s* sounds.

A spectrum shows the components of a complex wave or signal (here the Doppler signal), separated and arranged in order of increasing frequency (the so-called frequency domain). The **fast Fourier transform** (*FFT*) is the mathematic technique a Doppler system uses to derive the Doppler spectrum from the returning echoes (Fig. 5.31). The human auditory system performs a similar analysis of sound waves. The ear and brain break down the complex sounds we receive into the component frequencies contained in the sounds. Thus we can listen to a Doppler signal and recognize normal and abnormal flow sounds. Visual presentation of these sounds in the form of **spectral analysis** provides additional capability for recognition of flow characteristics and for diagnosis of disease.

Spectral analysis presents Doppler-shift frequencies in frequency order.

Various kinds of flow occur in blood vessels. Changes in vessel size, turns, and abnormalities such as the presence of plaque or stenoses can alter the flow character. We have seen that flow can be characterized as *plug, laminar, parabolic, disturbed*, and *turbulent*. Portions of the blood flowing within a vessel are moving at different speeds (even for normal flow) and sometimes in different directions (off-axis and/or out of plane flow components). Thus while the ultrasound beam intersects this flow and produces echoes, many different Doppler shifts are received from the vessel by the system, even from a small sample volume. These Doppler shifts can be analyzed to form the *Doppler-frequency spectrum* (Fig. 5.32).

The extent of the range of Doppler-shift frequencies generated depends on the character of the flow. For near-plug flow, a narrow range of Doppler-shift frequencies is received. FFTs can show **spectral broadening**, which is widening of the Doppler-shift spectrum (i.e., an increase in the range of Doppler-shift frequencies present) caused by a broader range of flow speeds and directions encountered by the ultrasound pulses (e.g., in connection with disturbed or turbulent flow).

Different flow conditions produce different spectral presentations.

ADVANCED CONCEPTS

The Fourier transform is defined as follows:

$$F(f) = \int_{-\infty}^{\infty} g(t)\,(\cos 2\pi ft - i \sin 2\pi ft)\,dt$$

where f is frequency, g(t) is the function of time to be analyzed, and i is the square root of −1.

The FFT is a computation that reduces the number of mathematical operations in the evaluation of the discrete Fourier transform:

$$F(\nu) = (1/n)\sum_{t=0}^{n-1} g(t)\,(\cos 2\pi\nu\tau - i \sin 2\pi\nu\tau)$$

where ν is related to frequency and τ is related to the time interval between sample points.

The FFT process includes sampling the complicated, multifrequency Doppler signal at a rate of approximately 25,600 times per second (or higher), which is a 25.6 kHz sampling rate. A 10 ms period of time (yielding 256 samples) is sufficient to provide a useful spectrum. Thus 100 such spectra can be produced per second. Each spectrum can include the amplitudes of 128 frequencies, the lowest of which is equal to the number of FFTs per second (100 Hz in this case) and the highest of which is equal to one-half the sampling rate (or 12.8 kHz in this case). This rapid sequence of FFT-generated spectra (100 per second) can be displayed in real time. Some current processors can calculate close to 1,000,000 FFTs per second.

The FFT is used to generate Doppler spectral displays.

Spectral Displays

The received Doppler signal is a combination of many Doppler-shift frequencies, yielding a complex waveform (see Figs. 5.31, B and 5.32). Applying the FFT algorithm separates these frequencies into a spectrum that can be presented on a two-dimensional display of Doppler frequency on the horizontal axis and power or amplitude of each frequency component on the vertical axis (an indication of the number of red blood cells moving at a given Doppler shift; see Fig. 5.31, A, C). Depending on the speed of the processor, approximately 100 to much more than 100,000 spectra can be generated per second. In the case of venous flow, such a spectral display usually would be rather constant. However, in the case of the pulsatile flow in the arterial circulation, such a presentation would change all the time, shifting to the right in systole as the blood accelerates and Doppler shifts increase, shifting to the left in diastole, and changing in

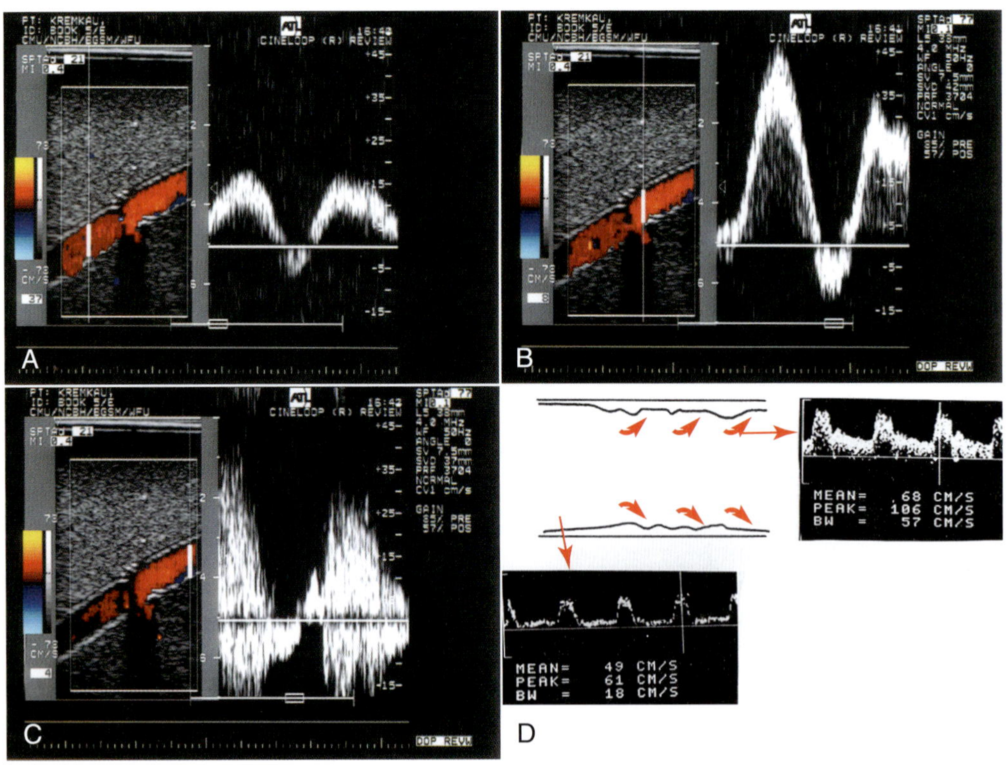

Fig. 5.32 Flow (*lower left to upper right*) in a tube with a stenosis in tissue-equivalent material. **A,** Proximal to the stenosis, a narrow spectrum is observed (indicating approximately plug [i.e., blunted] flow). **B,** At the stenosis, a reasonably narrow spectrum still is seen, but the Doppler shifts have tripled because of the high flow speed through the stenosis. **C,** Distal to the stenosis, a broad spectrum is observed, along with negative Doppler shifts, both of which are caused by turbulent flow. **D,** Spectral broadening produced by atheroma. (**D,** From Taylor KJW, Holland S: Doppler US. Part I. Basic principles, instrumentation, and pitfalls, *Radiology* 174:297–307, 1990.)

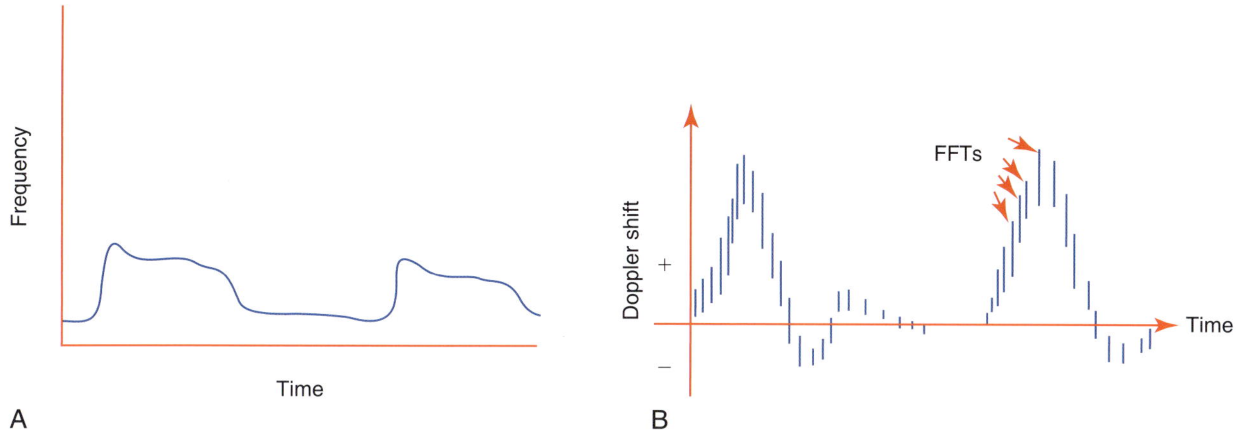

Fig. 5.33 **A,** A display of Doppler shift as a function of time for pure plug flow. The Doppler-shift frequency is represented on the vertical axis. The amplitude of the Doppler-shift frequency at each instant of time is represented by gray level or color. In this example, there is only a single shift frequency at each instant of time (i.e., no spectrum). **B,** A spectral display for nonplug flow is composed of thousands of fast Fourier transform (*FFT*) spectra arranged vertically next to each other across the time (horizontal) axis per second.

amplitude distribution over the cardiac cycle. Interpretation of this changing presentation would be very difficult; indeed, the character of the changes over the cardiac cycle could also be important.

Hence, all Doppler systems present this changing spectrum as a grayscale (or color)-encoded trace over time as shown in Figs. 5.31, D and 5.33. In these spectral displays, the vertical axis represents Doppler frequency (in Hz) or more commonly angle-adjusted velocities (in cm/s), and the horizontal axis represents time (e.g., Figs. 5.21–5.23, 5.27, and 5.28). The amplitude or power of each Doppler frequency component is now presented as brightness (grayscale; see Fig. 5.22,) or color (see Fig. 5.21). Doppler signal power is proportional to blood cell concentration (number of red blood cells per sample volume). A bright spot on a spectral display means that a strong Doppler shift component was received at that time (see Fig. 5.32). A dark spot means that the Doppler component at that point in time was weak or nonexistent. Intermediate values of gray shade or brightness indicate intermediate amplitudes or powers of these Doppler components at the given times. A strong signal at a particular frequency and time means that many scattering blood cells are moving at speeds and directions corresponding to that Doppler shift. A weak signal means that few cells are traveling at speeds and directions corresponding to that Doppler shift at that point in time.

The spectral display is a presentation of Doppler spectra versus time.

Spectral Broadening

Spectral displays provide information about flow that can be used to discern conditions at the site of measurement and at sites proximal or distal to it. Peak flow speeds and, to a lesser degree, spectral broadening are indicative of the degrees of stenosis. Spectral "broadening" is a vertical increase of the spectral trace (Fig. 5.32). If all the red blood cells were moving at the same speed, the spectral trace would be a thin line (see Fig. 5.33, A). As stated previously, though, this is not the case in practice. However, narrow spectra can be observed, particularly in large vessels during upstroke systole (Fig. 5.34). The narrowing of the spectrum while the blood accelerates in systole may not only be an indication of *plug* flow. A spectrum of consistent width will also appear to be thinner in a steep-rise portion of a curve, which may lead to misinterpretations (Fig. 5.35). These two effects cannot easily be separated.

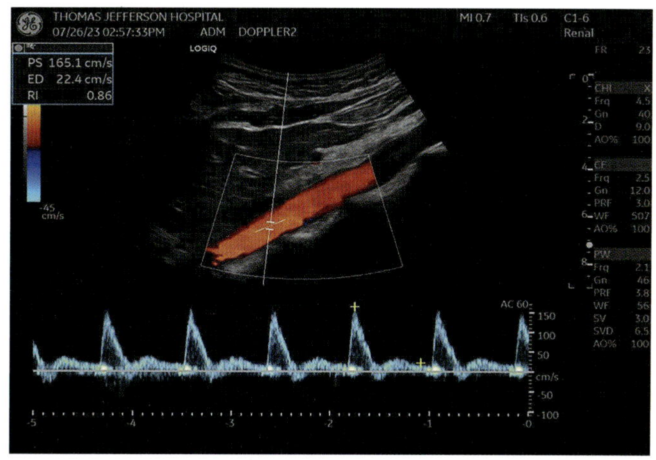

Fig. 5.34 Very narrow spectra can be observed during upstroke systole in the aorta, as demonstrated here. (Courtesy Corrine Wessner, MSc, RDMS, Thomas Jefferson University.)

Disturbed and/or turbulent flow induces greater variation in the velocities present within various portions of the flowing blood, which in turn produce a greater range of Doppler-shift frequencies. This results in a broadened spectrum in the spectral display (see Fig. 5.32, C–D). Thus spectral broadening is indicative of disturbed or turbulent flow and can be related to a pathologic condition. However, spectral broadening can also be produced artificially by excessive sample volume length (see Fig. 5.36, A–B) or by excessive Doppler gain (see Fig. 5.36, C). Additionally, some

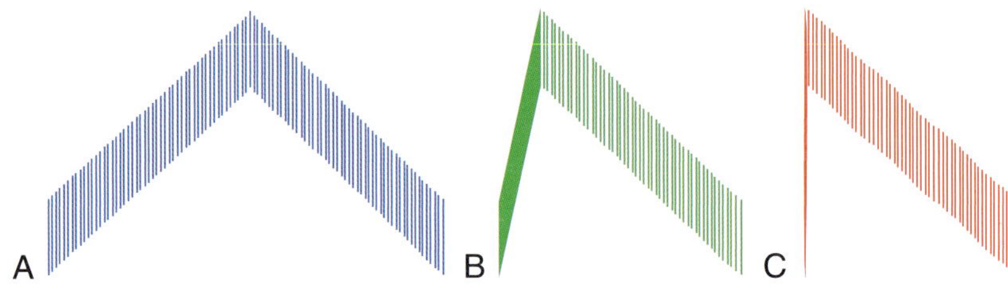

Fig. 5.35 Apparent spectral narrowing in rapidly accelerating flow. **A,** Slowly accelerating and decelerating flow shows that the spectral widths (bandwidths) are all equal. **B–C,** While the acceleration phase becomes steeper, the bandwidths appear to narrow. However, the *vertical lines* representing bandwidth in all cases are the same.

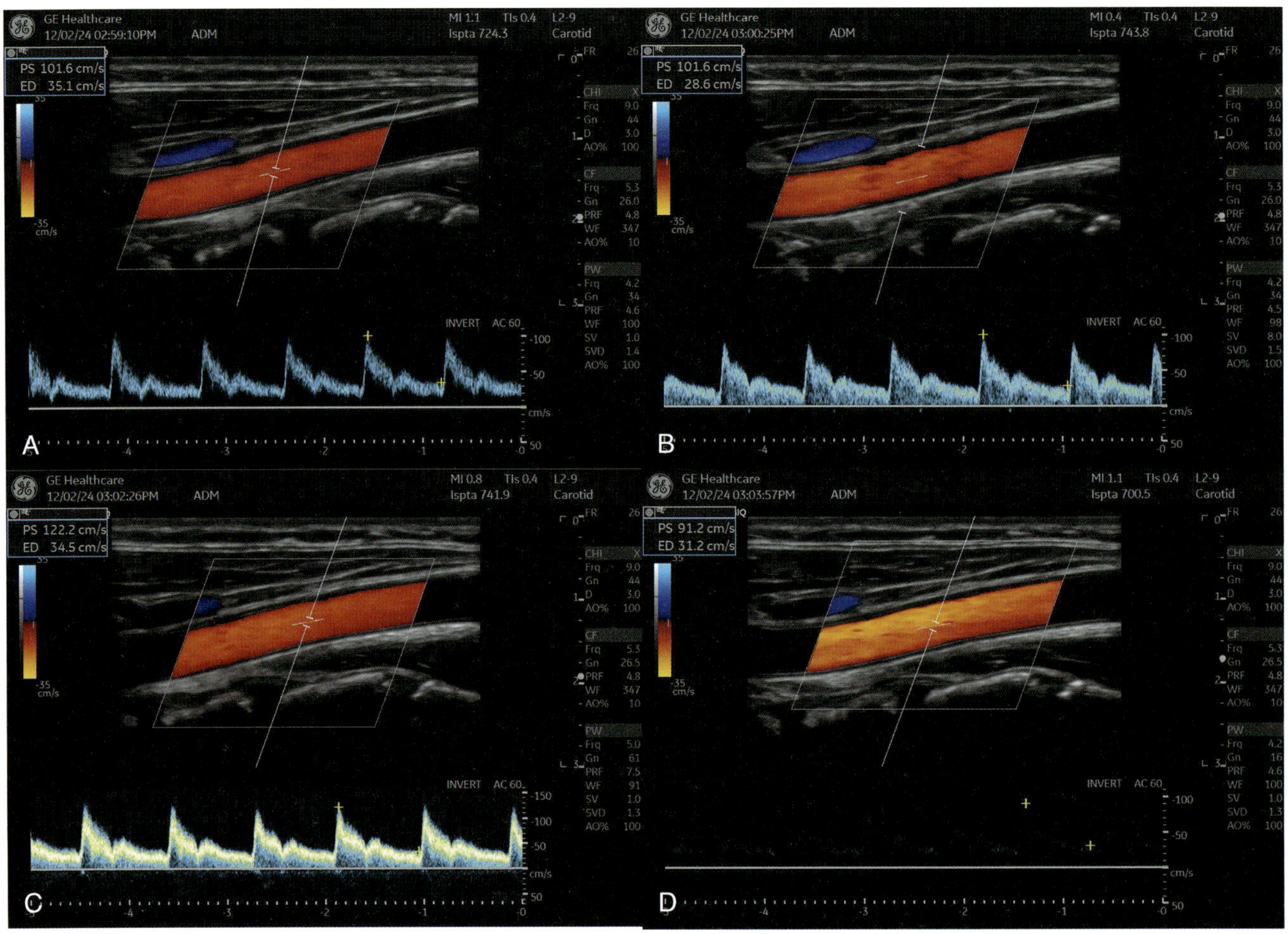

Fig. 5.36 **A,** Illustrating spectral broadening due to sample volume size—correct setting with a sample volume size of 1 mm. **B,** After increasing the sample volume size to 8 mm, extensive spectral broadening is seen. **C,** Spectral broadening due to a Doppler gain increase to 64 (relative to the 34 used in **A**). **D,** Almost complete elimination of spectral information by reducing the Doppler gain to 16.

spectral broadening is an artifact due to transit time broadening caused by a combination of beam width (sample volume size really) and the velocity of the moving blood (see Fig. 5.19, F).

ADVANCED CONCEPTS

Spectral broadening also occurs because of the finite size of the sample volume. This is called transit time broadening. The smaller the sample volume, the shorter time the propagating Doppler pulse has to interact with the blood flow. This shortens the returning Doppler-shifted echo, broadening its bandwidth.

The effective bandwidth of the Doppler echoes is a combination of the various contributions to spectral broadening: the bandwidth of the initial transmitted pulse, the range of flow speeds and angles encountered by the pulse, excessive Doppler gain, beam width, and the associated transit time broadening. Hence, trying to diagnose and assess a stenosis based on spectral broadening is not recommended.

Disturbed or turbulent flow conditions produce spectral broadening.

Downstream (Distal) and Upstream (Proximal) Conditions

Doppler flow measurements can yield information about downstream (distal) conditions. Flow reversal in early diastole and lack of flow in late diastole (see Fig. 5.7) indicate high resistance to flow downstream (e.g., because of vasoconstriction of arterioles). If flow resistance is reduced, because of vasodilation, significant differences in the spectral display are observed (Fig. 5.37). A comparison between low-resistance and high-resistance flow spectra is given in Fig. 5.38. Stenoses upstream (proximal) produce dampened spectral displays that have the so-called tardus-parvus character (see Fig. 5.38, C).

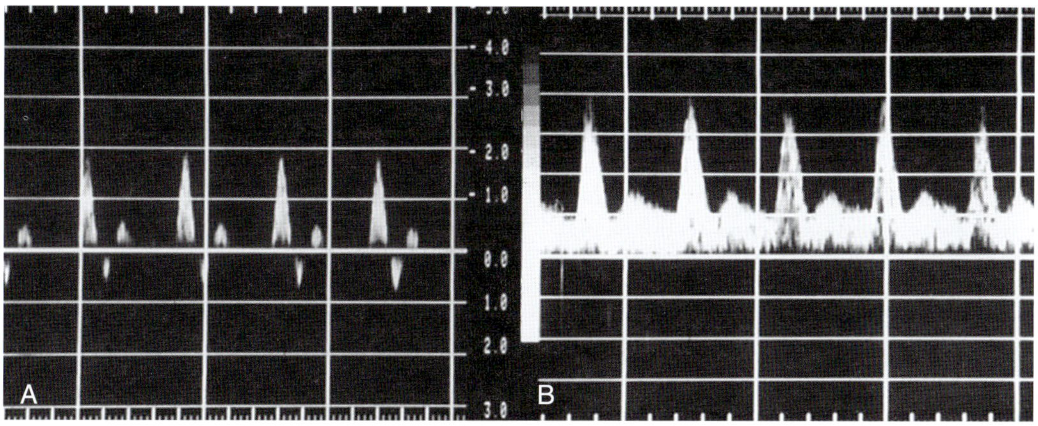

Fig. 5.37 **A,** High distal resistance flow in the popliteal artery with the patient's leg at rest. **B,** Low distal resistance flow is observed after exercise. (From Taylor KJW, Holland S: Doppler US. Part I. Basic principles, instrumentation, and pitfalls, *Radiology* 174:297–307, 1990.)

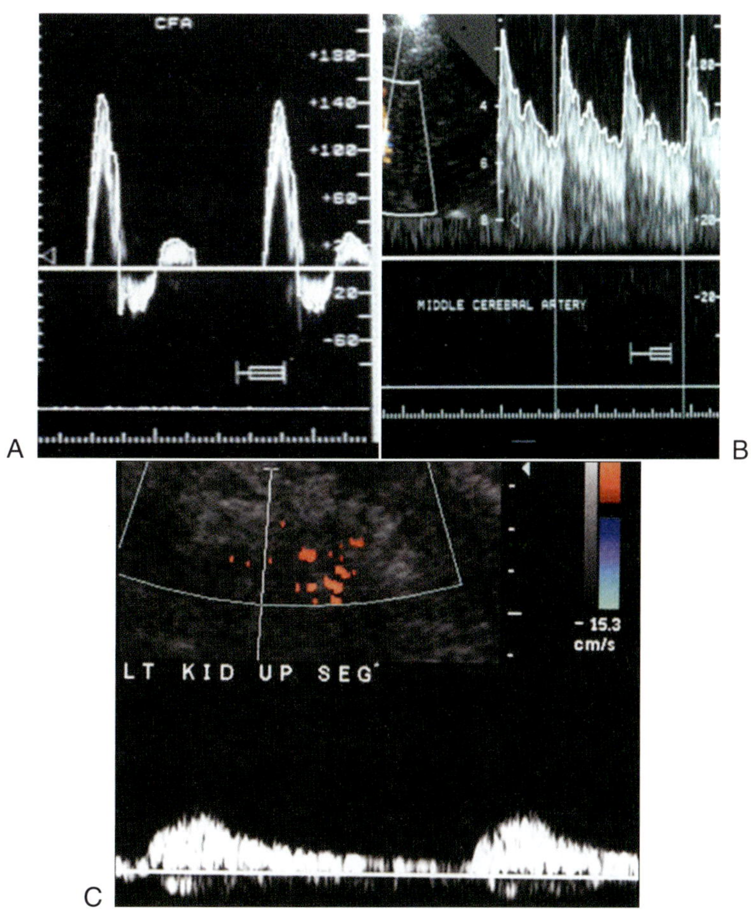

Fig. 5.38 **A,** High distal resistance flow is seen in the common femoral artery of the resting lower limb. **B,** Low distal resistance flow is seen in the middle cerebral artery. Although these spectral displays are very different, they are both normal for the locations and conditions given. **C,** *Tardus-parvus* waveform typical of flow with proximal stenosis.

Normal vessels can be occluded in diastole when pressure drops below the critical value for flow. When this happens, no diastolic Doppler shift is detected.

> High- and low-impedance conditions upstream and downstream give rise to spectral display changes that can aid in diagnosis.

COLOR DOPPLER DISPLAYS

While PW Doppler presents real-time blood flow information along with two-dimensional, cross-sectional, grayscale imaging, the flow information is limited to a small sample volume. Instead **Color Doppler imaging** (or CDI) presents two-dimensional, cross-sectional, real-time, relative blood flow, or tissue motion information along with two-dimensional, cross-sectional, grayscale imaging. Two-dimensional real-time presentations of flow information allow the observer to readily locate regions of abnormal flow, which can then undergo further quantitative evaluation by PW Doppler and spectral analysis. The direction of flow is readily appreciated and disturbed or turbulent flow is evident in two-dimensional flow maps. Color Doppler presents anatomic information in the conventional grayscale form but also rapidly depicts Doppler shifts at multiple locations along each Doppler **scan line**, presenting them as a color map overlaying the cross-sectional grayscale image.

Color Doppler Principle

CDI (sometimes called *color-flow imaging*) extends the use of the pulse-echo imaging principle to include color maps that indicate blood flow or tissue motion. Echoes returning from stationary tissues are detected and presented in grayscale at appropriate locations along each scan line. As usual, depth is determined by echo arrival time, and brightness is determined by echo intensity. Within a two-dimensional region of interest (ROI) or **color box**, a pulse train of Doppler pulses is transmitted along each scan line, and if a returning echo contains a different frequency from the transmitted frequency, a Doppler shift has occurred because the echo-generating object (typically the red blood cells within the flowing blood) was moving. All locations along the Doppler scan lines where Doppler shifts are detected are assumed to have a zero-degree Doppler angle, and arbitrary colors are assigned to the display pixels according to a chosen color assignment map.

Doppler-shifted echoes are recorded and presented in color at many locations along each scan line in the Doppler ROI (Fig. 5.39,

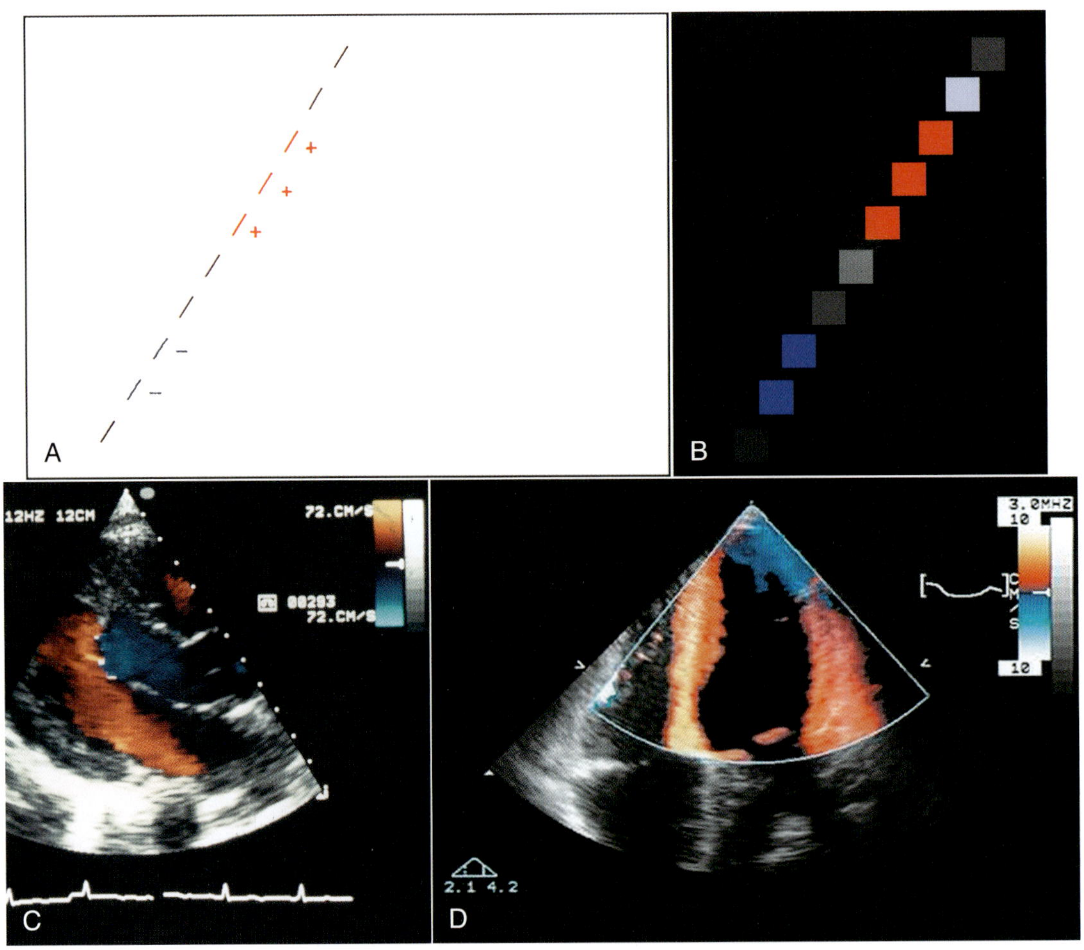

Fig. 5.39 A, Ten echoes are received as a pulse travels through tissues. Three (*red*) have positive Doppler shifts, and two (*blue*) have negative shifts. **B,** These echoes are shown (in this example) as red and blue pixels, respectively, on the color Doppler display. As in grayscale ultrasound imaging, a two-dimensional cross-sectional image is made up of many scan lines. **C,** A parasternal long-axis image of normal mitral valve blood flow. **D,** A parasternal short-axis view of myocardial tissue motion (*Tissue Doppler Imaging*).

A–B). This ROI or color box is overlaid on the regular B-mode (i.e., grayscale) image appearing as one cross-sectional image (see Fig. 5.39, C–D). Multiple images (frames) are presented each second, yielding real-time CDI.

> CDI shows 2D regions of blood flow or tissue motion in a color overlay on top of grayscale images.

Linear array presentation of color Doppler information is sometimes problematic when vessels run parallel to the skin surface, because the pulses (and scan lines) run perpendicular to the transducer surface, resulting in a 90-degree Doppler angle where the pulses intersect the flow in the vessel (assuming the flow is parallel to the vessel walls). A 90-degree Doppler angle yields no Doppler shift (i.e., $f_D = 0$) and hence no color within the vessel. To solve this problem, phasing is used to steer each transmitted Doppler pulse train from the array in a given direction (e.g., 20 degrees away from perpendicular). This steering results in a parallelogram presentation of the color Doppler ROI (or color box) on the display (Fig. 5.40).

Doppler-Shift Detection in Color Flow Mode

The signal processor receives the digitized samples (i.e., voltages) from the beam former that represent the echoes returning from the tissue over time. Regular (non-Doppler shifted) echoes are processed conventionally as in any pulse-echo system. Doppler-shifted echoes are commonly analyzed in the signal processor using a mathematical technique called **autocorrelation**, which rapidly (based on as few as three to four samples or Doppler scan lines) determines the mean and **variance** of the Doppler signal (Fig. 5.41) at each location along the Doppler scan line (i.e., at each echo arrival time). The autocorrelation technique estimates the sign, mean, and variance of the Doppler signal, and these are stored at appropriate locations in the memory corresponding to the anatomical sites where the Doppler shifts have been found. Typically, 100 to 400 Doppler samples (locations) per scan line are shown in a **color Doppler display**. Depending on the depth and width of the color box, typically 5 to 50

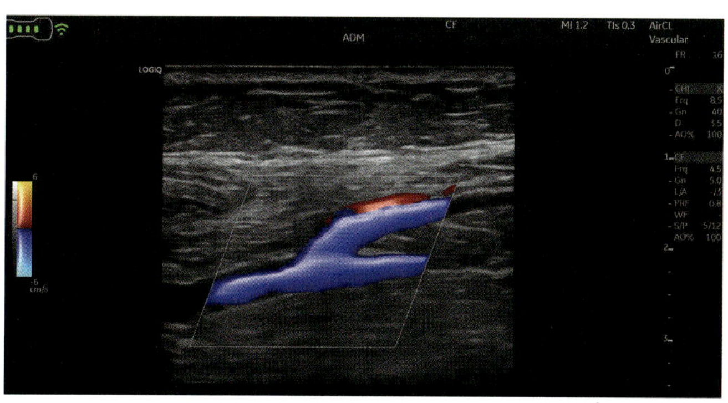

Fig. 5.40 A perpendicular Doppler angle is avoided in this image by electronically steering the color-producing Doppler pulses to the left of vertical as indicated by the angle of the color box. Notice that this Color Doppler imaging was obtained with a point-of-care ultrasound system. (Courtesy GE HealthCare.)

frames per second can be shown (when narrow transmit beams are used). Recall that in traditional grayscale mode, a single pulse produces one scan line. In color Doppler mode, multiple pulses are employed along each Doppler scan line within the color Doppler box, because they are required in the autocorrelation process. A three-pulse minimum is required for one blood flow estimate. More pulses are required in the Doppler pulse train for improved accuracy of the estimates, for variance determinations, or to improve detection of lower frequency mean Doppler shifts (slower flows). However, it is important to notice that the number of pulses transmitted along each scan line in color Doppler mode is typically an order of magnitude less than in PW Doppler systems, meaning the velocity estimates are inherently less accurate than with PW Doppler.

> Autocorrelation is the mathematical process commonly used to detect Doppler shifts in color Doppler instruments.

ADVANCED CONCEPTS

Autocorrelation is a mathematical process that compares a function with itself, in this case the Doppler signal phase at different times. Autocorrelation is a measure of similarity (or non-randomness) of the function at the different times. Autocorrelation is the cross-correlation of a signal with a time-delayed version of itself. Autocorrelation is useful for finding repeating patterns in a signal, such as determining the presence of a periodic signal that has been hidden by noise. For our purpose, autocorrelation determines the phase shift that has occurred over some short time interval. This phase shift is a measure of the Doppler shift and thus flow velocity as well as providing an indicator of the motion of a reflector (i.e., red blood cell) over the time interval.

Color Controls

Color controls include gain, color box location, width and depth, steering angle, color-map inversion, **wall filter**, **priority**, **baseline shift**, velocity range (i.e., indirect choice of *PRF*), color map selection, variance, smoothing, and **ensemble length**. Steering angle control permits 90-degree beam-to-vessel angles to be avoided (Fig. 5.42). The wall filter allows elimination of clutter caused by tissue and wall motion (Fig. 5.43). However, one must take care not to set the wall filter too high, or slower blood flow signals will be removed (see Fig. 5.43, C). It should be noted that wall filter controls are less and less likely to be available on newer scanners, where this setting is often controlled internally by the selected scanning preset.

Direct control of the *PRF* is not available in grayscale mode, but when operating in color Doppler mode, the operator controls *PRF* with the scale control (or velocity range). This control sets the *PRF* and the limit at the color bar extremes. Decreasing the value permits observation of slower flows (smaller Doppler shifts) (see Fig. 5.43, F) but increases the probability of an artifact, called aliasing, occurring for faster flows (aliasing is described in Chapter 7). Color Write Priority selects the grayscale echo strength below which color, instead of gray level, will be displayed at a given pixel location (Fig. 5.44). Baseline control and color map selection allow shifting the baseline up or down to correct for aliasing and changing the color scheme

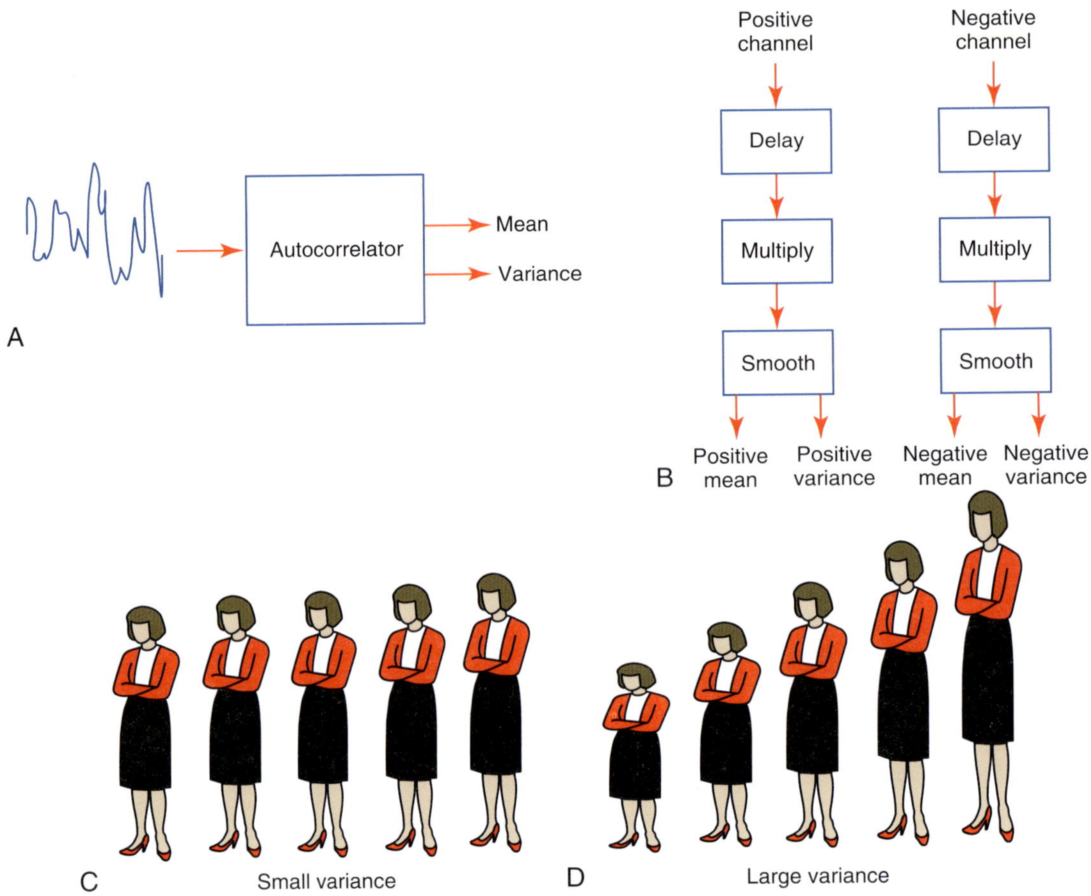

Fig. 5.41 A, The autocorrelator rapidly performs Doppler demodulation on the complicated echo signal (entering at left). The outputs of the autocorrelator yield the magnitude of the mean and the variance of Doppler shifts at each location in the scanned cross-section. These items of information are stored in each pixel location in the memory. Color assignments are selected appropriately to indicate these items of information two-dimensionally on the display. **B,** After splitting the Doppler signal into positive and negative Doppler-shift channels, each signal is multiplied by a version of itself delayed by one pulse repetition period. High-frequency variations are filtered out (smoothed) to yield the mean and variance of Doppler shifts. Variance is a measure of data spread around a mean and is equal to the standard deviation squared. **C–D,** Two groups of women with equal mean heights but unequal variances.

used for depicting flow direction and speed (including alternating the color assignments on either side of the zero-Doppler-shift baseline; see Fig. 5.42, D–E).

Smoothing (also called persistence) provides frame-to-frame averaging to reduce noise (Fig. 5.45). Ensemble length is the number of pulses used along each color Doppler scan line. The minimum is 3 with 15 to 30 being common (when narrow transmit beams are used). Greater ensemble lengths provide more accurate estimates of mean Doppler shift, improved detection of slow flows within an organ or gland (see Fig. 5.45), and more complete representation of flow within a vessel but at the expense of longer time per scan line and per frame and therefore lower frame rates. Wider color windows (viewing areas) also reduce frame rates because more scan lines are required for each frame.

It should be noted that many of these subjective parameter optimizations, performed by the operator of the ultrasound scanner (typically the sonographer), can now be automatically adjusted by the single button optimization functions available on many high-end scanners.

Doppler-Shift Displays

Doppler-shifted echoes are presented as hue, saturation, and luminance according to a choice of color schemes. The selected color display scheme is presented on the display as a color map (Fig. 5.46). The map allows the observer to interpret the meaning of the hue, saturation, and luminance at each location in terms of the sign, magnitude, and variance of Doppler shifts. Hue indicates the sign of the Doppler shift. Changes in hue, saturation, or luminance up or down the map from the center indicate increasing Doppler shift magnitude (relative to each other not in absolute terms, since the Doppler angle is assumed to be zero throughout the imaging plane). When selected, variance is shown as a change in hue from left to right across the map.

> The color map, always shown on the display, is the key to understanding how image colors are related to Doppler characteristics.

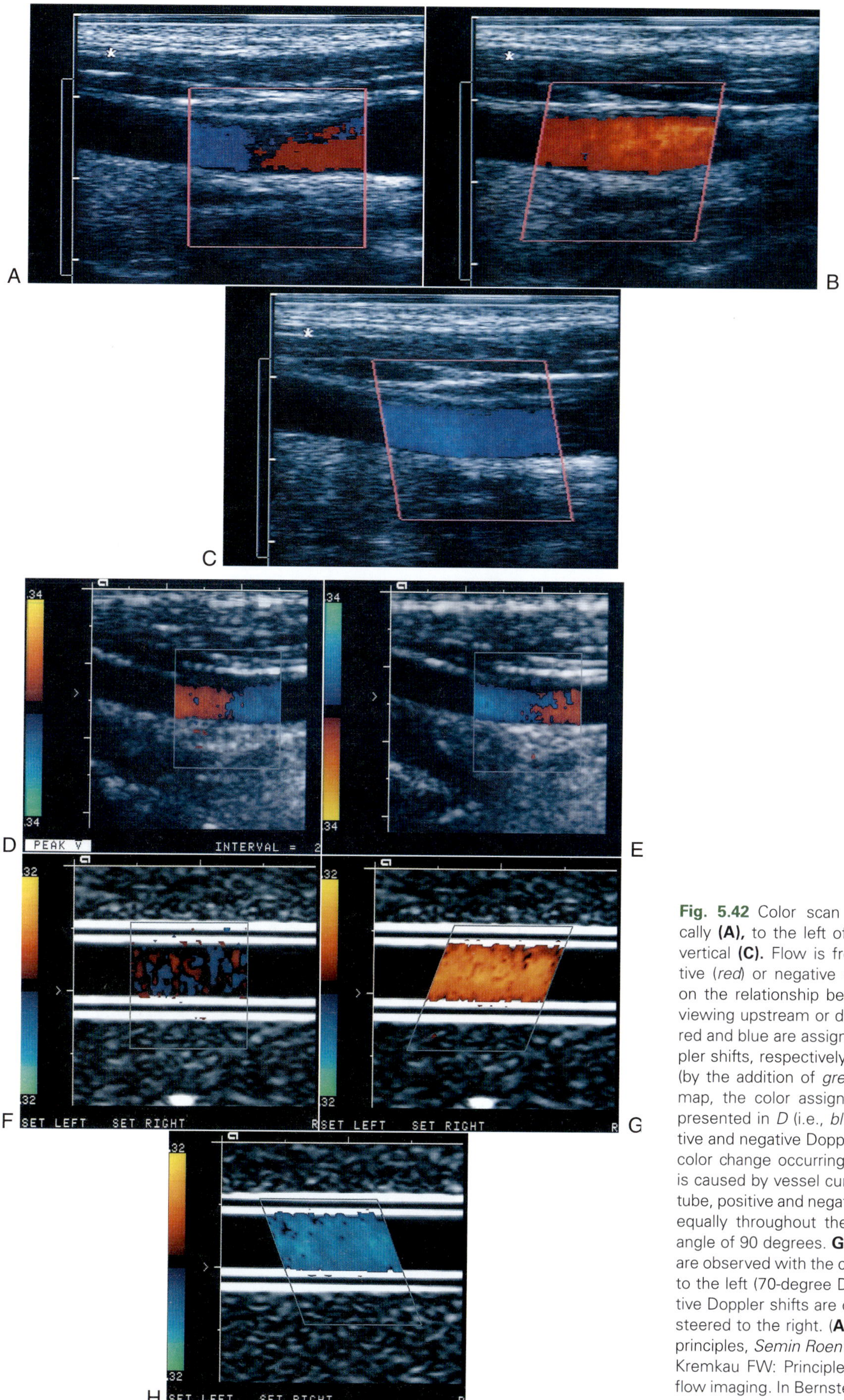

Fig. 5.42 Color scan lines are directed down vertically **(A),** to the left of vertical **(B),** and to the right of vertical **(C).** Flow is from left to right, producing positive (*red*) or negative (*blue*) Doppler shifts, depending on the relationship between scan lines and flow (i.e., viewing upstream or downstream). **D,** In this hue map, red and blue are assigned to positive and negative Doppler shifts, respectively, progressing to yellow and cyan (by the addition of *green*) at the map limits. **E,** In this map, the color assignments are inverted from those presented in *D* (i.e., *blue* and *red* are assigned to positive and negative Doppler shifts, respectively). Note the color change occurring within each color window. This is caused by vessel curvature. **F,** With flow in a straight tube, positive and negative Doppler shifts are distributed equally throughout the color window with a Doppler angle of 90 degrees. **G,** Uniform positive Doppler shifts are observed with the color window steered 20 degrees to the left (70-degree Doppler angle). **H,** Uniform negative Doppler shifts are observed with the color window steered to the right. (**A–C,** From Kremkau FW: Doppler principles, *Semin Roentgenol* 27:6–16, 1992. **D–E,** From Kremkau FW: Principles and pitfalls of real-time color-flow imaging. In Bernstein EF, editor: *Vascular diagnosis*, 4th ed, St. Louis, 1993, Mosby.)

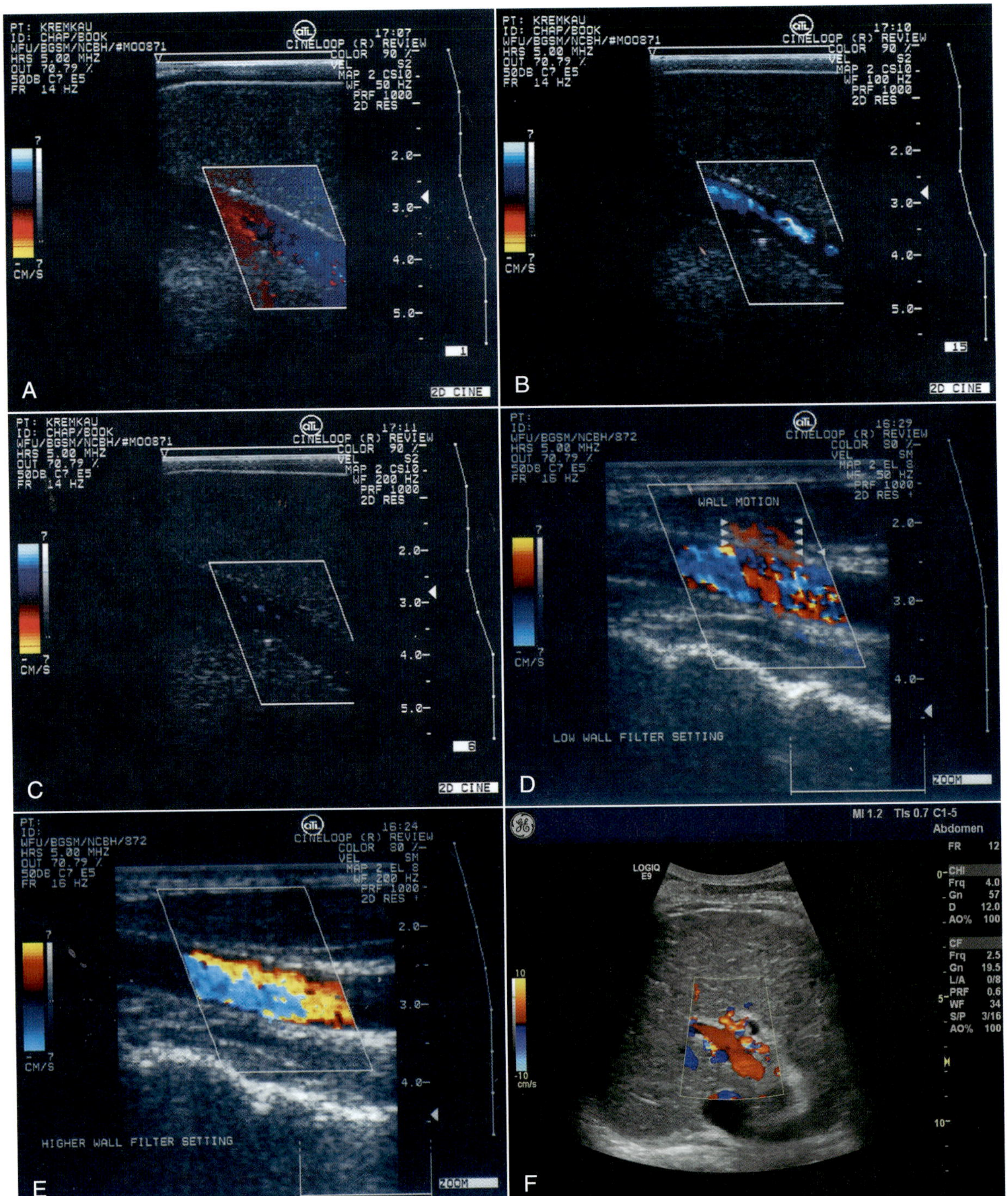

Fig. 5.43 **A,** Tissue motion causes clutter, obscuring the flow in the vessel and clouding the gray-scale tissue with color Doppler information. **B,** Wall filter has been increased to 100 Hz, thereby eliminating the color clutter. **C,** Wall filter has been increased (too much) to 200 Hz, eliminating virtually all the color Doppler information derived from the vessel. **D,** With a low wall filter setting (50 Hz), wall motion appears in color on the image. **E,** With a higher wall filter setting (200 Hz), this motion no longer appears in color. **F,** Slow portal flow imaged with low pulse-repetition frequency. (**A–C,** From Kremkau FW: Principles and pitfalls of real-time color-flow imaging. In Bernstein EF, editor: *Vascular diagnosis*, 4th ed, St. Louis, 1993, Mosby. **D–E,** From Kremkau FW: Principles and instrumentation. In Merritt CRB, editor: *Doppler color imaging*, New York, 1992, Churchill Livingstone.)

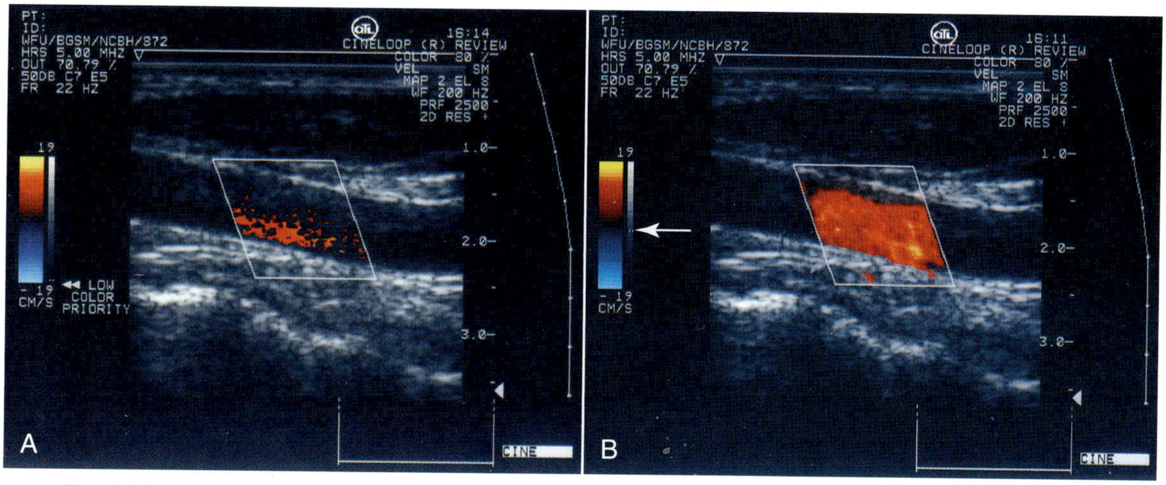

Fig. 5.44 A, With the color priority set low (*at the bottom of the gray bar*), weak, non-Doppler-shifted reverberation, and off-axis echoes within the vessel take precedence over the Doppler-shifted echoes, and little color is displayed. **B,** With a higher color priority setting (*halfway up the gray bar [arrow]*), the Doppler-shifted echoes (*color*) take precedence over the weaker gray-scale echoes. (From Kremkau FW: Principles and instrumentation. In Merritt CRB, editor: *Doppler color imaging*, New York, 1992, Churchill Livingstone.)

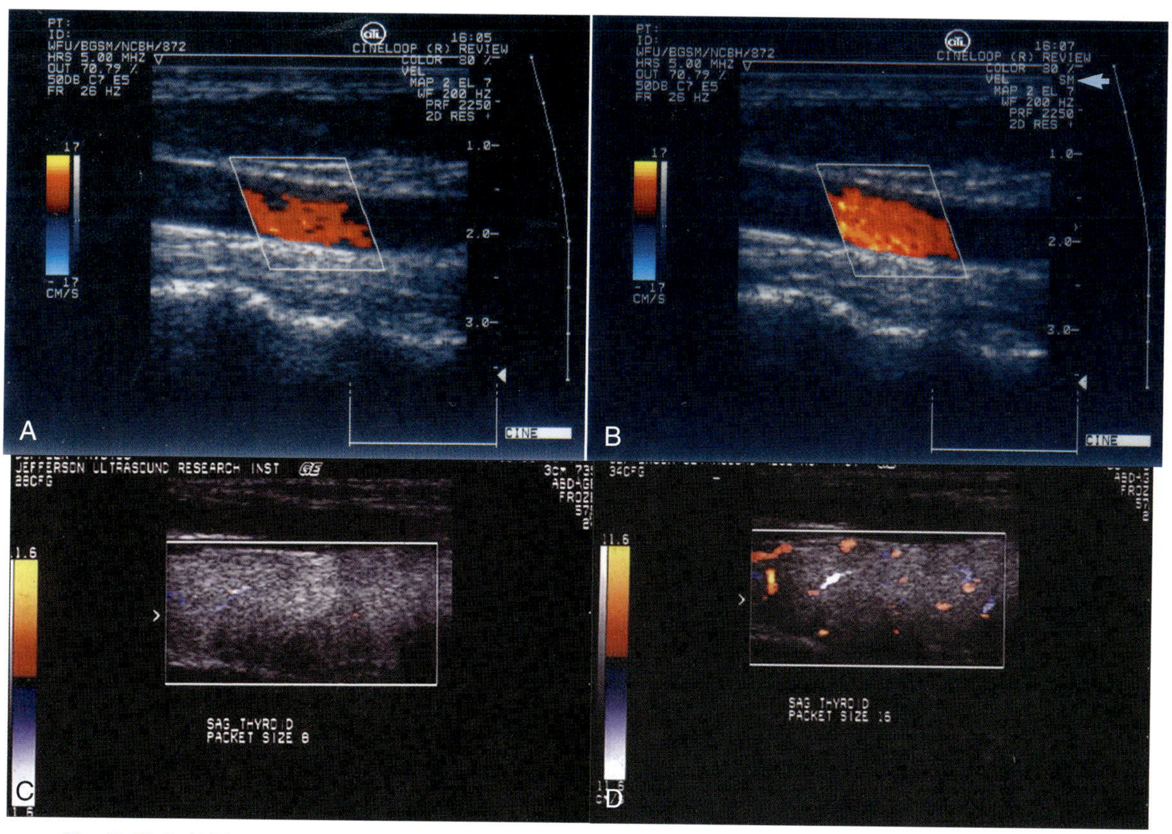

Fig. 5.45 A, With no smoothing (persistence), only the Doppler-shifted echoes received from the pulses generating an individual frame are shown. **B,** With smoothing, consecutive frames are averaged, filling gaps in the presentation and presenting a smoother but less detailed representation of flow. **C–D,** More accurate and complete detection of flow information within a thyroid is obtained with increasing ensemble lengths from 8 (see **C**) to 16 (see **D**). Note that this increase will decrease the frame rate by a factor of 2. (**A–B,** From Kremkau FW: Principles and instrumentation. In Merritt CRB, editor: *Doppler color imaging*, New York, 1992, Churchill Livingstone.)

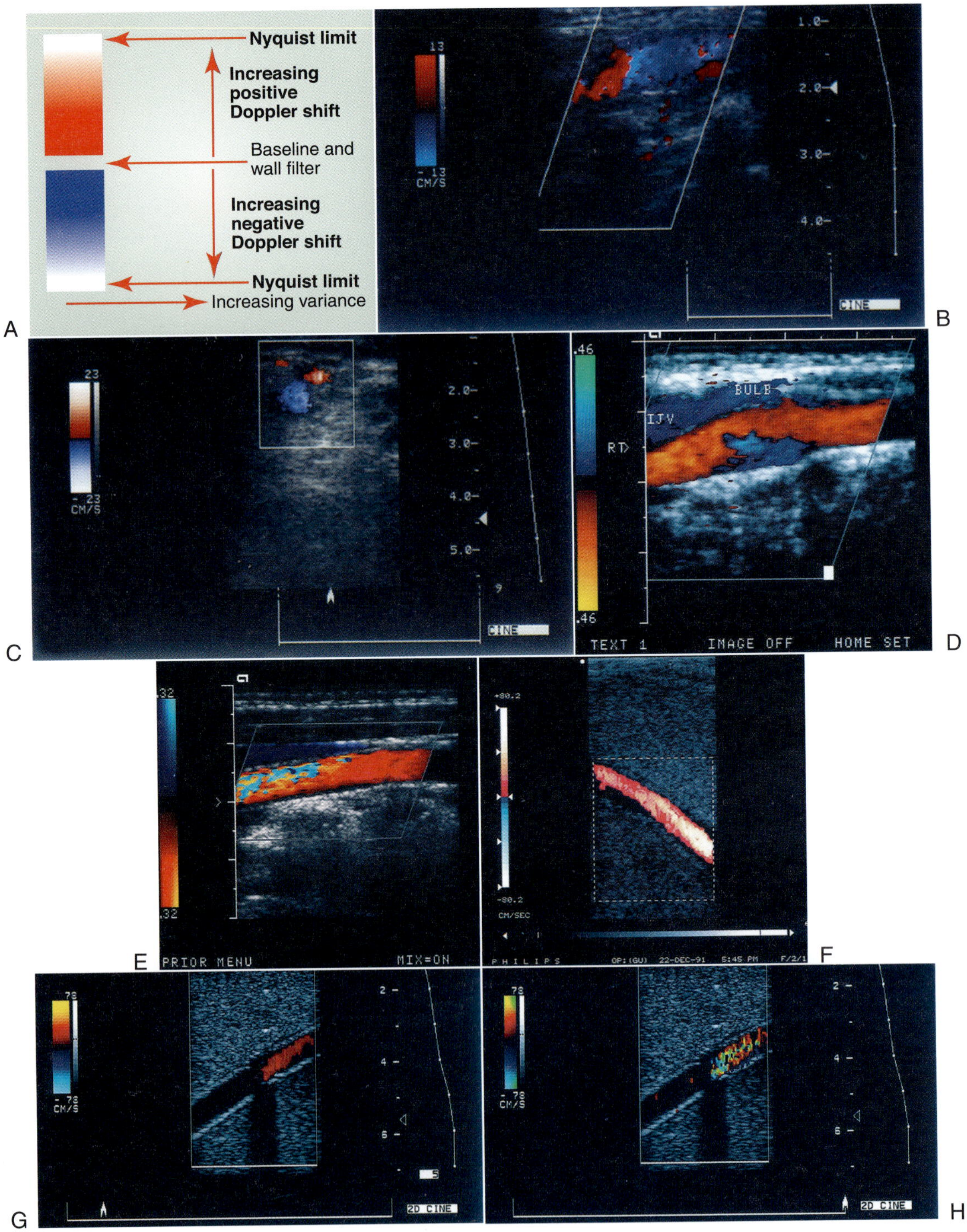

Fig. 5.46 Color map information. **A,** Diagram describing the information contained in a color map or color bar. **B,** A luminance map. Increasing luminance of red or blue indicates, respectively, increasing positive or negative mean Doppler shifts. **C,** A saturation map is used to show flow transversely in two vessels. Flow in the upper vessel is toward the transducer, yielding positive Doppler shifts (*red*). Flow in the lower vessel is away from the transducer, yielding negative Doppler shifts (*blue*). On this color map, red and blue progress to white (decreasing saturation, increasing luminance) with increasing positive and negative Doppler shift means, respectively. **D,** A hue map showing flow in the carotid artery (with reversal in the bulb) and jugular vein. Increasingly positive Doppler shifts progress from dark blue to bright cyan (*blue plus green*). Increasingly negative Doppler shifts progress from dark red to bright yellow (*red plus green*). **E,** A luminance (*dark blue and red to bright blue and red*) map with variance included. Increasing variance adds green to red or blue (*producing yellow or cyan*), progressing from left to right across the map. **F,** A saturation map. Red and blue progress toward white. **G,** A stenosis in a tube (*located at the shadow*) increases the flow speed. Proximal to (left of) the stenosis, flow speed is too slow to be detected, whereas distal to (right of) the stenosis, positive Doppler shifts are seen. **H,** The variance map shows spectral broadening (*green*) in the turbulent flow region distal to the stenosis. (**A,** From Kremkau FW: Principles and instrumentation. In Merritt CRB, editor: *Doppler color imaging*, New York, 1992, Churchill Livingstone. **B–F,** From Kremkau FW: Principles of color flow imaging, *J Vasc Technol* 15:104–111, 1991.)

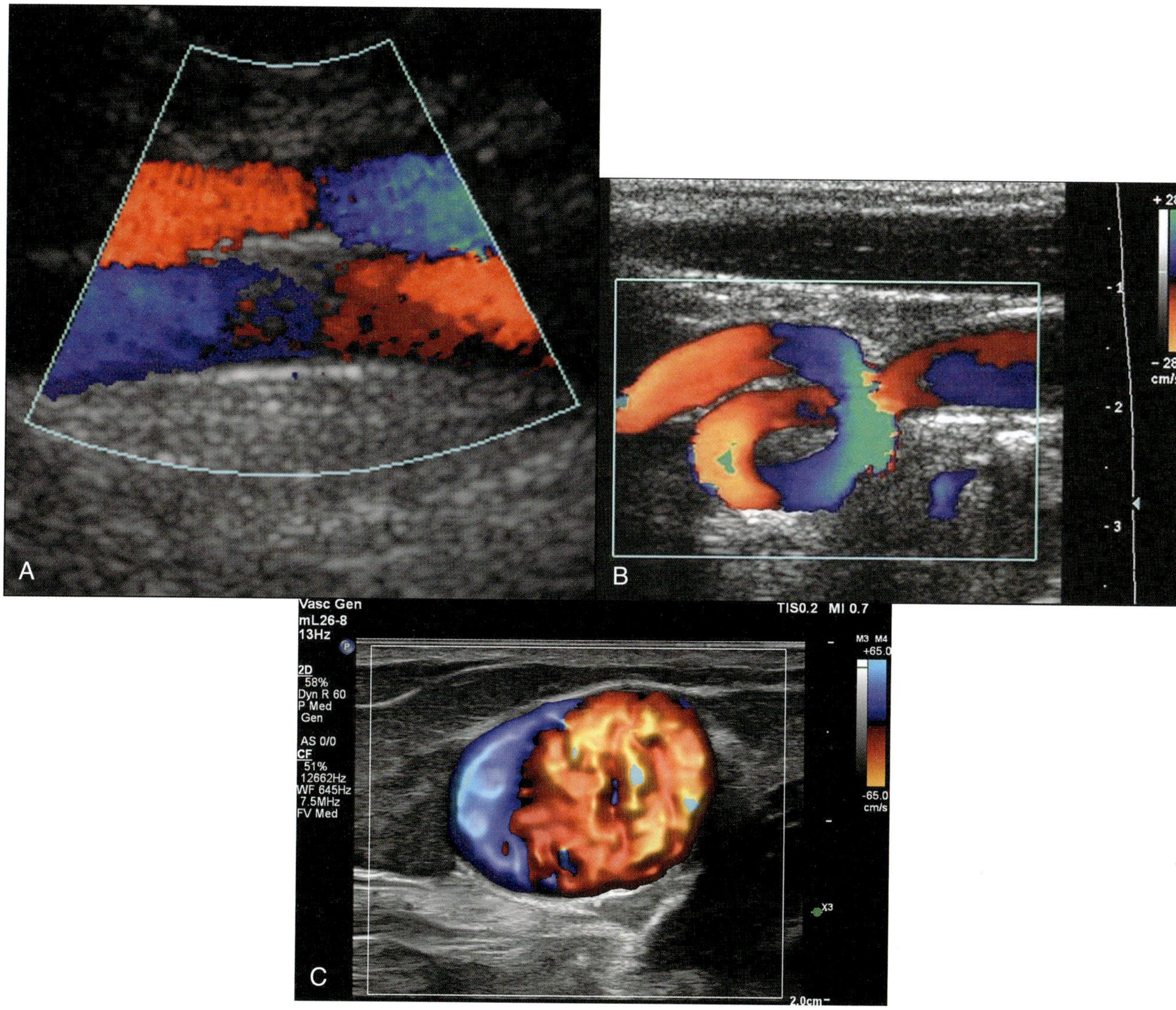

Fig. 5.47 Beam-to-vessel angle is important for any Doppler technique, but in color Doppler imaging, this is a critical parameter, since all Doppler shits are color coded relative to the position of the transducer. **A,** Two vessels imaged by a curvilinear array with the proximal vessel depicted with red on the left and blue on the right, while the distal vessel is the exact opposite (i.e., *blue* on the left and *red* on the right). The color changes are due to flow on the left in the top vessel being upstream (i.e., moving toward the transducer), while flow on the right is seen as being downstream (i.e., moving away from the transducer). At the 90-degree Doppler angle point, the color changes because the situation changes from upstream to downstream. Conversely, in the bottom vessel flow is from the right to the left. **B,** A linear-array transducer shows flow from right to left in this tortuous vessel. Initially flow is toward the transducer on the right (positive Doppler shifts are *blue* on this map) and away from the transducer further on the left (negative Doppler shifts are *red*), while the second color change is caused by the vessel curving upward before finally flowing away from the transducer at the extreme left (i.e., red Doppler shifts). **C,** A fistula with clockwise circulating flow demonstrating the angle dependency of color Doppler. (**C,** Courtesy of Philips Medical Systems).

Angle

Beam to vessel angle is important for any Doppler technique, but in CDI, this is a critical parameter, since all Doppler shits are color coded relative to the position of the transducer. Fig. 5.47 shows curvilinear and linear array views of vascular flow. The two vessels in Fig. 5.47, A are similar in appearance, but the proximal vessel presents with red on the left and blue on the right, while the distal vessel is the exact opposite (i.e., blue on the left and red on the right). How is this inconsistency explained? In fact, why does the color change at all, considering that there is no reason not to expect unidirectional flow in these vessels? The color changes in the vessel in Fig. 5.47, A, because, with the sector image format, pulses and scan lines travel in different directions away from the transducer. Thus they have different Doppler angles relative to the flow in the straight vessels. So pulses view the flow on the left in the top vessel as being upstream (i.e., moving toward the transducer) and flow on the right as being downstream (i.e., away from the transducer). At the 90-degree Doppler angle point, the color changes because the situation changes from upstream to downstream. Conversely, in the bottom vessel flow is from the right to the left. However, this is not the case in Fig. 5.47, B. All the pulses travel in the same direction (straight down) from this linear-array transducer. If the color change is not caused by changing scan-line directions, then it must be as a result of changing flow direction. Flow is from right to left in this tortuous vessel, so flow is toward the transducer on the right (positive Doppler shifts are blue on this map) and away from the transducer further on the left (negative Doppler shifts are red). A view further to the left reveals a second color change caused by the curve upward (from red to blue; see Fig. 5.47, B) before finally moving away from the transducer at the extreme left (i.e., red Doppler shifts). Fig. 5.47, C shows an example of circulating clockwise flow in a fistula demonstrating the angle dependency of CDI.

Another example of color Doppler angle impact is shown in Fig. 5.48, A of a splenic vein. We now understand that flow is going from the right to the left (from upstream to downstream) as indicated by the red to blue color shift (in this map red indicates flow toward the transducer or positive Doppler shifts). This assessment of flow conditions is confirmed by spectral Doppler showing positive and negative Doppler shifts on the right and left of the image, respectively (Fig. 5.48, B–C).

> All Doppler shifts are color coded relative to the position of the transducer.

In Fig. 5.49, some interesting questions arise. First, in part A, what is the blood flow direction? According to the color map in the upper left-hand corner of the figure, negative Doppler shifts are coded in red and yellow, whereas positive Doppler shifts are coded in blue and cyan. The color scan lines (and pulses) are steered to the left, and negative Doppler shifts (red and yellow) are received from the blood flowing within the vessel in the upper and lower portions of the figure. If we are looking to the left and seeing blood flowing away from us (negative Doppler shifts), the blood must be flowing from right to left in the upper and lower horizontal portions of the vessel. What about the central portion of the vessel? Clearly, the blood would have to be flowing from left to right there, but why are negative Doppler shifts also seen in this portion? The answer is that this portion of the vessel is not horizontal but is angled down, so even though the blood is flowing from left to right, it is also flowing away from the transducer because of the downward direction (more precisely, it is flowing from upper left to lower right). Thus negative Doppler shifts are found throughout the vessel in this scan. In other words, the flow direction

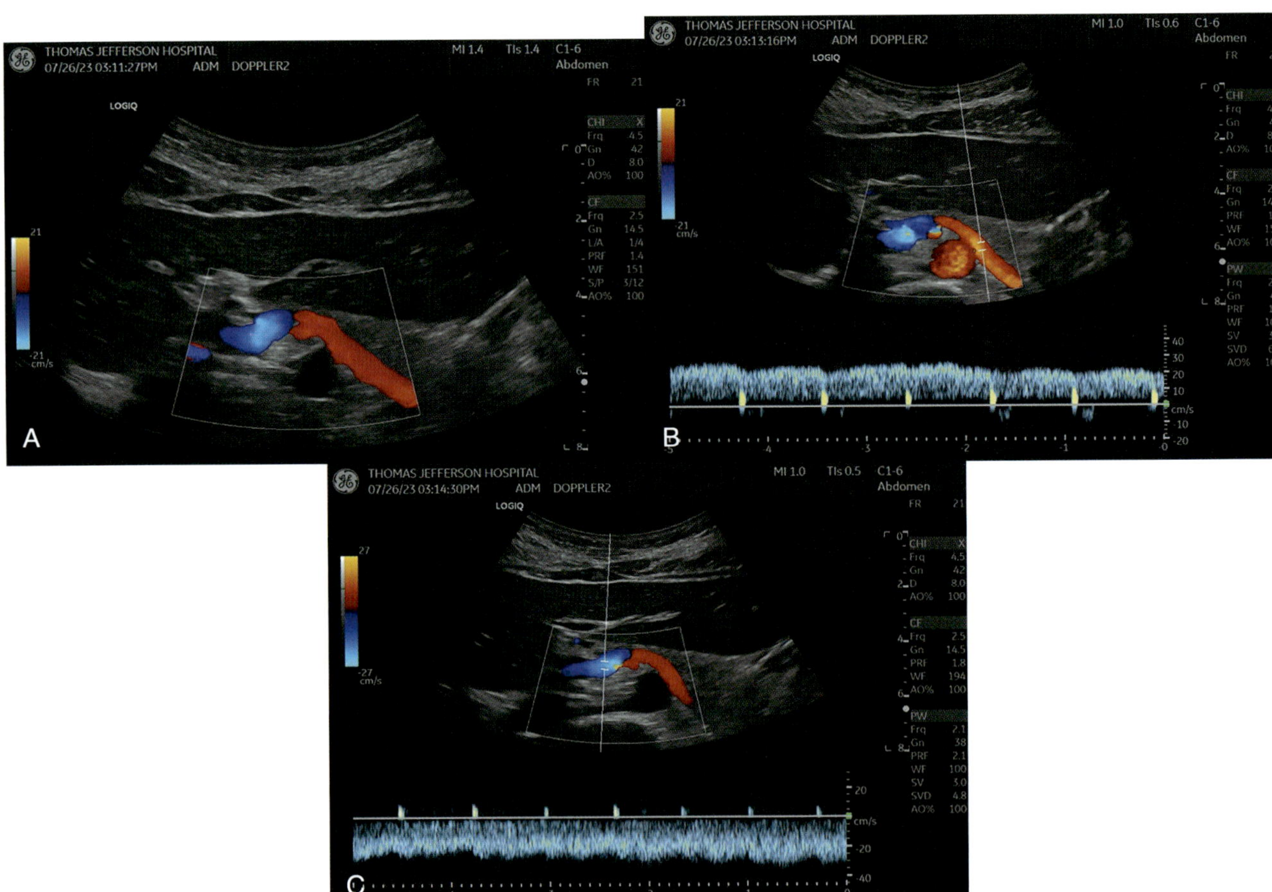

Fig. 5.48 **A,** Splenic vein with flow from the right to the left (from upstream to downstream) as indicated by the red to blue color shift (in this map *red* indicates flow toward the transducer or positive Doppler shifts). **B,** Spectral Doppler showing positive Doppler shifts on the right. **C,** Negative Doppler shifts on the left confirming the directional observations made in **A**.

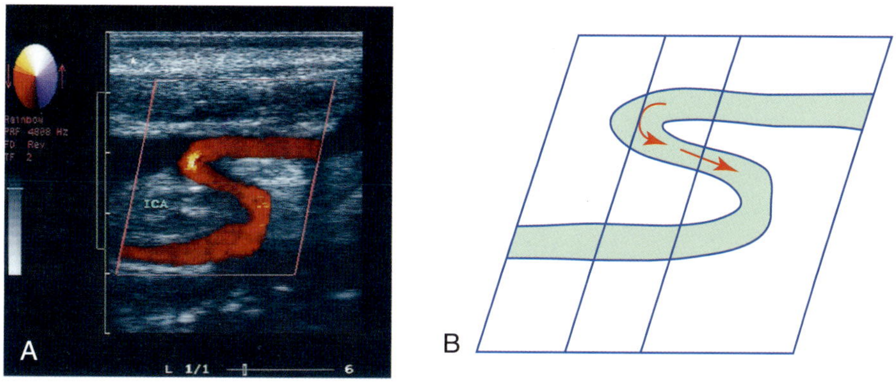

Fig. 5.49 **A,** A tortuous artery. **B,** This drawing shows the angle relationships depicted in **A.** (**A–B,** From Kremkau FW: Color interpretation, *J Vasc Technol* 16:215–216, 1992.)

gets close to, but never crosses, the perpendicular to the scan lines (see Fig. 5.49, B).

Another question arises with respect to Fig. 5.49, A. According to the color map, the yellow region in the bend at the upper left is where the highest negative Doppler shifts are generated. Does this indicate that the blood flow is the fastest at this location? The answer is no. The highest negative Doppler shifts are found in this region, because the smallest Doppler angles are encountered there, and not because high flow speeds are found there. In this region, the flow is approximately parallel to the scan lines (see Fig. 5.49, B), yielding Doppler angles of around zero. No evidence of vessel narrowing is present to explain increased flow speed. Hence, the increased Doppler shift can be explained purely on grounds of angle.

Color Doppler Limitations

The limitations of narrow transmit beam CDI include angle dependence, lower frame rates, and lack of detailed spectral information. Spectral Doppler presents the entire range of Doppler-shift frequencies received across the cardiac cycle. Color Doppler displays present only a single statistical representation of the complete spectrum at each pixel location. The sign, mean value, and, if chosen, the power or the variance of the spectrum are color-coded into combinations of **hue**, **saturation**, and **luminance** that are presented at each display pixel location. Some color Doppler displays were able to produce quantitative digital values for mean Doppler shifts (using so-called time domain cross-correlation algorithms; Fig. 5.50). However, none of these systems are currently commercially available.

Since color Doppler techniques require multiple pulses per scan line, frame rates are lower than those for grayscale imaging. Therefore, multiple foci are not used in CDI. Instead, the focus is at the mid-level of the color box (when narrow transmit beams are used). The relationship between penetration (pen, the depth to which the ultrasound is penetrating tissue; not necessarily the displayed depth on the instrument display), line density, and frame rate is the same as that presented in Chapter 4, except that ensemble length (n) replaces the number of foci. The maximum permissible frame rate (FR_m) is as follows:

$$FR_m\,(Hz) = \frac{77{,}000\,(cm/s)}{pen\,(cm) \times lines\ per\ frame\ (LPF) \times n}$$

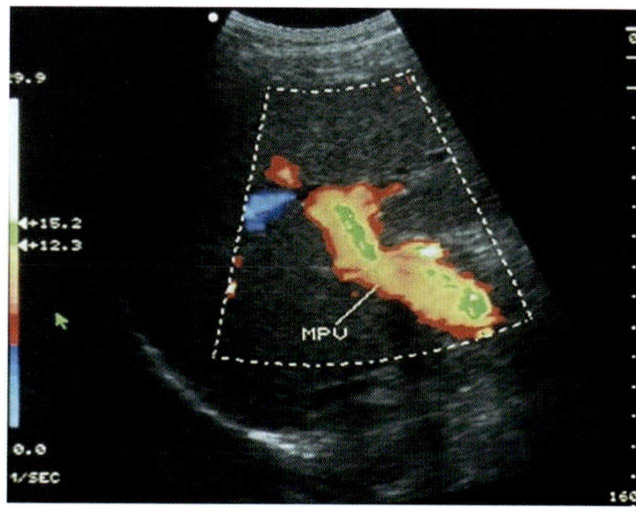

Fig. 5.50 Quantitative mean Doppler velocities (12–15 cm/s) measured along the center-line of the main portal vein (MPV) using a time domain cross-correlation algorithms.

> If ensemble length increases, frame rate decreases.

Tissue Doppler Imaging

Echocardiographic evaluation of myocardial function is a long-standing clinical application. **Tissue Doppler imaging** (TDI) can provide a quantitative evaluation of myocardial function. Blood flow in the heart results in high-frequency, low-amplitude Doppler-shifted signals, whereas myocardial motion produces low-velocity, high-amplitude signals. Thus TDI is achieved by inverting the low pass filter used in traditional Doppler processing into a high pass filter. There are both spectral (i.e., pulsed wave) and color TDI modes available (Fig. 5.51).

Power Doppler Imaging

CDI displays encode the mean Doppler shifts within a two-dimensional ROI according to the color map selected. **Power Doppler imaging** presents two-dimensional Doppler information by color coding the *strength* of the Doppler shifts. This approach eliminates aliasing, limits angle dependence, and is more sensitive to depicting slow flow as well as flow in small or deep vessels. Marketing names

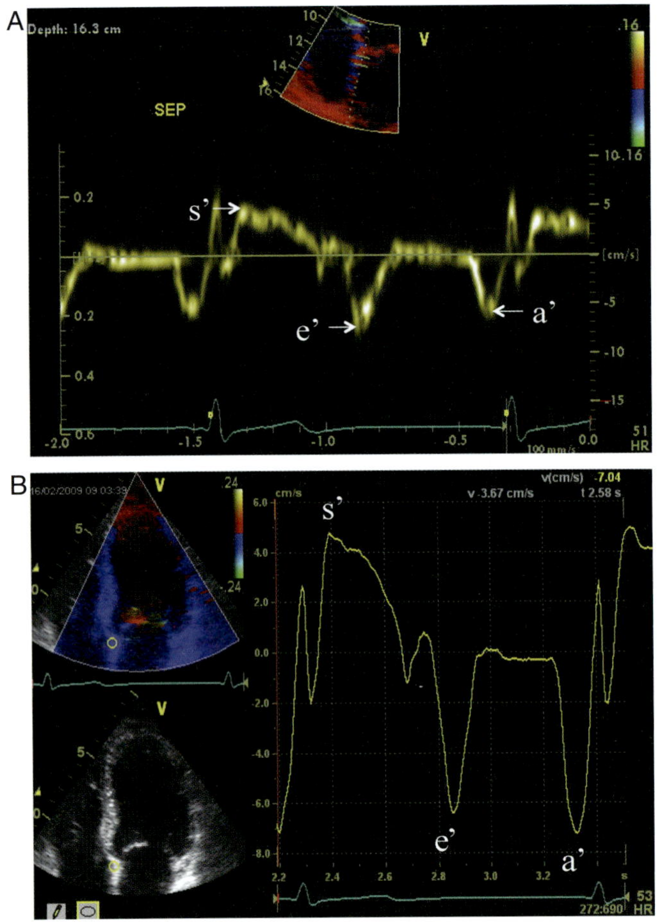

Fig. 5.51 Tissue Doppler imaging (*TDI*) examples from cardiology **A,** Pulsed wave TDI from the apical four-chamber view sampling from the septal mitral annulus. **B,** Color TDI from the apical four-chamber view sampling from the septal mitral annulus. (Reproduced from Kadappu KK, Thomas L: Tissue Doppler imaging in echocardiography: value and limitations, *Heart Lung Circ* 24:224–233, 2015.)

applied to this technique include *color power Doppler, ultrasound angio, color Doppler energy*, and *color power angio*. Rather than assigning various hue, saturation, and luminance values to mean Doppler frequencies, this technique assigns color values to Doppler shift *power* values. The power of Doppler shifts is determined by the *concentration* of moving scatterers producing the Doppler shifts and is independent of Doppler shift frequency and Doppler angle. Orange hues are often used in power Doppler maps, but obviously, there is a plethora of different maps available across different ultrasound imaging platforms.

Power Doppler imaging displays color-coded Doppler shift power values in the color box.

ADVANCED CONCEPTS

In **power Doppler displays**, a cross-correlation calculation yields the integral of power density with respect to time. Noise is less of a problem in power Doppler compared with color Doppler displays. This is because noise is spread evenly over all frequencies and thus interferes with all aspects of a color Doppler display, but noise is not spread across all amplitudes; it mostly exists at the weaker levels. Thus the stronger Doppler-shifted echoes are lifted out of the noise floor and are assigned colors different from the background noise. The result is that power Doppler imaging can show flow in slower, deeper, and smaller vessels than CDI can, but at the cost of eliminating flow direction and velocity information.

Conventional CDI is still very useful, since showing dynamic flow direction and characteristics over the cardiac cycle are critical pieces of diagnostic information in many applications. Conversely, power Doppler displays show only the presence of flow (and not dynamic changes over time). However, integration of the Doppler signal over time also improves the SNR in power Doppler imaging. These two color flow modes are complimentary.

The Doppler detector in color Doppler imaging scanners yields the sign, mean, variance, and amplitude and power of the **Doppler spectrum** (Fig. 5.52, A) at each of the hundreds of **sample volume** locations within the color box selected in an anatomical cross-section (i.e., a grayscale image). Traditionally, in CDI, the sign and mean Doppler shift, and sometimes variance (usually in cardiac applications), are color coded and displayed. These parameters depend on the Doppler angle and are subject to aliasing (Fig. 5.53, A and Chapter 7). Power Doppler integrates the area under the spectrum (see Fig. 5.52, B), which is independent of angle and aliasing, displaying the effects of neither (see Fig. 5.53, B). Thus one advantage of power Doppler is the uniform (angle-independent and alias-free) presentation of flow information, albeit accomplished by discarding direction, speed, and flow character information.

This uniformity of flow displays extends through regions of 90-degree Doppler angles (see Fig. 5.53, B–C, E), because even though the mean Doppler shift is zero (yielding a black region in CDI; see Fig. 5.53, A, D), the beam width ensures non-90-degree angles and, thus, a spectrum there has a nonzero area (see Fig. 5.52, B).

Power Doppler imaging is also essentially free of variations in flow speed (as in the cardiac cycle) and thus can be frame averaged to improve the SNR and sensitivity (Fig. 5.54). Because aliasing is not a problem in power Doppler, lower *PRF*s can be used to detect slow flows. Box 5.3 lists the advantages and disadvantages of power Doppler displays. In general, Doppler ultrasound can determine (1) the presence or absence of flow, (2) the direction and (3) speed of flow, and (4) the character of flow. Power Doppler imaging is superior in terms of the first but at the expense of the other three. Table 5.9 compares color Doppler displays.

Power Doppler does not display direction, speed, or flow character information. They are, however, insensitive to angle effects and aliasing, which means they can present slower flows as well as flows in deeper and/or tinier vessels than CDI.

Recall that motion mode (M mode) presents a depth versus time display to record motion of moving structures (see Fig. 4.31). Likewise, with a stationary beam, color Doppler presents a motion versus time display of Doppler shifts produced by moving tissue or blood flow (see Fig. 5.51). Table 5.10 compares three types of Doppler displays: (1) CDI, (2) power Doppler imaging, and (3) spectral Doppler.

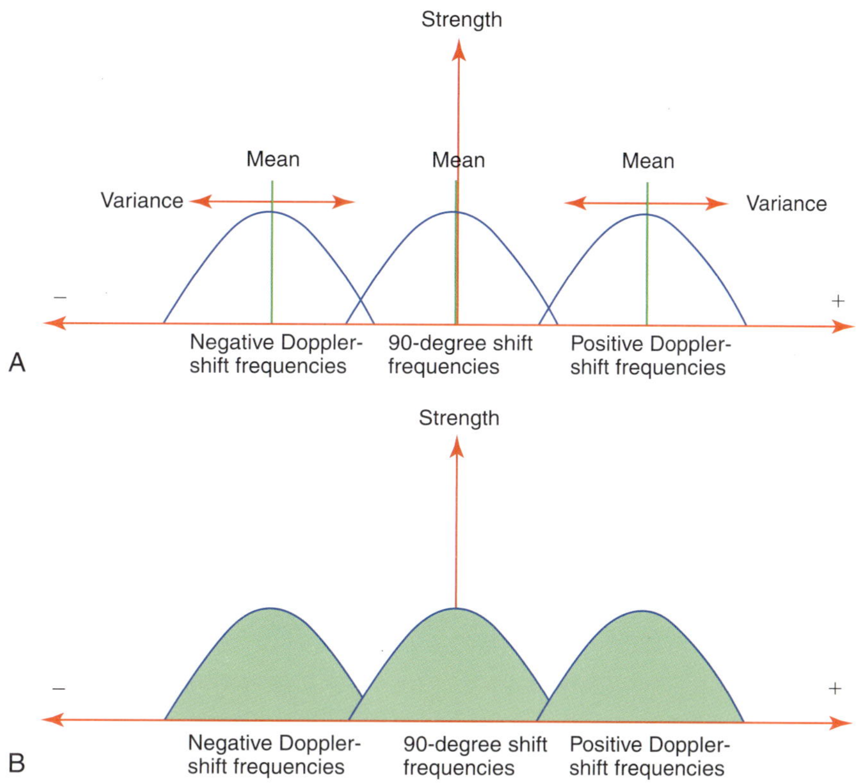

Fig. 5.52 **A,** Spectra for flow toward (positive) and away from (negative) the transducer and perpendicular (90 degrees) to the sound beam. Conventional color Doppler imaging determines and displays, in color-coded form, the sign and mean (and sometimes the variance) of the Doppler-shift frequency spectrum. **B,** Power Doppler imaging determines and displays, in color-coded form, the size of the area under the spectral curve. The axes of the spectral graph represent strength (amplitude, power, energy, or intensity) versus frequency.

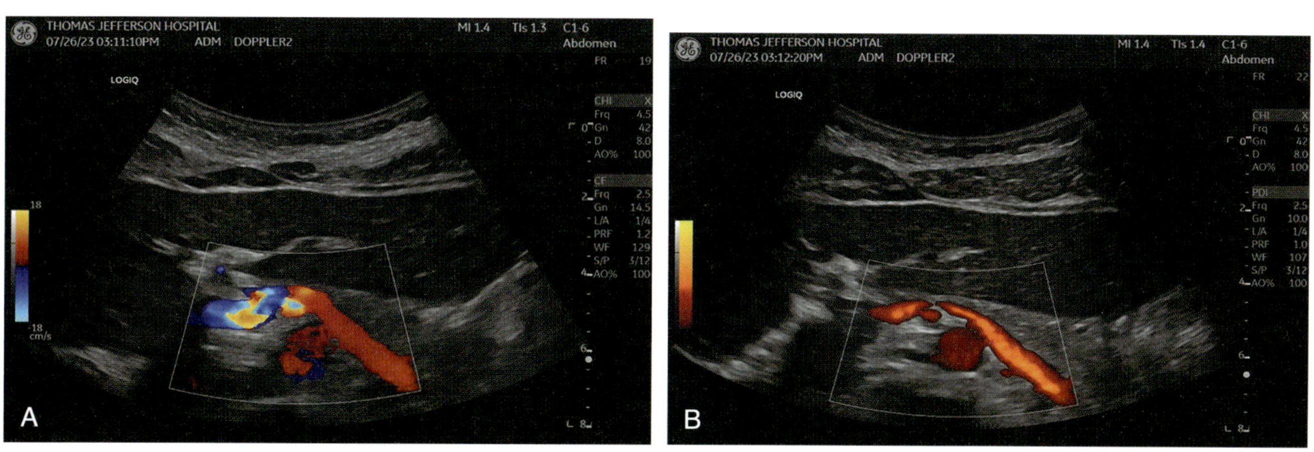

Fig. 5.53 **A,** A color Doppler image of flow in a splenic vein, acquired in sector format. The varying Doppler angle from left to right yields aliasing and positive, negative, and zero Doppler-shift regions. **B,** The same vessel shown in A imaged in power Doppler mode yields a uniform image, free of angle dependence and aliasing. However, it contains no directional, speed, or dynamic information.

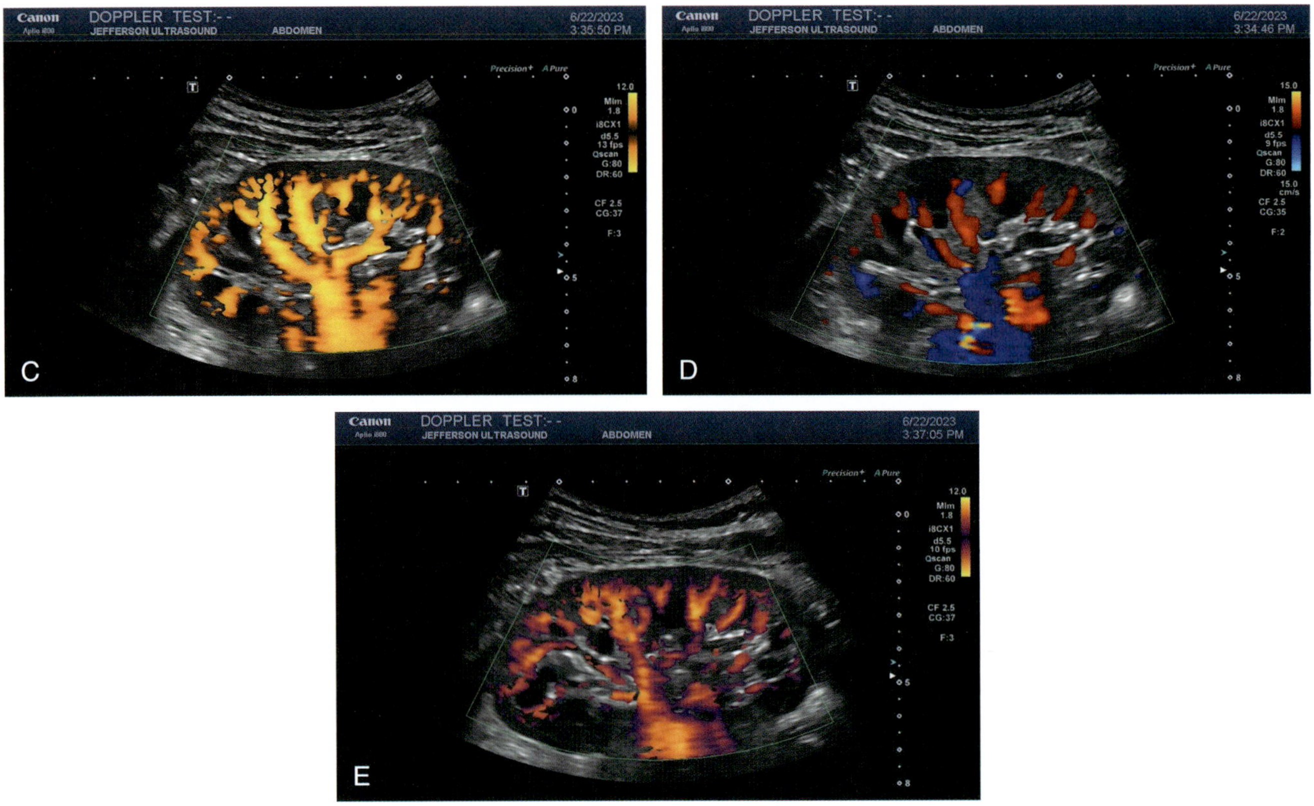

Fig. 5.53, cont'd C, Angle independence is seen with power Doppler imaging (*PDI*) of the kidney compared to **D,** the equivalent color Doppler imaging display. **E,** A different PDI map of the same kidney.

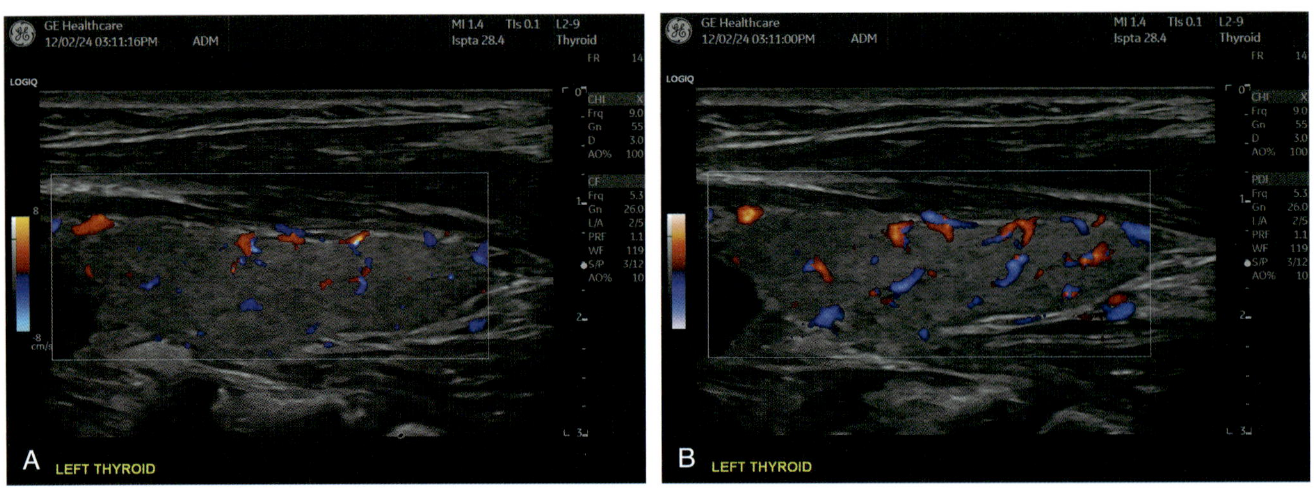

Fig. 5.54 A, Color Doppler imaging (*CDI*) of flow in a thyroid. **B,** Improved flow sensitivity with power Doppler compared with CDI (*shown in A*).

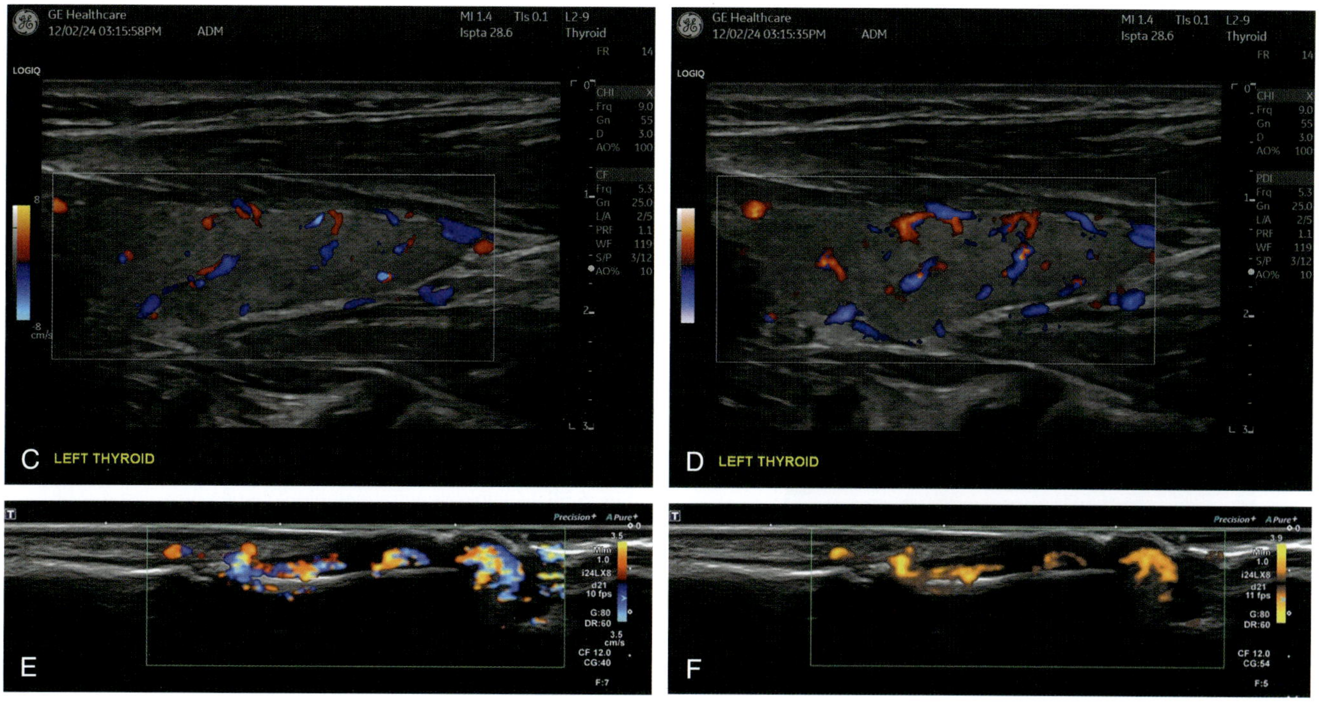

Fig. 5.54, cont'd **C,** Another thyroid example imaged in CDI mode **(D)** and in power Doppler imaging (PDI) mode. **E,** CDI of a finger. **F,** The same image in PDI mode showing better delineation of the vasculature (but not necessarily more vessels or improved flow sensitivity). (Courtesy Corrine Wessner, MSc, RDMS, Thomas Jefferson University.)

BOX 5.3 Advantages and Disadvantages of Power Doppler Compared to Color Doppler Displays

Advantages

- Less angle dependence
- No aliasing
- Improved sensitivity (deeper penetration, smaller vessels, slower flows)

Disadvantages

- No directional information
- No flow speed or character information
- More motion artifacts

TABLE 5.9 Comparison of Doppler-Shift Display and Doppler-Power Display

Presentation	Doppler Shift Display	Doppler Power Display
Quantitative	No	No
2D overview	Yes	Yes
Indication of perfusion	No	Yes

TABLE 5.10 Comparison of Doppler-Shift Display, Doppler-Power Display, and Spectral Display

Presentation	Color Doppler—Shift Display	Color Doppler—Power Display	Spectral Display
Quantitative	No	No	Yes
2D overview	Yes	Yes	No
Indication of perfusion	No	Yes	No

MOTION AND FLOW IMAGING WITH BROAD TRANSMIT BEAMS

In addition to the improvements to anatomical imaging that imaging with broad transmit beams provides, as discussed in Chapter 4, there are several improvements to Doppler flow imaging that becomes available with this technology. Primary among them is the fact that grayscale, color (or power) Doppler, and spectral Doppler (so-called triplex imaging) are implemented simultaneously rather than with time-sharing between them as required when using narrow transmit beams. The increased frame rates (up to 6000 Hz) possible with broad transmit beams (ultimately plane wave imaging) increase the speed with which these grayscale and Doppler calculations and presentations are updated. Doppler framerates from 80 to 250 Hz can be realized, an order of magnitude faster than those achievable with narrow transmit beams.

Vector velocity imaging is possible with broad transmit beams, where arrows show speed (by arrow length) and direction (by arrow direction), that is, complete velocity of flow at any point in the color box (Fig. 5.55). Moreover, the expanded requirements for memory and storage space required for broad transmit beam imaging also enable several seconds of complete

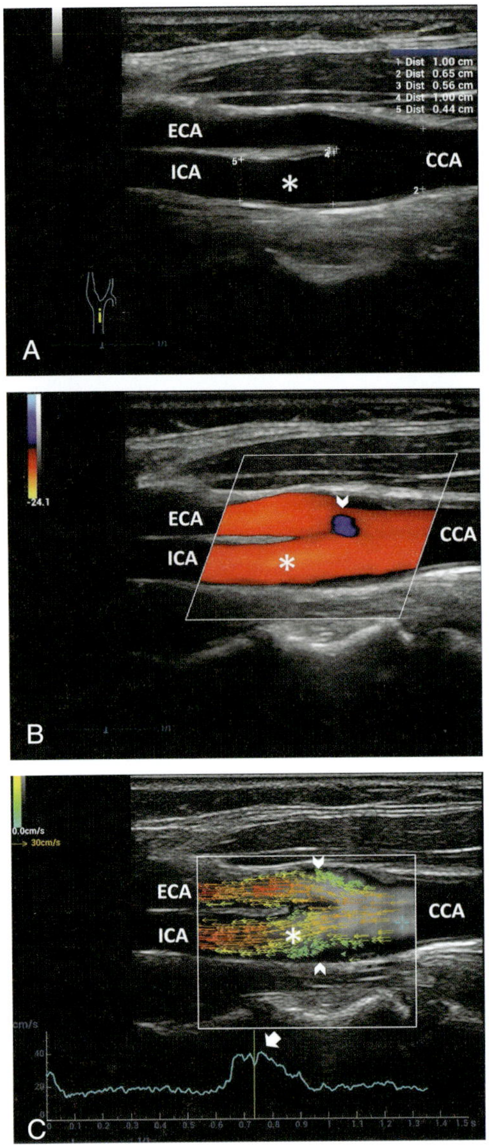

Fig. 5.55 Carotid example of vector flow compared to color Doppler imaging (*CDI*). **A,** B-mode of the carotid bifurcation from the CCA to ICA (*asterisk*) and ECA. **B,** CDI shows a uniformly colored flow pattern throughout the ICA (*asterisk*) with a small area of flow reversal seen at the entrance to the ECA (*arrowhead*). **C,** Vector flow imaging frame at the systolic peak (*arrow* on the velocity-versus-time curve) shows blood flowing upstream through the entire diameter in the ICA (parallel red/orange vectors; *asterisk*), while areas of flow separation area, without recirculation, are highlighted by slow green vectors (*arrowheads*). (Reproduced from Goddi A, et al: High–frame rate vector flow imaging of the carotid bifurcation in healthy adults: comparison with color Doppler imaging, *J Ultrasound Med* 37:2263–2275, 2018.)

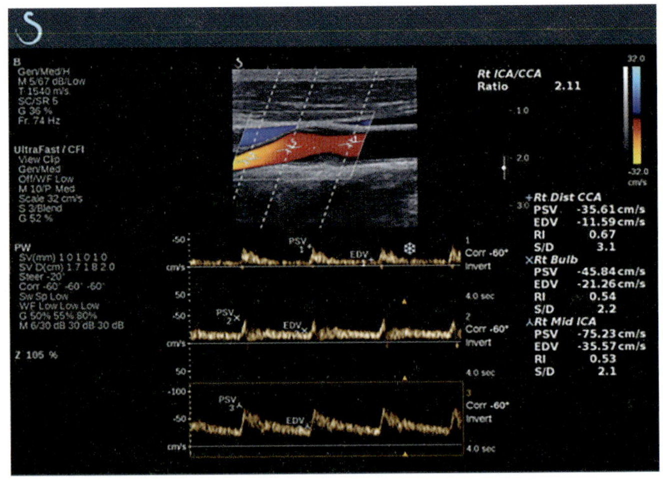

Fig. 5.56 Multiple spectral sample volumes showing 4 s of flow information from a stenosis in the carotid bulb using the stored Doppler data in the color box. Notice the color Doppler imaging frame rate is 74 frames per second. (Courtesy Supersonic Imagine.)

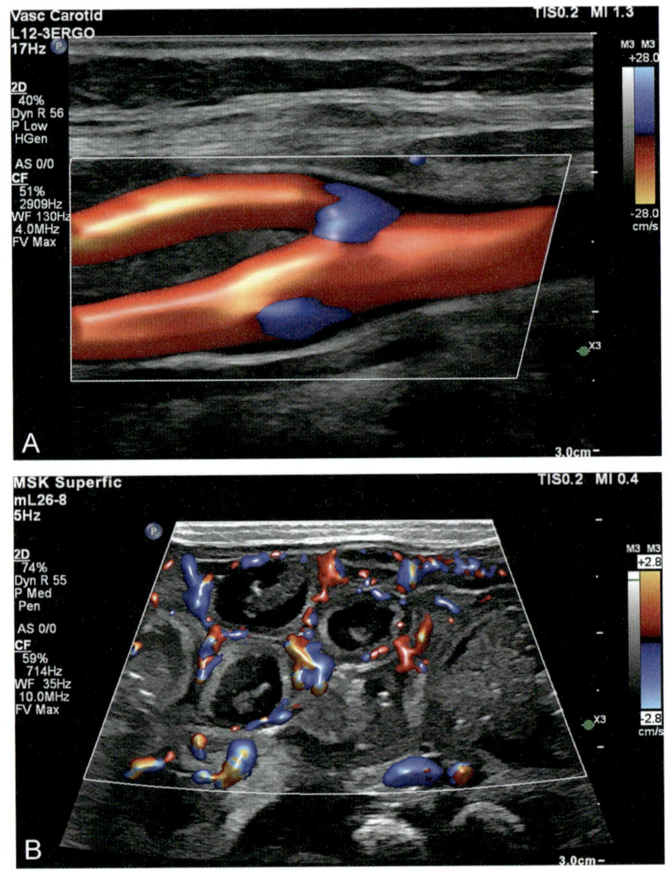

Fig. 5.57 Examples of broad transmit beam color Doppler. **A,** Flow through the carotid bifurcation showing two clear and distinct areas of flow separation (in *blue hues*). **B,** Flow in the bowel wall of a pediatric patient. (Courtesy Philips Medical Systems.)

imaging data to be stored in the scanner buffers. Fig. 5.56 shows an example of a retrospective Doppler examination; that is, after the patient has departed, data from three sample volumes are shown simultaneously with 4 seconds of Doppler spectra presented for each of spectral sample volume. Note that the color Doppler display is being acquired at 74 frames per second.

Ultrasound imaging in general, including flow imaging, is in a transition period in which systems fall into two classes of operation depending on whether they employ traditional narrow (focused) transmit beams or the more recent broad (unfocused) transmit beam schemes, which do result in dramatically different imaging capabilities. Unfocused beams can now produce images that have excellent detail resolution throughout the image, with significantly higher frame rates and improved imaging in nearly every aspect of image and Doppler characteristics (Fig. 5.57; Box 5.4).

BOX 5.4 Improvements in Doppler Operation With Broad Transmit Beams

- Simultaneous grayscale, color or power Doppler, and spectral Doppler (no time-sharing)
- Color flash (motion artifact) reduced or eliminated
- Flow velocity vector mapping
- Retrospective sample volume placement and analysis
- Automatic aliasing correction

Virtual beamforming enables simultaneous grayscale, color (or power) Doppler, and spectral Doppler presentations at high frame rates, vector flow, as well as multiple simultaneous sample volumes and spectral displays (retrospective as well as prospective).

REVIEW

The following key points are presented in this chapter:

- The heart provides the pulsatile pressure necessary to produce blood flow.
- Volumetric flow rate is proportional to the pressure difference at the ends of a tube.
- Volumetric flow rate is inversely proportional to flow resistance.
- Flow resistance increases with viscosity and tube length and decreases strongly with increasing tube diameter.
- Flow classifications include steady, pulsatile, plug, laminar, parabolic, disturbed, and turbulent.
- In a stenosis, flow accelerates, pressure drops (Bernoulli effect), and flow is disturbed or turbulent.
- Pulsatile flow is common in arterial circulation.
- Diastolic flow and/or flow reversal occur in some locations within the arterial system.
- The Doppler effect is a change in frequency resulting from motion.
- Blood flow and tissue motion are the sources of the Doppler effect in ultrasound imaging.
- The change in frequency of the returning echoes with respect to the emitted frequency is called the *Doppler shift*.
- For flow toward the transducer, the Doppler shift is positive.
- For flow away from the transducer, the Doppler shift is negative.
- The Doppler shift depends on the speed of the scatterers of sound, the Doppler angle, and the operating frequency of the Doppler system.
- Greater flow speeds and smaller Doppler angles produce larger Doppler shifts but not stronger Doppler-shifted echoes.
- Higher operating frequencies produce larger Doppler shifts.
- Typical ranges of flow speeds (10–100 cm/s), Doppler angles (30–60 degrees), and operating frequencies (2–18 MHz) yield Doppler shifts in the range of 100 Hz to 20 kHz for vascular studies.
- In Doppler echocardiography, in which zero angle and speeds of a few meters per second can be encountered, Doppler shifts can be as high as 30 kHz.
- CW Doppler systems provide motion and flow information, but without any depth selection capabilities.
- PW Doppler systems provide the ability to select the depth from which Doppler information is received.
- Spectral analysis provides visual information on the distribution of Doppler-shift frequencies resulting from the distribution of the scatterer speeds and directions encountered.
- The Doppler spectrum is generated by the range of scatterer velocities encountered by the ultrasound beam.
- The spectrum is derived electronically using the FFT and is presented on the display as Doppler shift versus time, with brightness indicating power.
- Flow conditions at the site of measurement are indicated by the width (vertical thickness) of the spectrum, with spectral broadening being indicative of disturbed and turbulent flows.
- CDI acquires Doppler-shifted echoes from a two-dimensional cross-section of tissue scanned by an ultrasound beam.
- Doppler shifts are presented in color and superimposed on the grayscale anatomic image of stationary echoes that were received during the scan.
- Flow echoes are assigned colors according to the color map chosen.
- Several pulses (the number is called ensemble length) are needed to generate a color scan line.
- Color controls include gain, map selection, variance on/off, persistence, ensemble length, color/gray priority, scale (*PRF*), baseline shift, wall filter, and color window angle, location, and size.
- Doppler-shift displays are subject to Doppler angle dependence and aliasing.
- Power Doppler displays color-coded Doppler-shift strengths into angle-independent, aliasing-independent, more sensitive presentations of flow information.
- With broad transmit beams operations, massive parallel processing with GPUs enables rapid image acquisition with exquisite detail resolution, contrast resolution, and very high frame rates, enabling excellent temporal resolution.
- Virtual beamforming enables simultaneous grayscale, color and spectral Doppler presentations, vector flow, and retrospective sample volumes with multiple spectral displays.

EXERCISES

Answers appear in the Answers to Exercises section at the back of the book.

1. Which of the following are parts of the circulatory system? (More than one correct answer.)
   a. heart
   b. cerebral ventricle
   c. artery
   d. arteriole
   e. capillary
   f. bile duct
   g. venule
   h. vein
2. The __________ are the tiniest vessels in the circulatory system.
   a. arteries
   b. arterioles
   c. capillaries
   d. bile ducts
   e. venules
   f. veins
3. In which of the following can Doppler ultrasound detect flow? (More than one correct answer.)
   a. the heart
   b. arteries
   c. arterioles
   d. capillaries
   e. venules
   f. veins
4. To flow is to move in a __________.
   a. direction
   b. container
   c. stream
   d. reversal
5. The characteristic of a fluid that offers resistance to flow is called __________.
   a. resistance
   b. viscosity
   c. inertia
   d. impedance
   e. density
6. Poise is a unit of __________.
   a. resistance
   b. viscosity
   c. inertia
   d. impedance
   e. density
7. Pressure is __________ per unit area.
   a. resistance
   b. viscosity
   c. inertia
   d. force
8. Pressure is __________.
   a. nondirectional
   b. unidirectional
   c. omnidirectional
   d. all of the above
   e. none of the above
9. Flow is a response to pressure __________ or __________.
   a. difference, gradient
   b. increase, decrease
   c. fore, aft
   d. presence, absence
10. If the pressure is greater at one end of a liquid-filled tube or vessel than it is at the other, the liquid will flow from the __________ pressure end to the __________ pressure end.
    a. higher, lower
    b. lower, higher
    c. depends on the liquid
    d. all of the above
    e. none of the above
11. The volumetric flow rate in a tube is determined by __________ difference and __________.
    a. resistance, pressure
    b. pressure, resistance
    c. diameter, length
    d. pressure, length
12. Flow increases if __________ increase(s).
    a. pressure difference
    b. pressure gradient
    c. resistance
    d. a and b
    e. all of the above
13. While flow resistance increases, volumetric flow rate __________.
    a. increases
    b. decreases
    c. is unchanged
    d. depends on pressure
14. If pressure difference is doubled, volumetric flow rate is __________.
    a. unchanged
    b. quartered
    c. halved
    d. doubled
    e. quadrupled
15. If flow resistance is doubled, volumetric flow rate is __________.
    a. unchanged
    b. quartered
    c. halved
    d. doubled
    e. quadrupled
16. Flow resistance in a vessel depends on __________.
    a. vessel length
    b. vessel radius
    c. blood viscosity
    d. all of the above
    e. none of the above
17. Flow resistance decreases with an increase in __________.
    a. vessel length

b. vessel radius
c. blood viscosity
d. all of the above
e. none of the above

18. Flow resistance depends most strongly on __________.
a. vessel length
b. vessel radius
c. blood viscosity
d. all of the above
e. none of the above

19. Volumetric flow rate decreases with an increase in __________.
a. pressure difference
b. vessel radius
c. vessel length
d. blood viscosity
e. c and d

20. When the speed of a fluid is constant across a vessel, the flow is called __________ flow.
a. volume
b. parabolic
c. laminar
d. viscous
e. plug

21. The type of flow (approximately) seen in Fig. 5.58, A is __________.
a. volume
b. steady
c. parabolic
d. viscous
e. plug

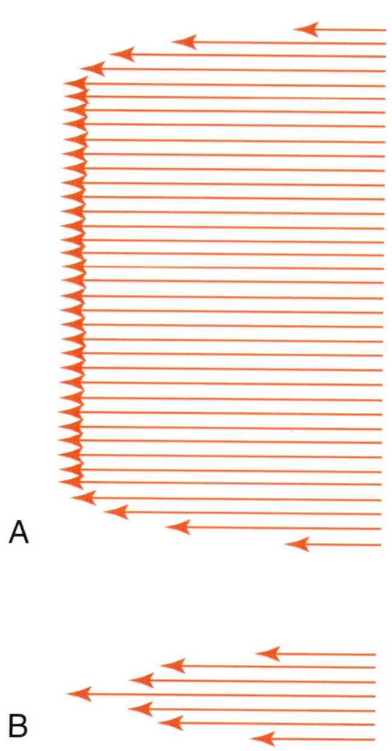

Fig. 5.58 Two types of flow patterns. Illustration to accompany Exercises 21 and 22.

22. The type of flow seen in Fig. 5.58, B is __________.
a. volume
b. steady
c. parabolic
d. viscous
e. plug

23. __________ flow occurs when straight parallel streamlines describing the flow are altered.
a. Volume
b. Turbulent
c. Parabolic
d. Disturbed

24. __________ flow involves random and chaotic flow patterns, with particles flowing in all directions.
a. Volume
b. Turbulent
c. Parabolic
d. Disturbed

25. Turbulent flow is more likely __________ to a stenosis.
a. proximal
b. distal

26. A narrowing of the lumen of a tube is called a __________.
a. stenosis
b. gorge
c. titer
d. kink

27. Proximal to, at, and distal to a stenosis, __________ must be constant.
a. laminar flow
b. disturbed flow
c. turbulent flow
d. volumetric flow rate
e. none of the above

28. For the answer to Exercise 27 to be true, flow speed in the stenosis must be __________ that proximal and distal to it.
a. greater than
b. less than
c. less turbulent than
d. less disturbed than
e. none of the above

29. Poiseuille equation predicts a(n) __________ in flow speed with a decrease in vessel radius.
a. increase
b. decrease

30. The continuity rule predicts a(n) __________ in flow speed with a localized decrease (stenosis) in vessel diameter.
a. increase
b. decrease

31. In a stenosis, the pressure is __________ the proximal and distal values.
a. less than
b. equal to
c. greater than
d. depends on the fluid
e. none of the above

32. Added forward flow and flow reversal in diastole can occur with __________ flow.
a. volume
b. turbulent

c. laminar
d. disturbed
e. pulsatile

33. While stenosis diameter decreases, __________ pass(es) through a maximum.
a. flow speed at the stenosis
b. flow speed proximal to the stenosis
c. volumetric flow rate
d. the Doppler shift at the stenosis
e. a and d

34. In Fig. 5.59, at which point is pressure the lowest?
a. P
b. S
c. D
d. P and D
e. None of the above

35. In Fig. 5.59, at which point is flow speed the lowest?
a. P
b. S
c. D
d. P and D
e. None of the above

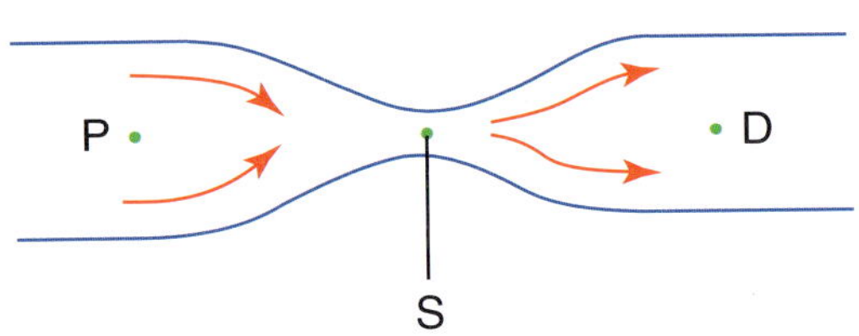

Fig. 5.59 Proximal to (*P*), at (*S*), and distal to (*D*) a stenosis. Illustration to accompany Exercises 34–37. (From Kremkau FW: Fluid flow, *J Vasc Technol* 17:153–154, 1993.)

36. In Fig. 5.59, at which point is volumetric flow rate the lowest?
a. P
b. S
c. D
d. P and D
e. None of the above

37. In Fig. 5.59, at which point is pressure energy the greatest?
a. P
b. S
c. D
d. P and D
e. None of the above

38. The __________ effect is used to detect and measure __________ in vessels.
a. Bernoulli, blood
b. Poiseuille, pressure
c. Poiseuille, flow
d. Doppler, flow

39. Motion of an echo-generating structure causes an echo to have a different __________ from that of the emitted pulse.
a. form
b. strength
c. amplitude
d. frequency

40. If the incident frequency is 1 MHz, the propagation speed is 1600 m/s, and the reflector speed is 16 m/s toward the source, the Doppler shift is __________ MHz, and the reflected frequency is __________ MHz.
a. −0.02, 1.02
b. 0.02, 1.02
c. 0.026, 1.026
d. −0.026, 1.026

41. If 2 MHz ultrasound is reflected from a soft tissue boundary moving at 10 m/s toward the source, the Doppler shift is __________ Hz.
a. 20.020
b. 0.020
c. 0.026
d. 20.026

42. If 2 MHz ultrasound is reflected from a soft tissue boundary moving at 10 m/s away from the source, the Doppler shift is __________ MHz.
a. 20.020
b. 0.020
c. 0.026
d. 20.026

43. The Doppler shift is the difference between __________ and __________ frequencies.
a. operating, emitted
b. echo, received
c. fundamental, harmonic
d. received, emitted

44. When incident sound direction and reflector motion are not parallel, calculation of the reflected frequency involves the __________ of the angle between these directions.
a. sine
b. cosine
c. tangent
d. cotangent

45. If the angle between incident sound direction and reflector motion is 60 degrees, the Doppler shift and reflected frequency in Exercise 40 are __________ and __________ MHz.
a. 0.02, 1.02
b. 0.01, 1.01
c. −0.02, 1.02
d. −0.026, 1.026

46. If the angle between incident sound direction and reflector motion is 90 degrees, the cosine of the angle is __________, and the reflected frequency in Exercise 40 is __________ MHz.
a. 0.02, 1.02
b. 0.01, 1.01
c. 0.0, 1.00
d. 0.0, −1.00

47. For an operating frequency of 2 MHz, a flow speed of 10 cm/s toward, and a Doppler angle of 0 degrees, calculate the Doppler shift (kHz).
a. −0.026
b. 0.026

c. −0.26
d. 0.26

48. For an operating frequency of 6 MHz, a flow speed of 50 cm/s, and a Doppler angle of 60 degrees, calculate the Doppler shift (kHz).
a. 1.95
b. 9.15
c. 5.91
d. 5.19

49. For blood flowing in a vessel with a plug flow profile, the Doppler shift is ___________ across the vessel.
a. constant
b. variable
c. parabolic
d. circular

50. Which Doppler angle yields the greatest Doppler shift?
a. 290
b. 245
c. 0
d. 45
e. 90

51. To proceed from a measurement of Doppler-shift frequency to a calculation of flow speed, ___________ ___________ must be known or assumed.
a. pressure amplitude
b. peak frequency
c. Doppler angle
d. average intensity

52. If operating frequency is doubled, the Doppler shift is ___________.
a. halved
b. unchanged
c. doubled
d. quadrupled

53. If flow speed is doubled, the Doppler shift is ___________.
a. halved
b. unchanged
c. doubled
d. quadrupled

54. If Doppler angle is doubled, the Doppler shift is ___________.
a. doubled
b. halved
c. increased
d. decreased

55. The functions of a Doppler detector include ___________.
a. amplification
b. phase quadrature detection
c. Doppler-shift detection
d. sign determination
e. all of the above

56. An earlier gate time means ___________ sample volume depth.
a. a later
b. a shallower
c. a deeper
d. a stronger
e. none of the above

57. Doppler signal power is proportional to ___________.
a. volume flow rate
b. flow speed
c. the Doppler angle
d. cell concentration
e. more than one of the above

58. Doppler ultrasound provides information about flow conditions only at the site of measurement. True or false?

59. Stenosis affects ___________.
a. peak systolic flow speed
b. end diastolic flow speed
c. spectral broadening
d. window
e. all of the above

60. Spectral broadening is a ___________ of the spectral trace.
a. vertical thickening
b. horizontal thickening
c. brightening
d. darkening
e. horizontal shift

61. If all the cells in a vessel were moving at the same constant speed, the spectral trace would be a ___________ line.
a. thin horizontal
b. thin vertical
c. thick horizontal
d. thick vertical
e. none of the above

62. Disturbed flow produces a narrower spectrum. True or false?

63. Turbulent flow produces a narrower spectrum. True or false?

64. As stenosis progresses, which of the following increase(s)?
a. lumen diameter
b. systolic Doppler shift
c. diastolic Doppler shift
d. spectral broadening
e. more than one of the above

65. Higher flow speed always produces a higher Doppler shift on a spectral display. True or false?

66. Flow reversal in diastole indicates ___________.
a. a stenosis
b. an aneurysm
c. high distal resistance
d. low distal resistance
e. more than one of the above

67. Decreased distal resistance normally causes end diastolic flow to ___________.
a. increase
b. decrease
c. be disturbed
d. become turbulent
e. more than one of the above

68. If angle correction is set at 60 degrees but should be zero degrees, the display indicates a flow speed of 100 cm/s. The correct flow speed is ___________ cm/s.
a. 25

b. 50
c. 100
d. 200
e. 400

69. If angle correction is set at zero degrees but should be 60 degrees, the display indicates a flow speed of 100 cm/s. The correct flow speed is __________ cm/s.
a. 25
b. 50
c. 100
d. 200
e. 400

70. If a 5 kHz Doppler shift corresponds to 100 cm/s, then a 2.5 kHz shift corresponds to __________ cm/s.
a. 100
b. 75
c. 50
d. 25

71. Which of the following is increased if Doppler angle is increased?
a. aliasing
b. Doppler shift
c. effect of angle error
d. b and c
e. none of the above

72. Color Doppler instruments present two-dimensional, color-coded images representing __________ that are superimposed on grayscale images representing __________.
a. flow, anatomy
b. motion, flow
c. anatomy, frequency
d. amplitude, frequency

73. Which of the following on a color Doppler display is (are) presented in real time?
a. grayscale anatomy
b. flow direction
c. Doppler spectrum
d. a and b
e. all of the above

74. Color Doppler instruments use an __________ technique to yield Doppler information in real time.
a. automatic
b. autocorrelation
c. autonomic
d. autocratic

75. The information in Exercise 74 includes __________ Doppler shift, __________, __________, and __________.
a. peak, sine, variables, intensity
b. mean, sign, variance, power
c. median, direction, deviation, amplitude
d. mean, sine, tangent, variance

76. The angle dependencies of color and power Doppler displays are different. True or false?

77. Do the different colors appearing in Fig. 5.47, B indicate that flow is going in two different directions in the vessel? Yes or no?

78. In color Doppler systems, color is used only to represent flow direction. True or false?

79. In practice, approximately __________ pulses are required to obtain one line of color Doppler information.
a. 1
b. 10
c. 100
d. 1000

80. About __________ frames per second are produced in conventional Color Doppler imaging.
a. 10
b. 20
c. 40
d. 80
e. More than one of the above

81. Color Doppler imaging displays are not dependent on Doppler angle. True or false?

82. If a color Doppler image shows two colors in the same vessel, it always means flow is occurring in opposite directions in the vessel. True or false?

83. A region of bright color on a CDI display always indicates the highest flow speeds. True or false?

84. Increasing the ensemble length __________ the frame rate.
a. increases
b. decreases
c. doubles
d. triples

85. The __________ technique is commonly used to detect Doppler shifts in color Doppler mode.
a. automatic
b. autocorrelation
c. autonomic
d. autocratic

86. Which of the following reduces the frame rate of color Doppler imaging? (More than one correct answer.)
a. Wider color window
b. Longer color window
c. Increased ensemble length
d. Higher transducer frequency
e. Higher priority setting

87. Lack of color in a vessel containing blood flow may be attributable to __________. (More than one correct answer.)
a. Low color gain
b. A high wall filter setting
c. A low-priority setting
d. Baseline shift
e. Aliasing

88. Increasing ensemble length __________ color sensitivity and accuracy and __________ frame rate.
a. improves, increases
b. degrades, increases
c. degrades, decreases
d. improves, decreases
e. none of the above

89. Which control can be used to help with clutter?
a. wall filter

b. gain
c. baseline shift
d. PRF
e. smoothing

90. Color map baselines are always represented by ___________.
a. white
b. black
c. red
d. blue
e. cyan

91. Doubling the width of a color window produces a(n) ___________ frame rate.
a. doubled
b. quadrupled
c. unchanged
d. halved
e. quartered

92. Steering the color window to the right or left produces a(n) ___________ frame rate.
a. doubled
b. quadrupled
c. unchanged
d. halved
e. quartered

93. Autocorrelation produces ___________. (More than one correct answer.)
a. the color of the Doppler shift
b. the mean value of the Doppler shift
c. variance
d. spectrum
e. peak Doppler shift

94. Steering the color window to the right or left changes ___________.
a. frame rate
a. PRF
b. the Doppler angle
c. the Doppler shift
d. more than one of the above

95. Color Doppler frame rates are ___________ grayscale rates.
a. equal to
b. less than
c. more than
d. depends on color map
e. depends on priority

96. In a single frame, color can change in a vessel because of ___________.
a. vessel curvature
b. sector format
c. helical flow
d. diastolic flow reversal
e. all of the above

97. Angle is not important in transverse color Doppler views through vessels. True or false?

98. Compared with CDI, PDI is ___________.
a. more sensitive
b. angle independent
c. aliasing independent
d. speed independent
e. all of the above

99. Power Doppler imaging indicates (with color) the ___________ of flow.
a. presence
b. direction
c. speed
d. character
e. more than one of the above

100. Color Doppler imaging indicates (with color) the ___________ of flow.
a. presence
b. direction
c. speed
d. character
e. more than one of the above

101. Broad transmit beam flow imaging improves sensitivity in part by reducing frame rates. True or false?

102. Multiple Doppler sample volumes are ___________.
a. a pipedream
b. possible today with all Doppler systems
c. only possible with broad transmit beams
d. not that clinically useful

6

Advanced Techniques

LEARNING OBJECTIVES

After reading this chapter, the student should be able to do the following:

- Discuss the purposes of coded excitation, harmonic imaging, high-sensitive Doppler, and fusion imaging.
- Describe the clinical utility of point-of-care ultrasound.
- Describe how elastography differs from conventional grayscale anatomical imaging.
- Explain what ultrasound contrast agents are and how they are used in contrast-enhanced ultrasound imaging.
- Describe the possibilities of artificial intelligence algorithms in diagnostic ultrasound.

CHAPTER OUTLINE

KEY TERMS

Acoustic radiation force impulse (ARFI) imaging
Amplitude modulation
Artificial intelligence (AI)
Attenuation imaging
B-flow
Capacitive micromachined ultrasound transducer (CMUT)
Cardiac strain imaging
Contrast agent
Contrast harmonic imaging
Contrast-specific imaging
Deep learning
Elastography
Frequency compounding
Fusion imaging
Harmonics
High-sensitive Doppler
Intravenous (IV)
Machine learning (ML)
Metabolic dysfunction–associated steatotic liver disease (MASLD)
Microbubbles
Nonlinear propagation
Panoramic imaging
Picture archiving and communication systems (PACS)
Piezoelectric micromachined ultrasound transducer (PMUTs)
Point-of-care ultrasound (POCUS)
Pulse inversion
Quantitative ultrasound (QUS)
Shear wave
Shear wave elastography
Spatial compounding
Speckle
Stiffness
Time-intensity curves
Tissue harmonic imaging
Transient elastography
Ultrasound computed tomography
Young's modulus

TRANSDUCER AND IMAGING TECHNOLOGIES

In Chapters 4 and 5, we discussed how scanners receive and process echoes from the transducer and display them in the form of anatomical and/or flow (or motion in general) images. Diagnostic ultrasound systems are pulse-echo instruments that receive echo information using the traditional narrow transmit beams or the more recent concept of unfocused broad transmit beams and process this information to produce the final display. In this chapter we describe the main imaging modes and technologies beyond simple grayscale and Doppler imaging that are employed to improve image quality as well as provide new qualitative and quantitative physiological data.

Tissue Harmonic Imaging

Filtering of received ultrasound echoes is a common technique to improve image quality (see Chapter 4). It is also possible to improve image quality by using **tissue harmonic imaging**, which transmits at the fundamental frequency but filters the received echoes to retain only (or mainly) the echoes at the second harmonic frequency (i.e., double the fundamental frequency as discussed in Chapter 2). A bandpass filter centered at the second harmonic frequency with an appropriate bandwidth will keep any echoes generated through **nonlinear propagation** within the high-intensity parts of the ultrasound pulse as it travels through the tissues (Fig. 6.1, A–C). Tissue harmonic imaging improves the image quality in three primary ways:

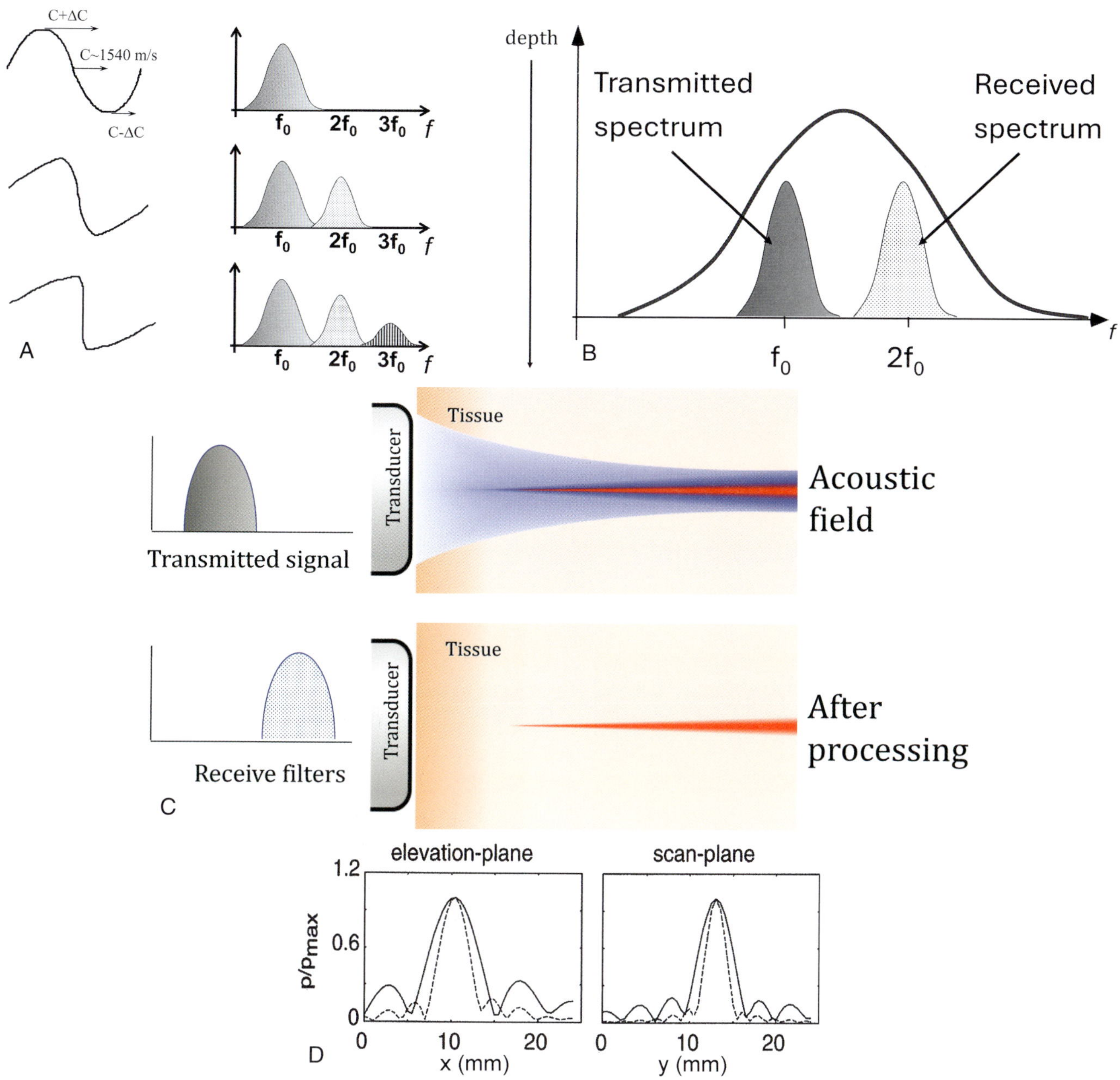

Fig. 6.1 Principle of tissue harmonic imaging. **A,** When transmitting a sinusoidal pulse, local areas of higher pressures (i.e., areas of compression) will also experience higher sound speeds. Conversely, areas of rarefaction will experience lower sound speeds. Over time (i.e., as the pulse travels deeper into the tissue), the sinusoidal pulse will be distorted and resemble a swap-tooth pulse, thus generating higher harmonic, nonlinear signals (at double the fundamental frequency, at triple the fundamental frequency, etc.). **B,** Fundamental and second harmonic echo bandwidths are depicted. On reception, a bandpass filter eliminates the fundamental frequency echoes and retains the second harmonic echoes. **C,** This processing results in a harmonic beam that is much narrower than the fundamental. **D,** The fundamental beam in the elevation and scan plane (*solid line*) becomes narrower and with lower side lobes in tissue harmonic mode (*dashed line*). (D - Courtesy Dr. Brian Fowlkes.)

- The harmonic beam is at a higher frequency and much narrower, improving axial and lateral resolution, because harmonics are generated only in the highest-intensity portion of the beam (see Fig. 6.1, C).
- Grating and side lobe artifacts (discussed later) are eliminated because these areas of acoustic signals are not sufficiently strong to generate harmonics (see Fig. 6.1, D).
- Because the harmonic signals are generated deeper in the tissues, some of the near-field problems (e.g., superficial reverberations or phase aberrations breaking up the wave front) are reduced or eliminated.
- In essence, tissue harmonic imaging is a sophisticated form of beam forming.

Because the fundamental and second harmonic bandwidths must fit within the overall transducer bandwidth (see Fig. 6.1, B), they must either be reasonably narrow or the transducer must have a wider bandwidth (which is becoming the norm for state-of-the-art transducers). The improved resolution (finer speckle pattern) and depiction of vessel margins are demonstrated in Fig. 6.2.

> Tissue harmonic imaging improves image quality by transmitting pulses at a given fundamental frequency into the body but then receiving echoes at double that frequency to form the displayed images.

Coded Excitation

In Chapter 2, the concept of the penetration/resolution tradeoff was described. One way around this dilemma involves more complicated driving voltage-pulse forms, so-called coded excitation. This approach enables multiple functions such as multiple transmission foci, separation of harmonic echo bandwidth from transmitted pulse bandwidth, increased penetration, speckle reduction (for improved contrast resolution), and grayscale imaging of blood flow (called ***B-flow***). In straightforward pulsing, the pulse generator drives the transducer through the pulse delays with one voltage pulse per transmitted beam (so per scan line in traditional narrow transmit beam systems). In coded excitation, ensembles of driving voltage pulses are applied to the transducer to generate a single transmit pulse or beam. For example, instead of a single pulse, a series (such as three pulses followed by a missing pulse [a gap], then two pulses followed by another gap, and then two pulses) could be used. Other examples are shown in Fig. 6.3, A–B. A decoder in the reception portion of the beam former recognizes and disassembles the coded sequence in the returning echoes and stacks up the individual pulses in the sequence to make a short, high-intensity echo voltage out of them (i.e., this decode recaptures the axial resolution that would otherwise be lost by using a much longer pulse).

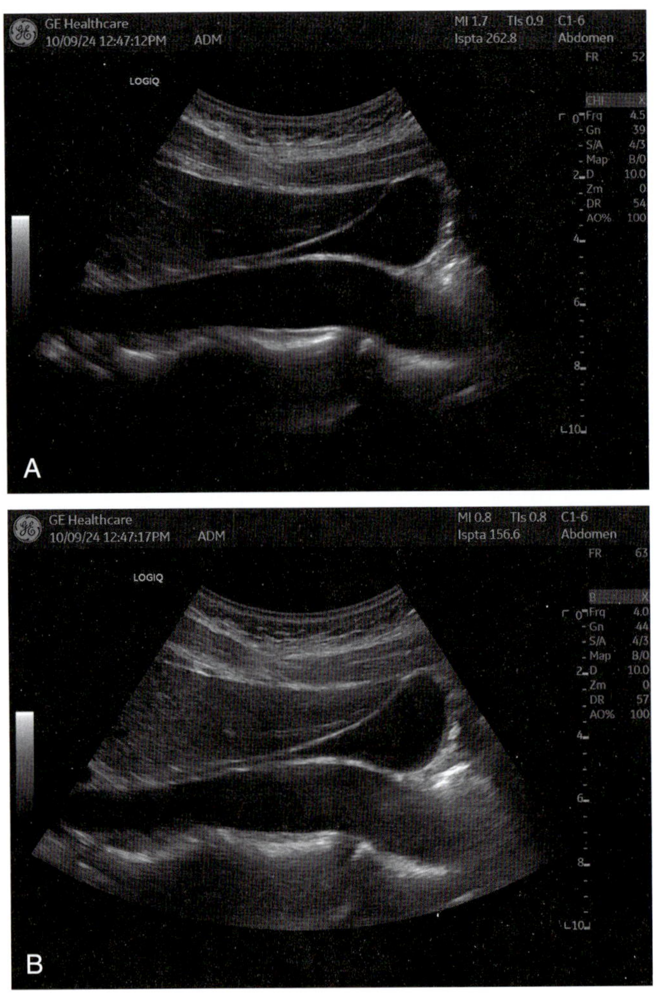

Fig. 6.2 Example of tissue harmonic imaging (THI) showing the gallbladder and aorta with **(A)** and without THI **(B)**. Notice how the noise in the aorta is cleaned up in **(A)** compared to **(B)**.

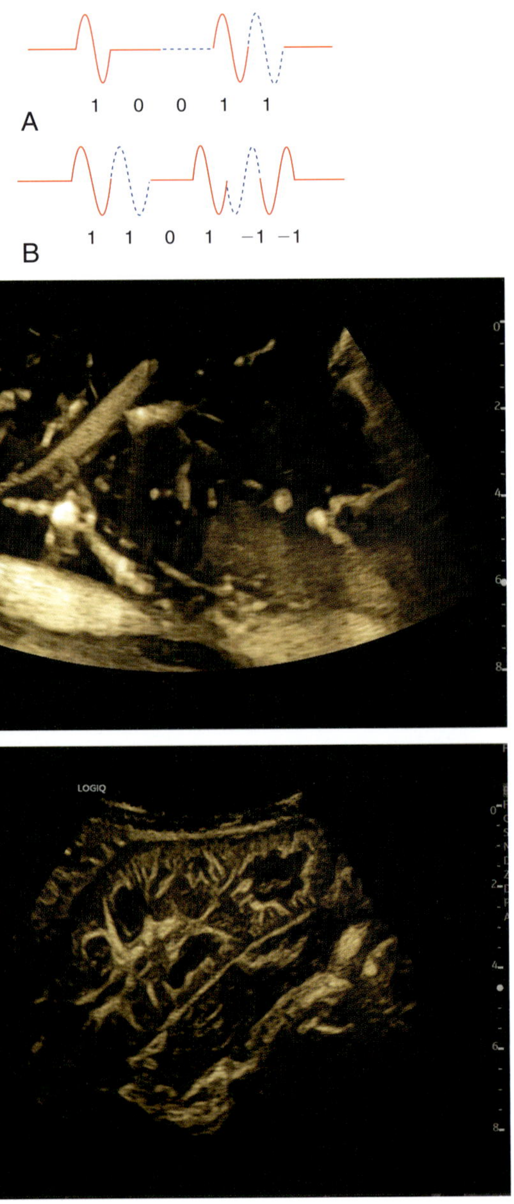

Fig. 6.3 Examples of coded pulse sequences. Each pulse consists of a cycle of pressure variation. **A,** This sequence includes a pulse, two gaps, and two final pulses. **B,** This sequence includes two pulses, a gap, and one pulse followed by two inverted pulses. **C,** Blood flow imaging, in which weak echoes from flowing blood in the liver are depicted. **D,** Example of B-flow imaging of a kidney. (Courtesy GE HealthCare.)

The result is equivalent to having a much higher-intensity driving pulse or a much more sensitive receiving system. Thus, for example, weak echoes from blood flow can be detected and imaged in colorized grayscale mode (see Fig. 6.3, C).

> Coded excitation uses a series of pulses and gaps rather than a single driving pulse.

ADVANCED CONCEPT

Coded excitation has been applied in radar for decades. A coded pulse is one that has internal amplitude, frequency, or phase modulation used for pulse compression. Pulse compression is the conversion, with use of a matched filter, of a relatively long coded pulse to one of short duration, improved resolution, and equivalent high intensity and sensitivity. A matched filter maximizes the signal-to-noise ratio of the returning signal. The longer the coded pulse, the higher will be the signal-to-noise ratio in matched-filter implementations. Intrapulse coding is chosen to attain adequate axial resolution, and pulse duration is chosen to achieve the desired sensitivity. The matched-filter decoding process can be thought of as a sliding correlation of the parts of the coded pulse with the matched filter. The result of this process is, in effect, a shorter and stronger pulse (Fig. 6.4) yielding good resolution and sensitivity, while conforming to the transmitted pulse amplitude and intensity limitations imposed by technologic and safety considerations. Such coding schemes are called *Barker codes*. An even better match can be achieved by *Golay codes*, which use pairs of transmitted pulses. The second pair is a bipolar sequence in which the latter portion of the pulse is the inverse of the first. This approach shortens the effective pulse length (improving axial resolution) and increases its amplitude (improving sensitivity). As a trade-off, the frame rate is reduced (degrading temporal resolution) because two pulses are required for each scan line.

Other forms of coded excitation that improve image quality include (1) frequency compounding (described later on in more detail), where echo information is acquired and combined from an anatomic region at two different frequencies; and (2) frequency modulation, where, in a relatively long transmitted pulse, the frequency is increased or decreased within the pulse—that is, the frequency is not constant within the pulse.

Panoramic Imaging

Panoramic imaging provides a way to produce an image that has a wider field of view than what is available on an individual frame from a transducer. Panoramic imaging is an example of preprocessing and is achieved by manually sliding the transducer in a direction parallel to the scan plane, thus extending it. The old echo information from previous frames is retained, allowing new echoes to be matched and added to the image in the direction in which the scan plane is moving. The result is a larger field of view allowing presentation of large organs and regions of anatomy on one image (Fig. 6.5). During the acquisition process, while the transducer is being moved, it is important to properly locate the new echoes relative to those previously received. This match is accomplished by correlating the locations of echoes common to adjacent frames (i.e., the overlap) so that the new information on the new frame is incorporated properly into the panoramic image.

> Panoramic imaging expands the image beyond the normal limits of the field of view of the transducer.

Fusion Imaging

Fusion imaging is the combined real-time and synchronous presentation of grayscale ultrasound images with another imaging form (typically computed tomography [CT] or MRI, but positron emission tomography [PET] has also been used) in the same anatomical cross-sectional ultrasound imaging plane (Fig. 6.6). Other ultrasound imaging technologies (e.g., elastography, color Doppler, or contrast-enhanced ultrasound [CEUS]) have also been merged with CT/MRI/PET for better localization and characterization.

Typically, fusion imaging is performed with a magnetic console placed approximately 5 to 12 cm above the patient (although other tracking systems such as optical systems have also been employed). Changes to the magnetic field are used to track the ultrasound transducer orientation and position in three-dimensional (3D) space (some systems can also account for respiratory motion). Previously acquired CT or MRI sequences (typically) are uploaded onto the ultrasound scanner and aligned with the ultrasound imaging planes. For alignment, a sonographer has to select locations (commonly three to five anatomical landmarks) in the tissue (i.e., organ) of interest and match each of these points to the corresponding CT or MR to fuse the imaging plane. This coregistration can be challenging, but once achieved, ultrasound images and the prior cross-sectional imaging can be viewed side by side or in an overlay mode in real time (see Fig. 6.6).

> Fusion imaging is the real-time and synchronous presentation of ultrasound images together with cross-sectional images from CT, MRI, or PET in the same anatomical imaging plane.

For example, fusion imaging has been widely used in the liver for both biopsy and treatment guidance (such as radiofrequency ablation) as well as for post ablation monitoring (Fig. 6.7). There are even examples of physicians performing biopsies on lesions high in the dome of the liver that were completely isoechoic on ultrasound (i.e., invisible), merely guided by the fused CT/MRI images.

High-Sensitive Doppler Modes

Since the mid-2010s a number of manufacturers of ultrasound scanners have introduced new Doppler flow modes with high sensitivity to slow flow in small vessels (despite the poor signal-to-noise ratios and overwhelming clutter signals associated with traditional Doppler flow imaging; as described in Chapter 5). Generally, these techniques use advanced adaptive clutter suppression to extract flow signals from large to small vessels and

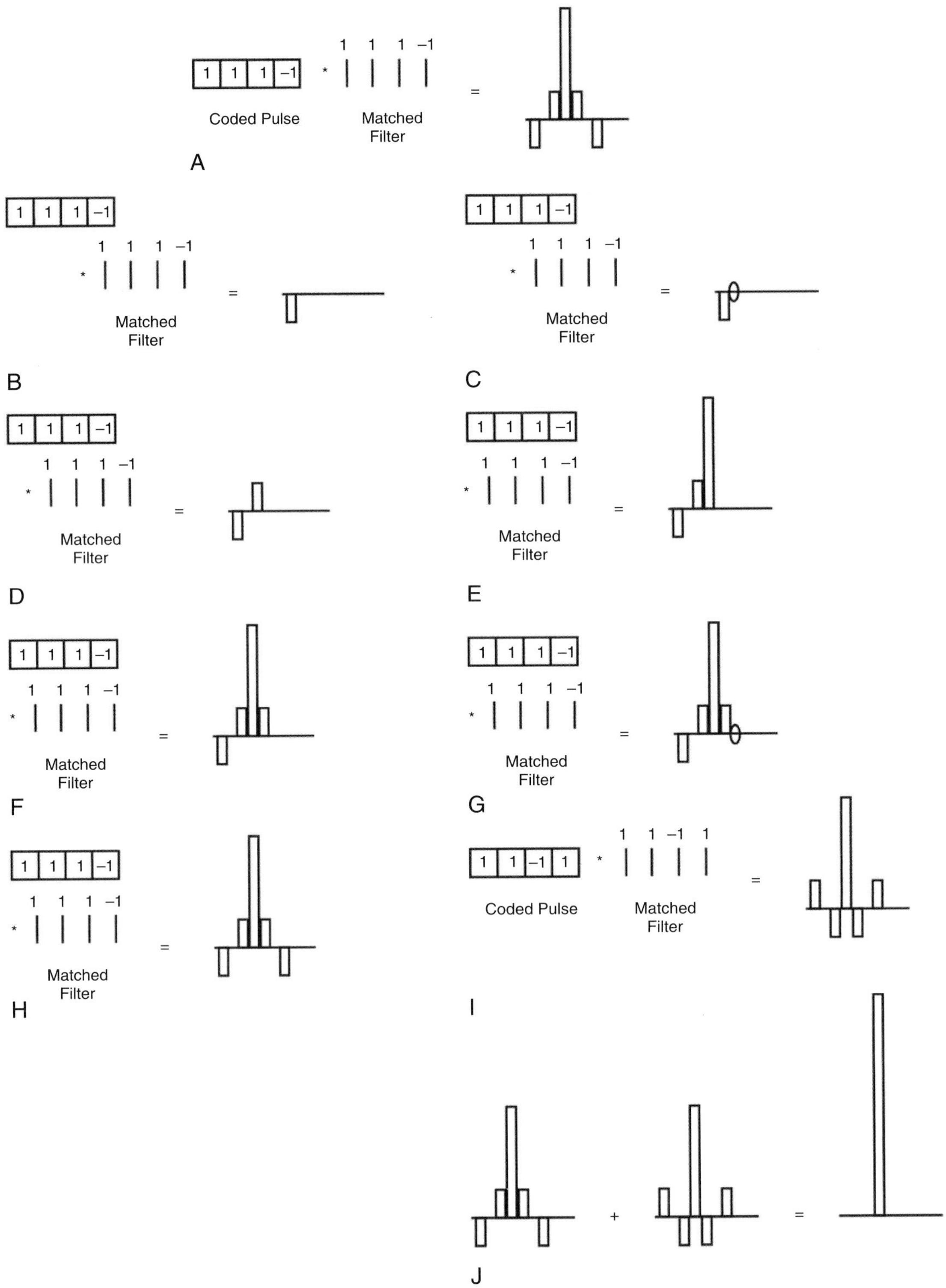

Fig. 6.4 Matched filter decoding of coded pulse. **A,** Correlation (*) of the coded pulse with the matched filter yields a result that has a peak amplitude 4 times (16 times for intensity) that for a comparable uncoded pulse. This is accomplished by sliding the coded pulse in time over the matched filter characteristic and multiplying the two. **B,** Multiplying the first part of the coded pulse (−1) with the first part of the matched filter (+1) yields the result of −1, seen to the right of the equals sign. **C,** With the coded pulse slid more to the right (two portions overlap), there are two multiplications (−1 × +1 and +1 × +1). Summing the results yields 0. **D,** Sliding farther to the right yields three multiplications, the sum of which is +1. **E,** The sum of four multiplications [(−1) × (−1), 1 × 1, 1 × 1, 1 × 1] is 4. **F, G** and **H,** The next results are +1, 0, and −1. To make the result even stronger and sharper, a pair of codes (called a Golay code pair) can be used. The appropriate coded sequence to use with **A** is shown in **I. J,** When the two results (**A** and **I**) are summed, there is a sharp, strong result (amplitude 8 compared with the individual amplitudes of 1 in the coded sequence and the amplitude of 4 in the result in **A**).

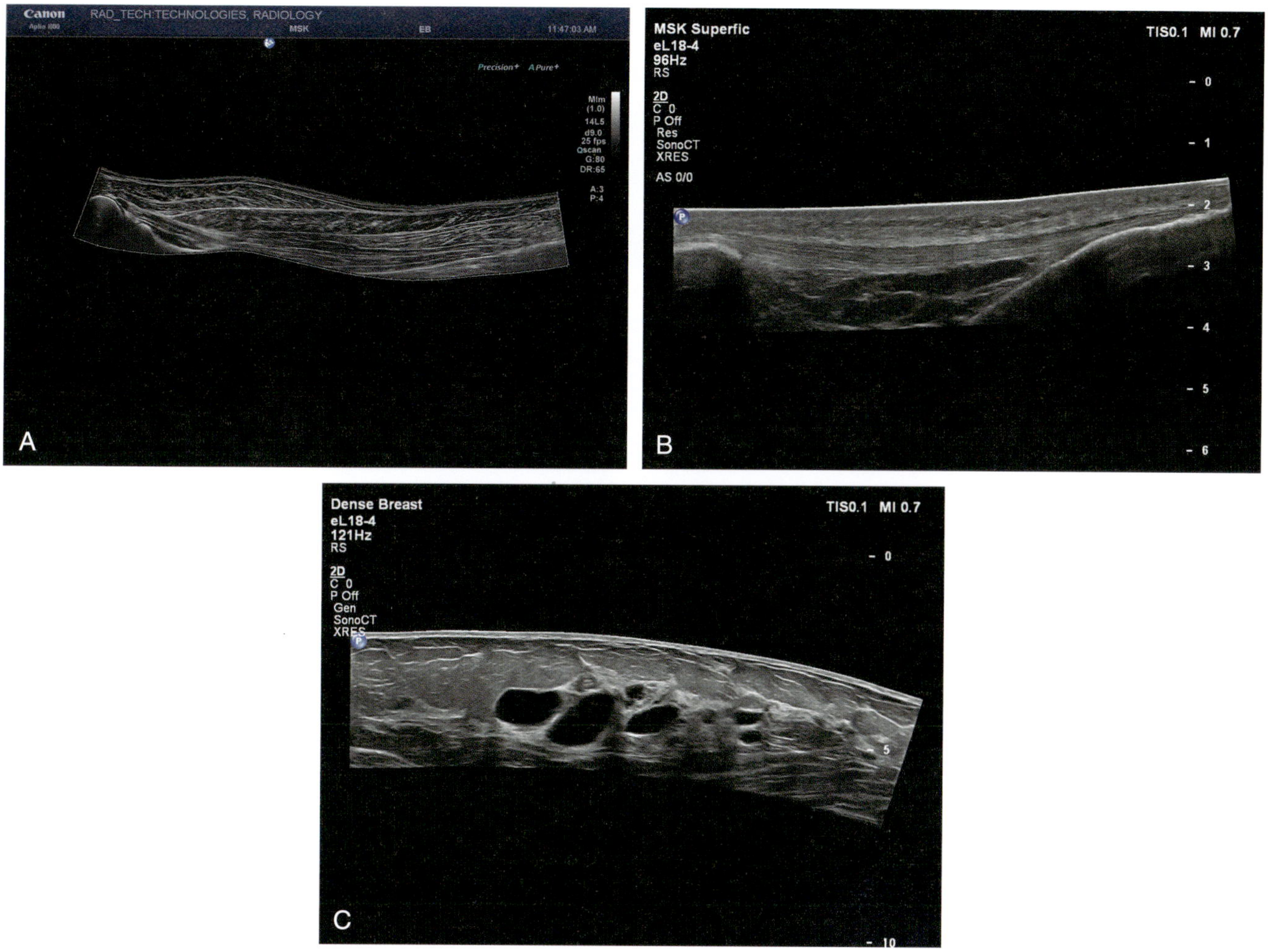

Fig. 6.5 Examples of panoramic imaging. **A–B,** Tendons in muscoloskeletal applications. **C,** Breast cysts in a dense breast. Panoramic imaging is accomplished by adding new information to one end of an image, spatially correlating the overlapping old echoes to properly locate the new ones. (**A,** Courtesy Canon Medical Systems USA. **B–C,** Courtesy Philips Medical Systems.)

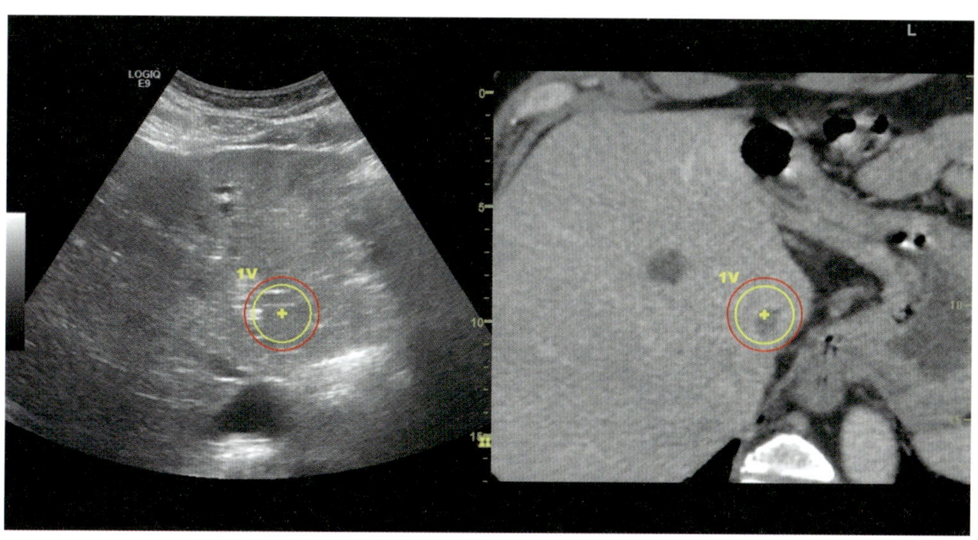

Fig. 6.6 Fusion imaging example. (Courtesy GE Healthcare.)

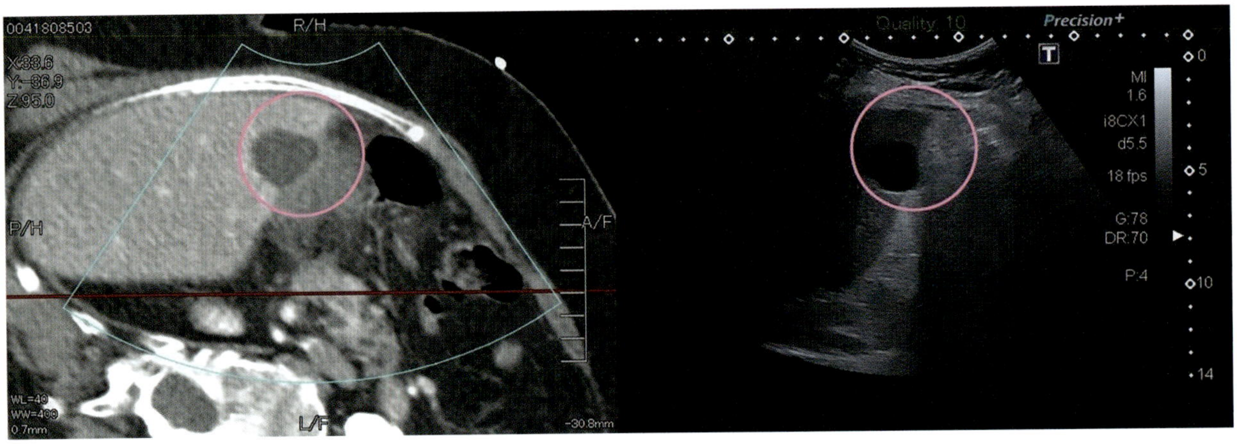

Fig. 6.7 More fusion imaging of a liver lesion. (Courtesy Canon Medical Systems USA.)

depict this information at high frame rates as a color overlay image (although grayscale maps of flow are also available). **High-sensitive Doppler** modes appear to outperform traditional power Doppler imaging (PDI) in the depiction of small vessels across a number of different vascular beds.

Examples of high-sensitive Doppler images demonstrate significantly improved depiction of thyroid vascularity compared to PDI (Fig. 6.8), as well as slow flow associated with plaque neovascularity and the testes (cf., Fig. 6.9).

Quantitative Ultrasound Techniques

Deriving quantitative information related to the underlying acoustic properties of different tissues has been a long sought-after goal in diagnostic ultrasound imaging. The umbrella term for such measurements is **quantitative ultrasound (QUS)**. As a matter of fact, elastography and contrast kinetics derived from contrast-enhanced images can be considered special cases of QUS. However, due to their ubiquitousness, these techniques are described separately and in more detail later in this chapter.

Here we will focus on measurements of attenuation, backscatter, scatterer spacing, and speed of sound, which have lately become available on a number of ultrasound platforms. Of these parameters, the most well established is the attenuation coefficient calculated in decibel per centimeter per megahertz (dB/cm/MHz; as described in Chapter 2). Diagnosing ***metabolic dysfunction–associated steatotic liver disease (MASLD)*** is a major worldwide health problem and estimates of the attenuation coefficient have been shown to be higher among fatty versus nonfatty livers compared to the clinical reference standards of liver biopsy and MRI fat quantification and may even be able to estimate the severity of hepatic steatosis (i.e., MASLD; Fig. 6.10).

Ultrasound on a Chip

A whole new class of transducers, based on silicon wafer manufacturing technologies, has recently become commercially available. These transducers are called **capacitive micromachined ultrasound transducers (CMUTs)** and are suitable for high-volume production using semiconductor technologies, which also allows for easy integration with beam-former electronics on application-specific integrated circuits—essentially an ultrasound scanner on a chip (Fig. 6.11).

CMUTs contain miniature elements that are comprised of two electrically conducting layers facing each other, one of which is fixed and the other is a flexible membrane. An insulating layer and a vacuum-sealed gap separate the two layers. When an alternating voltage is applied to the two layers, the flexible membrane vibrates toward and away from the fixed layer, producing an ultrasound pulse (Fig. 6.12, A–D). CMUT elements have advantages over PZT elements including broader bandwidth (1–40 MHz), improved detail resolution, ability to be integrated with electronic circuits, miniaturization, facilitating 3D imaging with two-dimensional (2D) element arrays, and cost-effectiveness. Examples of 2D and 3D renal and hepatic images are presented in Fig. 6.13.

Related technologies centered around **piezoelectric micromachined ultrasound transducers (PMUTs)** are also under development. The advantage of PMUTs is mainly for lower frequencies (0.4–1.0 MHz), which makes it more likely that CMUTs will dominate in medical imaging applications.

ADVANCED CONCEPT

CMUTs are composed of thousands of microscopic silicon drums that include thin, suspended membranes. Pulse generation is accomplished by applying a voltage to the drum. The voltage creates an electrostatic force on the membrane, causing it to vibrate and emit a pulse of ultrasound. Conversely, echoes arriving at the element cause the membrane to vibrate, producing the corresponding voltage that represents the echo in the electronics (cf., see Fig. 6.12). One major advantage of CMUTs is that their impedance is much lower than that of ceramic elements (such as PZT), easing the impedance-matching challenge and enabling broader bandwidth pulses (exceeding 100%) to be transmitted into tissues. Another advantage is that with semiconductor-based technology, the elements and electronics are combined in silicon. Thus more of the electronic components can be housed in the probe assembly, allowing more of the signal processing to be accomplished before sending the electric signals through the probe cable to the rest of the scanner. As a matter of fact, it is possible to contain the entire scanner electronics in just the transducer handle (see Fig. 4.1, D–F). A third advantage is that less energy is lost in the damping material, because the pulse is coupled better to the tissues. This makes the transducer more efficient. Finally, the CMUT approach may allow flexible transducers to be fabricated that will conform to the surface of the patient more effectively and will allow a broader area of acoustic coupling to the tissues. In summary, CMUTs will enable more efficient production and coupling of broader band pulses to the patient.

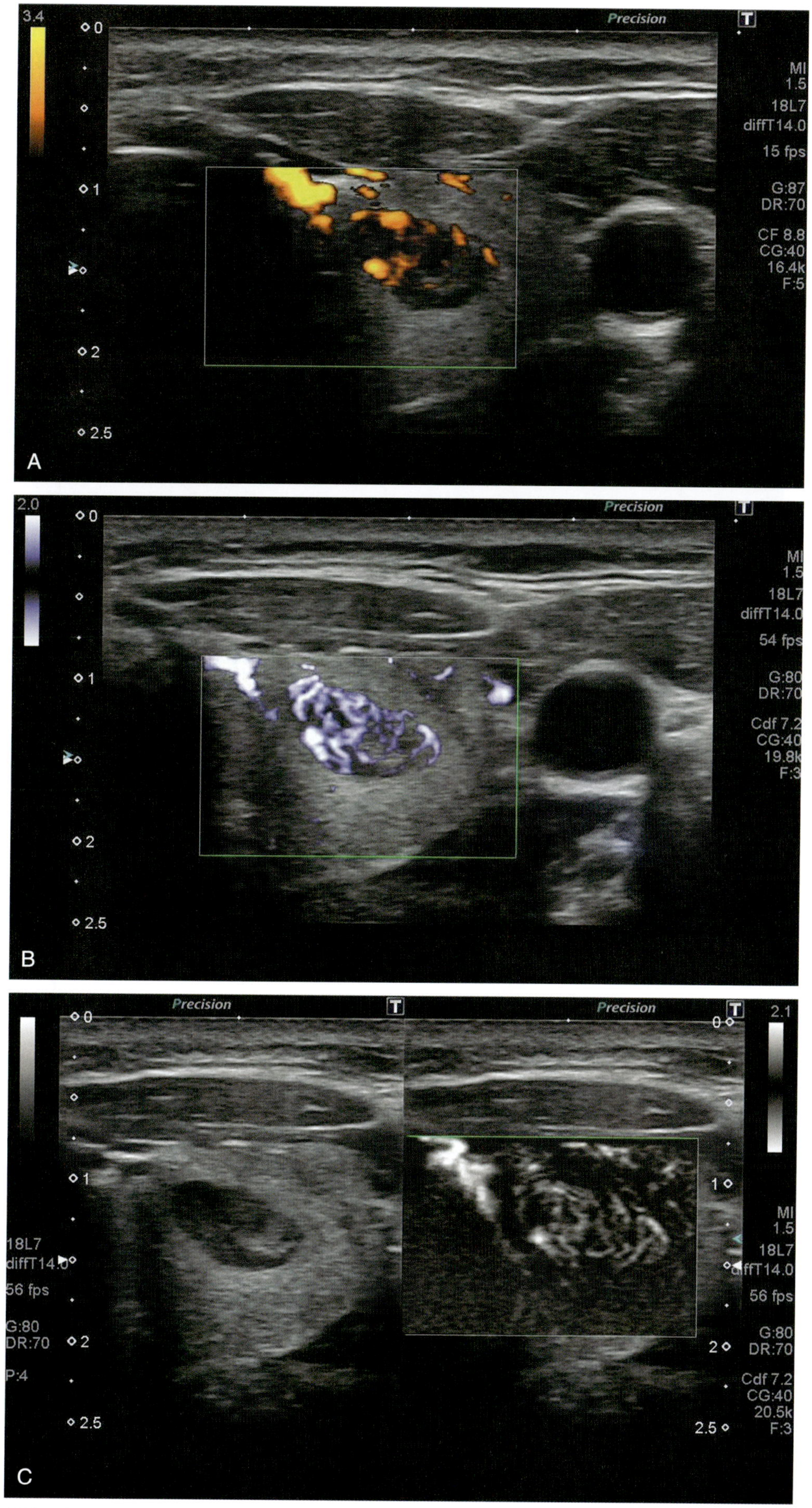

Fig. 6.8 Thyroid lesion seen in **(A)** power Doppler imaging mode, **(B)** high-sensitive Doppler mode as a color overlay, and **(C)** high-sensitive, grayscale Doppler mode (shown as dual imaging with anatomical grayscale on the left).

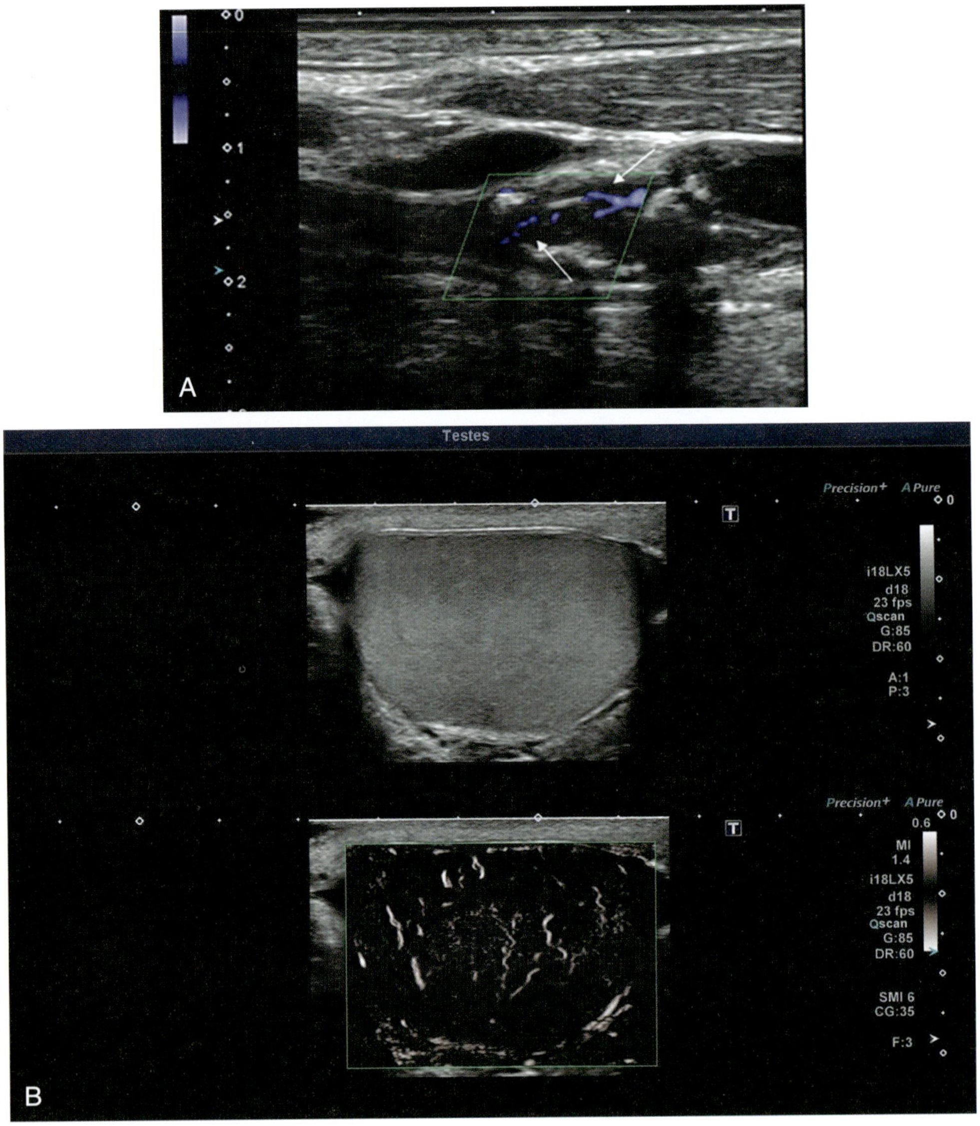

Fig. 6.9 Examples of high-sensitive Doppler imaging. **(A)** Plague neovessels. **(B)** Testicular flow. (**B,** Courtesy Canon Medical Systems USA.)

Point-of-Care Ultrasound

Point-of-care ultrasound or POCUS refers to clinicians (typically not radiologists) performing studies at the bedside (in the ED or in the OR), at a sporting event, among underserved and/or inaccessible communities, or just anywhere else where patients can be found, and quick decision-making based on ultrasound imaging is required (Fig. 6.14). POCUS does not replace traditional diagnostic ultrasound imaging but rather expands the use of ultrasound across many specialities for initial assessments that may (or may not) be followed up by more traditional comprehensive ultrasound examinations using more versatile, state-of-the-art ultrasound equipment.

It bears mentioning that POCUS is also making important inroads at medical schools and other training facilities, where future physicians and other specialists are being introduced to the benefits of ultrasound imaging with real-time depiction of anatomy from the get-go.

POCUS requires portable ultrasound scanners, which is why handheld devices such as those based on CMUTs are commonly used. The applications for POCUS are wide ranging but typically attempt to answer a few specific questions to confirm or rule out a suspected diagnosis or guide an interventional procedure in real time. The POCUS information then supplements data gathered from traditional physical examinations, patient history, and other tests. Examples of POCUS applications include looking for pericardial effusion, pulmonary embolism, or just cardiac output in cardiology. In vascular ultrasound of the lower extremities trying to rule out deep vein thrombosis with POCUS, or screening patients for aortic aneurysms. POCUS is employed by anesthesiologists to do ultrasound-guided nerve blocks or to place central venous catheters, while ER physicians use POCUS to triage trauma patients. However, the most consequential use of POCUS is probably the emergence of lung ultrasound as the method of choice in connection with the COVID-19 pandemic.

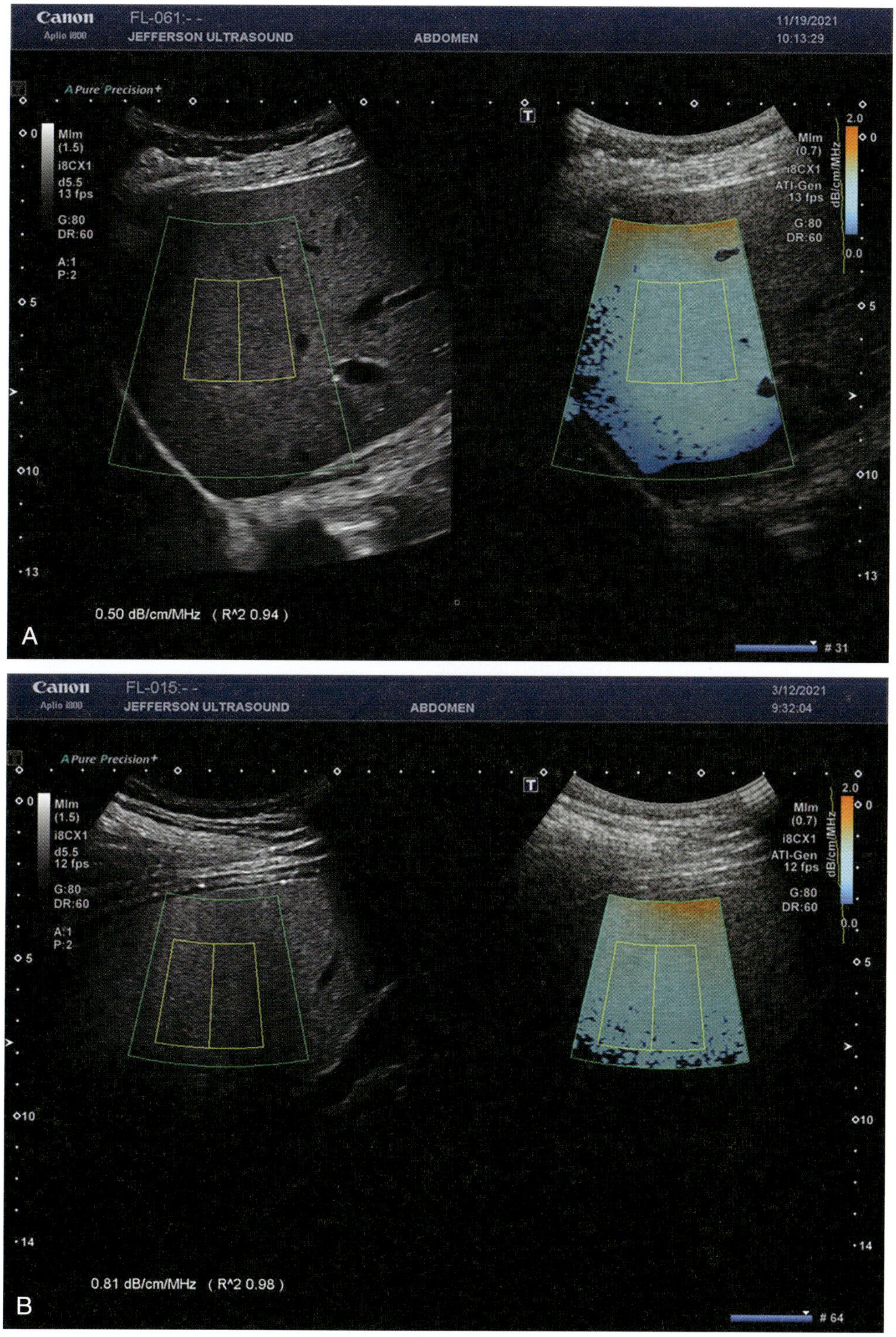

Fig. 6.10 Mapping the tissue attenuation (known as **attenuation imaging**) in **(A)** a normal liver with a 0.50 dB/(cm MHz) attenuation coefficient (fat fraction by MRI: 3%) and **(B)** in a liver suffering from steatosis with a 0.81 dB/(cm MHz) attenuation coefficient (fat fraction by MRI: 32%). (Courtesy Dr. Kibo Nam, Thomas Jefferson University.)

POCUS can detect signs of acute respiratory failure, often secondary to pneumonia, bronchitis, or asthma exacerbation with typical findings including bilateral B-lines, confluent B-lines, consolidations, and pleural line abnormalities (Fig. 6.15).

An international expert consensus statement on the clinical utility of POCUS in patients with COVID-19 recommended its use for diagnosing COVID-19 pneumonia with appropriate integration of clinical information. It is important to note that pulmonary capillary hemorrhage in connection with lung ultrasound scans has been reported and that recent recommendations from the American Institute of Ultrasound in Medicine highlight that prudent use of lung ultrasound requires mechanical index (MI) values at or below 0.3. This specific safety aspect will be discussed in more detail in Chapter 9.

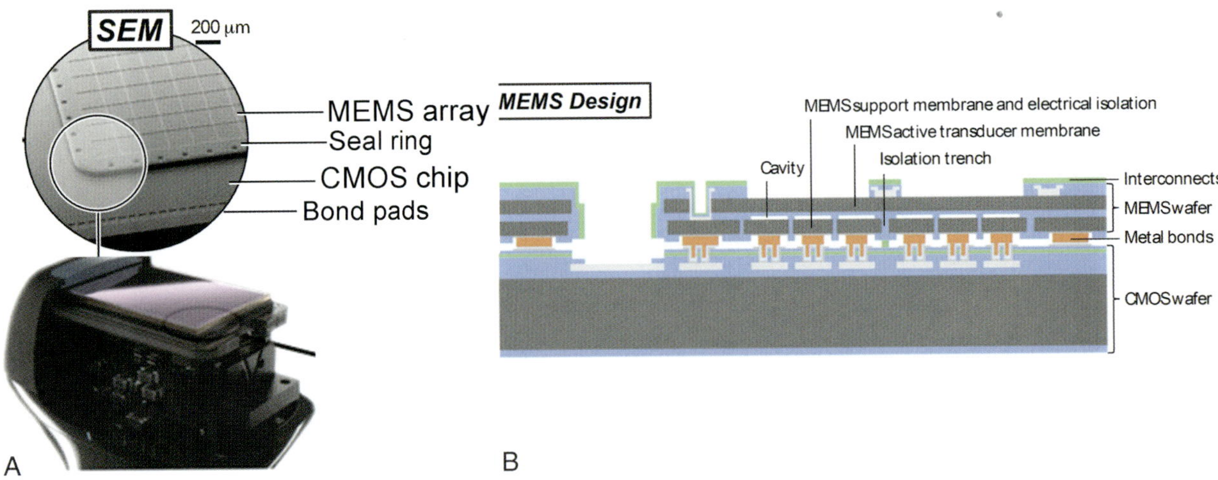

Fig. 6.11 **A,** An ultrasound-on-a-chip design with 8960 microelectromechanical systems (MEMS) ultrasound sensors. **B,** The design of an individual MEMS. SEM: scanning elctron microscope. (From *Rothberg JM, et al: Ultrasound-on-chip platform for medical imaging, analysis, and collective intelligence, Proc Natl Acad Sci U S A 118(27):e2019339118, 2021.*)

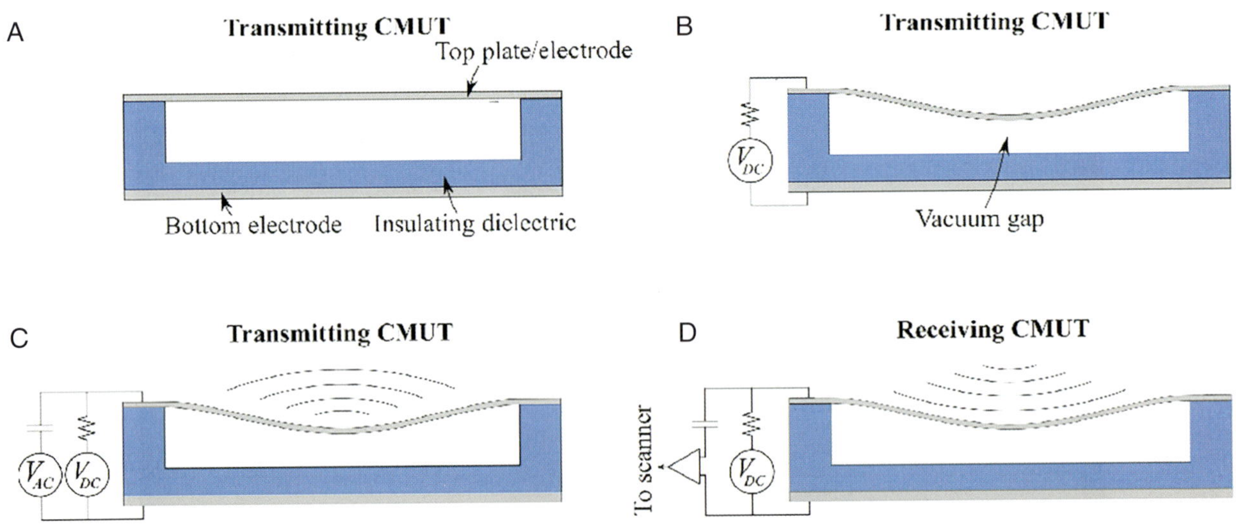

Fig. 6.12 Example of capacitive micromachined ultrasound transducer (*CMUT*) (**A**) acting as an air-backed transducer with a flexible membrane surface (**B**). When an alternating voltage is applied to the layers, the flexible membrane vibrates toward and away from the fixed layer, transmitting an ultrasound pulse (**C**). Conversely, on reception, the flexible membrane induces an alternating voltage (**D**). (From *Holbek S, et al: 3D vector flow using a row-column addressed CMUT array. In Medical imaging 2016: ultrasonic imaging and tomography, vol 9790, 2016, International Society for Optics and Photonics, pp 979005.*)

As more clinicians integrate POCUS into their medical practices, the benefits of improved diagnoses, faster time to diagnosis, and, thus, treatment as well as safer POCUS-guided interventional procedures are becoming obvious.

SPECKLE-REDUCTION TECHNIQUES

Ultrasound imaging inherently suffers from speckle, which limits low-resolution image contrast and may even obscure true structures in high-contrast regions, due to the intensity variations induced by constructive and destructive interference between tissue echoes (as described in Chapter 2). Many different techniques for speckle reduction have been proposed, but two in particular have been adopted by multiple vendors.

Spatial Compounding

The technique that is implemented on most scanners (under a plethora of trademarked names) is real-time spatial compounding. Spatial compounding is another example of preprocessing. Multiple images of an object are acquired from different directions by phasing (Fig. 6.16). These spatially independent scans are then averaged in real time assembling a final multi-angle compound image. The quality of the final compounded image is improved in several ways (Fig. 6.17):

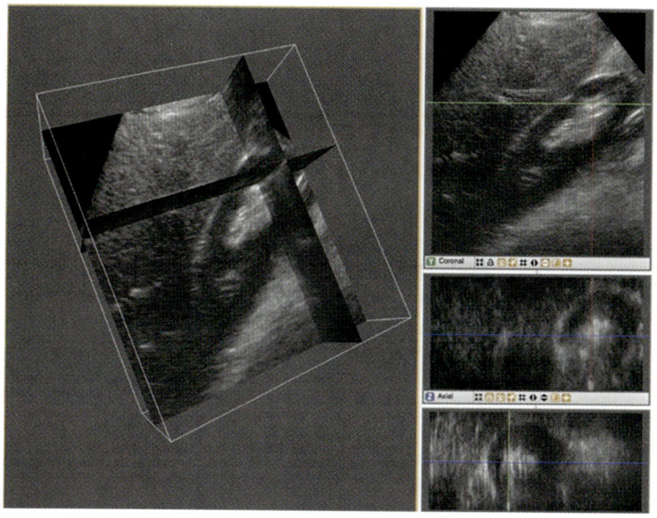

Fig. 6.13 Hepatic and renal two- and three-dimensional imaging examples acquired with a capacitive micromachined ultrasound transducer probe. (From *Rothberg JM, et al: Ultrasound-on-chip platform for medical imaging, analysis, and collective intelligence, Proc Natl Acad Sci U S A 118(27):e2019339118, 2021.*)

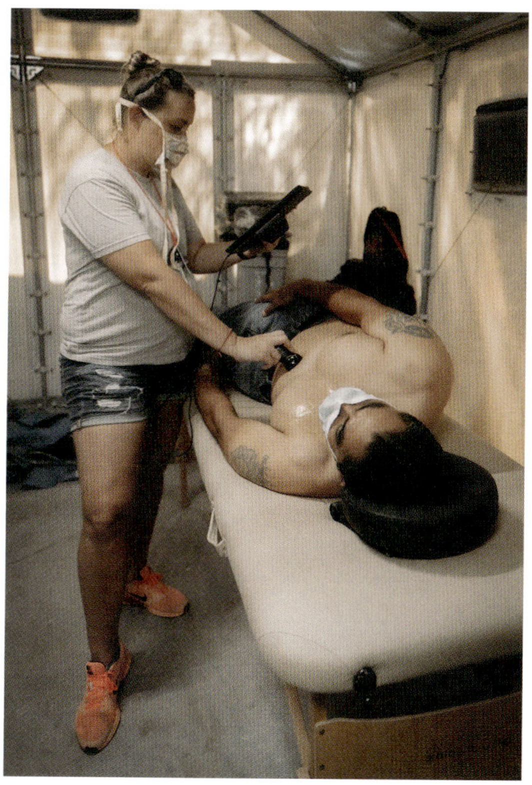

Fig. 6.14 Point-of-care ultrasound being used among people from underserved communities in Central America. (Courtesy Butterfly Network.)

- The detectability of low-contrast structures shows marked improvement mainly due to the decorrelation between individual images, which can reduce speckle markedly.
- Clutter caused by artifacts is reduced.
- Smooth (specular) surfaces are presented more completely because they are interrogated at more than one angle, increasing the probability that close to 90-degree incidence is achieved (which is necessary to receive echoes from them).

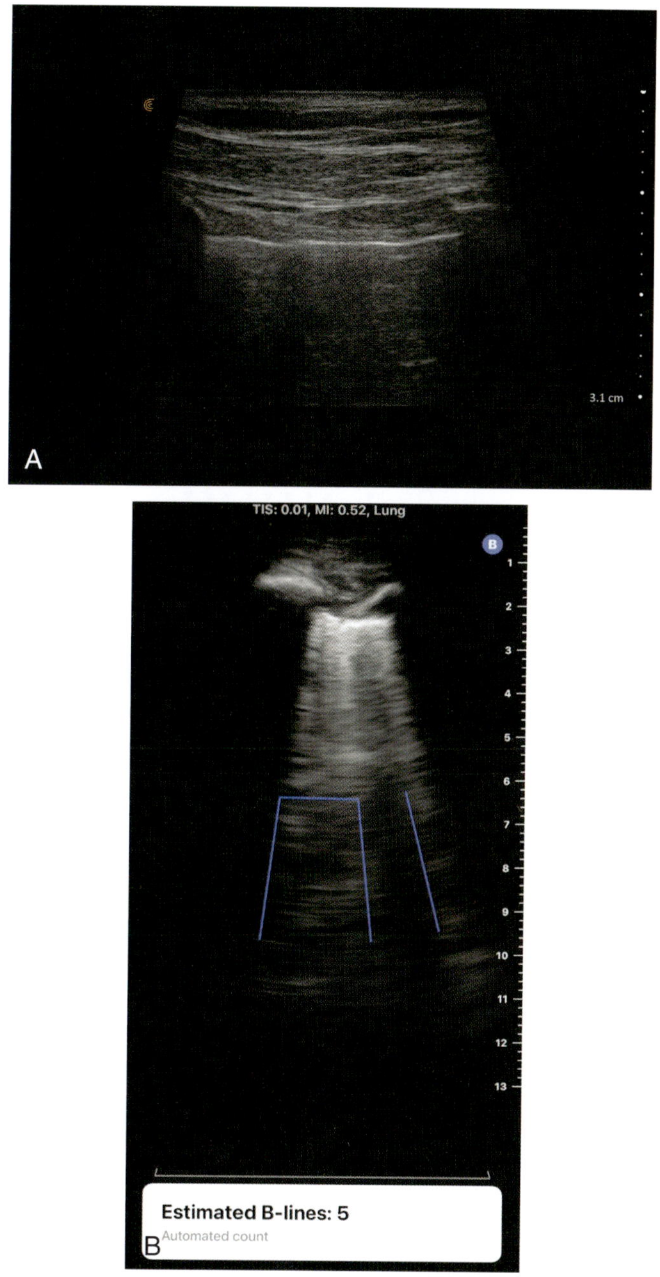

Fig. 6.15 Examples of point-of-care ultrasound lung scans. **A,** Shallow depiction of a normal lung. **B,** Automatic detection of 5 lung B-lines. (**A,** Courtesy Clarius. **B,** Courtesy Butterfly Network.)

- Structures previously hidden beneath highly attenuating objects can be visualized.

> **ADVANCED CONCEPT**
>
> Spatial compounding is the averaging of multiple frames acquired of the same object from different angles.

Spatial compounding is limited by the physical directions the beams can be steered in across a transducer aperture (i.e., surface). Thus spatial compounding is not possible very close to the transducer (i.e., at shallow depths) and becomes progressively more difficult to accomplish as the imaging depth increases (Fig. 6.18).

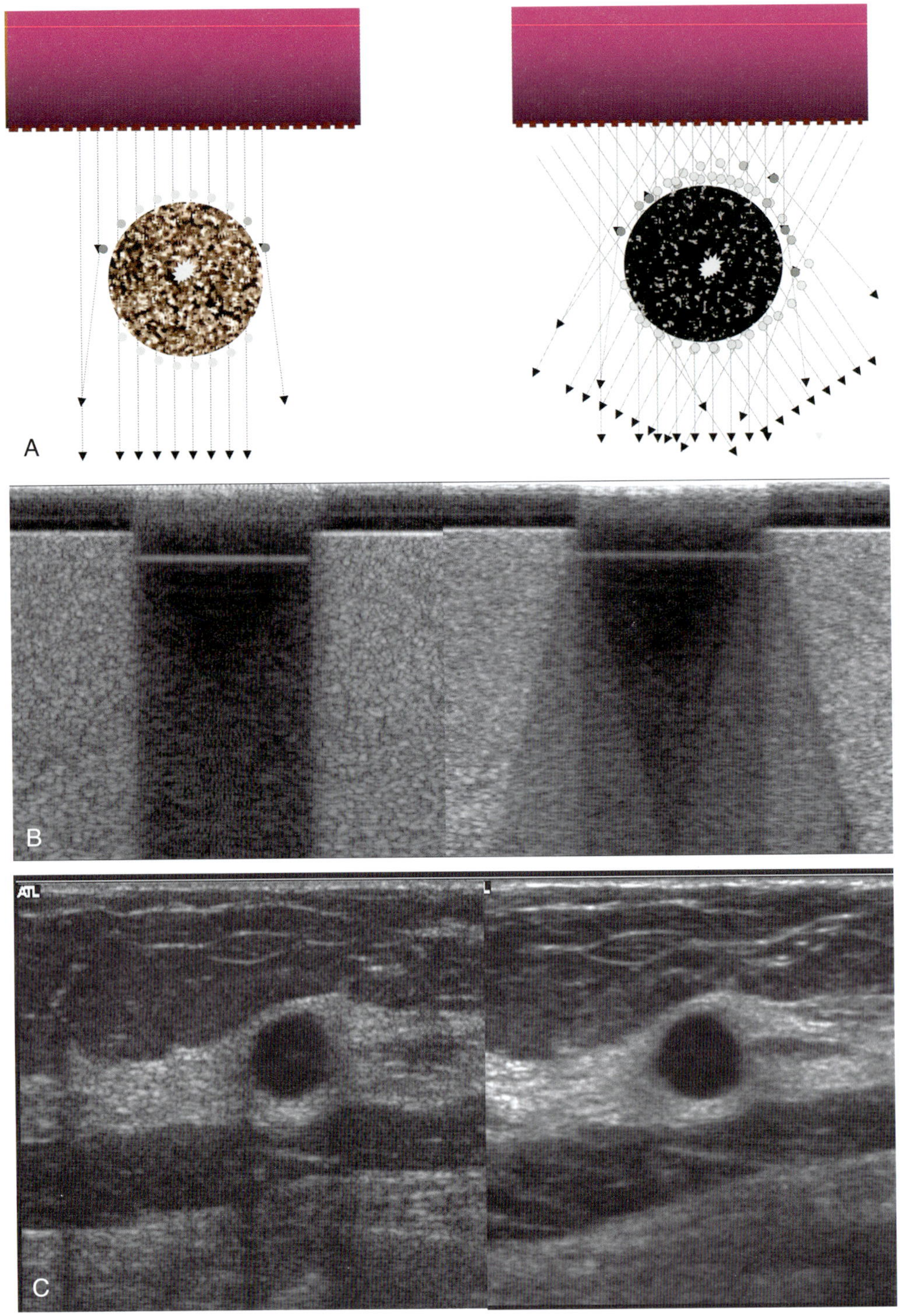

Fig. 6.16 Conventional scan lines (*left*) and spatial compounding (*right*) as (**A**) an illustration, (**B**) in phantom images, and (**C**) in depicting a breast cyst. Notice the improvement in image quality with finer speckle pattern and better echo continuity.

Frequency Compounding

Just like a compounded image can be assembled (in real time) across different directions in space, so can **frequency compounding** be applied by averaging across different frequency bands (Figs. 6.19 and 6.20). Producing images in different frequency bands is achieved in one of two ways:

- Transmitting multiple ultrasound beams at different frequencies
- Transmitting a broad bandwidth beam and then passing the resulting data through a bank of bandpass filters centered at different frequencies

The second option is less likely to impact frame rates and is, therefore, the most common technique employed. The advantage of frequency compounding over spatial compounding is that the speckle reduction that can be achieved is not depth dependent (cf., see Fig. 6.18).

ADVANCED CONCEPT

Frequency compounding is the averaging of multiple images obtained at different frequencies (most commonly from different bandpass filters).

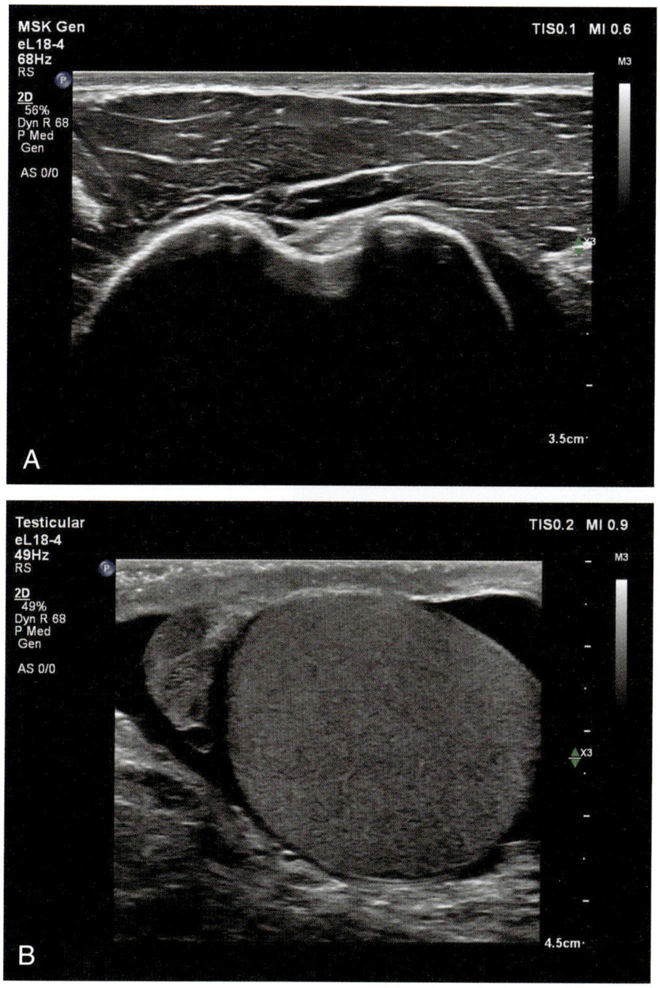

Fig. 6.17 Examples of improved image quality with spatial compounding depicting **(A)** the bicep tendon and **(B)** a testicle. (Courtesy Philips Medical Systems.)

ELASTOGRAPHY

Conventional grayscale images display representations of the scattering properties of the imaged tissues. Alternatively, information regarding the mechanical tissue properties (in other words, the **stiffness**, hardness, or softness of tissue) can be imaged using an ultrasound mode known as **elastography**. Elastography provides an imaging means of performing (noninvasive) "palpation" and can be qualitative or quantitative in its evaluation of tissue hardness.

If a material, such as tissue, is subjected to a stress (a force per unit area) that compresses or stretches the material, the ratio of the applied stress to the resulting strain (the increase or decrease of the length of a segment of the material divided by its original length) is called **Young's modulus** and is a measure of the stiffness (hardness or softness) of the material. Thus soft materials have a small Young's modulus (i.e., a given stress results in a large strain), whereas a large Young's modulus corresponds to hard or stiff materials for which a given stress results in little strain. As evidenced by the success of manual palpation for centuries, tissue hardness may be an indicator of normality or abnormality. Various approaches to elastography have been implemented commercially and some of the most common will be described in the following sections.

Transient Elastography

It is possible to obtain a relative measure of tissue stiffness by applying an external force to the tissue and tracking the movement of the tissue by spatial correlation, since soft tissues will compress more than hard ones. This external force can be initiated by the sonographer physically pushing on the transducer or by an external vibration source. Relative stiffness is commonly shown as a color overlay on top of the anatomical, grayscale image (Fig. 6.21) and is referred to as an *elastogram*.

Transient elastography has been used clinically for cancer detection, characterization of small parts (breast, thyroid, and prostate—see Fig. 6.22), assessment of the viability of the myocardium, and monitoring of therapies that alter tissue composition, such as ablation procedures. While this mode of elastography is relatively simple to implement, it is

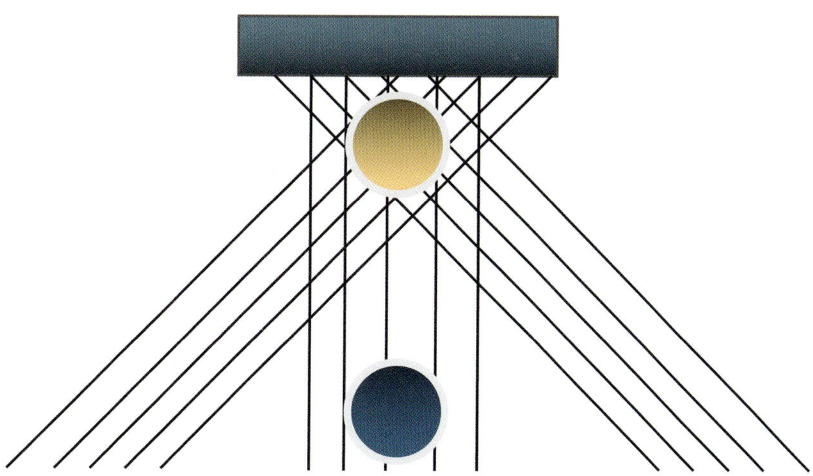

Fig. 6.18 The depth dependency of spatial compounding illustrated. Notice how shallow and large depths are less amenable to spatial compounding.

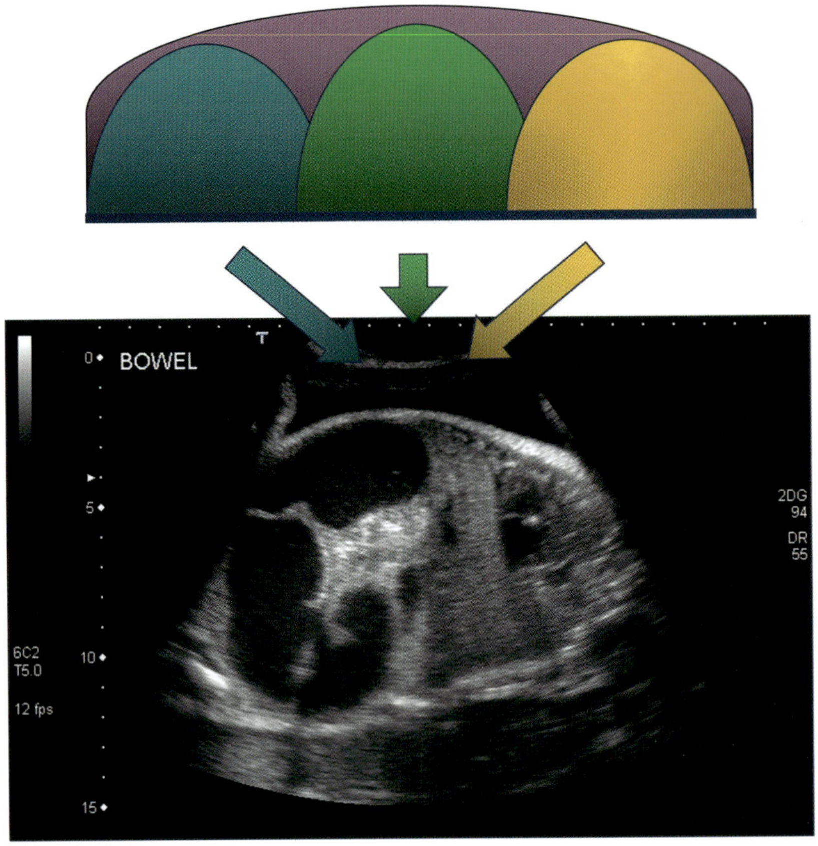

Fig. 6.19 The principle of frequency compounding illustrated with the overall transducer bandwidth being split into three sub-spectra (*top*) and then averaged resulting in the bowel image (*below*).

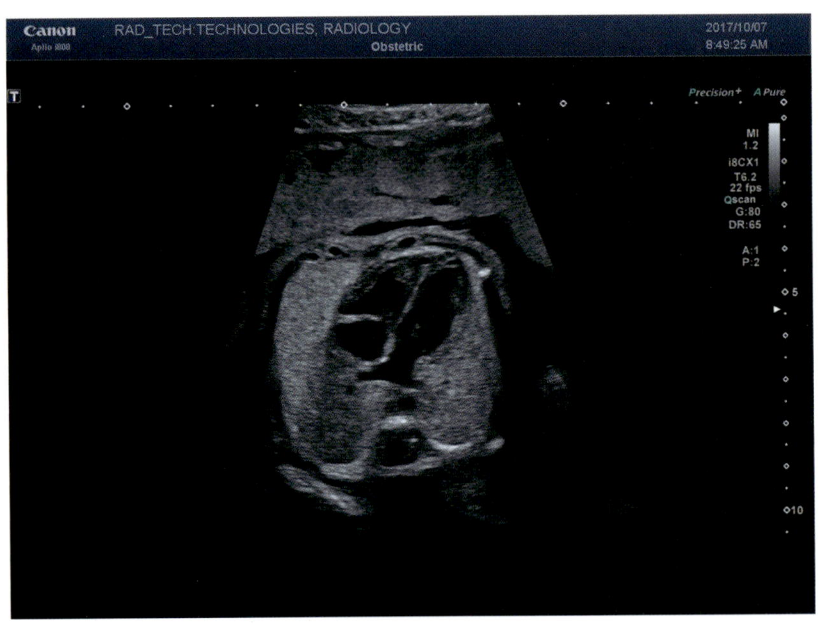

Fig. 6.20 Example of frequency compounding in obstetrics. (Courtesy Canon Medical Systems USA.)

fundamentally qualitative in that it shows relative hardness of various anatomic regions in relation to that of adjacent regions. Moreover, transient elastography suffers from significant variability, because it is very operator dependent. Finally, the Young's modulus cannot be calculated, because the applied stress is unknown.

Shear Wave Elastography

To obtain quantitative measurements of Young's modulus (i.e., tissue stiffness), **shear wave elastography** (SWE) is used. A long "push-pulse" (on the order of 100 μs) is transmitted into the tissue in the form of a longitudinal wave (i.e., a standard ultrasound pulse but longer and with greater intensity). The

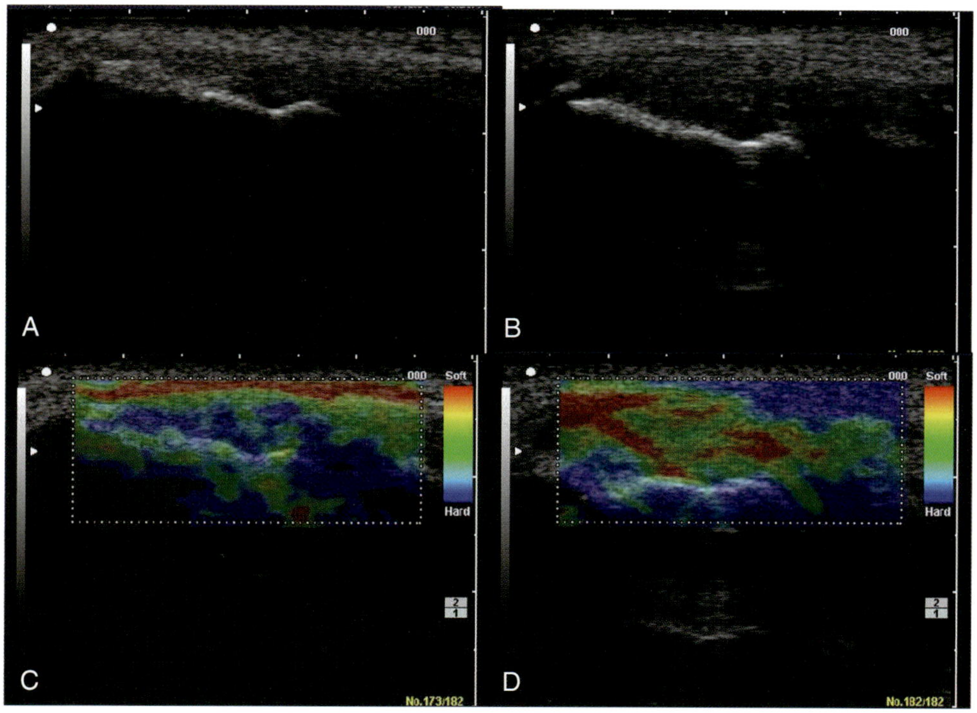

Fig. 6.21 **A,** Grayscale of the left common extensor tendon. **B,** Grayscale of the right symptomatic common extensor tendon. **C,** Transient elastography image of the left tendon with red colors signifying soft tissues and blue colors signifying hard tissue. The designations "soft" and "hard" are relative to the maximum stiffness found in the image. **D,** Transient elastography image of the right (symptomatic) tendon. Notice the tendon on the right is much softer with a preponderance of green and red colors compared to the left side shown in **C**.

force of this pulse initially produces a compressional strain that travels with a high propagation speed, but through a phenomenon called *radiation force*, some of the energy is converted into shear waves (also called *transverse waves* and described in Chapter 2) that travel at much slower speeds (0.5–10 m/s vs. 1440–1640 m/s for compressional waves) in directions perpendicular to the travel of the compressional wave. The shear displacements of the slower propagating shear wave can be tracked by transmitting ultrafast "tracking pulses" at high frame rates (100s to 1000s of frames per second making SWE particularly amenable to scanners using broad transmit beams) to determine the shear wave propagation speed (in m/s). Imaging the stiffness in this way is called **acoustic radiation force impulse imaging**.

The **shear wave** propagation speed is quantitatively related to other material characteristics such as Young's modulus. Thus these SWE methods provide the means to determine tissue hardness quantitatively. Recall that Young's modulus is stress divided by strain. Strain is unitless, because it is a change in length divided by the original length. Hence, the units for stress, which is kilopascal (kPa), and Young's modulus are identical. Young's modulus values for soft tissue range from approximately 1 kPa for fat to 300 kPa for a fibrotic liver. Young's modulus (E) is related to the shear wave propagation speed (c_s) as follows:

$$c_s = [E/3\rho]^{1/2}$$

where ρ is the density of the propagating medium (soft tissue in our case). SWE techniques measure shear wave speed directly, and therefore it has become common to express the stiffness in shear wave speed units (m/s) as well as in Young's modulus units (kPa).

There are two general SWE modes: point SWE (sometimes referred to as pSWE), where a region-of-interest is placed on the grayscale image within which the tissue is perturbed and the resulting shear wave speeds measured and 2D SWE where elasticity values are displayed as a color-coded overlay on top of the grayscale image. The color scale is often set as softer tissue in blue and harder tissue in red, but this is an arbitrary choice. The color scale is quantitative with values expressed in either m/s or kPa. Examples of SWE measurements and images from the breast and liver are presented in Figs. 6.23 and 6.24.

The Quantitative Imaging Biomarkers Alliance (QIBA) has taken the lead in establishing imaging setups that will lead to reproducible SWE measurements across units and manufacturers, which should expand the clinical utility of SWE.

> Elastography is an imaging technique that depicts qualitative or quantitative tissue stiffness information.

Cardiac Strain Imaging

In elastography, the hardness (stiffness) of the tissue is imaged and/or quantitatively determined by producing a strain in the tissue by an external force or by radiation force. However, the heart is a four-chambered muscle that functions as

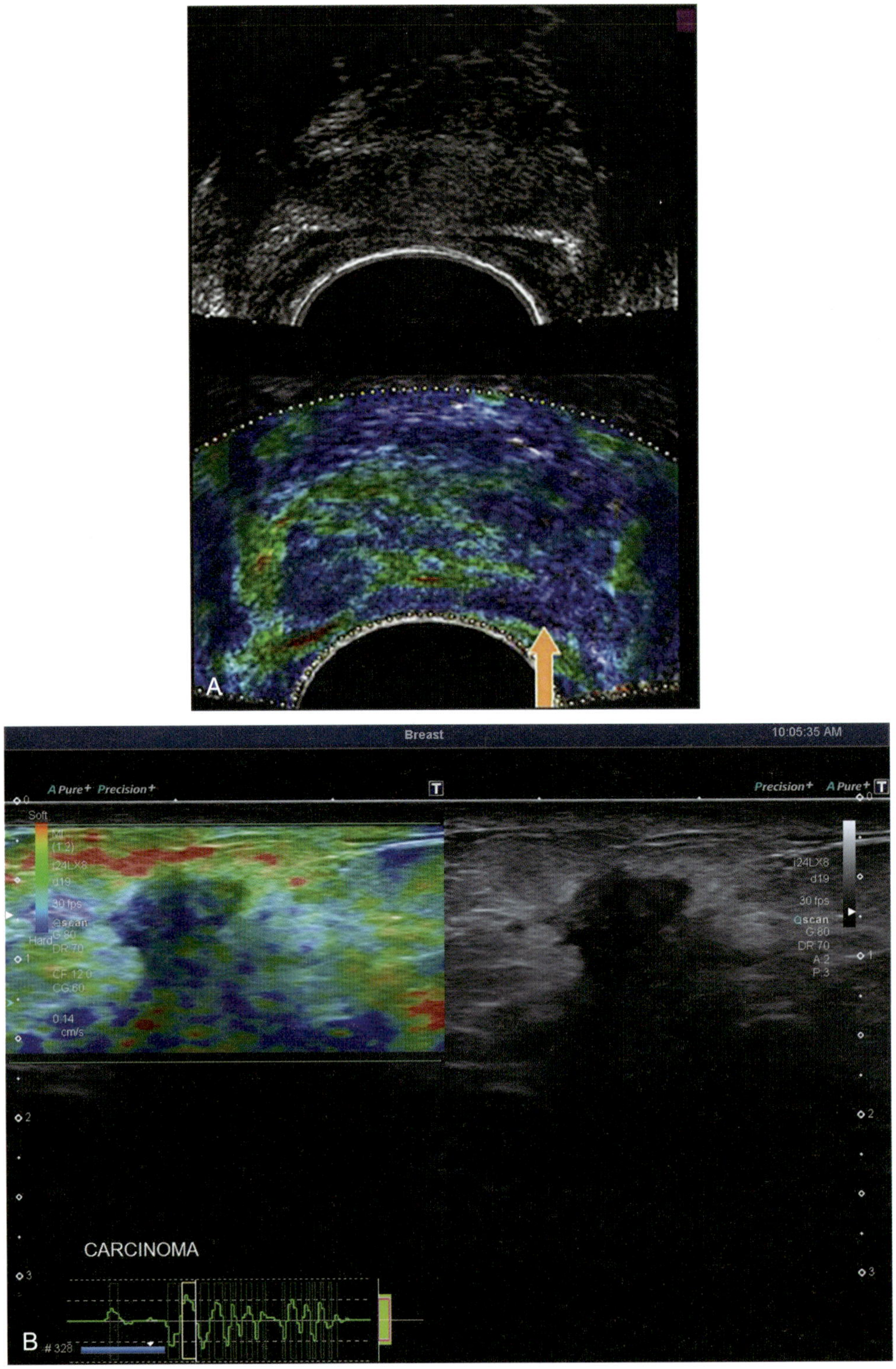

Fig. 6.22 A, Example of grayscale (*top*) transient elastography (*bottom*) of a Gleason 6 prostate cancer in the left apex (*arrow*). **B,** Transient elastography of a malignant breast mass, which is clearly harder than the surrounding normal breast tissue. Notice the curve at the bottom left, which indicates the relative pressure applied and, thus, the consistency of the *elastogram*. (Courtesy Canon Medical Systems USA.)

a mechanical pump forcing blood circulation by contracting and relaxing. Therefore this is a case in which strain occurs in the contracting muscle (myocardium) because of its electrical stimulation rather than a strain in response to an external force (as discussed in the previous section). Strain and strain rate are indicators of the effectiveness of the myocardial function and are useful diagnostic parameters. Strain and strain rate can be determined by 2D speckle-tracking techniques (which track the movement of specific portions of the myocardium) and from tissue Doppler imaging techniques (discussed in Chapter 5). Examples of **cardiac strain imaging** are shown in Fig. 6.25.

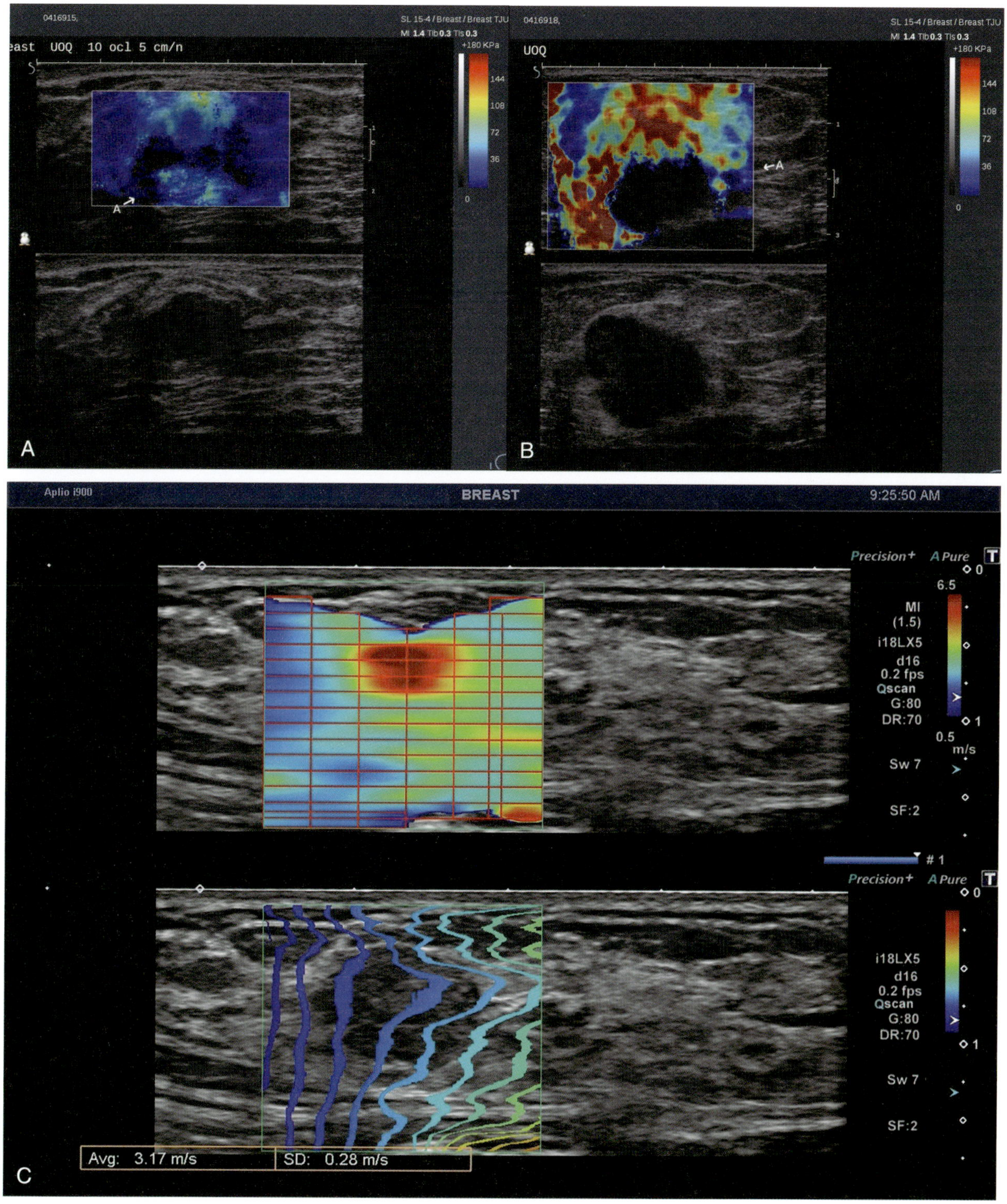

Fig. 6.23 Breast shear wave elastography examples. **A,** Fibroadenoma with stiffness values below 40 kPa according to the color scale (calibrated in kPa for Young's modulus stiffness units). **B,** Invasive ductal carcinoma with a soft necrotic center (E < 36 kPa) and a very hard periphery (E > 170 kPa). **C,** Measurements of the shear wave speed obtained simultaneously from over 80 regions of interest (*top*) with the overall average shear wave speed and standard deviation calculated (3.17 ± 0.28 m/s). The curves *below* indicate the shear wave speed dispersion and are an indication of the quality of the measurements.

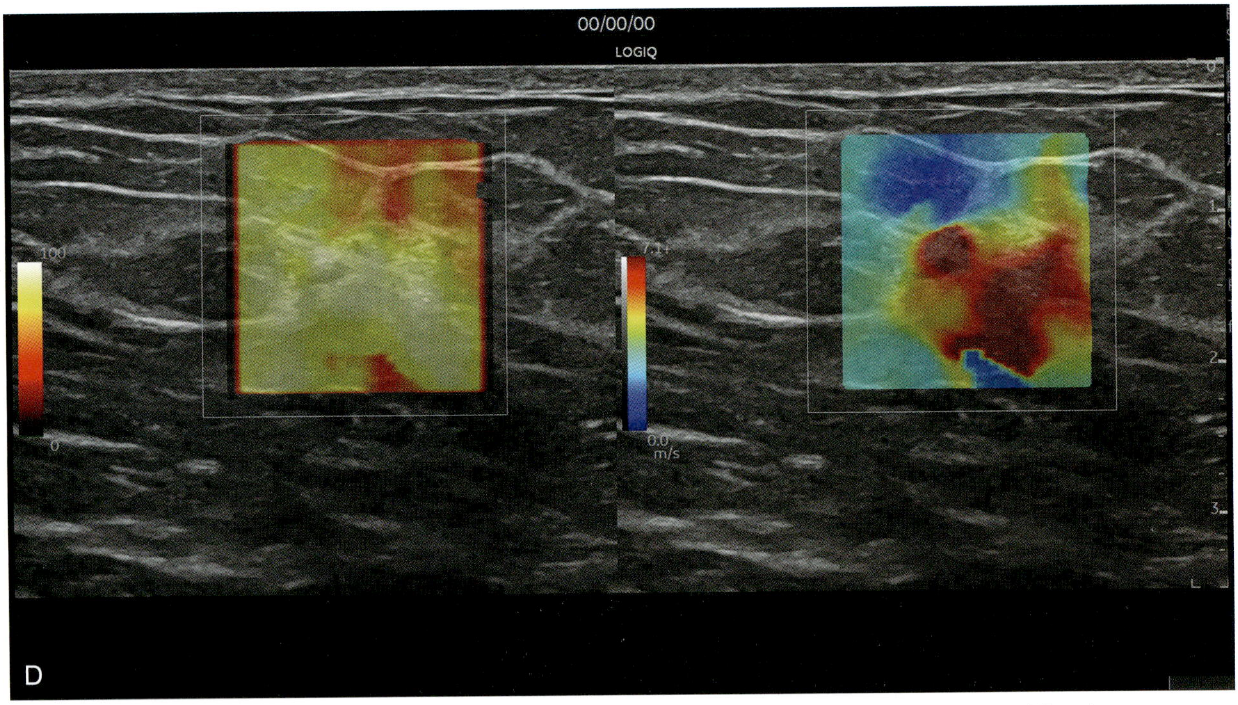

Fig. 6.23, cont'd D, Shear wave images expressed as stiffness in kPa (*left*) and shear wave speed (in m/s; on the *right*). (**C,** Courtesy Canon Medical Systems USA. **D,** Courtesy GE HealthCare.)

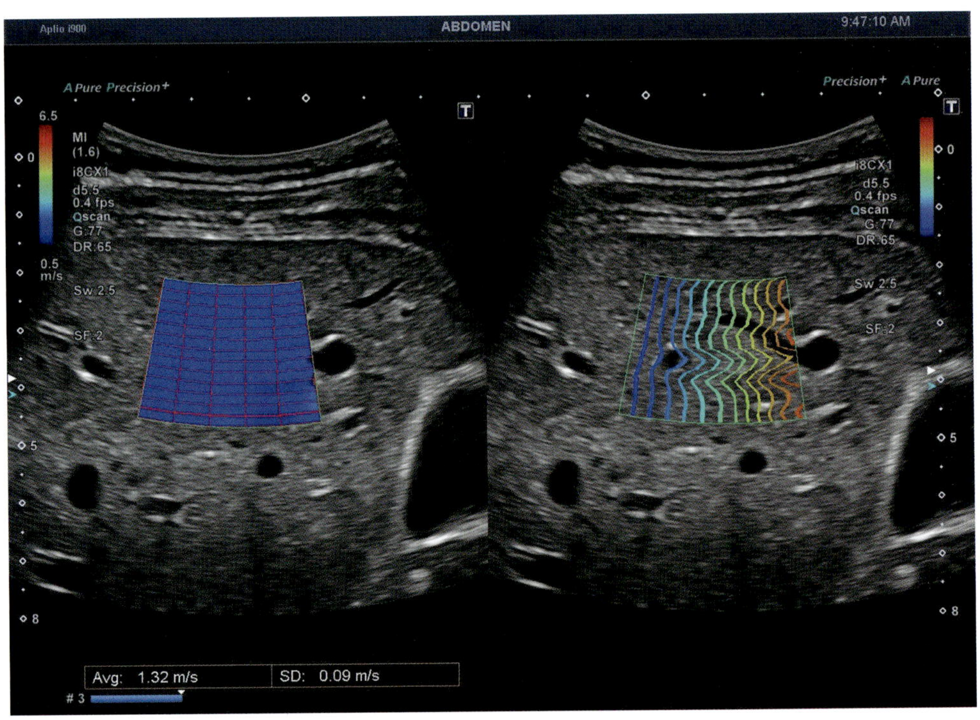

Fig. 6.24 Liver shear wave elastography where the color scale is calibrated in m/s (i.e., shear wave propagation speed). Measurements are obtained simultaneously from 65 regions of interest (*left*) with the average and standard deviation of the shear wave speed calculated (1.32 ± 0.09 m/s). The curves on the *right* indicate the shear wave speed dispersion and are an indication of the data quality. (Courtesy Canon Medical Systems USA.)

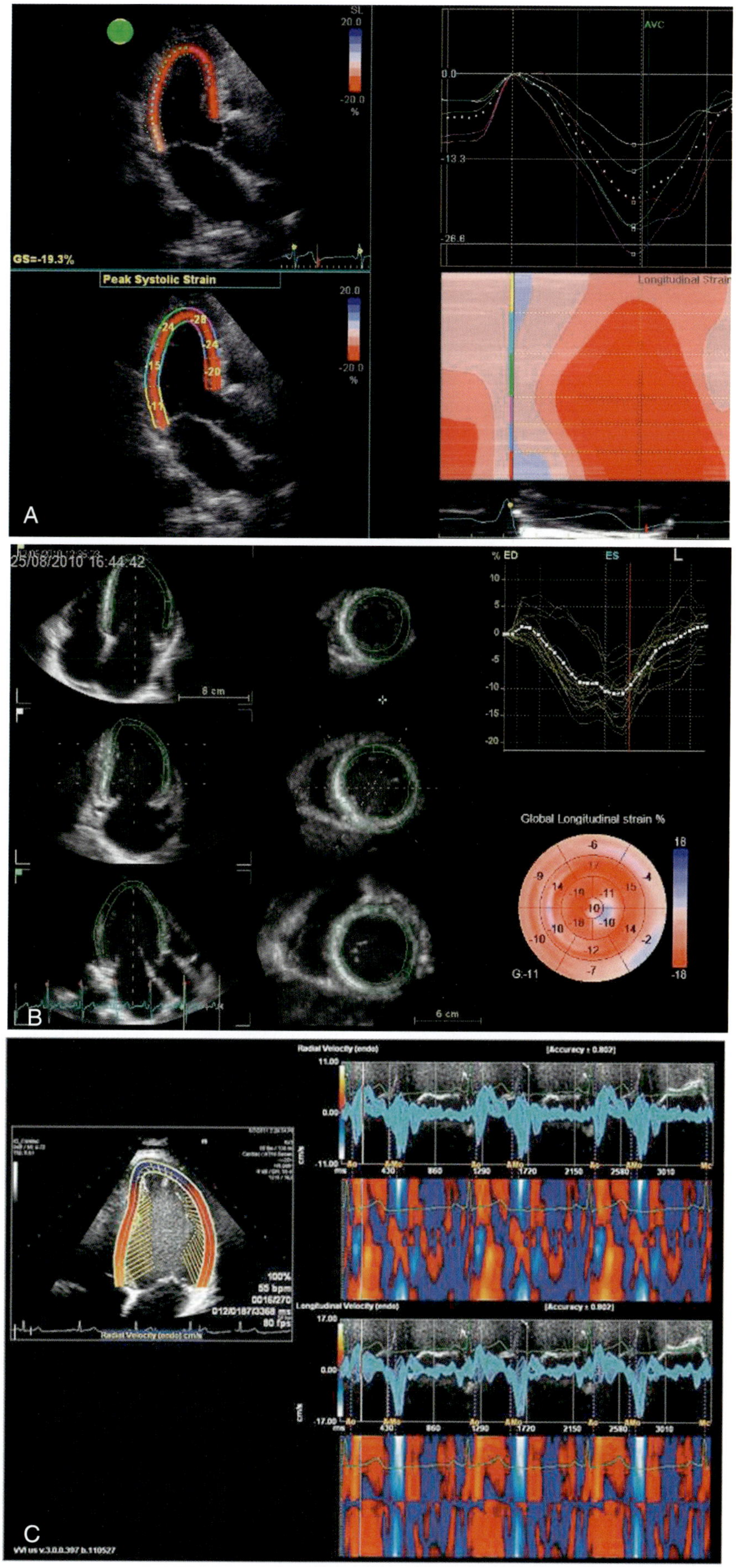

Fig. 6.25 **A–C,** Cardiac strain examples. (Courtesy Philips Medical Systems.)

Cardiac strain imaging presents information regarding contraction and relaxation strain and strain rate information for the myocardium of the beating heart.

CONTRAST-ENHANCED ULTRASOUND IMAGING

The value of enhancing imaging modes through the **intravenous (IV)** injection of a contrast medium is well established for CT and MRI. In the United States, it is really only in the last decade or two that the use of contrast agents in diagnostic ultrasound imaging has become clinically available (although contrast echocardiography has been around for much longer). With the development of better **CEUS imaging** modes and the approval of several ultrasound **contrast agents** for cardiology as well as radiology applications in adults and in children, CEUS is finally making an impact in day-to-day clinical practice, requiring more and more sonographers to become IV certified.

Contrast Agents

Ultrasound contrast agents consist of gas-filled **microbubbles**, 1 to 10 μm in diameter that are stabilized by a protein, lipid, or polymer shell (Fig. 6.26, A). Encapsulation of the gas slows its diffusion back into solution, lengthening the duration of the contrast effect. To further slow diffusion, low-solubility gases such as perfluorocarbons are used. Following IV injection these agents (i.e., bubbles) pass through the lungs and enhance echogenicity from vessels (even capillaries) and perfused tissues in grayscale and Doppler ultrasound modes by up to 30 dB for 3 to 6 minutes (or longer if they are not imaged continuously). Contrast agents produce such large echoes because of the impedance mismatch between the microbubbles and the surrounding medium (i.e., blood).

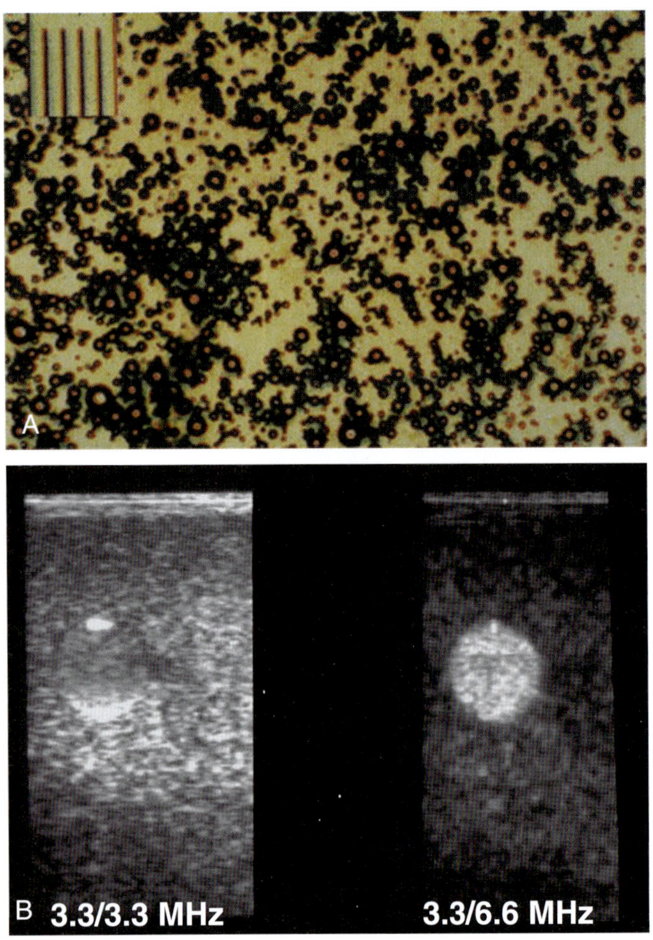

Fig. 6.26 A, Microscope images of microbubbles (size marker is 10 μm). **B,** Fundamental and second harmonic imaging (transmitting/receiving at 3.3/3.3 and 3.3/6.6 MHz, respectively, of bubbles in a tune within a tissue-mimicking phantom. (**A,** Courtesy Dr. Margaret Wheatley, Drexel University.)

The safety of ultrasound contrast agents has been investigated in numerous studies involving millions of patients and the adverse event rates are generally below 0.01% (further details can be found in Chapter 9). State-of-the-art, real-time CEUS-specific imaging modes operate at MIs under 0.2 and no bioeffects have been encountered at those levels.

Ultrasound contrast agents are made up of small gas-filled and encapsulated microbubbles about the same size as red blood cells.

Contrast Harmonic Imaging

Contrast agents not only enhance the backscattered ultrasound signals but, at sufficient acoustic pressures, also act as nonlinear oscillators. These oscillations generate significant nonlinear energy components in the received echo signals, which span the range of possible frequency emissions from subharmonics (half of the fundamental frequency; $f_0/2$) through higher **harmonics** (multiple of the fundamental frequency; $2f_0$, $3f_0$, ..., or even and odd harmonics). These nonlinear bubble echoes can be separated from tissue echoes and used to create **contrast-specific imaging** modalities such as **contrast harmonic imaging** (transmitting at the fundamental frequency but receiving at double that; cf., Chapter 4), which is commercially available on most state-of-the-art ultrasound scanners.

An example from a tissue-mimicking phantom demonstrates the improvement in contrast-to-noise ratio and overall image quality by using microbubbles and contrast harmonic imaging (see Fig. 6.26, B).

Pulse Inversion and Amplitude Modulation

CEUS image quality can be improved markedly by using multipulse imaging techniques. One such technique is **pulse inversion** that uses two pulses per scan line rather than one. The second pulse is the inverse of the first (i.e., 180 degrees out of phase). The echo sequences from the two pulses (Fig. 6.27, A–B) are combined to yield the resulting scan line. Fundamental frequency echoes are canceled, and the second harmonic echoes remain (see Fig. 6.27, B). This technique allows broad-bandwidth, short pulses to be used so that detail resolution is not degraded (see Fig. 6.27, C). Instead, the frame rate is reduced somewhat, with some degradation of temporal resolution, especially in narrow transmit beam systems.

Amplitude modulation is a similar multipulse CEUS technique with the same end-goal: to suppress fundamental echoes and retain the nonlinear echoes from contrast microbubbles to

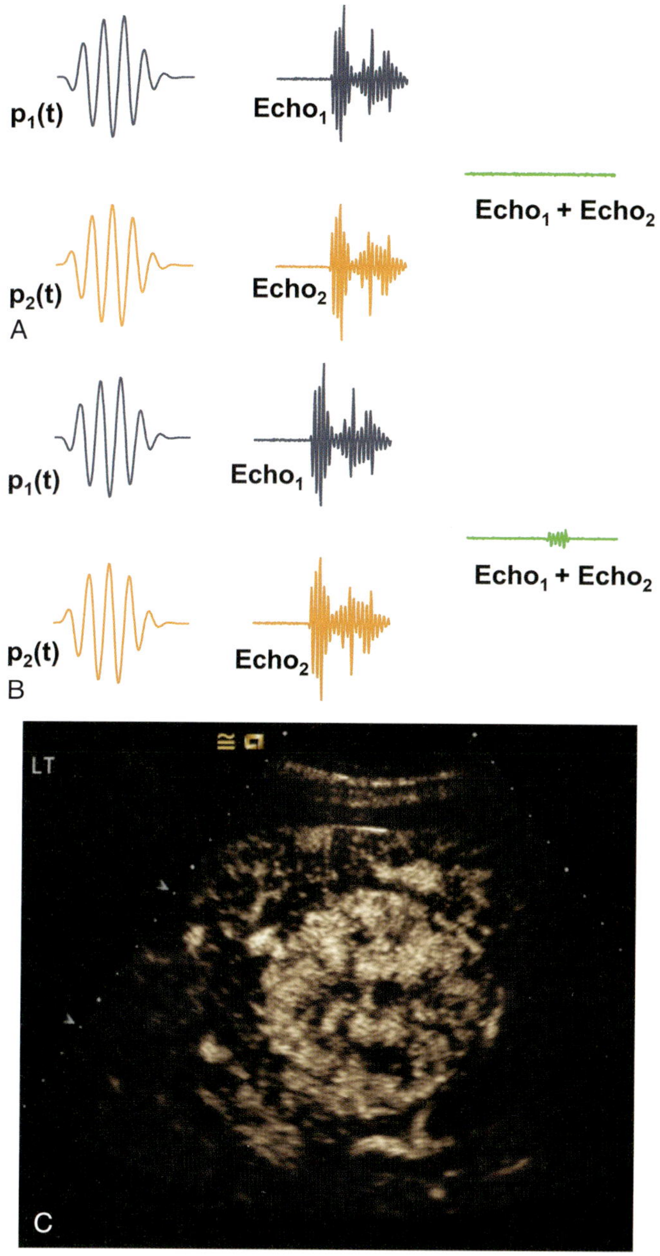

Fig. 6.27 A, In pulse inversion contrast-enhanced ultrasound (*CEUS*) imaging, two pulses 180 degrees out of phase are transmitted along each scan line so that the fundamental frequency echoes can be eliminated and the nonlinear ones retained. For linear scattering the echoes from the pulses are inverse copies and summing them will cancel everything out (i.e., fundamental echoes are suppressed) **B,** Under nonlinear scattering conditions the two pulse-inverted echoes are summed, the fundamental frequency echoes cancel, but nonlinear echoes are kept. **C,** Liver lesion on CEUS imaging in pulse inversion harmonic imaging mode.

improve CEUS image quality. In this scheme, two pulses are transmitted with one being half the amplitude of the other and the returned echoes from this pulse are scaled up and subtracted from the other pulse echoes. There are even three pulse techniques that combine pulse inversion and amplitude modulation into one firing scheme on top of contrast harmonic imaging. As before, the trade-off is between improved CEUS image quality and reduced frame rates. 2D and 3D contrast-specific multipulse imaging examples from the liver are shown in Fig. 6.28.

> CEUS-specific imaging modes aim to remove fundamental (linear) echoes and retain only echoes from nonlinear bubble signals. Multipulse imaging techniques markedly improve CEUS image quality (at the cost of somewhat reduced frame rates).

Quantitative Contrast-Enhanced Ultrasound Measurements

Contrast kinetics have been explored in other cross-sectional imaging modes and similar considerations apply to CEUS with the biggest differences being the real-time imaging frame rates and the true vascular tracers (since microbubbles stay in the blood flow and do not extravasate). As an example, the characterization of liver lesions relies on contrast wash-in and wash-out as well as the enhancement during the arterial and portal venous phases. The change in contrast enhancement as a function of time (so-called **time-intensity curves**) is used to evaluate such parameters and many scanners have built-in software packages for these calculations and to create parametric images (Fig. 6.29).

Ultrasound pulses of sufficiently high-pressure amplitude can rupture the microbubbles, allowing the gas to dissolve and eliminating the contrast effect. Subsequent low-amplitude imaging then can show the return of the bubbles, which provide an indication of tissue perfusion (in mL/min per gram of tissue). This is called destruction/reperfusion imaging.

OTHER CONCEPTS

This section deals with concepts that are of general interest but which will not appear on any ultrasound physics tests for a while to come.

Ultrasound Computed Tomography

Similar to CT, **ultrasound computed tomography** attempts to solve the acoustic inverse problem that arises when collecting echoes from 360 degrees around an object and wanting to determine sound speed and density at all points inside. Given that ultrasound does not travel in a straight line, this is a much more difficult problem to tackle than that of x-ray CT. Nonetheless, given advances in computing power, it is now possible to produce simultaneous breast images mapping speed of sound, attenuation, reflection (acoustic impedance), and/or stiffness (Fig. 6.30).

Artificial Intelligence

Artificial intelligence (AI) and related technologies, such as ***Deep Learning*** and ***Machine Learning*** (ML), are rapidly being deployed in medical instruments including ultrasound scanners. AI algorithms rely on large volumes of curated, high-quality annotated data with robust clinical validations. Moreover, successful deployment of an AI algorithm into the clinical practice of radiology and ultrasound requires extensive, interdisciplinary collaborations between computational scientists, signal processing engineers, and radiologists. These are obviously not trivial issues to resolve, but nonetheless, more and more AI algorithms are being approved by the FDA for augmenting ultrasound imaging.

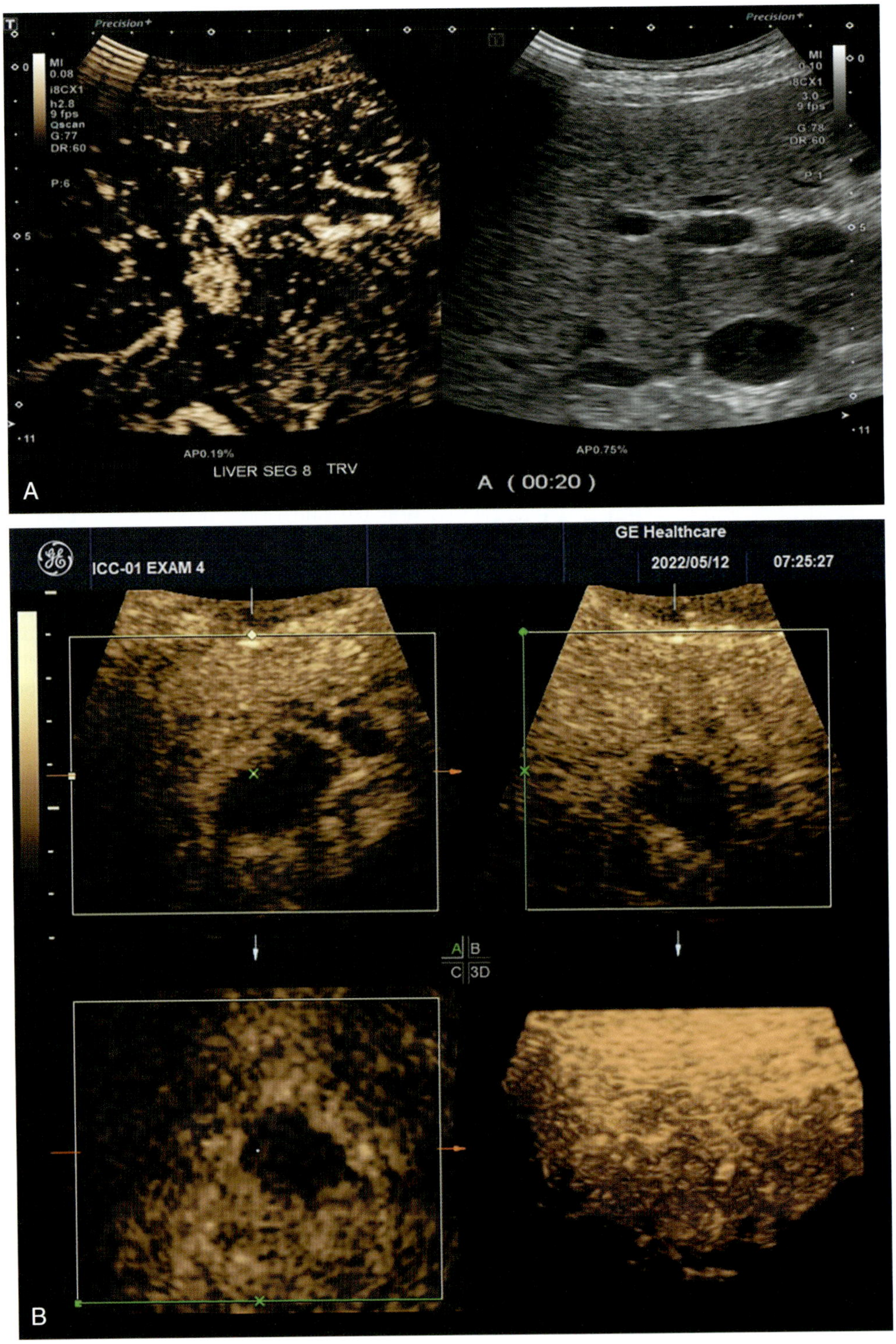

Fig. 6.28 Examples of contrast-enhanced ultrasound liver imaging using different nonlinear contrast-specific imaging modes in **(A)** two- and **(B)** three-dimensional display formats. (Courtesy Corinne Wessner, Thomas Jefferson University.)

Currently, there are AI algorithms providing scanning guidance and helping select standard imaging planes as well as identifying organs and other structures (e.g., bladder volume measurements and lung B-line counting). Improving image quality (e.g., through improved beam forming) and providing adjunct diagnoses (e.g., lesion characterization or level of suspicion indications) are also well developed. Examples of ultrasound AI are presented in Figs. 6.15, B and 6.31.

AI has the potential to improve the accuracy, efficiency, workflow, and productivity of diagnostic imaging, especially in resource-poor regions of the world. As this technology gets progressively more and more incorporated into medical imaging,

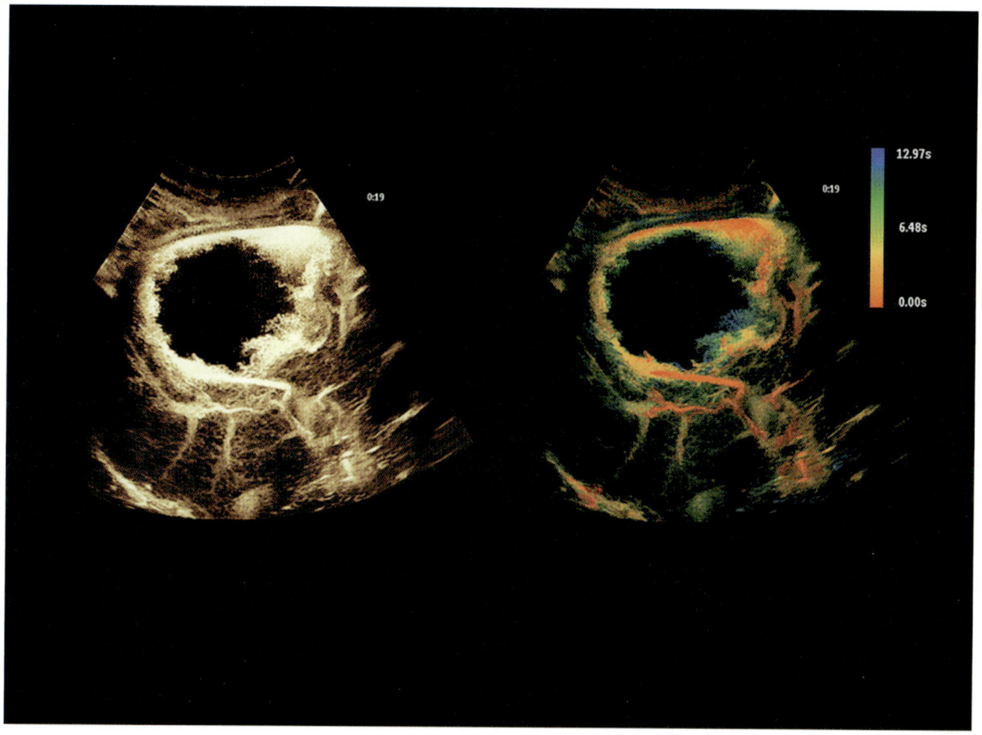

Fig. 6.29 Contrast-enhanced ultrasound of hemangioma in the liver (*left*) and a map of the wash-in time of arrival of the contrast microbubbles (*right*). (Courtesy Philips Medical Systems.)

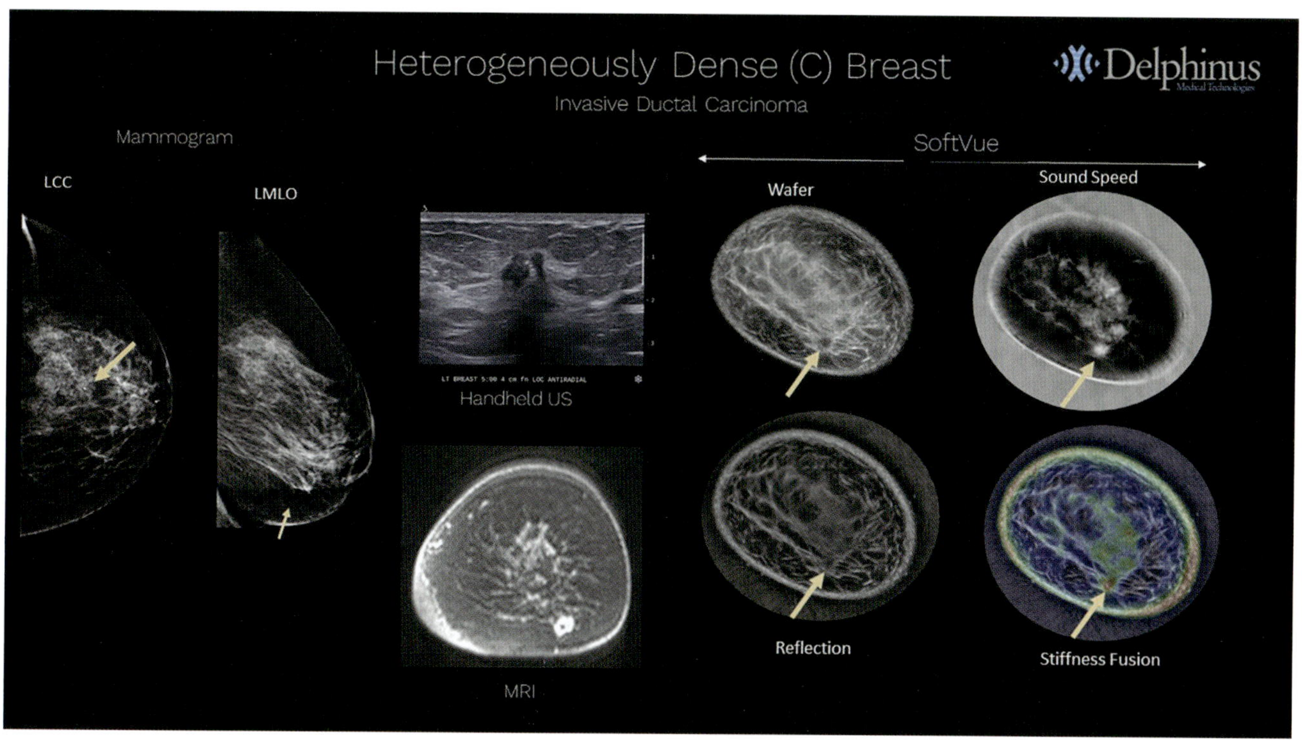

Fig. 6.30 Ultrasound tomography breast example. (From https://www.delphinusmt.com.)

regulatory, legal, and ethical issues will have to be addressed. As witnessed by the enthusiasm that has greeted ChatGPT and other AI-based chatbots, it is clear that public acceptance is probably a minor concern (and no, this section was not written by an AI chatbot). As long as we are sending ultrasound into the body and receiving ultrasonic echoes, these will be ultrasound systems, but the ever-expanding incorporation of AI and ML into ultrasound scanners means that what we do with the returning echoes will be radically different depending on the processing employed.

Output Devices and Systems

Diagnostic ultrasound scanners can export images and other information to external devices such as computer workstations (Fig. 6.32). Image information flows in digital form (numbers) to an internal memory and externally to a computer and/or a **picture archiving and communication system (PACS)** to be stored in digital format, just as it is in the image memory of the instrument. Such storage involves no loss of quality and allows postprocessing, measurements, and any other function that can be applied to a stored (frozen) image in the system memory.

Various standard protocols are used for communicating and storing digital images, for example, JPEG (Joint Photographic Experts Group), TIFF (tagged image file format), video clips (e.g., AVI [audio video interleave]), and MPEG (Moving Picture Experts Group). Quality depends on the number of pixels per image and the amount of compression used (image compression is a process that reduces digital file size, while retaining the data essential for acceptable image quality). Ultrasound images are not collections of random echo data and, thus, their repeating patterns allow shortened coding, called *lossless compression*, to reduce file size. Lossless compression reduces file size to approximately one-half its usual size without altering the image. Lossy compression involves visually similar, but not identical, images. The JPEG file is a compressed image file (file extension .jpg). File size is a trade-off with quality. The TIFF file (file extension .tif) has better quality than JPEG but creates larger files. The same is true for MPEG (file extension .mpg) video clips compared with AVI (file extension .avi) ones. Newer iterations of the MPEG standard (MPEG-4, MPEG-7, etc.) are steadily making AVI files more or less obsolete.

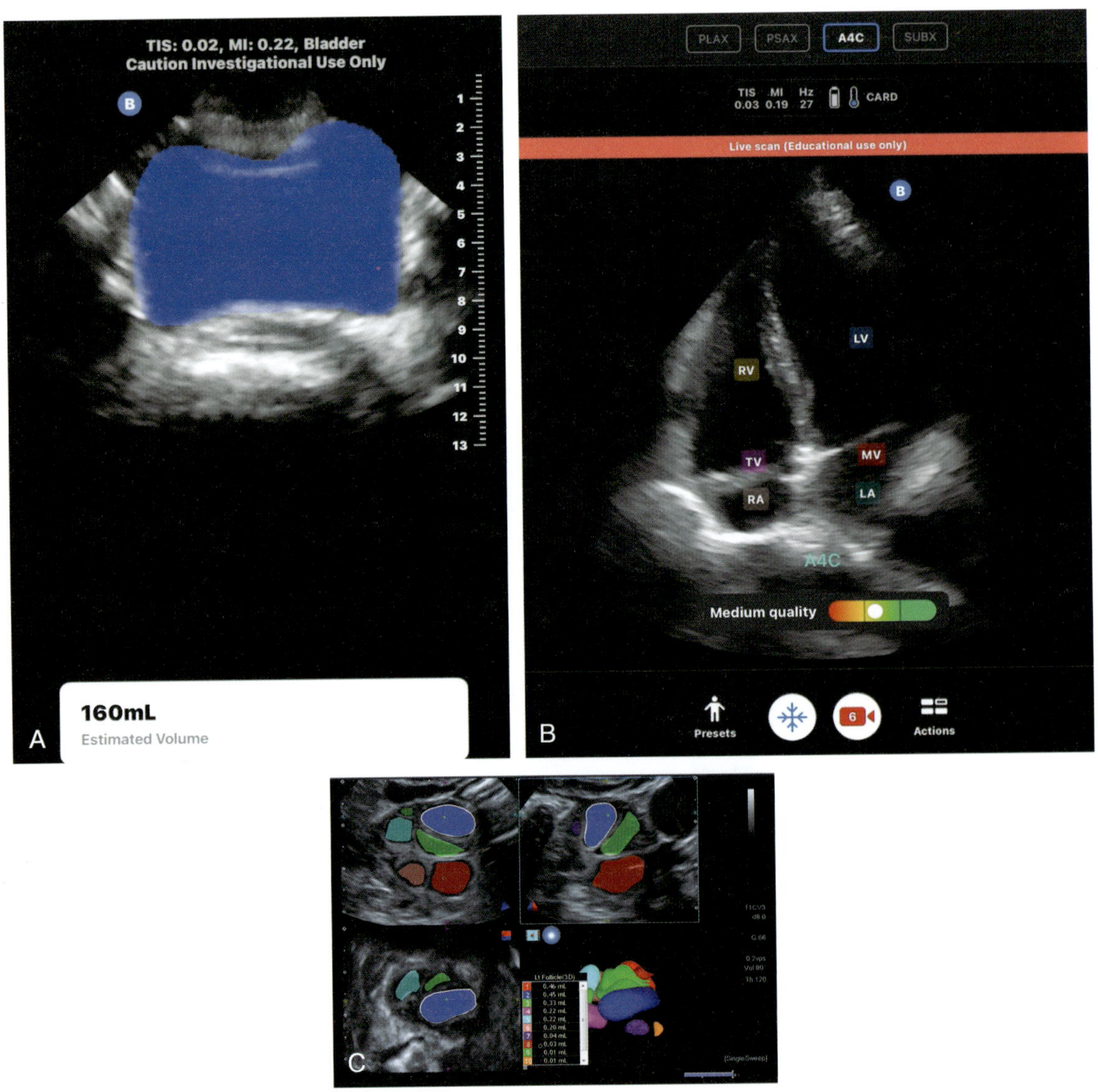

Fig. 6.31 Examples of artificial intelligence (*AI*)–assisted ultrasound imaging. **A,** Automatic bladder volume calculation on a point-of-care ultrasound device. **B,** AI identification of the cardiac chambers in a four-chamber view. **C,** AI-assisted identification of ovarian cysts with automated cyst volume calculations.

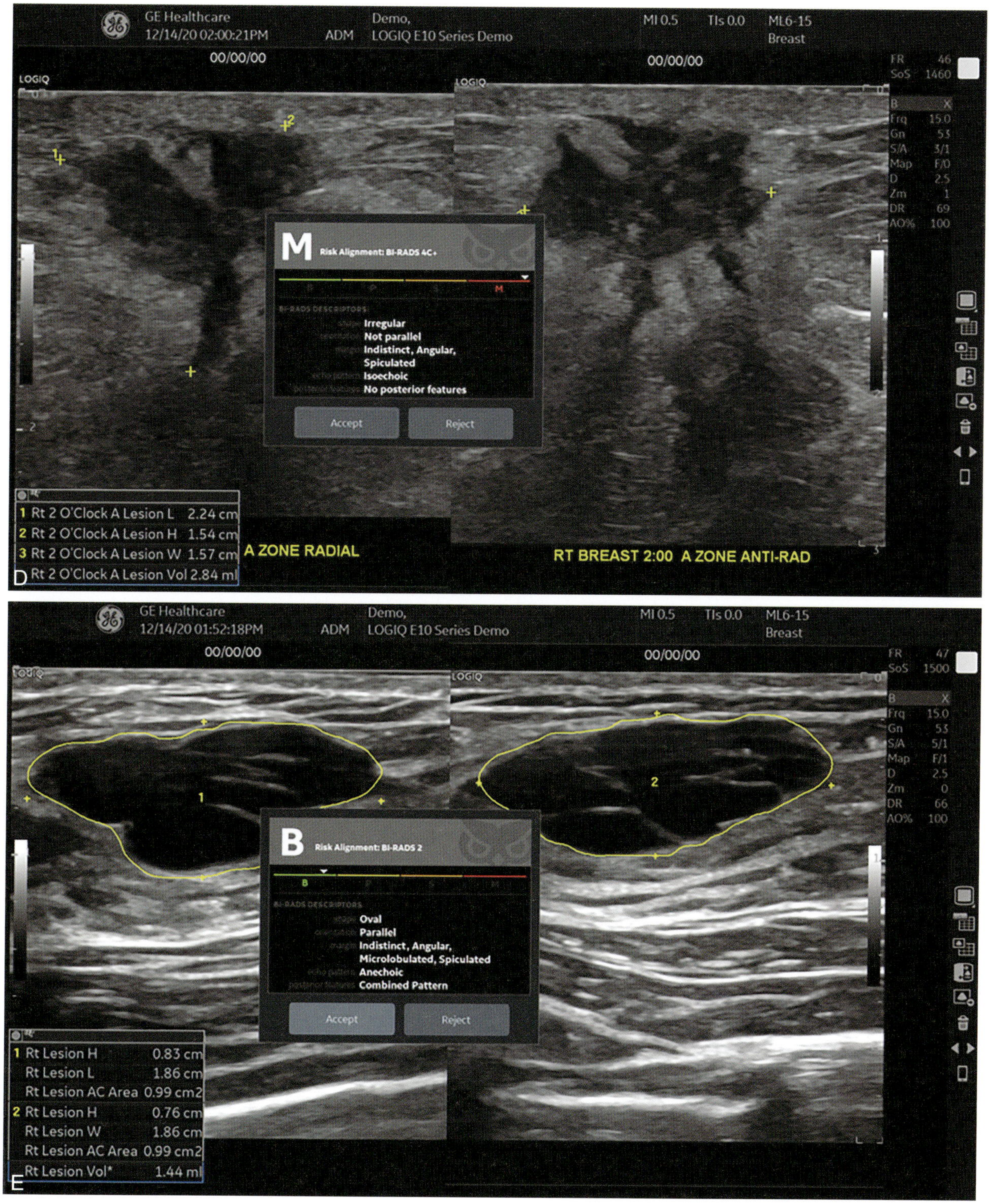

Fig. 6.31, cont'd D, Malignant breast lesion assessed by AI software to assist breast imagers in lesion characterization. **E,** Benign breast lesion assessed by AI software. (**A–B,** Courtesy Butterfly Network. **C,** Courtesy Canon Medical Systems USA. **D–E,** Courtesy GE HealthCare.)

While scanners with DVD drives and USB ports are still plentiful, ultrasound image files can be (and are) transmitted to anywhere in the world through the internet as more and more storage facilities are cloud based (similar to your iPhone storage). PACS is used with all digital imaging modes, including ultrasound. The protocols for communicating images and associated information between imaging devices and workstations have been standardized in the Digital Imaging and Communications in Medicine (DICOM) standard. This standard specifies a hardware interface, a minimum set of software commands, and a consistent set of data formats. This standard promotes communication of information, regardless of manufacturers of the linked devices, including the sonographic instrument, the PACS reading station, and other hospital/clinic information systems. The DICOM standard also enables the creation of diagnostic information databases that can be interrogated by a wide variety of geographically distributed devices.

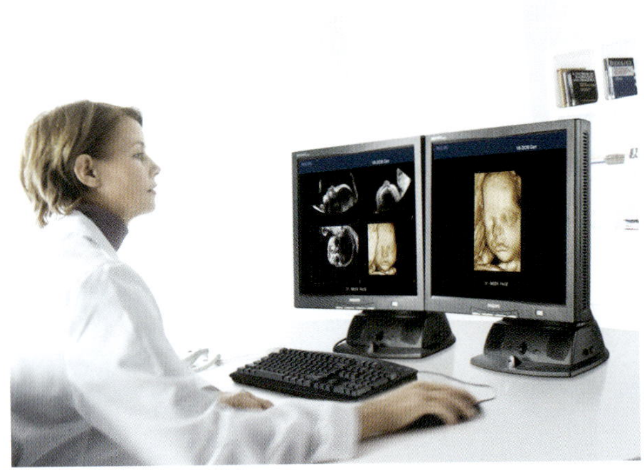

Fig. 6.32 A picture archiving and communications system workstation.

REVIEW

The following key points are presented in this chapter:

- Harmonic frequencies are generated while sound travels through tissue.
- Tissue harmonic imaging is a sophisticated form of beam forming.
- Coded excitation uses a series of pulses and gaps (as 1s and 0s) rather than a single driving pulse.
- A matched filter disassembles the coded sequence in the returning echoes improving image quality and sensitivity.
- Fusion imaging is the combined real-time and synchronous presentation of grayscale ultrasound images with another cross-sectional imaging mode (CT, MRI, or PET typically).
- QUS methods estimate parameters such as attenuation, backscattering, and speed of sound.
- Portable POCUS systems based on silicon wafer technologies are rapidly changing many specialities (emergency medicine, anesthesiology, etc.).
- Spatial and frequency compounding are the two most common speckle-reduction techniques.
- Elastography is an imaging method that presents qualitative or quantitative tissue stiffness (hardness or softness) information on the anatomical display.
- Quantitative elastography measurements require shear wave tracking.
- Cardiac strain imaging presents information regarding contraction and relaxation strain and strain rate information for the myocardium of the beating heart.
- Ultrasound contrast agents are made up of microbubbles about the same size as red blood cells.
- CEUS-specific imaging modes aim to remove fundamental (linear) echoes and retain only echoes from nonlinear bubble signals.
- Multipulse imaging techniques can markedly improve CEUS image quality.

EXERCISES

Answers appear in the Answers to Exercises section at the back of the book.

1. A high-intensity wave traveling into tissue will generate ___________.
   a. quadratic signals
   b. harmonic signals
   c. attention
   d. attenuation
2. Tissue harmonic imaging is a form of ___________.
   a. pulse shaping
   b. flow imaging
   c. beam forming
   d. a and b
   e. a and c
3. Coded excitation is a way to bypass the ___________ trade-off.
   a. penetration/resolution
   b. penetration/attenuation
   c. attenuation/pulsation
   d. attenuation/time of flight
4. Stitching ultrasound images together is known as ___________ imaging.
   a. X
   b. long
   c. panoramic
   d. fusion
5. Combining CT/MRI with ultrasound is ___________.
   a. a waste of time
   b. impossible except in the liver
   c. useful for biopsies
   d. useful for B-lines

6. Which of the following is not a quantitative ultrasound parameter?
   a. attenuation
   b. backscatter
   c. line density
   d. speed of sound
7. CMUT transducer frequencies cover ___________ MHz.
   a. 0.4–1.0
   b. 1.0–40.0
   c. 10.0–40.0
   d. 1.0–30.0
8. POCUS is useful ___________.
   a. at the bedside
   b. at a sporting event
   c. in the OR
   d. in the ER
   e. all of those locations
9. Lung ultrasound gained clinical acceptance during the ___________.
   a. COVID pandemic
   b. black death pandemic
   c. Ebola pandemic
   d. mad cow diseasepandemic
10. Compounding improves ___________ and ___________.
    a. frame rates and detail resolution
    b. image quality and interest payments
    c. detail resolution and bandwidth
    d. penetration and speckle reduction
11. Frequency compounding is better than spatial compounding over ___________.
    a. time
    b. space
    c. depth
    d. power
12. In elastography, the display presents qualitative or quantitative information on ___________.
    a. stress
    b. stiffness
    c. strain rate
    d. stress rate
13. Shear wave speeds range from _________ to _________ m/s.
    a. 1440, 1640
    b. 330, 1540
    c. 5, 25
    d. 0.5, 10
14. Transient and shear wave elastography both rely on ___________.
    a. a push-pulse
    b. ultra-high frame rates
    c. transducer motion
    d. changes in stiffness
15. Cardiac strain and strain measured by transient elastography are due to ___________.
    a. the liver and the heart
    b. frequency changes in stiffness and contractility
    c. muscle contractions and external force
    d. external force and stiffness
16. The average size of a contrast microbubble is _________ μm.
    a. 1–10
    b. 4–10
    c. 1–4
    d. 2–6
17. Microbubble oscillations can be _________.
    a. linear
    b. destructive
    c. nonlinear
    d. all of the above
18. The second harmonic of 3 MHz is ___________ MHz.
    a. 2
    b. 3.2
    c. 6
    d. 9
19. Nonlinear propagation means that ___________.
    a. the sound beam does not travel in a straight line
    b. propagation speed depends on frequency
    c. harmonics are not generated
    d. the waveform changes shape while it travels
20. In nonlinear propagation, additional frequencies appear that are ___________ and ___________ multiples of the fundamental frequency. They are called ___________.
    a. double, triple, harmonics
    b. double, triple, subharmonics
    c. odd, even, harmonics
    d. odd, even, subharmonics
21. Multipulse CEUS imaging modes are ___________.
    a. none of the below
    b. a nuisance
    c. a must
    d. a fad
22. Parameters derived from time-intensity curves include ___________.
    a. perfusion and dispersion
    b. curves and straight lines
    c. wash-in and wash-up
    d. wash-out and perfusion
23. Problems in ultrasound computed tomography include ___________.
    a. radiation and reconstruction
    b. processing requirements and straight lines of travel
    c. the inverse problem and curved lines of travel
    d. the multiverse problem and reconstruction
24. ChatGPT is among the tools being used to ___________.
    a. count lung B-lines
    b. improve image quality
    c. characterize breast lesions
    d. none of the above
25. The role of artificial intelligence in ultrasound imaging is ___________.
    a. constrained by the need for large, annotated data sets
    b. confused by large, annotated data sets
    c. to prepare for world domination
    d. expanding and contracting

7

Artifacts: Pitfalls and Misdiagnoses

LEARNING OBJECTIVES

After reading this chapter, the student should be able to do the following:

- List reasons for artifacts involving anatomical structures in grayscale images.
- List reasons for artifacts involving flow information in spectral and color Doppler displays.
- List reasons for artifacts involving contrast-enhanced ultrasound imaging.
- Describe how specific artifacts can be recognized.
- Explain how to avoid the pitfalls and misdiagnoses artifacts can cause.

CHAPTER OUTLINE

KEY TERMS

Aliasing
Anechoic
Comet tail
Cross-talk
Enhancement
Hypoechoic
Mirror image
Near field signal loss
Nyquist limit
Pseudo-enhancement
Pseudo-washout
Range ambiguity
Reverberation
Shadowing
Slice thickness
Speckle
Speed error

In previous chapters, we have covered the principles relevant to grayscale and Doppler ultrasound. We have seen how these techniques are intended to function. However, there is always the possibility of errors occurring. In medical imaging, an artifact is any situation where a factor (or a combination of factors) results in the imaged structures or function (such as blood flow) being displayed incorrectly. An artifact is caused by some problematic aspect of the imaging technique. In addition to some helpful artifacts, several hinder correct interpretation and diagnosis. Thus these artifacts should be avoided or at least handled properly when encountered.

Artifacts are incorrect representations of anatomy or function. Artifacts in grayscale images occur as apparent structures that have one of the following characteristics:

1. Not real
2. Missing
3. Misplaced
4. Of incorrect brightness, shape, or size

Some artifacts are produced by improper scanner settings (e.g., incorrect gain or TGC). Other artifacts are inherent in the imaging methods of ultrasound systems and can occur even with proper technique. Conversely, this chapter will also describe a number of artifacts that are becoming much rarer to encounter in today's clinical practice, due to the improved processing techniques implemented on state-of-the-art ultrasound scanners.

The assumptions inherent in the design of ultrasound scanners include the following:

- Sound travels in straight lines.
- Echoes originate only from objects located on the beam axis.
- Echo amplitudes are related directly to the scattering properties of reflecting objects.
- The distance to reflecting objects is proportional to the round-trip travel time (13 μs/cm of depth).

If any of these assumptions are violated, a grayscale ultrasound imaging artifact may occur. Possible artifacts are listed in Box 7.1.

Several artifacts are unique to Doppler ultrasound resulting in incorrect display of Doppler flow information (in color or spectral Doppler modes). The most common of these is **aliasing**. Other artifacts include **range ambiguity** and spectrum **mirror image**. There are also artifacts associated specifically with CEUS

BOX 7.1 Grayscale Ultrasound Imaging Artifacts

Propagation Group
- Comet tail
- Grating lobe
- Mirror image
- Range ambiguity
- Refraction
- Reverberation
- Ring-down
- Slice (section) thickness
- Speckle
- Speed error

Attenuation Group
- Enhancement
- Focal enhancement
- Refraction (edge) shadowing
- Shadowing

imaging, such as signal loss due to bubble destruction, pseudo-enhancement, and spectral Doppler velocity changes.

PROPAGATION

Slice Thickness

Limited detail resolution can introduce artifacts, because two adjacent structures may be visualized as one structure. This is becoming less and less of an issue as broad transmit beams combined with virtual beamforming assure the best possible detail resolution at any given pixel location. Nonetheless, there are still many systems using narrow transmit beams and more conventional beamforming technologies, where this can still be an issue. Moreover, the beam width perpendicular to the scan plane (the third dimension; Fig. 7.1,A) results in slice-thickness artifacts, for example the appearance of false debris in a simple, echo-free cyst (see Fig 7.1,B). These artifacts occur because of the finite thickness of the interrogating beam used in narrow transmit beam scanners to scan the patient. Echoes originate not only from the center of the main beam but also from off center (the **slice thickness**). These echoes are all collapsed into a zero-thickness, two-dimensional image that is composed of echoes that have come from a not-so-thin tissue volume scanned by the beam. The slice-thickness artifact is also called the *partial-volume* artifact.

Tissue harmonic imaging can resolve this artifact, because the sound beam in this mode is narrower than in the normal grayscale mode (see Fig 7.1,C). Finally, as mentioned, broad transmit beam systems reduce or eliminate this artifact by generating the thinnest (virtual) slices.

> Non-zero beam width perpendicular to the scan plane causes the slice-thickness artifact.

Speckle

The detailed echo pattern seen in grayscale images is often not related directly to the scattering properties of tissue (called

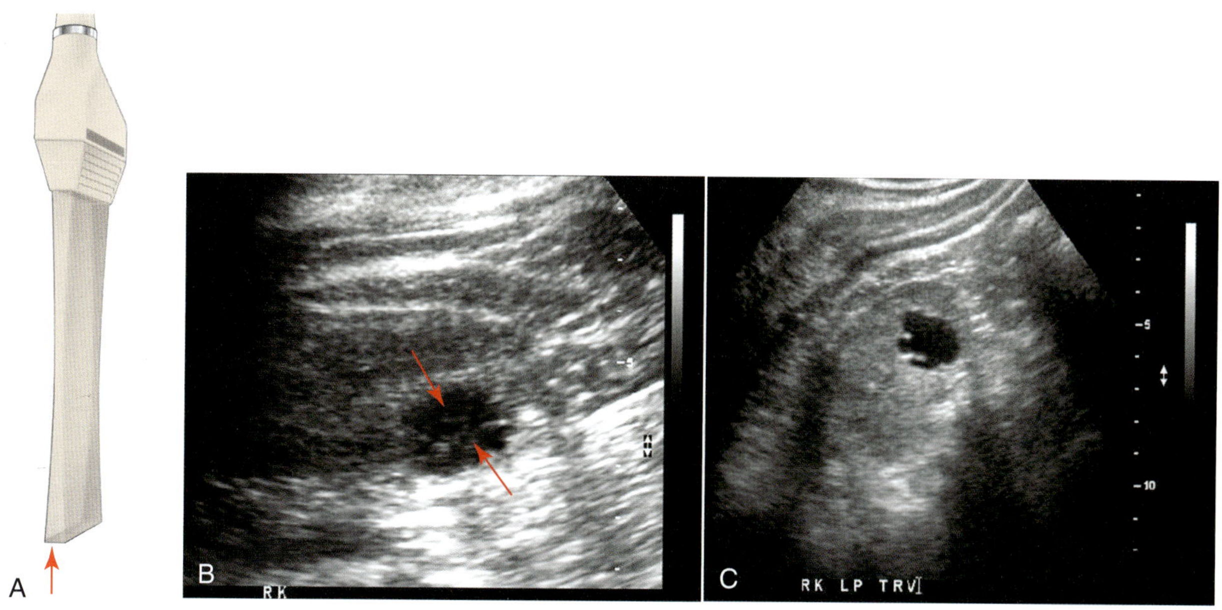

Fig. 7.1 **A**, The scan "plane" through the tissue is really a three-dimensional volume. Two dimensions (axial and lateral) are in the scan plane, but there is a third dimension (called *slice thickness* or *section thickness*). The third dimension *(arrow)* is collapsed to zero thickness when the image is displayed in two-dimensional format. **B**, A simple renal cyst that should be echo free is filled with echoes *(arrows)*, which could indicate a solid renal lesion. These off-axis echoes are a result of scan-plane slice thickness. **C**, When tissue harmonic imaging (*THI*) is activated (resulting in a narrower beam-profile), the slice-thickness artifact disappears. (**B–C**, Courtesy Patrick O'Kane, Thomas Jefferson University.)

tissue texture) but is a result of the constructive and destructive interference effects between echoes originating from the distribution of all the scatterers within the imaged tissue (i.e., **speckle**). These echoes are associated with the many small scatterers (smaller than the wavelength) included in the ultrasound pulse at any time (as discussed in Chapters 2 and 6). Speckle (Fig 7.2) is not an artifact in some sense, because it results from the underlying distribution of scatterers, but as it may obstruct the detection of low-contrast objects in an otherwise homogenous background, this distinction is really more academic. As discussed in Chapter 6, most ultrasound scanners have implemented spatial or frequency compounding (or some variation thereof) to markedly limit the effects of speckle.

Speckle is the granular appearance of ultrasound images caused by the interference between echoes from scatterers smaller than the wavelength.

Reverberation

Multiple reflections (**reverberations**) can occur between two strong reflectors or between the transducer and a strong reflector (Fig 7.3,A). When these multiple echoes are received by the scanner, they may be sufficiently strong to be detected and displayed by the scanner. This may cause confusion in the interpretation of the displayed image (although the equidistant set of echoes that progressively gets weaker should provide a strong hint).

The process by which reverberations are produced is shown in Fig 7.3,B. Reverberations will appear in the image as additional reflectors that do not represent real structures (Fig 7.4). Multiple reflections are displayed beneath the real reflector at intervals equal to the distance between the transducer and the real reflector. Each subsequent reflection is weaker than the one before, but this drop in echo strength is counteracted (at least partially) by the TGC function (compensating for attenuation). The **comet tail** artifact is a particular case of reverberation, in which two closely spaced surfaces generate a series of closely spaced, discrete echoes (Fig 7.5).

Reverberations are multiple reflections between a structure and the transducer, or between two structures, or within a structure.

Mirror Image

The mirror-image artifact is also a form of reverberation, but this artifact can be a lot more confusing. Essentially, structures that exist on one side of a strong reflector is being displayed on the other side of this reflector as well. Fig 7.6 shows how the extended travel path caused by echoes bouncing off a strong reflector is likely to end up being displayed elsewhere in the image and provides some examples. Mirror-image artifacts are common around the diaphragm and pleura, because of the reflection from the air-filled lungs, and they occasionally occur in other locations. Sometimes the mirrored structure is not in the unmirrored scan plane (see Fig 7.6,C).

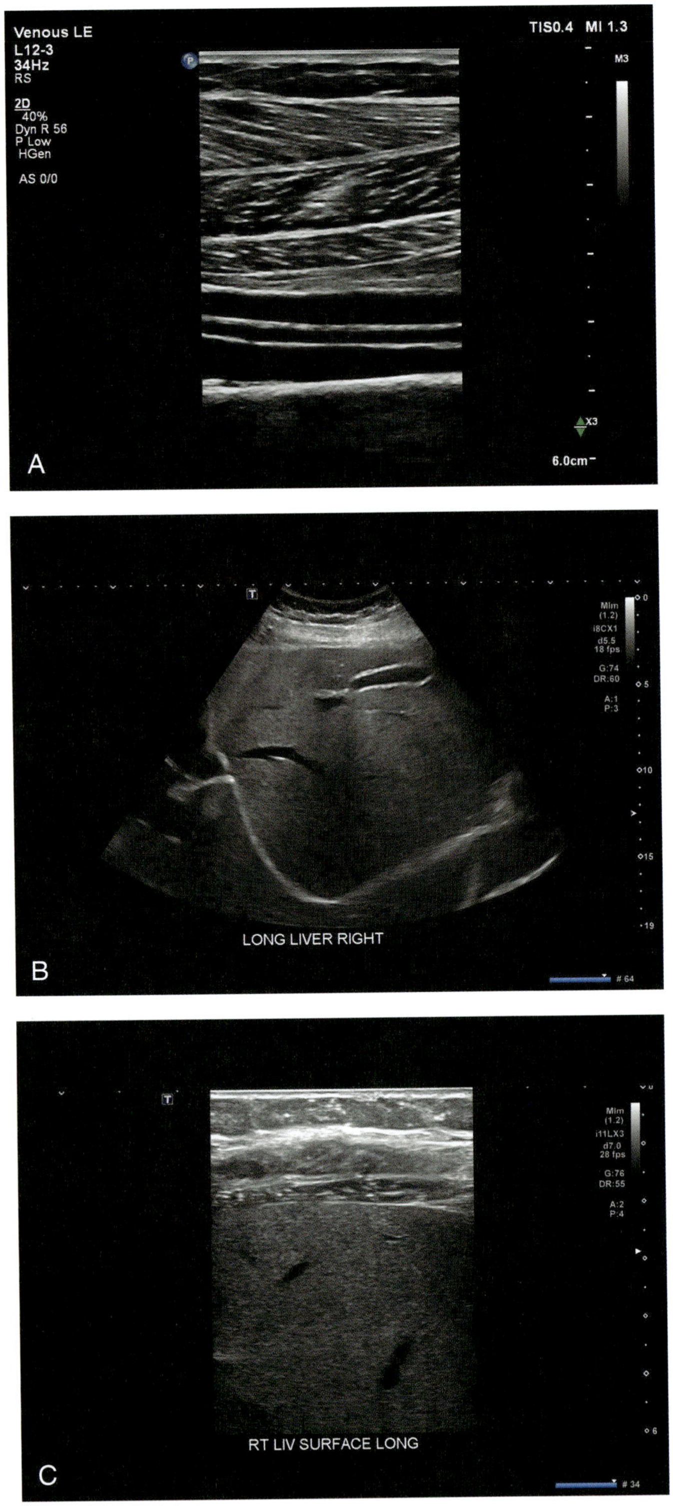

Fig. 7.2 A–C, Three examples of the typically grainy appearance of ultrasound images that is not primarily the result of detail resolution limitations but rather of speckle (**A** depicts calf veins, while **B–C** are from liver imaging with a curvi-linear and a linear array, respectively). Speckle is the interference pattern resulting from constructive and destructive interference of echoes returning simultaneously from many scatterers within the propagating ultrasound pulse at any instant.

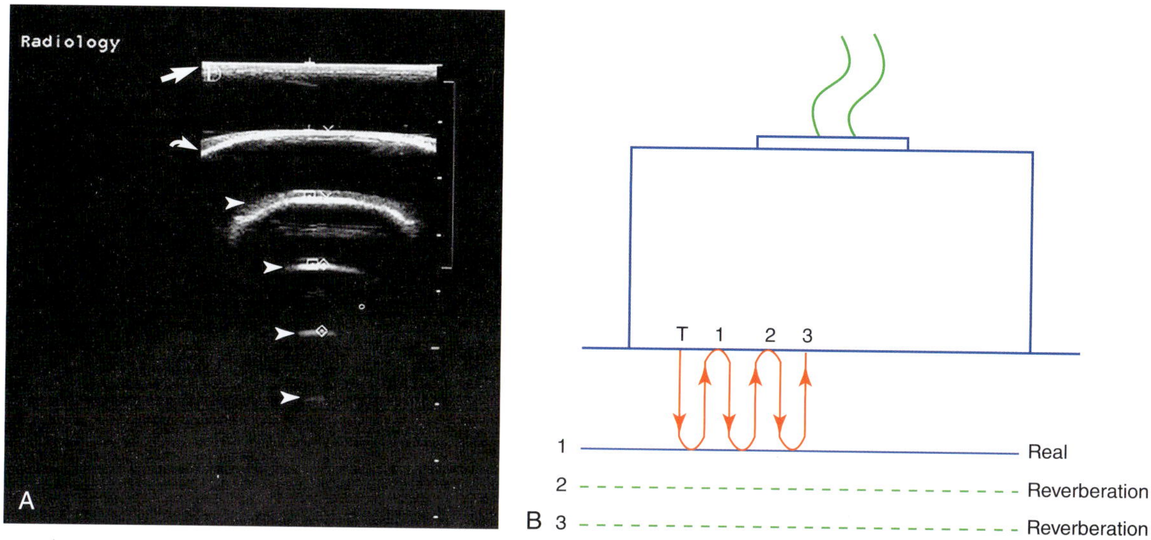

Fig. 7.3 **A**, Reverberation *(arrowheads)* resulting from multiple reflection through a water path between a linear array transducer *(straight arrow)* and the surface of an apple *(curved arrow)*. **B**, The behavior in A is explained as follows: A pulse *(T)* is transmitted from the transducer. A strong echo is generated at the real reflector and is received *(1)* at the transducer, allowing correct imaging of the reflector. However, the echo is reflected partially at the transducer so that a second echo *(2)* is received, as well as a third *(3)*. Because these echoes arrive later, they appear deeper on the display, where there are no reflectors. The lateral displacement of the reverberating sound path is for figure clarity. In fact, the sound repeatedly travels down and back on the same path.

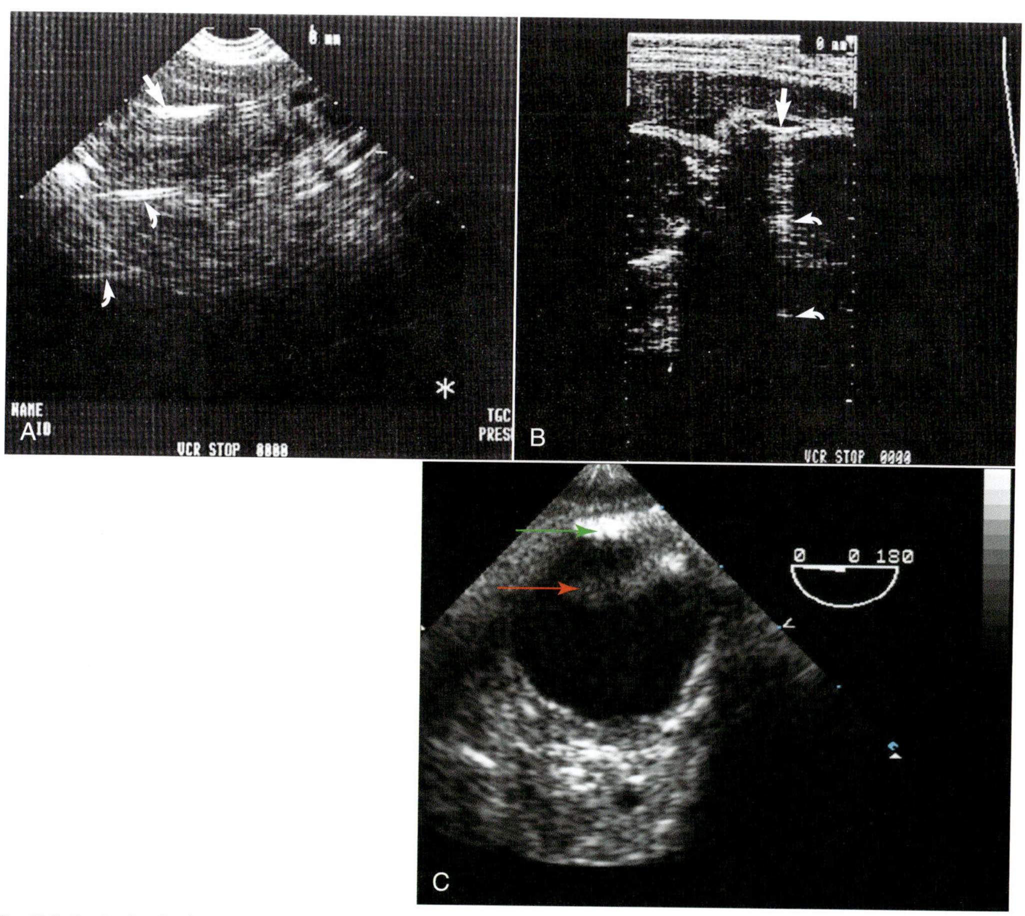

Fig. 7.4 **A**, A chorionic villi sampling catheter *(straight arrow)* and two reverberations *(curved arrows)*. **B**, A fetal scapula *(straight arrow)* and two reverberations *(curved arrows)*. **C**, Reverberation *(red arrow)* from hyperechoic region *(green arrow)* in transesophageal scan of the ascending aorta.

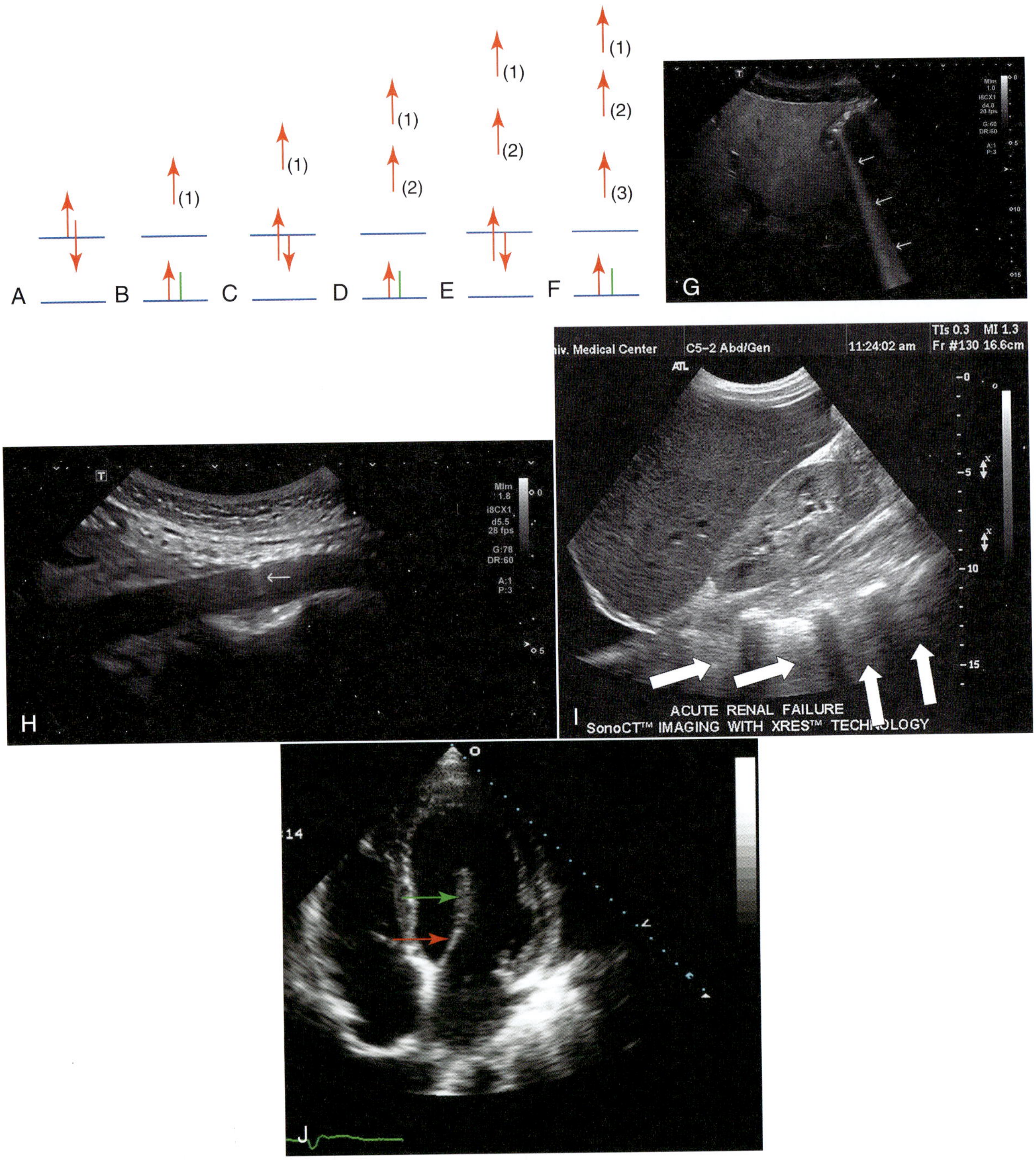

Fig. 7.5 Generation of comet-tail artifact (closely spaced reverberations). Action progresses in time from left to right. **A**, An ultrasound pulse encounters the first reflector, is reflected partially, and is transmitted partially. **B**, Reflection and transmission at the first reflector are complete. Reflection at the second reflector is occurring. **C**, Reflection at the second reflector is complete. Partial transmission and partial reflection are again occurring at the first reflector as the second echo passes through. **D**, The echoes from the first *(1)* and second *(2)* reflectors are traveling toward the transducer. A second reflection (repeat of B) is occurring at the second reflector. **E**, Partial transmission and reflection are again occurring at the first reflector. **F**, Three echoes are now returning—the echo from the first reflector *(1)*, the echo from the second reflector *(2)*, and the echo from the third reflector *(3)*—that originated from the back side of the first reflector **(C)** and reflected again from the second reflector **(D)**. A fourth echo is being generated at the second reflector (F). G, Comet-tail artifact from bowel gas (*arrows*). **H**, Comet-tail artifact from calcification in the wall of the aorta (*arrow*). Notice that this is also an example of the slice thickness artifact as evident by the low-level echoes in the aorta (since rouleaux formation would not be expected in an artery such as the aorta). **I**, Comet tail *(arrows)* from diaphragm. **J**, Apical four-chamber view of comet tail artifact *(green arrow)* in the left ventricle. The artifact is connected to anterior mitral leaflet *(red arrow)*.

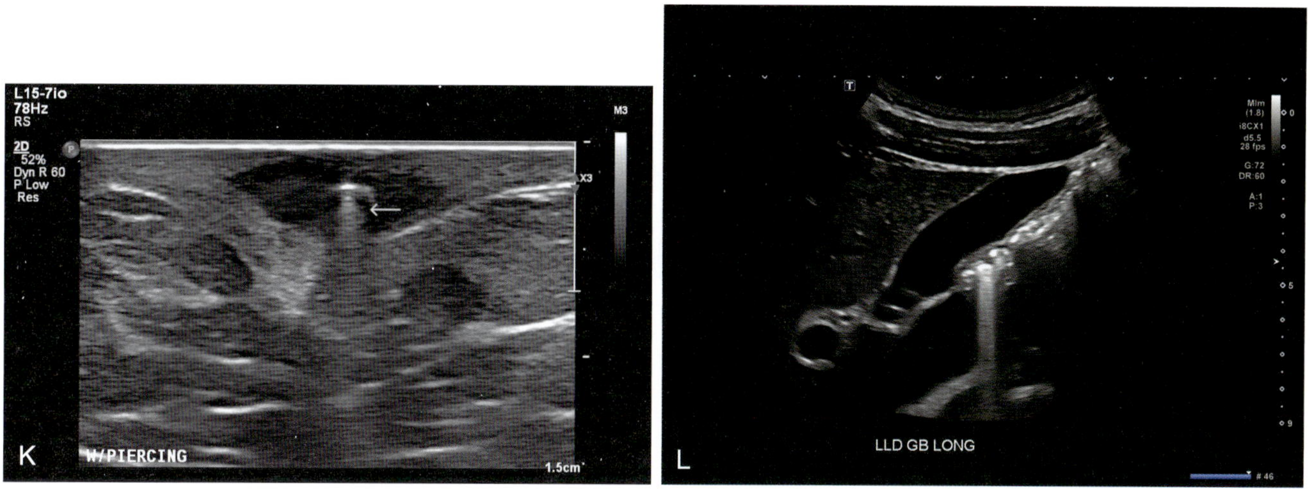

Fig. 7.5 cont'd K, Inflamed belly button piercing generating a comet tail (*arrow*), **L,** Comet tail from the gallbladder.

The mirror-image artifact duplicates a structure on the opposite side of a strong reflector.

Refraction

Refraction of light enables lenses to focus and distorts the presentation of objects, as shown in Fig 7.7. Refraction can cause a reflector to be improperly positioned to a lateral location in the image (Fig 7.8). This can occur, for example, when the transducer is placed on the abdominal midline (see Figs. 7.8,C and 7.9), producing doubling of single objects. Beneath are the rectus abdominis muscles, which are surrounded by fat. These tissues present refracting boundaries because of their different

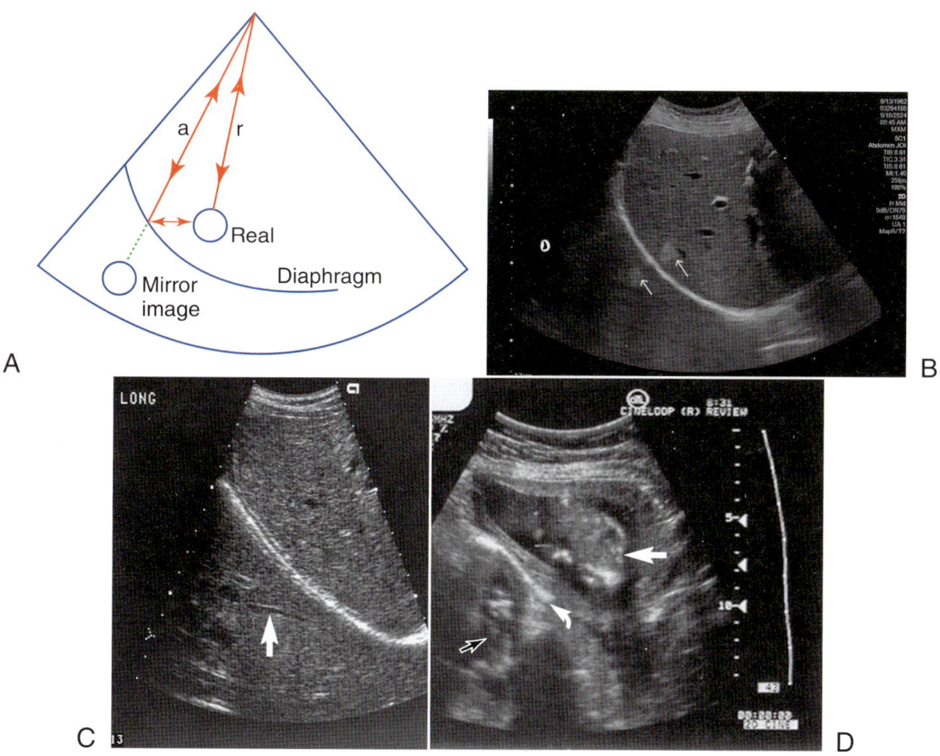

Fig. 7.6 A, When pulses encounter a real hepatic structure directly *(scan line r)*, the structure is imaged correctly. If the pulse first reflects off the diaphragm *(scan line a)* and returns along the same path, the structure is displayed on the other side of the diaphragm. **B**, Liver mass with its mirror image *(arrows)*. **C**, A vessel is mirror-imaged *(arrow)* superior to the diaphragm but does not appear inferior because it is outside the unmirrored scan plane. **D**, A fetus *(straight arrow)* also appears as a mirror image *(open arrow)*. The mirror *(curved arrow)* is probably echogenic muscle.

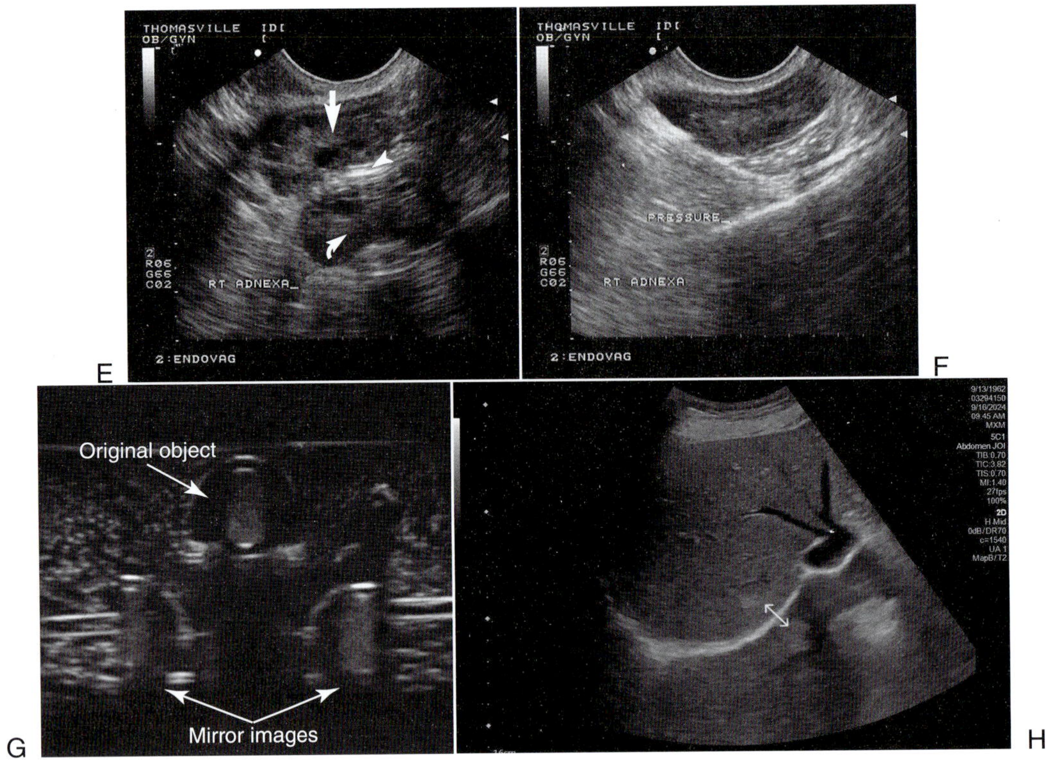

Fig. 7.6 cont'd **E**, Ovary *(arrow)* with mirror image *(curved arrow)* that could be mistaken for an adnexal mass or ectopic pregnancy. Bowel gas *(arrowhead)* is apparently the mirror in this case. **F**, Applying external abdominal pressure displaces the gas, eliminating the mirror image seen in **E**. **G**, Mirror image of a thick-walled vessel in a tissue-equivalent phantom. The echoes are being reflected from the echogenic scatterers used in the circulating fluid and the vessel wall resulting in two mirror images split on either side of the center line *(arrows)*. **H**, Liver lesion with its mirror image below the diaphragm (*arrow*).

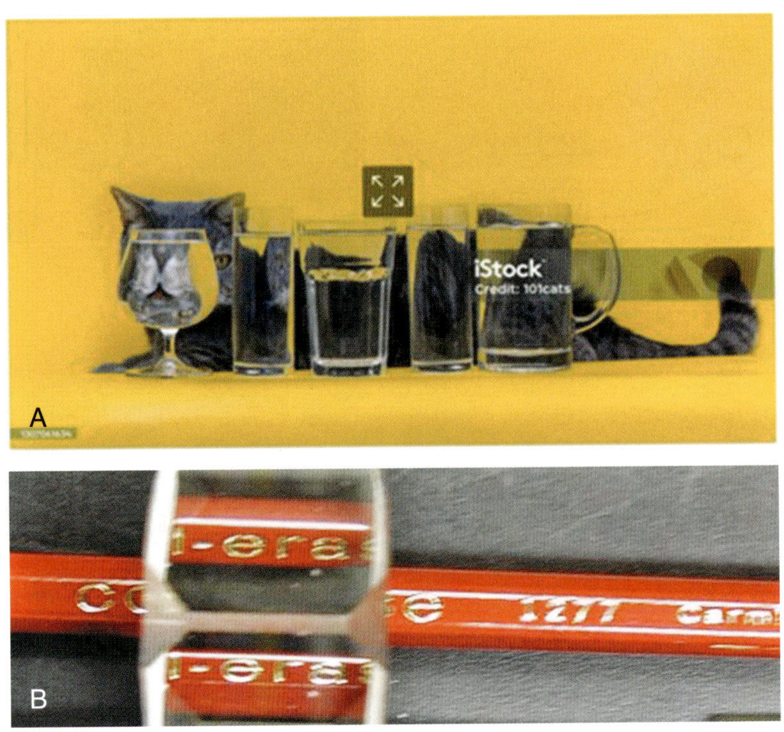

Fig. 7.7 **A**, Refracted light through a series of water-filled glasses distorts the appearance of the cat behind them. **B**, A pencil beneath a prism appears to be split in two.

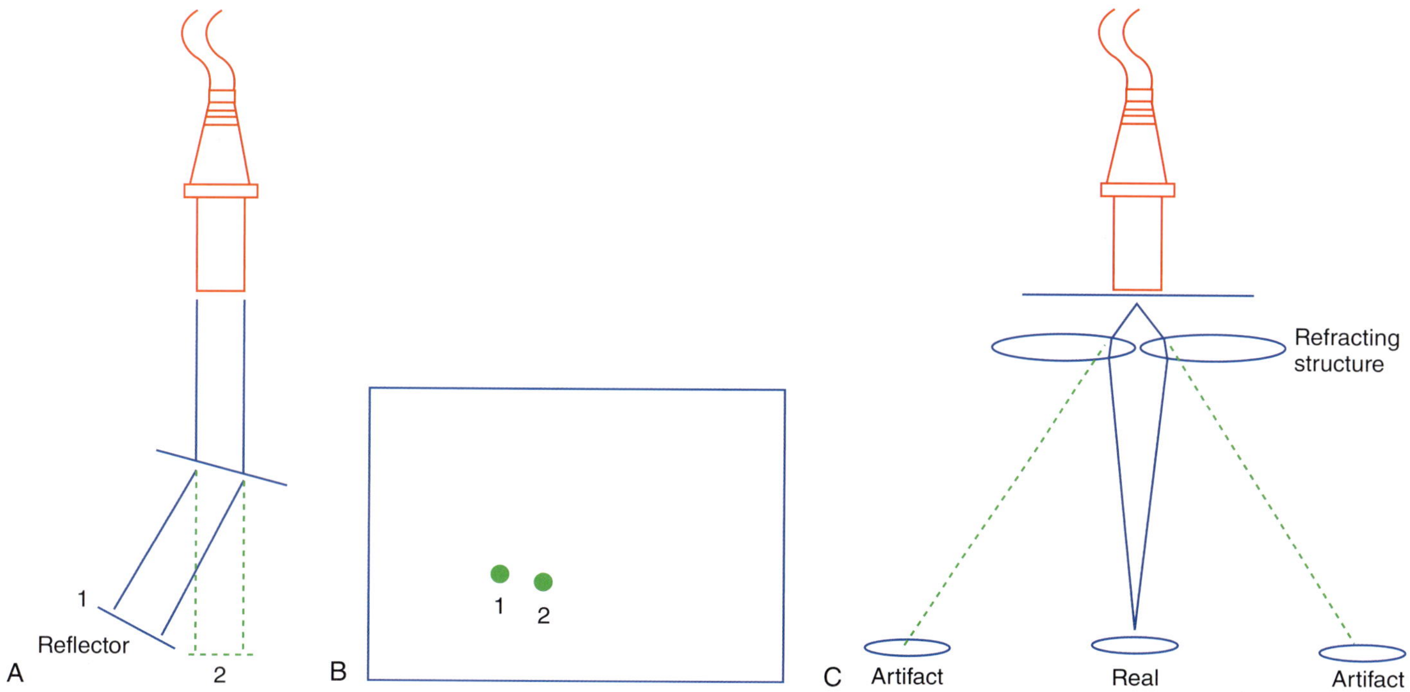

Fig. 7.8 Refraction (**A**) results in improper positioning of a reflector on the display (**B**). The system places the reflector at position 2 (because that is the direction from which the echo was received), when in fact the reflector is actually at position 1. **C**, One real structure is imaged as two artifactual objects, because of the refracting structure close to the transducer. If unrefracted pulses can propagate to the real structure, a triple presentation (one correct, two artifactual) will result.

propagation speeds (higher in muscle, lower in fat). However, better sound speed correction algorithms limit this artifact on many scanners and the use of a broad transmit beam will completely eliminate it.

Refraction displaces structures laterally from their correct locations.

Grating Lobes

Side lobes and grating lobes are weaker beams that propagate from a transducer in directions different from the primary or main beam. A very old example of grating lobes is shown in Fig. 7.10. The reason for showing such an old image of a grating lobe is that they are (almost) nonexistent in modern scanners. Whether due to 1.5D or 2D array technology or due to the use of amalgamated narrow transmit beam pulses that will be focused (on transmission) across most of the imaging depth (see Fig. 3.23) or tissue harmonic imaging or a combination of these factors, or, of course, the use of broad transmit beams with virtual beam forming, such artifactual beams are not an issue in clinical practice.

Nonetheless, the diligent student still needs to know what these artifacts looked like. So, if grating lobes encountered a strong reflector (e.g., bone or gas), their echoes might be displayed, particularly if they fell within an **anechoic** region. If so, they would appear in incorrect locations, such as in the examples of Figs. 7.11 and 7.12,A. Compare Fig. 7.12,A to the more modern image in Fig. 7.12,B of a breast cyst with calcifications, which would seem likely to generate grating lobe, slice thickness, and comet tail artifacts but doesn't.

Grating lobes duplicate structures laterally to the true ones (but are very rarely a problem in clinical practice these days).

Speed Error

Propagation **speed error** occurs when the assumed value for the speed of sound in soft tissues (1.54 mm/μs, leading to the 13 μs/cm rule) is incorrect. If the propagation speed in a region is greater than 1.54 mm/μs, the calculated distance to the reflector is too small, and the display will place the reflector too close to the transducer (Fig. 7.13) and vice versa if the actual speed is less than 1.54 mm/μs (Fig. 7.14), because the echoes arrive later. Refraction and propagation speed error can also cause a structure to be displayed with an incorrect shape.

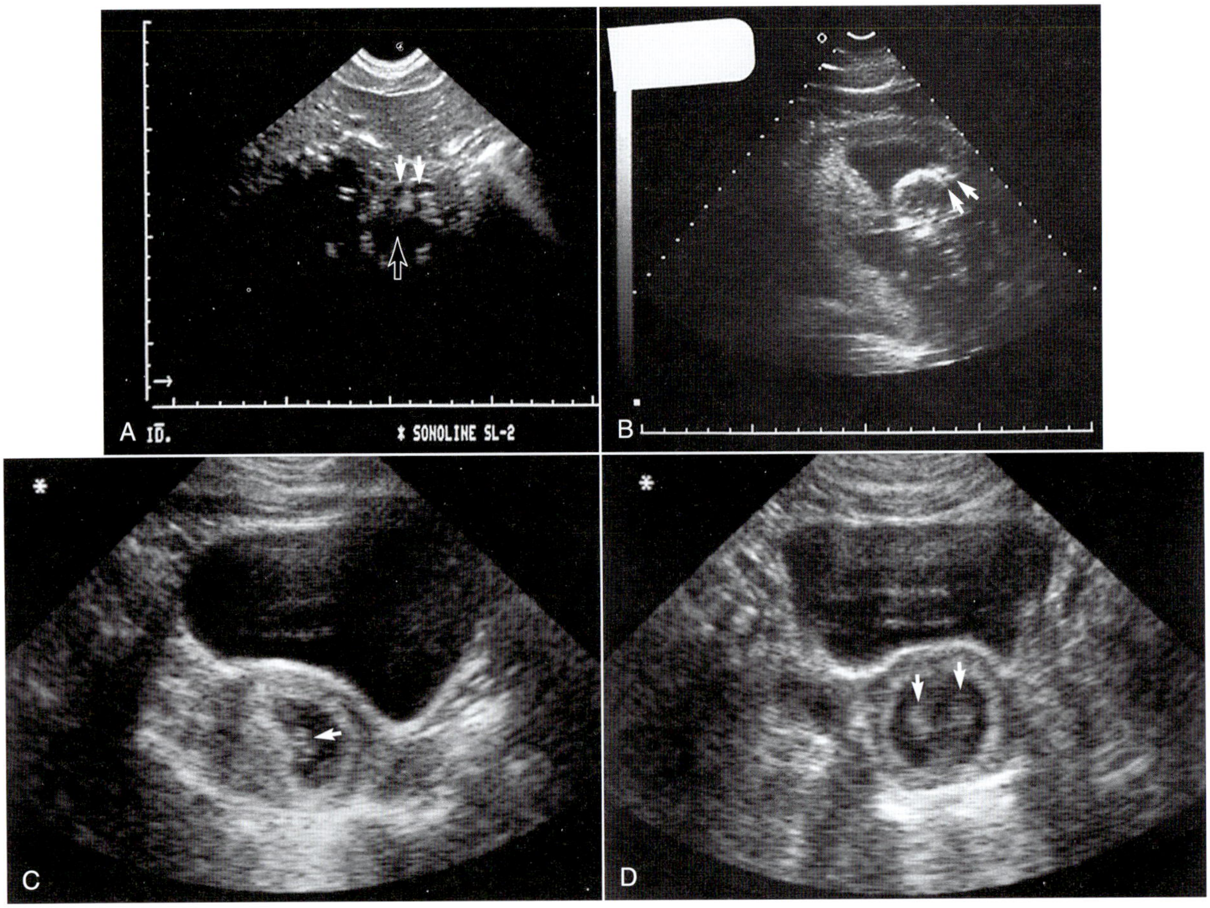

Fig. 7.9 **A**, Refraction (probably through the rectus abdominis muscle) has widened the aorta *(open arrow)* and produced a double image of the celiac trunk *(arrows)*. **B**, Refraction has produced a double image of a fetal skull *(arrows)*. Refraction also may cause a single gestation (**C**) to appear as a double gestation (**D**).

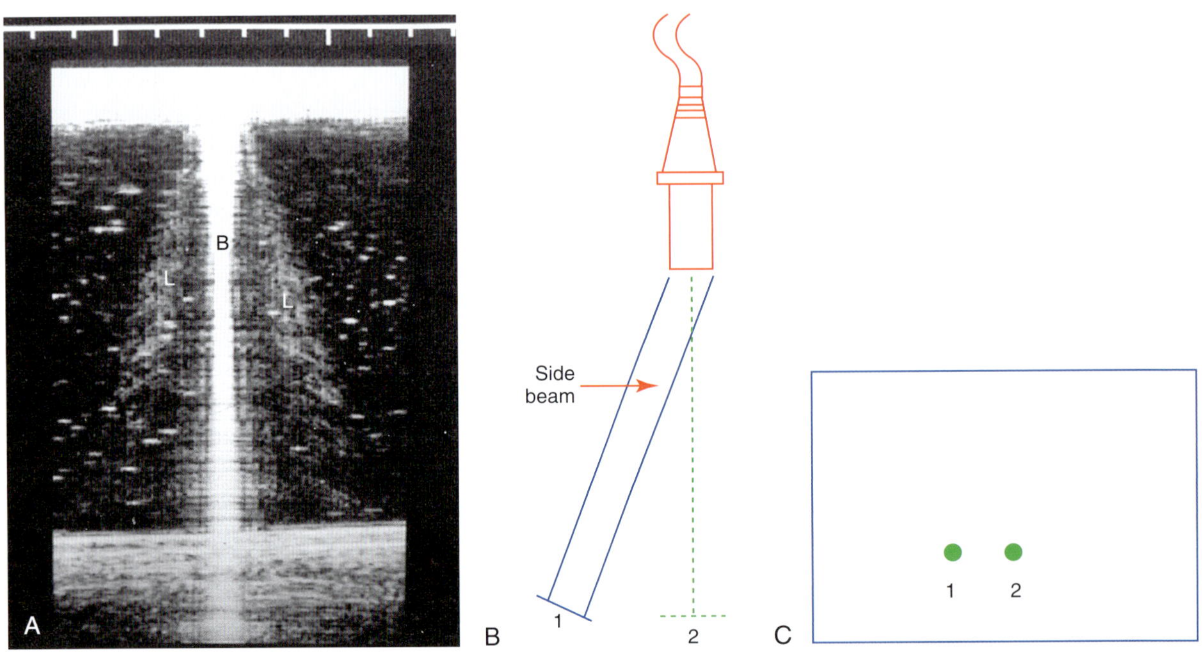

Fig. 7.10 **A**, The primary beam *(B)* and grating lobes *(L)* from a linear array transducer. **B**, A side lobe or grating lobe can produce and receive a reflection from a "side view." **C**, This will be placed on the display at the proper distance from the transducer but in the wrong location (direction) because the instrument assumes that echoes originate from points along the main beam axis. The instrument shows the reflector at position 2 because that is the direction in which the main beam travels. The reflector is actually in position 1.

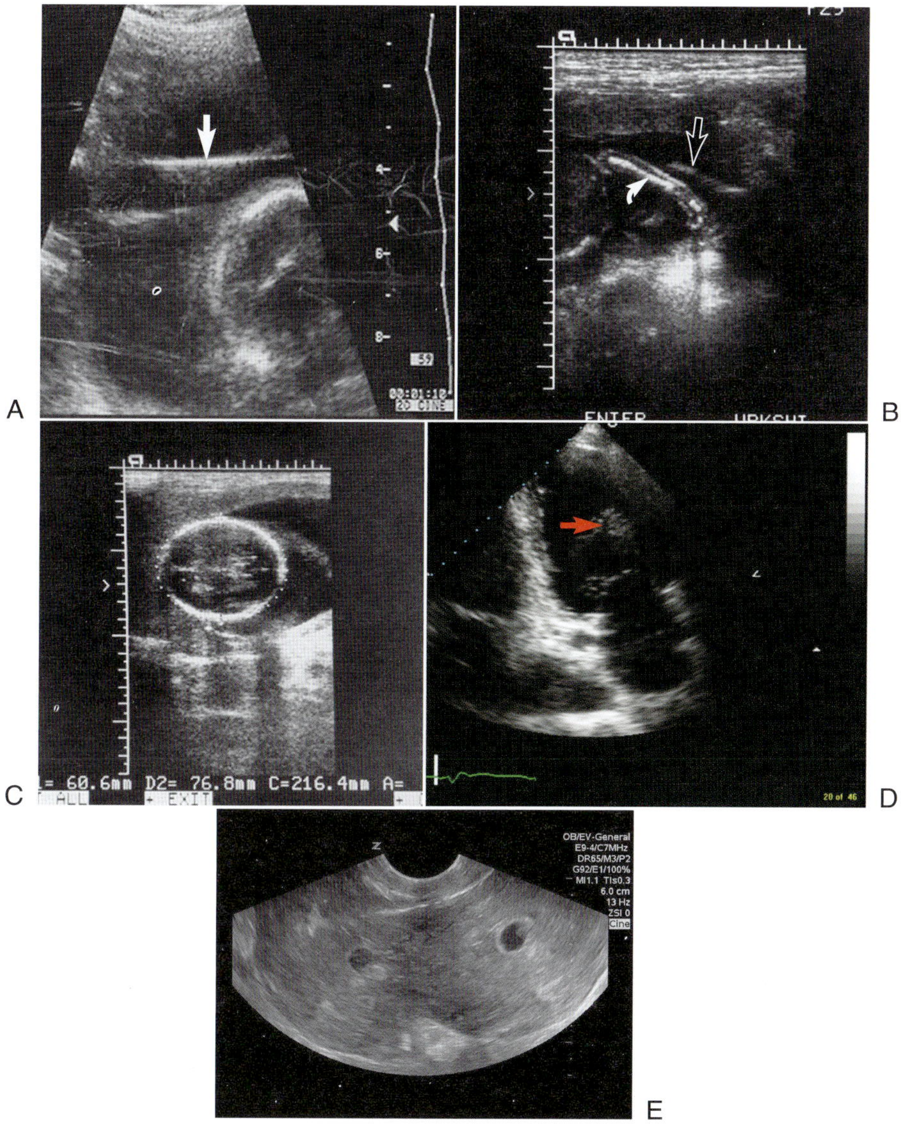

Fig. 7.11 Grating lobe examples. **A**, A real amniotic sheet *(arrow)*. **B**, Grating lobe duplication *(open arrows)* of fetal bones *(curved arrows)* resembles amniotic bands or sheets. C, Grating lobe duplication of a fetal skull. **D**, Apical two-chamber view of grating-lobe artifact *(arrow)* in left ventricle. E, At first glance, this seems to be a mirror image artifact, similar to what is seen in abdominal imaging (see Figure 7.6,**A–C**). However, it is not, for two reasons: (1) there is no apparent echogenic mirror, and (2) the repeat on the left side is not horizontally reversed as would be the case with mirroring. Rather, it is a less echogenic repeat of what is on the right. Therefore this is a grating-lobe duplication. Such duplications appear laterally and with less brightness than the correct presentation. (**E**,Courtesy David Bahner, MD, RDMS, College of Medicine, Ohio State University.)

However, measurements of speed of sound have lately become available on a number of ultrasound platforms (as mentioned in Chapter 6) rendering this artifact much more rare in today's clinical practice.

Propagation speed error displaces structures axially but is becoming more infrequent in practice.

Range Ambiguity

In ultrasound imaging with narrow transmit beams, it is assumed that for each pulse, all echoes are received before the next pulse is emitted. If this was not the case, error could result (Figs. 7.15 and 7.16). The maximum depth imaged correctly by an instrument is determined by its pulse-repetition frequency (PRF). To avoid range ambiguity, PRF is automatically reduced in deeper imaging situations. This also causes a reduction in frame rate.

The use of broad transmit beam systems effectively eliminates the possibility of this artifact occurring, since frame rates in the hundreds to thousands of Hz are possible.

The range-ambiguity artifact places structures much closer to the surface than they should be.

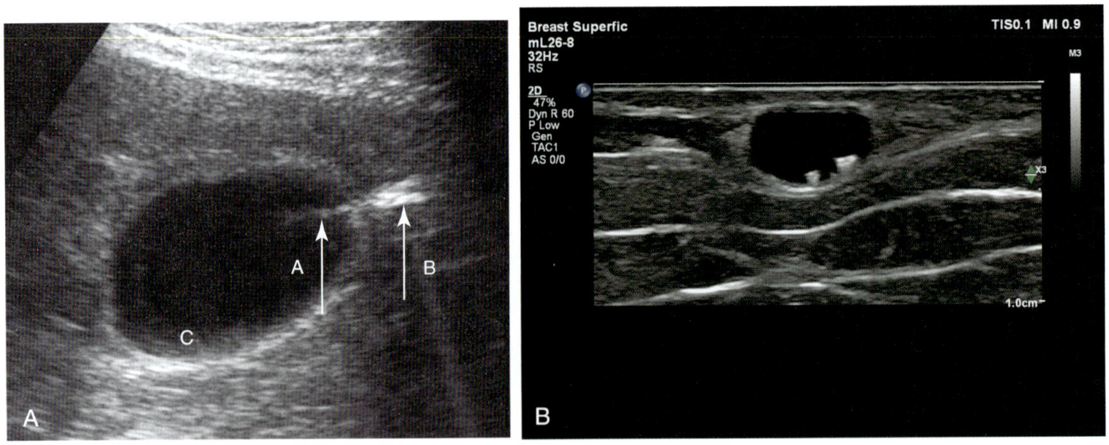

Fig. 7.12 **A,** Needle tip *(A arrow)* is correctly seen in a cyst for aspiration, whereas grating lobes show the out-of-plane body of the needle *(B arrow)*. In this example, there is also a slice-thickness artifact depicting nonexistent sludge in the cyst *(C)*. ***B,*** *Breast cyst with microcalcifications and none of the artifacts, which might have plagued an older image (i.e.,* grating lobes, slice thickness, and comet tails).

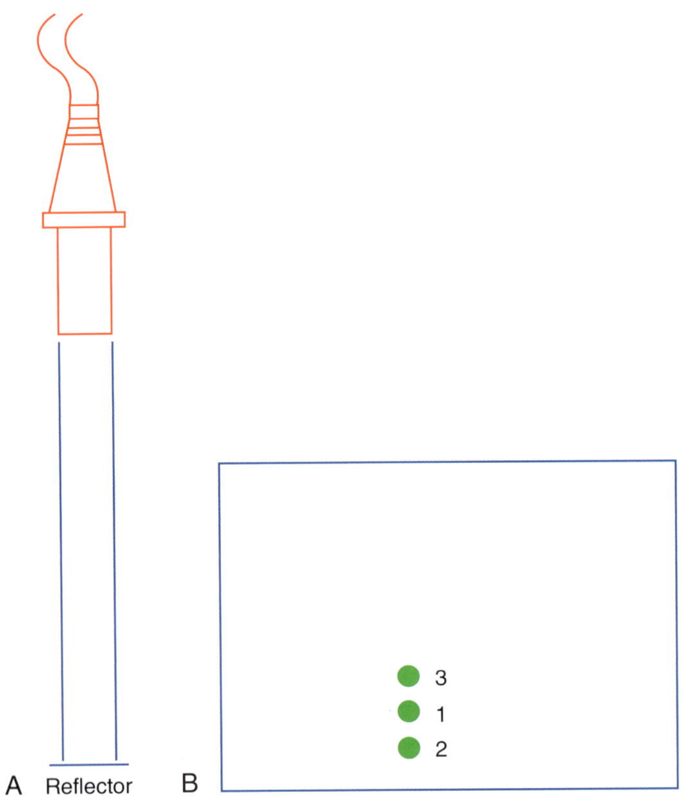

Fig. 7.13 The propagation speed over the traveled path (**A**) determines the reflector position on the display (**B**). The reflector is actually in position 1. If the actual propagation speed is less than that assumed, the reflector will appear in position 2. If the actual speed is more than that assumed, the reflector will appear in position 3.

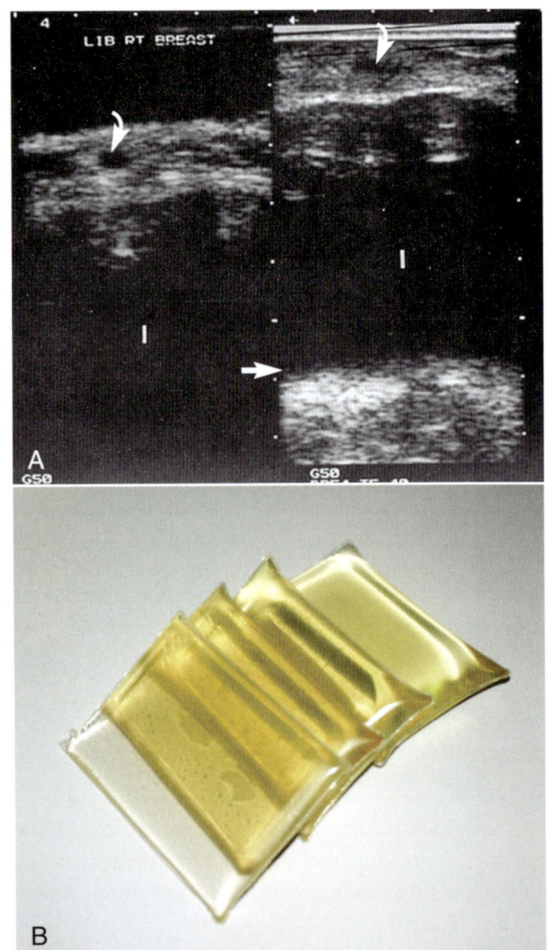

Fig. 7.14 The low propagation speed in a silicone breast implant *(I)* causes the chest wall (*straight arrow*) to appear deeper than it should (**A**). Note that a cyst (*curved arrow*) is shown more clearly on the left image than on the right because a gel standoff pad (**B**) was placed between the transducer and the breast moving the beam focus closer to the cyst.

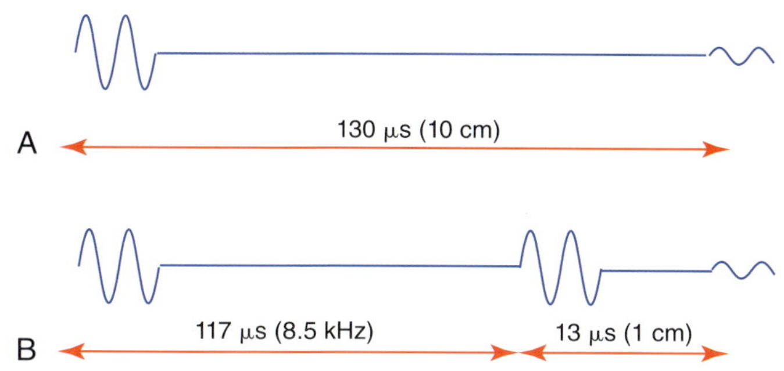

Fig. 7.15 **A**, An echo (from a depth of 10 cm) arrives 130 µs after pulse emission. **B**, If the pulse repetition period were 117 µs (corresponding to a PRF of 8.5 kHz), the echo in A would arrive 13 µs after the next pulse was emitted. The instrument would place this echo at a 1-cm depth rather than the correct value. This range location error is known as the *range-ambiguity artifact.*

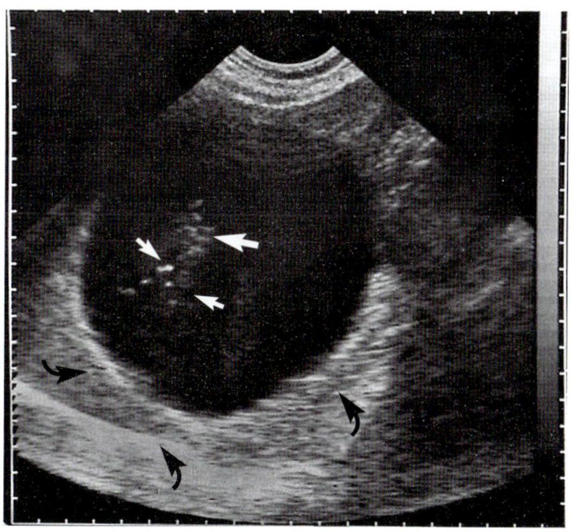

Fig. 7.16 A large renal cyst (diameter approximately 10 cm) contains artifactual range-ambiguity echoes *(white arrows)*. They are generated from structures below the display. These deep echoes arrive after the next pulse is emitted. Because the time from the emission of the last pulse to echo arrival is short, the echoes are placed closer to the transducer than they should be. Echoes arrive from much deeper (later) than usual in this case because the sound passes through the long, low-attenuation paths in the cyst. These echoes may have come from bone or a far body wall. Low attenuation in the cyst is indicated by the enhancement below it *(curved black arrows)*.

Sometimes two artifacts combine to present even more challenging cases. An example involving range ambiguity is shown in Fig. 7.17.

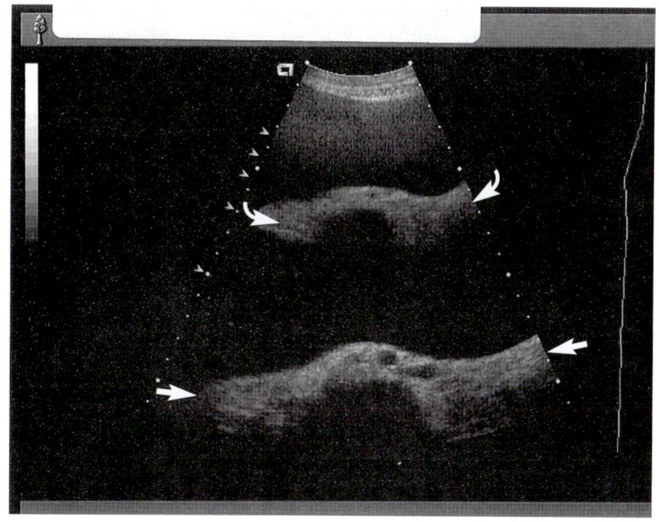

Fig. 7.17 Abdominal ascites produces a large echo-free region in this scan. A structure is located at a depth of approximately 13 cm *(straight arrows)*. Located in the anechoic region at a depth of approximately 6 cm is a structure *(curved arrows)* shaped like the structure at 13 cm. How could this artifact appear closer than the actual structure, implying that these echoes arrived earlier than those from the correct location? It turns out that the artifact is actually a combination of two: reverberation and range ambiguity. The artifact seen is a reverberation from the deep structure and the transducer. But a reverberation should appear at twice the depth of the actual structure, that is, at about 26 cm. However, the arrival of the reverberation echoes occurs approximately 78 µs after the next pulse is emitted, so that they are placed at a depth of 6 cm. Single artifacts are difficult enough. Fortunately, combinations like this occur infrequently.

ATTENUATION

Shadowing

Shadowing is the reduction in echo amplitude from reflectors that lie behind a strongly reflecting or attenuating structure (Fig. 7.18). A strongly attenuating or reflecting structure weakens the sound distal to it, causing echoes from the distal region to be weak and thus to appear darker, like a shadow. Of course, the returning echoes must also pass through the attenuating structure, adding to the shadowing effect. Examples of shadowing structures include calcified stones (see Fig. 7.18,A), loops of bowel (see Fig. 7.18,B), as well as stones (Fig. 7.19,A).

Shadowing can also occur behind the edges of objects that are not necessarily strong attenuators (Fig. 7.20). In this case, the cause may be the defocusing action of a refracting curved surface. Alternatively, it may be attributable to destructive interference caused by portions of an ultrasound pulse passing through tissues with different propagation speeds and subsequently getting out of phase. In either case, the intensity of the beam decreases beyond the edge of the structure, causing echoes to be weakened.

The almost universal implementation of speckle reduction techniques in general and spatial compounding in particular have rendered shadowing less of an issue. Obtaining images from multiple insonation angles makes it more likely that tissues behind strong reflectors or at the edge of objects can still be imaged correctly. This may uncover structures (especially pathological ones) that were not previously imaged (i.e., they were effectively invisible), because they were located in the shadows. Today what we do in the shadows is much less of a mystery. Nonetheless, imaging through air-filled structures, such as lungs or bowel, or through narrow rib spaces, continues to be a problem in diagnostic ultrasound.

Shadowing is the weakening of echoes distal to a strongly attenuating or reflecting structure or from the edges of a

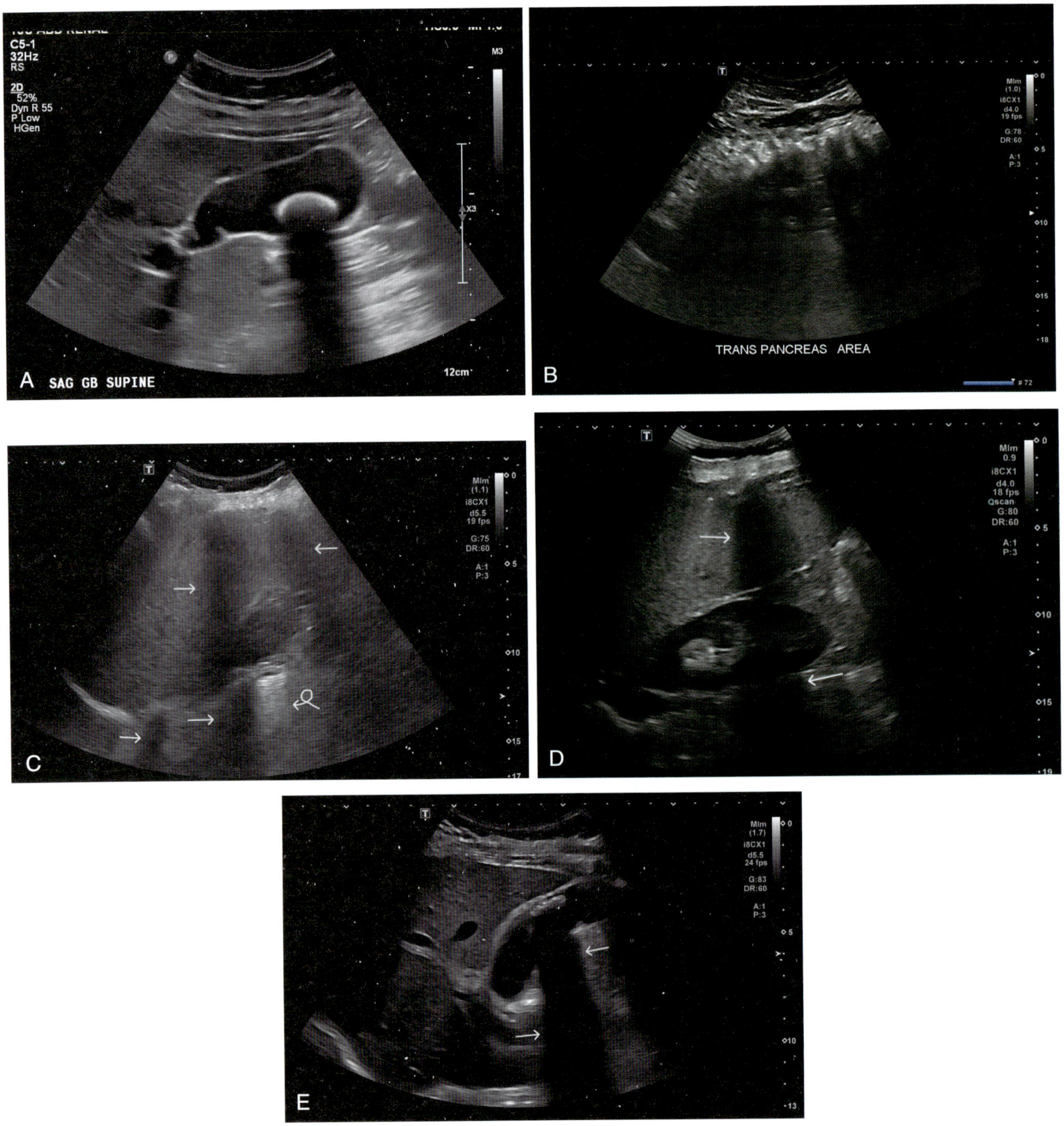

Fig. 7.18 **A**, Shadowing from a high-attenuation calcified stone in the gall bladder. **B**, Shadowing from loops of bowel across the pancreas. **C–E**, Examples of shadowing *(arrows). Enhancement in C is indicated by a curly arrow.*

refracting structure. Speckle reduction algorithms have greatly reduced the occurrence of this artifact.

Enhancement

Enhancement is the strengthening of echoes from reflectors that lie behind a weakly attenuating structure (see Figs. 7.16 and 7.19). Shadowing and enhancement result in reflectors being displayed on the image with amplitudes that are too low and too high, respectively (occasionally they occur together; see Figs. 18,C and 19,D). Brightening of echoes also can be caused by the increased intensity in the focal region of a beam because the beam is narrow there. This is called *focal enhancement* or *focal banding* (Fig. 7.21) and will, obviously, only occur when using narrow transmit beam systems.

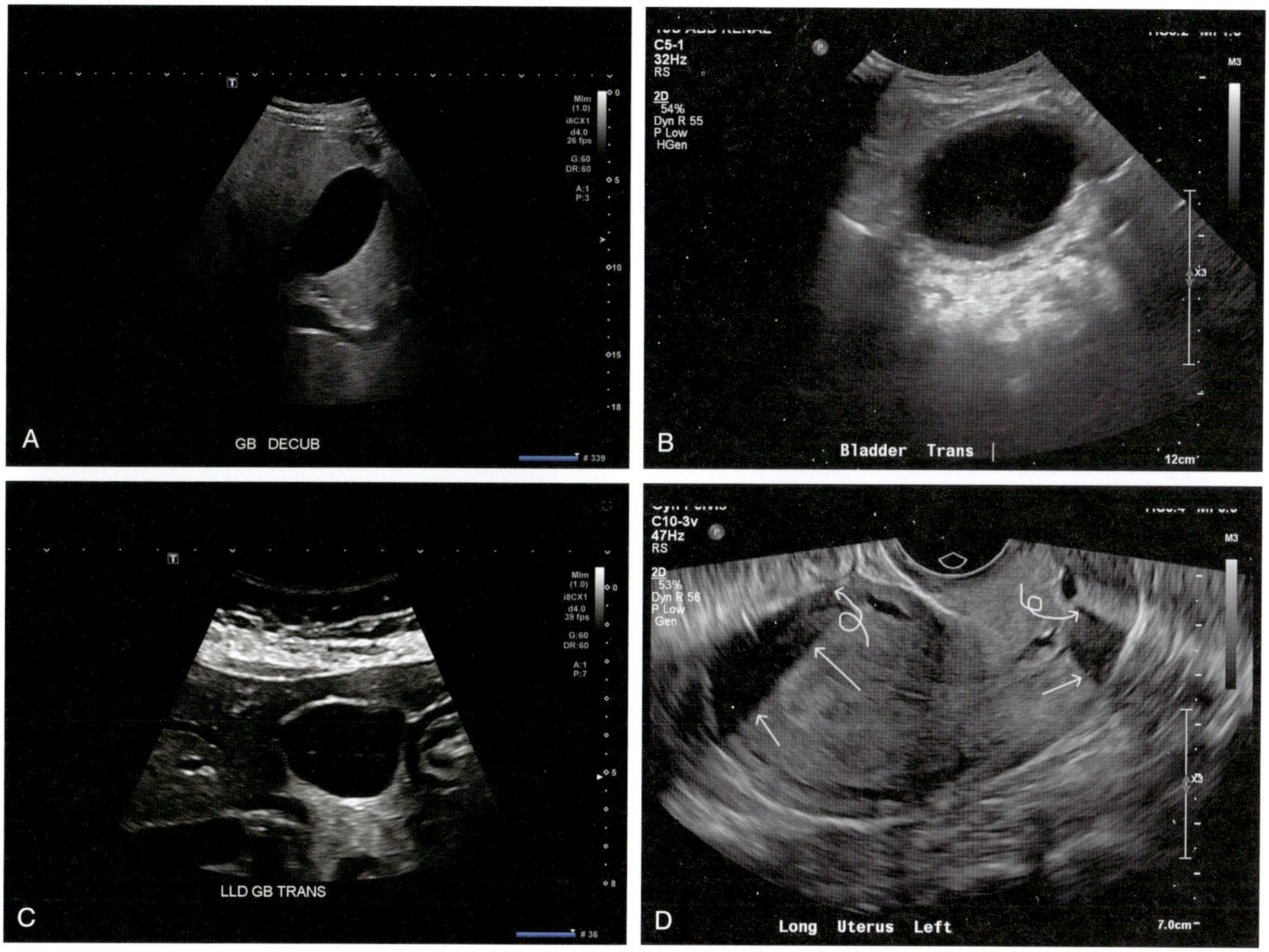

Fig. 7.19 **A**, Enhancement from the low attenuation of bile in the gallbladder. **B–C**, Examples of enhancement. ***D***, Transvaginal scan of a uterus showing areas of both enhancement *(curly arrows)* and shadowing (arrows).

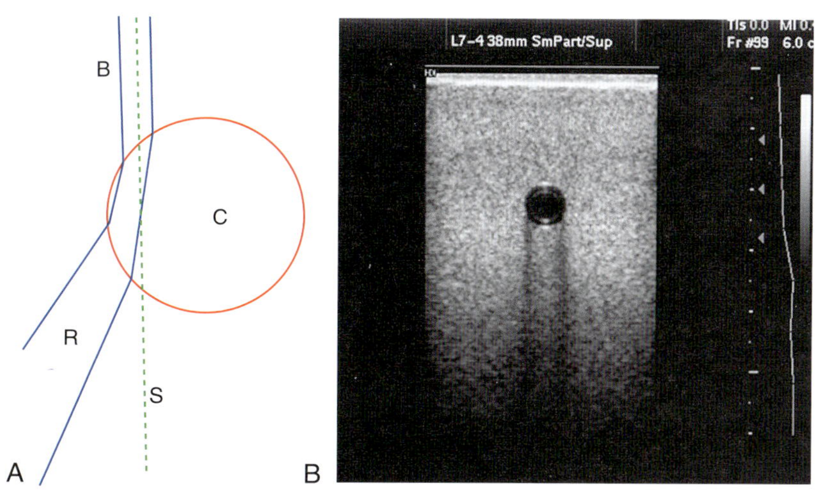

Fig. 7.20 **A**, When a sound beam *(B)* enters a circular region *(C)* of higher propagation speed, it is refracted, and refraction occurs again while it leaves. This causes spreading of the beam with decreased intensity. The echoes from region *R* are presented deep to the circular region in the neighborhood of the dashed line. Because of beam spreading, these echoes are weak and thus cast a shadow *(S)*. **B**, Edge shadows from a tube (shown in transverse view) embedded in tissue-equivalent material in a flow phantom.

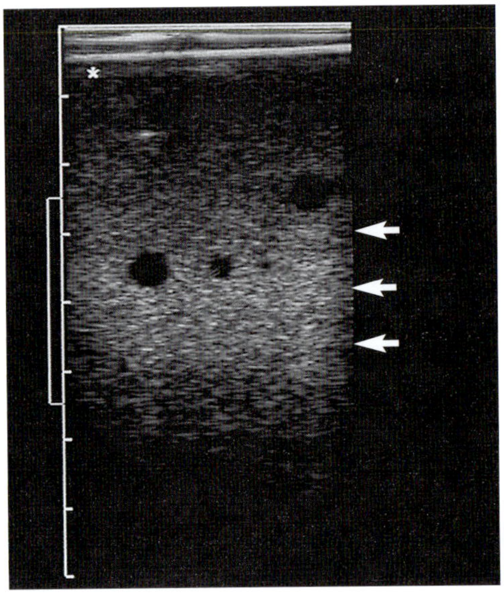

Fig. 7.21 Focal banding *(arrows)* is the brightening of echoes around the focus, where intensity is increased by the narrowing of the beam.

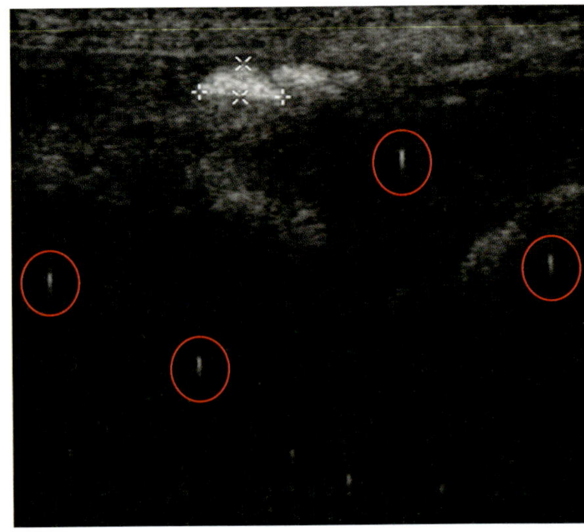

Fig. 7.22 Interference *(circled random white specks)* from nearby electronic equipment seen below a small lymph node.

Shadowing and enhancement artifacts can be useful for determining the nature of masses and structures, which is why their reduction is one of the few occasions where practitioners missed an artifact. As mentioned above, shadowing and enhancement are reduced with spatial compounding (and other speckle reduction techniques), because several imaging approaches to each anatomic site form the final image, allowing the beam to avoid the attenuating or enhancing structure.

Enhancement is the strengthening of echoes distal to a weakly attenuating structure. Speckle reduction algorithms have greatly reduced the occurrence of this artifact.

External interferences can also produce artifacts. For example, electronic equipment adds unwanted noise to the image as shown in Fig. 7.22.

SPECTRAL DOPPLER ARTIFACTS

Aliasing

Aliasing is the most common artifact encountered in Doppler ultrasound and indicates incorrect reconstruction based on a signal that has been sampled insufficiently. The sampling can be spatial or temporal, but in spectral Doppler, it is the latter that matters.

Nyquist Limit

Pulsed wave Doppler instruments are sampling instruments. Each emitted pulse (in narrow transmit beam systems) or frame (in broad transmit beam systems) yields a sample—hopefully of the desired Doppler shift (until the patient breathes, coughs, moves, or something). The highest Doppler shift that can be detected properly by a spectral Doppler system is called the **Nyquist limit** (f_{NL}). If the received Doppler shift frequency exceeds half of the PRF (which is typically in the 5–30 kHz range for pulsed Doppler), aliasing occurs:

$$f_{NL} = \frac{PRF}{2} \text{ (in kHz)}$$

Incorrect Doppler shift information (depicting the wrong direction of flow or wrong absolute velocities) occurs when the Nyquist limit is exceeded. Similarly, an optical form of temporal aliasing occurs in motion pictures when wagon wheels appear to rotate at various speeds and in reverse direction.

Higher PRFs (Table 7.1) not only permit higher Doppler shifts to be detected but also increase the chance that the range-ambiguity artifact will occur. Continuous wave Doppler instruments do not experience aliasing (the internal clock speed is too high relative to the Doppler shifts/velocities encountered in the human body). However, recall that CW Doppler systems do not provide depth resolution (due to their lack of a localized sample volume), which makes them much less useful clinically. It is important to note that broad transmit beam systems will (under almost all circumstances) eliminate aliasing, since the sampling frequency is equal to the frame rate—that is, encompassing the entire image instead of just an individual beam.

Aliasing is the depiction of incorrect Doppler spectral information (i.e., flow direction and/or speed).

Figs. 7.23 and 7.24 illustrate aliasing in the carotid artery and in the aorta. Also illustrated is how aliasing can be corrected or eliminated (Box 7.2) by increasing the PRF (i.e., shifting f_{NL} higher), increasing the Doppler angle (which decreases the Doppler shift for a given flow) or by shifting the baseline (thus

TABLE 7.1 Aliasing and Range-Ambiguity Artifact Values

PRF (kHz)	Doppler Shift Above Which Aliasing Occurs (kHz)	Range Beyond Which Ambiguity Occurs (cm)
5.0	2.5	15
10.0	5.0	7
15.0	7.5	5
20.0	10.0	3
25.0	12.5	3

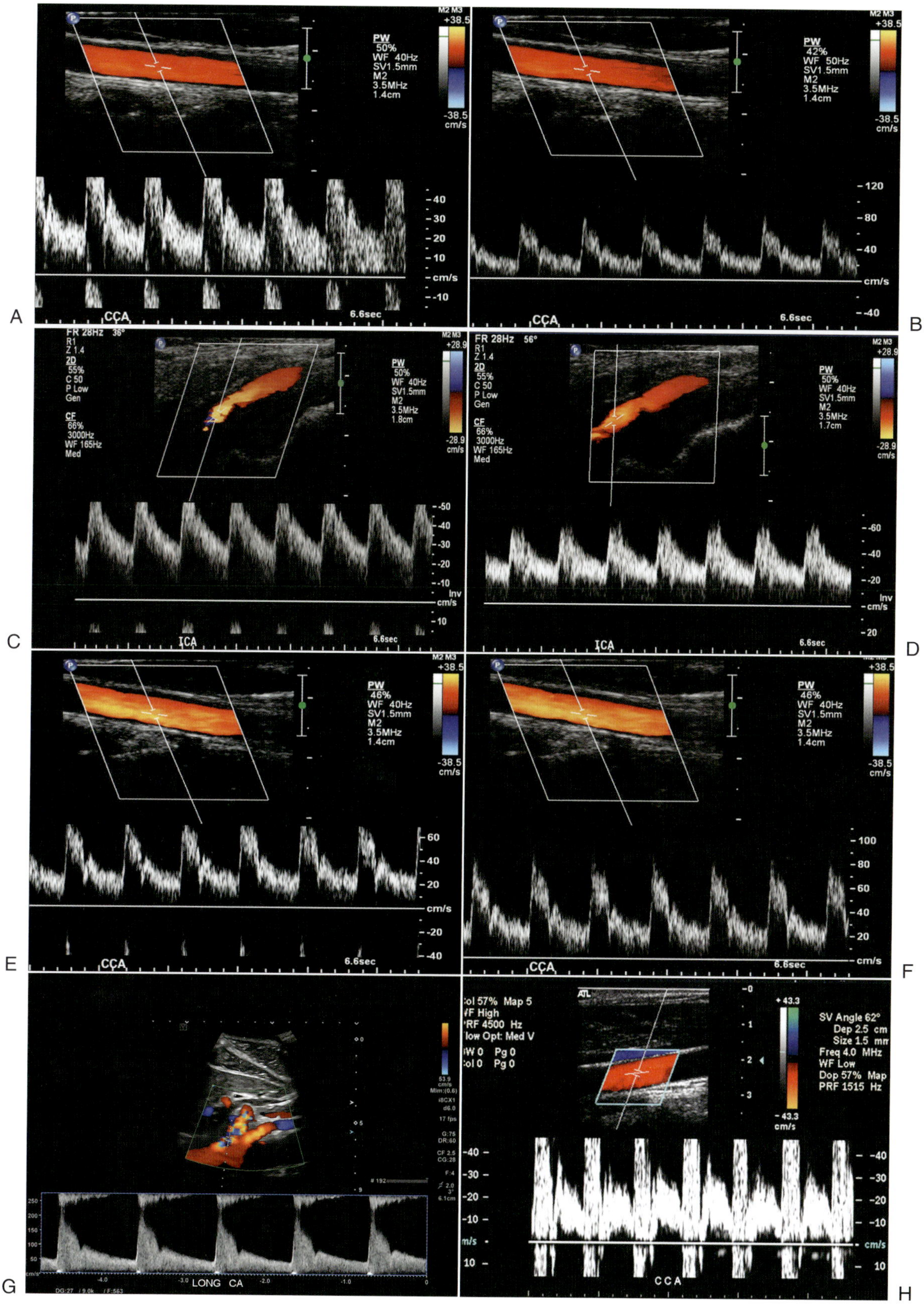

Fig. 7.23 **A**, Aliasing in the common carotid artery *(CCA)*. **B**, Pulse-repetition frequency (scale control) is increased to eliminate the aliasing. **C**, Aliasing in the internal carotid artery at a 36-degree Doppler angle. **D**, When the Doppler angle is increased to 56 degrees, the aliasing is resolved. **E–F**, Baseline is shifted down to correct for aliasing in the CCA. **G**, An example of too large baseline shift introducing aliasing. **H**, An example in which baseline shifting would not be helpful.

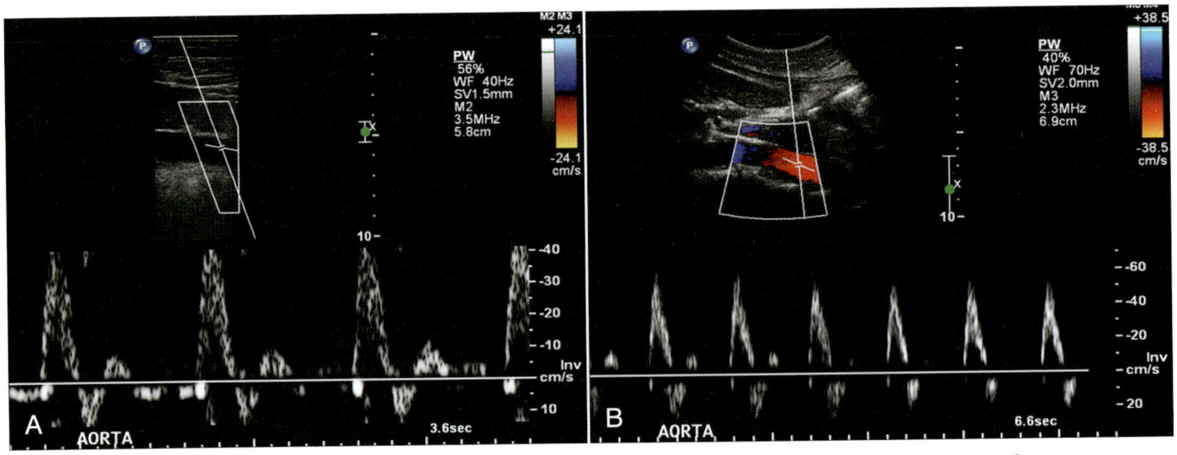

Fig. 7.24 Aliasing in the aorta when imaged at 3.5 MHz (**A**) can be eliminated by imaging at a lower frequency of 2.3 MHz (**B**) in which the Doppler shifts are reduced to less than the Nyquist limit.

BOX 7.2 Methods for Correcting or Eliminating Aliasing

1. Shift the baseline.
2. Increase the pulse-repetition frequency.
3. Increase the Doppler angle.
4. Use a lower operating frequency.
5. Use CW mode.

depicting more flow in one direction). The technique can be successful as long as there are no genuine Doppler shifts in the other direction. If there are legitimate Doppler shifts, they will be moved to an incorrect location along with resolving the aliasing peaks. Baseline shifting is not helpful if the desired information (e.g., peak systolic Doppler shift) is buried in another portion of the spectral display or if the shift is too large (see Fig. 7.23G–H). Other approaches to eliminating aliasing include changing to a lower frequency (see Fig. 7.24) or switching to CW Doppler operation. Single-button autocorrect algorithms can automate these corrections, while more sophisticated scanners (so-called high-end systems) may just do these steps prior to display.

Aliasing occurs in pulsed Doppler mode, because the received Doppler-shifted echoes must be sampled (to overcome the inherently poor signal-to-noise ratio). If samples are acquired often enough, the correct result is achieved as demonstrated in Fig. 7.25. Sufficiently frequent sampling yields the correct result and, conversely, sampling insufficiently often produces an incorrect result. To reiterate, if the highest Doppler shift frequency present in a signal exceeds half the PRF, aliasing will occur (Fig. 7.26).

Aliasing is caused by under-sampling of the Doppler shifts.

Aliasing is commonly corrected by shifting the baseline, increasing the PRF, or both.

Reducing the operating frequency or switching to CW mode to correct for aliasing is used less often than the other approaches. Operating frequency reduction reduces the Doppler shift, and CW mode does not provide range discrimination, both of which are less desirable outcomes in practice.

Range Ambiguity

When attempting to solve the aliasing problem by increasing the PRF, one can encounter the range-ambiguity artifact mentioned previously. This artifact occurs when a pulse is emitted before all the echoes from the previous pulse have been received. When this happens, early echoes from the last pulse are received simultaneously with late (i.e., deep) echoes from the previous pulse. The system is unable to determine whether an echo is an early one (superficial) from the last pulse or a late one (deep) from the previous pulse (Fig. 7.27). This artifact is caused by the scanner simply assuming that all echoes are derived from the last pulse and that these echoes originate from depths determined by the 13-μs/cm rule. As long as all echoes are received before the next pulse is sent out, this is true. However, with high PRFs, this may not be the case.

Therefore, Doppler flow information may come from locations other than the assumed one (the sample-volume location). In effect, multiple gates or sample volumes are operating at different depths. Table 7.1 lists, for various PRFs, the ranges beyond which ambiguity occurs. Table 7.2 lists, for various depths, the maximum Doppler-shift frequency (f_{NL}) that avoids aliasing and the range-ambiguity artifact. Maximum flow speeds that avoid aliasing for given angles are also listed. Instruments have been known to increase the PRF (to avoid aliasing) into a range in which range ambiguity occurs. In this quite rare occurrence, multiple sample volumes are shown on the display to indicate this situation.

Range ambiguity can be completely avoided if the ultrasound scanner is able to identify each transmitted pulse individually (e.g., using coded excitation) or uses broad transmit beams, which pushes the limit for range ambiguity much higher.

High PRF causes Doppler-range ambiguity (and is therefore rarely used in clinical practice).

Mirror Image

The mirror-image artifact described previously can also occur with Doppler systems. This means that an image of a vessel and a source of Doppler-shifted echoes can be duplicated on the

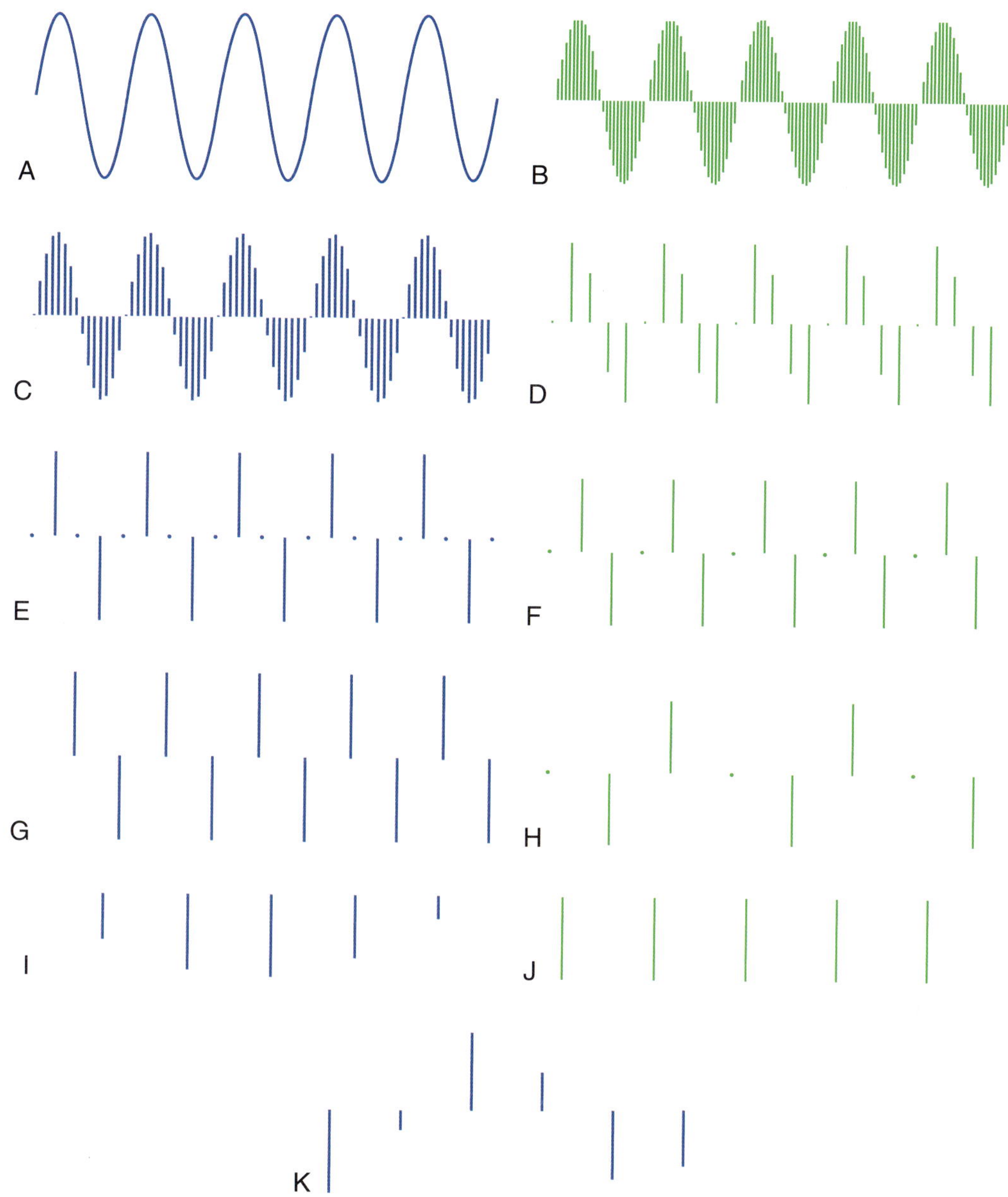

Fig. 7.25 Decreasing sampling rate leads to aliasing. Sampling of a five-cycle voltage (**A**) is progressively decreased from 25 samples per cycle (**B**), to 15 samples per cycle (**C**), to five samples per cycle (**D**), to four samples per cycle (**E**), to three samples per cycle (**F**), to two samples per cycle (**G**), and finally to successive sampling of one sample per cycle (**H–K**). In the last four cases, aliasing occurs.

opposite side of a strong reflector. The duplicated vessel containing flow could be misinterpreted as an additional vessel that has a spectrum identical to that of the real vessel. Fig. 7.28 shows an example of image and spectrum duplication of the subclavian artery. The strong reflector in this case is the air at the pleural boundary.

A mirror image of a Doppler spectrum can appear on the opposite side of the baseline when, indeed, flow is unidirectional and should appear only on one side of the baseline. This is an electronic duplication of the spectral information. The duplication can occur when Doppler gain is set too high (causing overloading in the amplifier and leakage, called **cross-talk**, of the signal from the proper channel into the other channel; Fig. 7.29). Moreover, duplication can also occur when the Doppler angle is near 90 degrees (Fig. 7.30,A). In this situation, the duplication is not an artifact, but due to the beam-to-vessel angle being not quite 90° at the beam edges, so one edge of the beam is angled upstream, and the other edge downstream or, alternatively, that the vessel being imaged is angled slightly within the imaging plane (see Fig. 7.30,B).

Spectral mirror image is the appearance of spectral information on both sides of the baseline. It occurs at high Doppler gains or Doppler angles near 90°.

Doppler spectra have a speckle quality similar to that observed in grayscale imaging, discussed previously. Electromagnetic interference from nearby equipment can cloud the

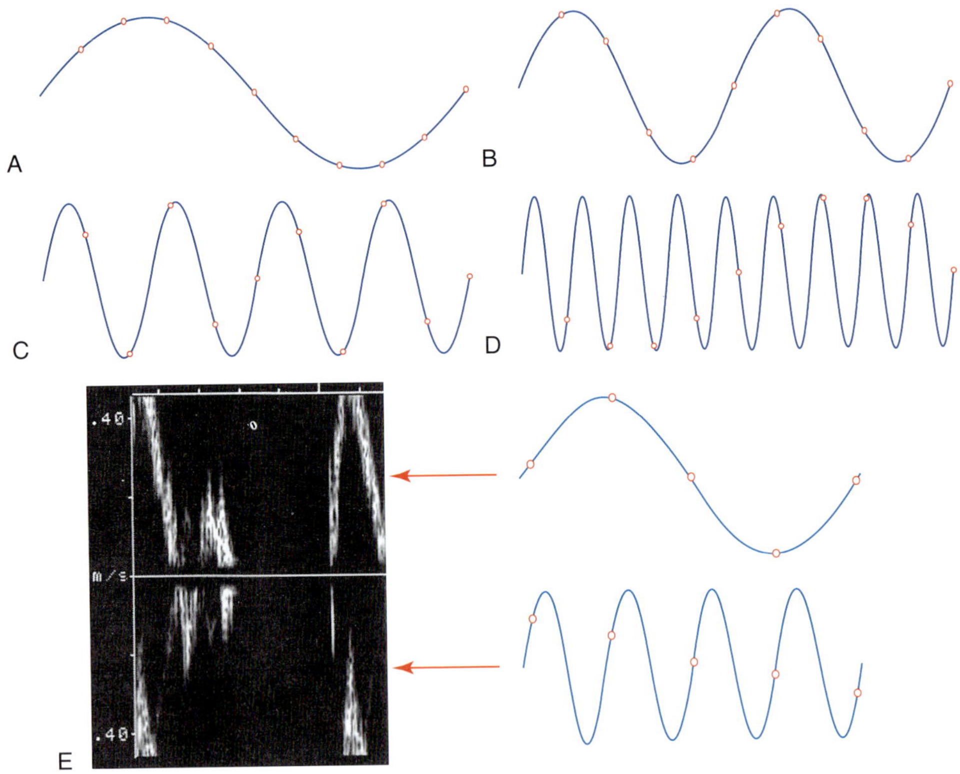

Fig. 7.26 Increasing frequency leads to aliasing. Signal voltages are sampled at 10 points *(red circles)*: (**A**) one cycle, (**B**) two cycles, (**C**) four cycles, and (**D**) nine cycles. As signal frequency is increased, aliasing occurs when the Nyquist limit is exceeded (in this case, beyond five cycles). Thus D is an example of aliasing. It can be seen that connecting the circles would yield a one-cycle representation of what is actually a nine-cycle signal voltage. **E**, In this spectral display, the presentation above the baseline is correct (unaliased, five samples per cycle), whereas the systolic peaks appear incorrectly below the baseline (aliased, one sample per cycle).

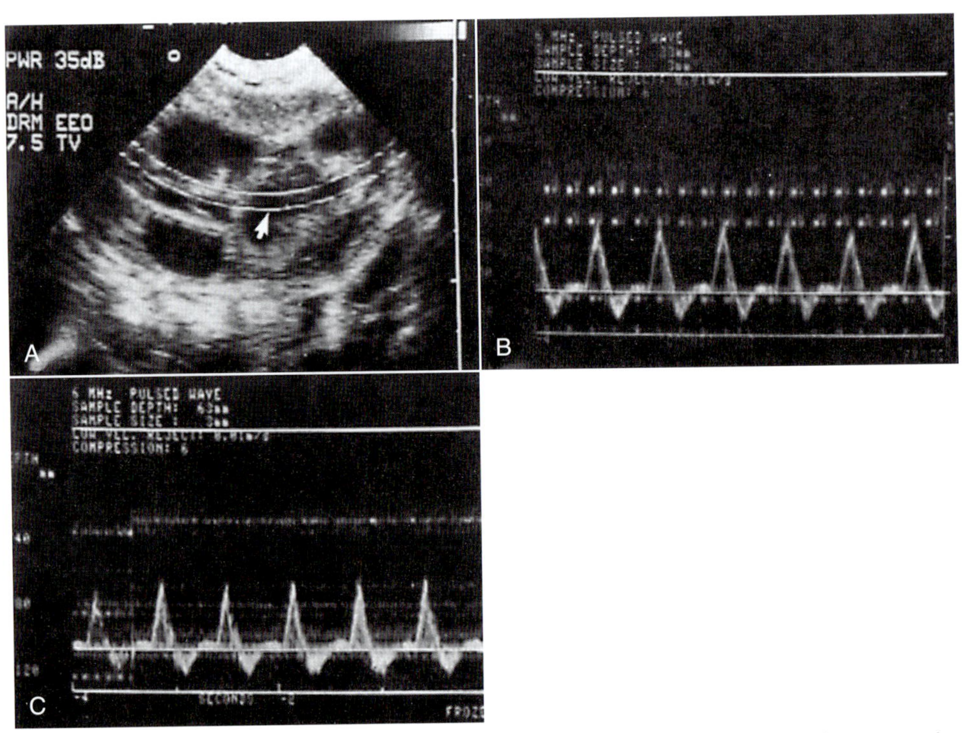

Fig. 7.27 Ambiguity is caused by sending out a pulse before all echoes from the previous pulse are received. **A**, This transvaginal image shows the pulsed Doppler sample volume or range gate *(arrow)* set at 33 mm within an ovary. **B**, The resulting Doppler spectrum shows a waveform typical of the external iliac artery. **C**, A signal identical to that shown in B was obtained when the range was increased to 63 mm, proving that the signal actually originated from the external iliac artery at this depth.

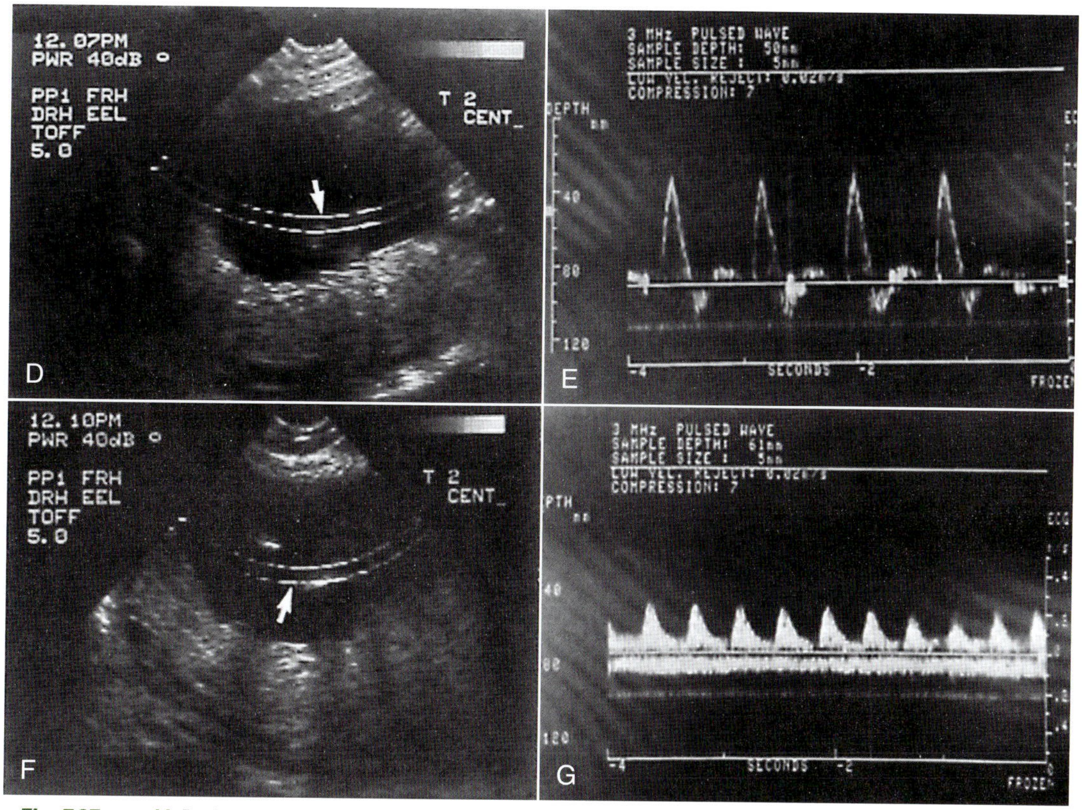

Fig. 7.27, cont'd **D**, A sample volume *(arrow)* placed at a depth of 50 mm in the uterus of a pregnant woman (16 weeks' gestation) produces signals typical of the external iliac artery as shown in **E**. **F**, In the same patient, a slight adjustment of the sample volume *(arrow)* produced the desired umbilical artery signal of G eliminating the range ambiguity artifact. (From Gill RW, Kossoff MB, Kossoff **G**, Griffiths KA: New class of pulsed Doppler US ambiguity at short ranges, *Radiology* 173:272, 1989.)

TABLE 7.2 Aliasing and Range-Ambiguity Limits

			MAXIMUM VELOCITY (CM/S) FOR THREE DIFFERENT BEAM-TO-VESSEL ANGLES		
Depth (cm)	**Maximum PRF (kHz) for Avoiding Range Ambiguity**	**Nyquist Limit (kHz) for Avoiding Aliasing**	**0°**	**30°**	**60°**
1	77.0	38.5	593	685	1186
2	38.5	19.2	296	342	593
4	19.2	9.6	148	171	296
8	9.6	4.8	74	86	148
16	4.8	2.4	37	43	74

Assuming a 5-MHz operating frequency.

spectral display with lines or "snow" (Fig. 7.31). Given the improvements to shielding implemented in state-of-the-art ultrasound scanners, this is unlikely to happen in practice and would almost certainly indicate a failing system (but is retained in this edition for historical and exam related issues).

COLOR DOPPLER ARTIFACTS

Artifacts observed with color Doppler imaging (CDI) are 2D color representations of artifacts seen on grayscale or spectral Doppler displays. The most common of which is aliasing. However, others, including anatomical mirror imaging, Doppler angle effects, shadowing, and clutter, also occur.

Aliasing

Aliasing occurs when the Doppler shift exceeds f_{NL} (Fig. 7.32), which happens more often in color Doppler than in spectral Doppler, because of the reduced PRFs used in the former relative to the latter assuming the imaging is conducted with narrow transmit beams. Color aliasing results in incorrect flow

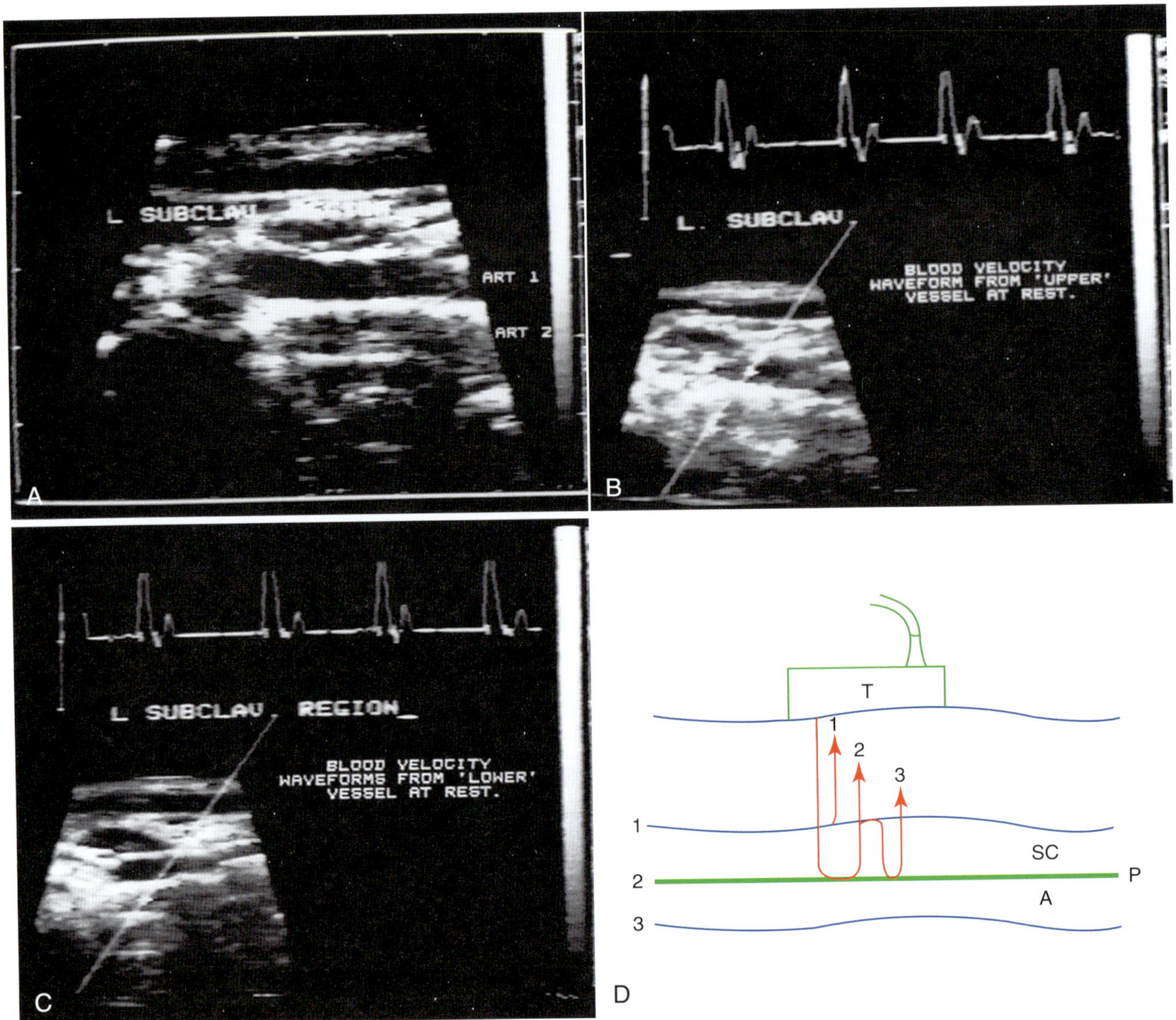

Fig. 7.28 **A**, The subclavian artery *(ART 1)* and its mirror image *(ART 2)*. **B**, Flow signal from artery. **C**, Flow signal from the mirror image of the artery. **D**, Multiple reflections produce a mirror image. Paths *1* and *2* are legitimate, but path *3* arrives late, producing the artifactual deep arterial wall. *A*, Artifactual artery; *P*, pleura; *SC*, subclavian artery; *T*, transducer. (***D*** from Kremkau FW: Principles and pitfalls of real-time color-flow imaging. In Bernstein EF, editor: *Vascular diagnosis, ed 4,* St. Louis, 1993, Mosby.)

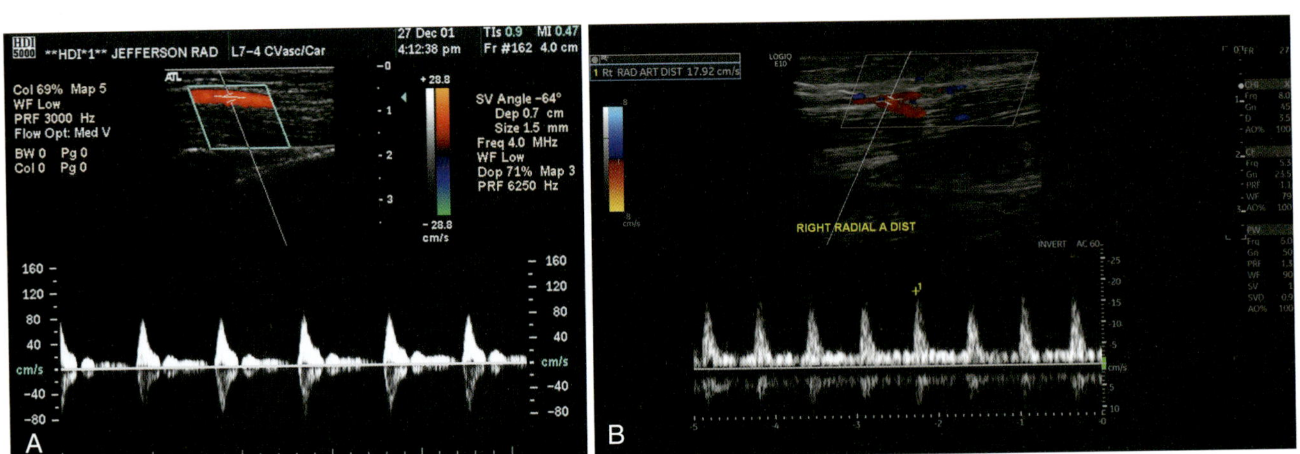

Fig. 7.29 **A**, **B**, Examples of mirror images of the carotid and radial artery spectra below the baseline.

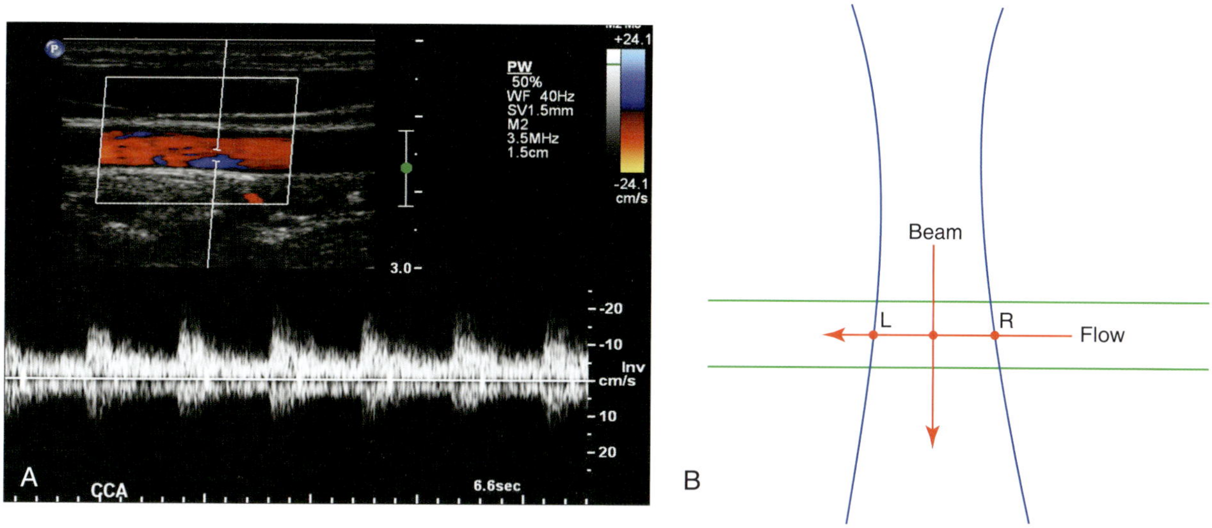

Fig. 7.30 **A**, The Doppler angle is nearly 90 degrees in the common carotid artery, which produces a spectral mirror image with flow on both sides of the baseline. **B**, Because beams are focused and not cylindrical, portions of the beam (R) can experience flow toward the transducer, whereas other portions (L) can experience flow away when the central beam axis intersects the flow at 90 degrees. In a broad transmit beam system with multiple angles of insonation this artifact will not occur.

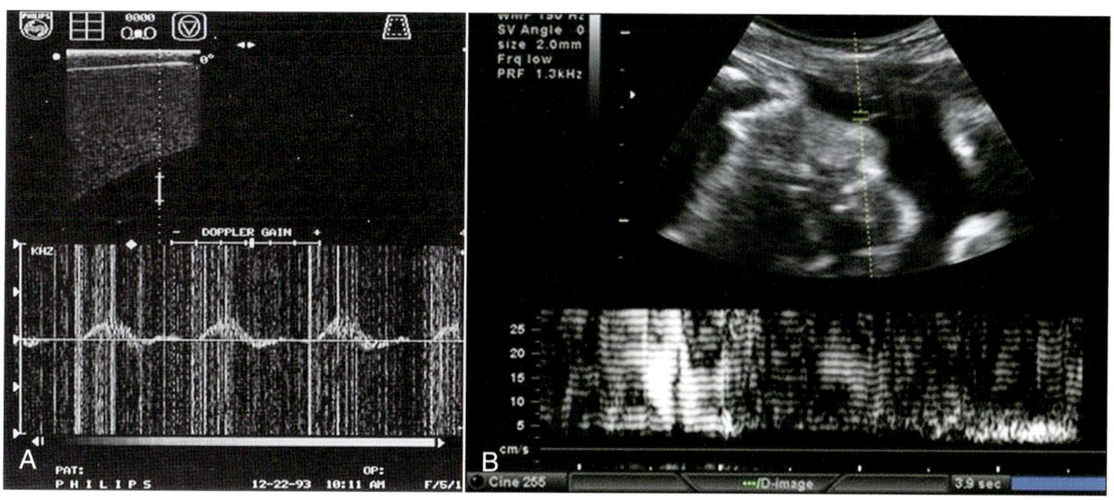

Fig. 7.31 **A**, Interference from nearby electrical equipment clouds the spectral display with electric noise (the vertical "snow" lines). **B**, External interference produces bands of frequency that are fairly constant with time.

direction being displayed on the CDI image (Fig. 7.33). Increasing the flow speed range (which is actually an increase in PRF) can solve the problem (see Figs. 7.33,E–F and 7.34). However, setting the range too high can cause loss of flow information, particularly if the wall filter is set high. This artifact can also be eliminated (or at least reduced) by angling the color box, that is, changing the beam-to-vessel angle (see Fig. 7.33,C–D). Baseline shifting can also decrease or eliminate the effect of aliasing (see Fig. 7.33,G–H), as described above for spectral Doppler displays.

It is important to note that broad transmit beam systems will eliminate almost all aliasing, since the sampling frequency is equal to the frame rate, which is both very high (up to thousands of Hz) and applies to the entire image instead of just an individual beam.

Aliasing in CDI mode appears as an incorrect color from the opposite side of the baseline on the color map.

A related artifact is the multiple-angle artifact—the Doppler angle in color-Doppler displays is assumed (unrealistically) to be zero. Hence, the color overlay is coded relative to the location of the transducer, which can lead to somewhat confusing displays (demonstrated, e.g., in Fig. 5.47). In Fig. 7.35,A, the region of the portal vein shown in red hues indicates positive Doppler shifts according to the color map albeit with a small region in blue that has exceeded the positive aliasing limit. The blood flow in the rest of the vessel is generating negative Doppler shifts

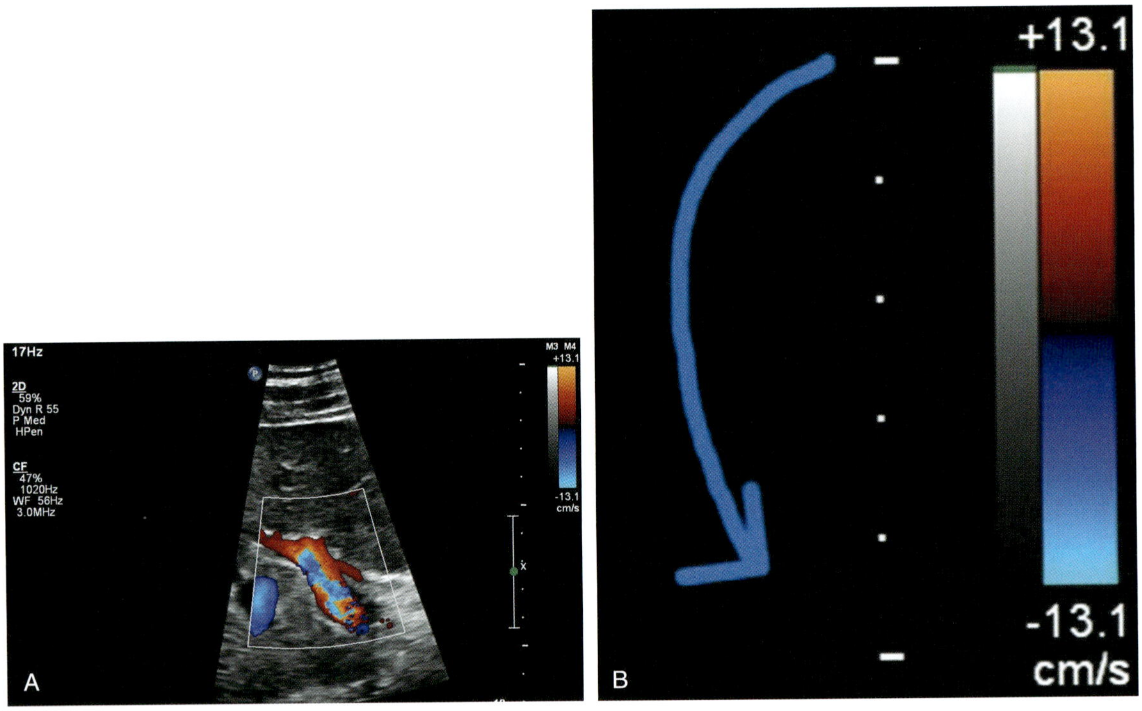

Fig. 7.32 **A**, Negative *(blue)* Doppler shifts are shown in the flow in this image. These are actually positive Doppler shifts that have exceeded the higher Nyquist limit (converted here to the equivalent flow speed: +13.1 cm/s) and are wrapped around to the negative portion of the color bar (**B**). (Similarly, negative shifts that exceed the −13.1 cm/s limit would alias to the positive side.)

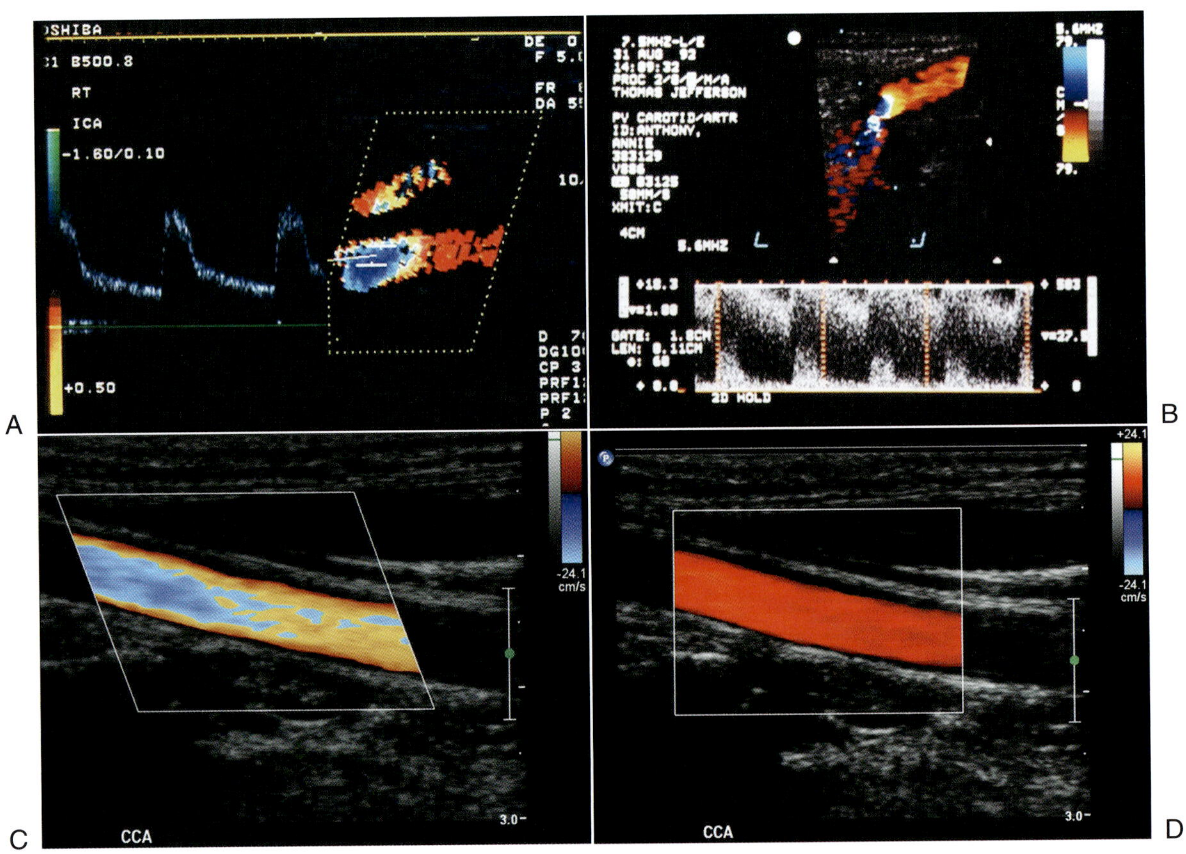

Fig. 7.33 **A**, A color Doppler image with aliasing. The blue colors demonstrate aliasing, whereas the higher pulse-repetition frequency *(PRF)* associated with the spectral Doppler ensures that the spectral display is not aliased. **B**, An example in which both the color and spectral displays of the carotid are aliasing. **C**, Aliasing in the common carotid artery with a color box angled incorrectly. **D**, Adjusting the angle of the color box eliminates the aliasing.

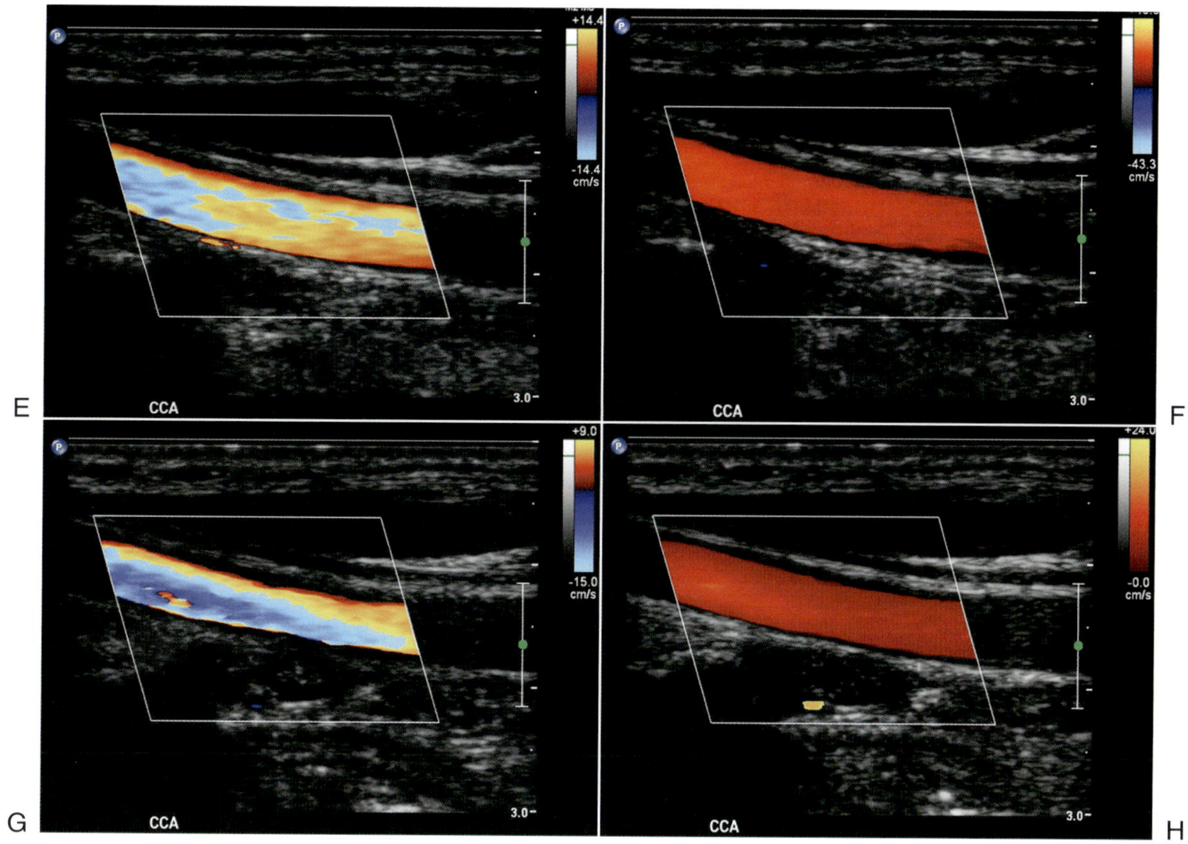

Fig. 7.33, cont'd E–F, Increasing the color scale from 14.4 cm/s to 43.3 cm/s resolves the aliasing. **G–H**, Color correction can also be achieved by changing the baseline from covering –15 to 9.0 cm/s to covering the 0 to 24 cm/s range.

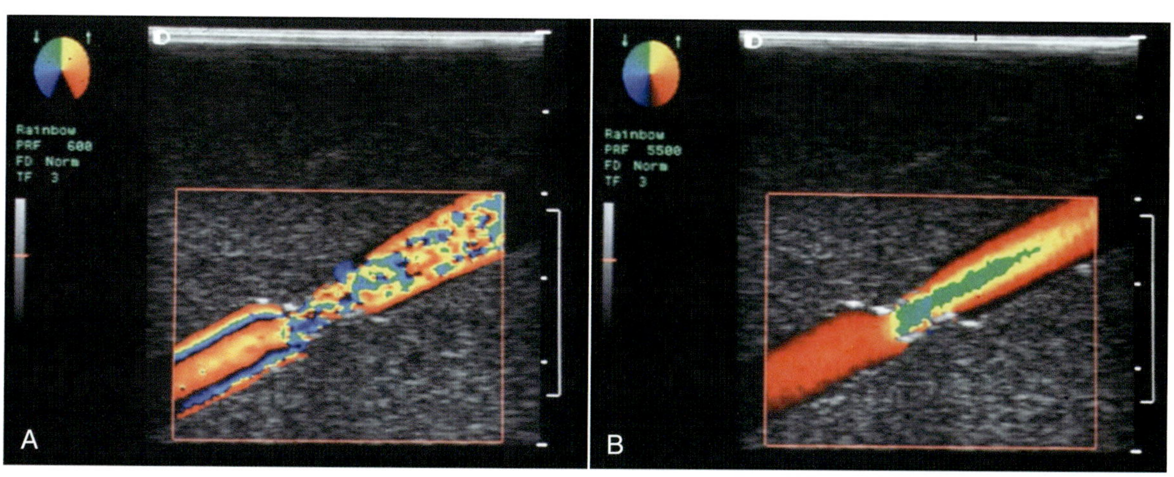

Fig. 7.34 A, Flow in this phantom with an 80% stenosis is toward the upper right, producing positive Doppler shifts. The pulse-repetition frequency (600 Hz) and Nyquist limit (300 Hz) are too low, resulting in aliasing (negative Doppler shifts) at the edge of the vessel as well as at the center of the flow in the vessel (positive Doppler shifts). **B**, With the PRF increased to 5500 Hz, the aliasing has been eliminated except for right in the stenosis, where the aliasing outlines the stenotic jet.

(blue hues) indicating that we are looking downstream, seeing flow away from the transducer; likewise in Fig. 7.35,B showing tortuous and, therefore, multicolored flow in the pancreas.

Proper understanding of the effects of angle on the Doppler shift is necessary to interpret complex images properly.

Mirror Image, Shadowing, Enhancement, Clutter, and Noise

In the mirror (or ghost) artifact (Fig. 7.36), an image of a vessel can be duplicated and appear on the opposite side of a strong reflector (e.g., pleura or diaphragm). This is the CDI version of the grayscale artifact of Figs. 7.6 and 7.28. Shadowing is the weakening or elimination of Doppler signals beyond a shadowing object, just as occurs with grayscale echoes (Fig. 7.37,A). Conversely, lack of attenuation or just too high a Doppler gain can lead to excess color (noise), which may confuse the interpretation of color flow presentations (see Fig. 7.37,B–D). Color signals can overwrite tissue and mimic flow, particularly in **hypoechoic** or anechoic regions if the gain settings are too high. Another example of color noise is the "twinkling artifact" that can appear in the shadow region distal to strongly reflecting objects with rough surfaces (e.g., kidney stones). This artifact is dependent on instrument settings and is a presentation of electronic noise from the instrument appearing as randomly alternating colors in the hypoechoic region.

Clutter, also known as the flash artifact, results from tissue motion producing strong Doppler shifted signals (Fig. 7.38). Such clutter can be eliminated by wall filters that remove the lower-frequency Doppler shifts from moving tissue.

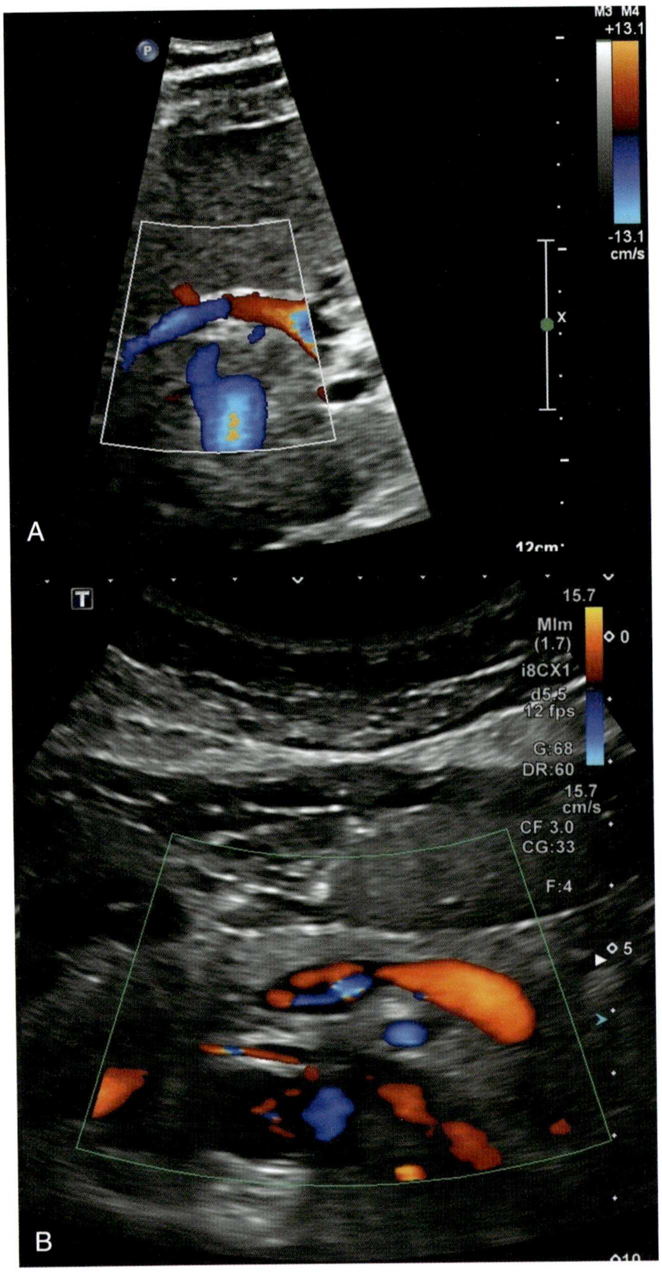

Fig. 7.35 **A**, Flow from the right to the left in the portal vein. Thus the flow is upstream from the transducer in the right half of the image (thus coded *red*) and downstream in the left half of the image (color-coded *blue*). **B**, The same effect can be observed in tortuous vessels in the pancreas.

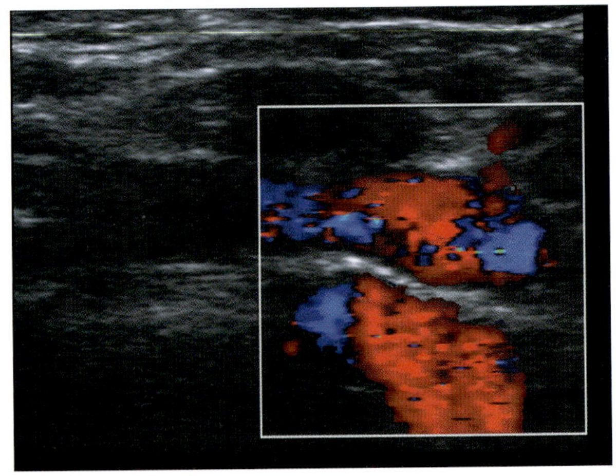

Fig. 7.36 Longitudinal color Doppler image of the subclavian vein. The pleura causes the mirror image. The diagram in Figure 7.28,D shows how this artifact occurs.

CEUS ARTIFACTS

While contrast agent artifacts are in a class of their own, it is important to note that CEUS-induced artifacts are not currently on the sonographer registration tests.

Near Field Signal Loss

Contrast agent microbubbles are susceptible to destruction at higher acoustic powers (typically MI values above 0.3–0.4), which can be exploited in flash imaging modes and for destruct-reperfusion studies (as discussed in Chapter 6). However, it is also possible to induce unintended bubble destruction—especially in the near field where the impact of attenuations on the pulse is limited (see Fig. 7.39). When **near-field signal loss** occurs, the bubbles in the shallowest part of the image will be destroyed first and the gradual change to the near-field enhancement pattern should catch the eye of the operator. The easiest

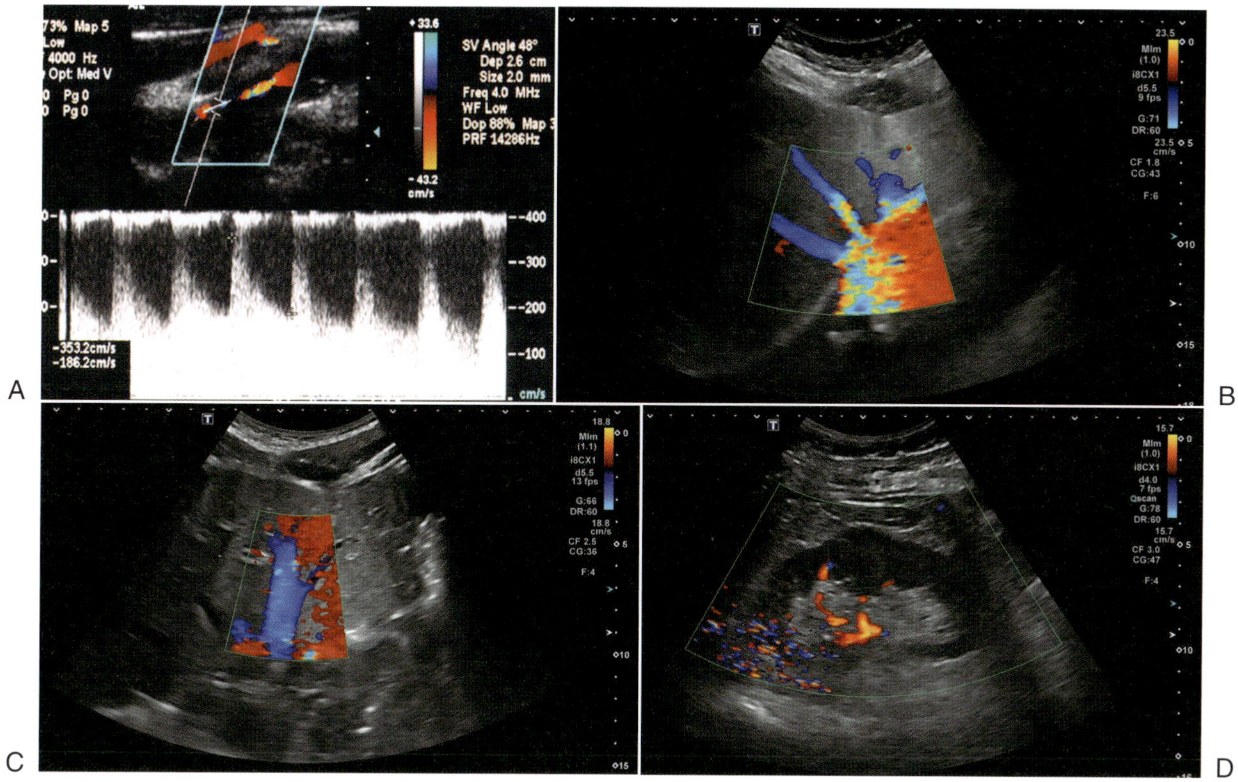

Fig. 7.37 **A**, Shadowing from calcified plaque follows the grayscale scan lines straight down. Notice how the color aliases. **B–D**, Color appears as noise in areas where non-Doppler-shifted echoes are weak or absent if the color gain is too high.

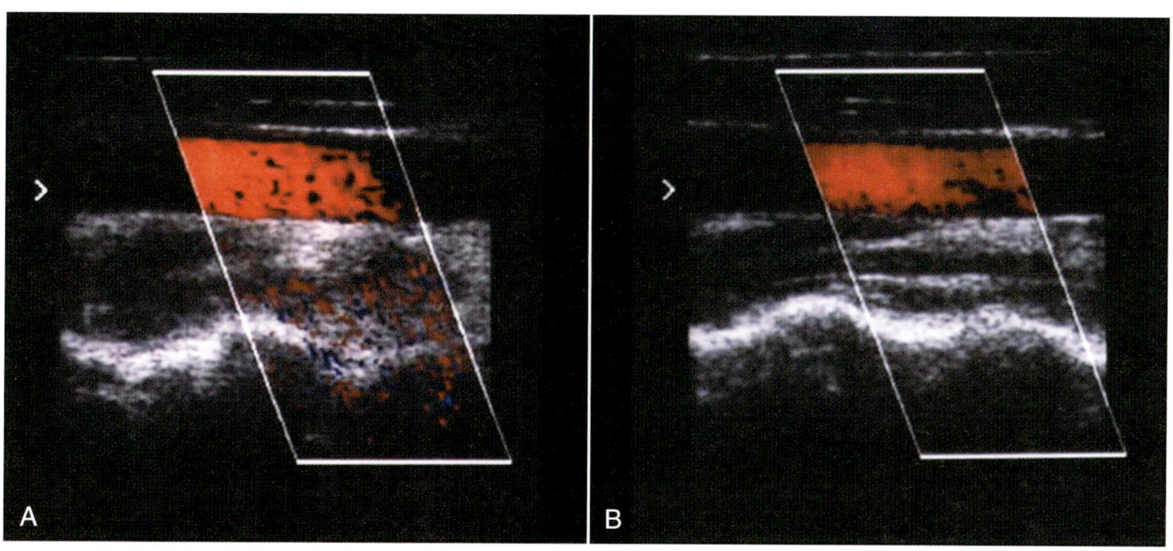

Fig. 7.38 **A**, Clutter from tissue motion (i.e., flash artifact) in the neck (caused by speaking) appears as color Doppler below the common carotid artery. **B**, When the speaking stops, the clutter is gone, revealing the underlying tissue.

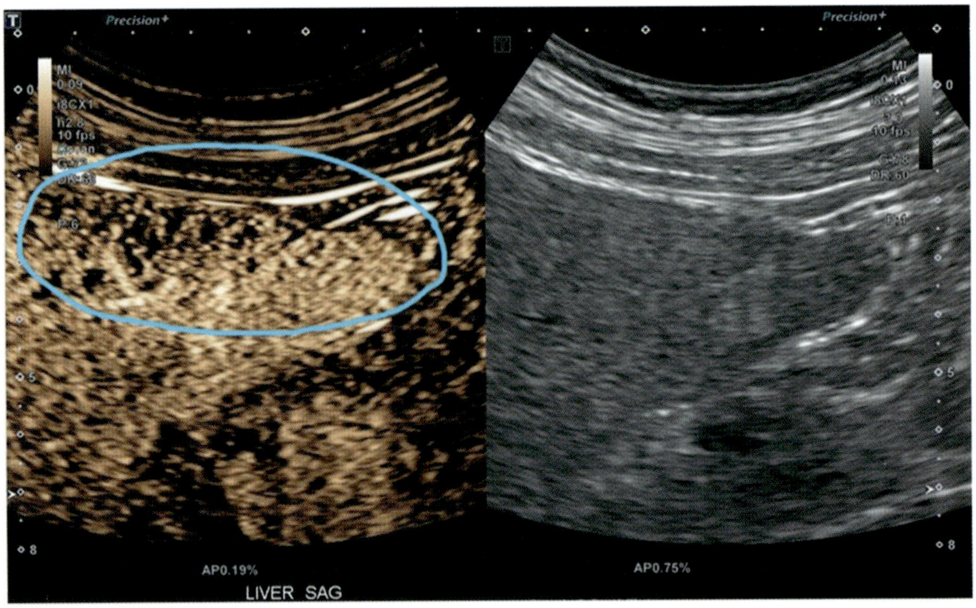

Fig. 7.39 Near field signal loss (*blue ellipsoid*) in CEUS liver examination. (Courtesy Corinne Wessner, MS, RDMS, Thomas Jefferson University.)

remedy is obviously to turn the output power down, but that may prevent adequate enhancement deeper in the image. In that case, ignoring this unavoidable artifact is probably the simplest way to deal with it.

Pseudo-Enhancement and Pseudo-Washout

When the region of interest of the CEUS examination contains highly echogenic tissue or when an excessive amount of contrast has been administrated, it is possible that **pseudo enhancement** will occur. Even areas with no flow can appear as enhanced (see Fig. 7.40) where an HCC that was successfully ablated (i.e., no internal flow whatsoever) still present as enhanced. Careful consideration of the optimal contrast agent dose and awareness of the clinical history are really the only ways to deal with this artifact.

A very similar artifact is **pseudo-washout**, where the internal vascularity of a lesion or other area of interest will appear to washout over time (see Fig. 7.41). During the late phases of enhancement (so >3 minutes after contrast injection), it may seem like washout, but in reality, it is just the bubble signal decreasing over time. The key to understanding this artifact is to always compare the area of interest to normal tissue at the

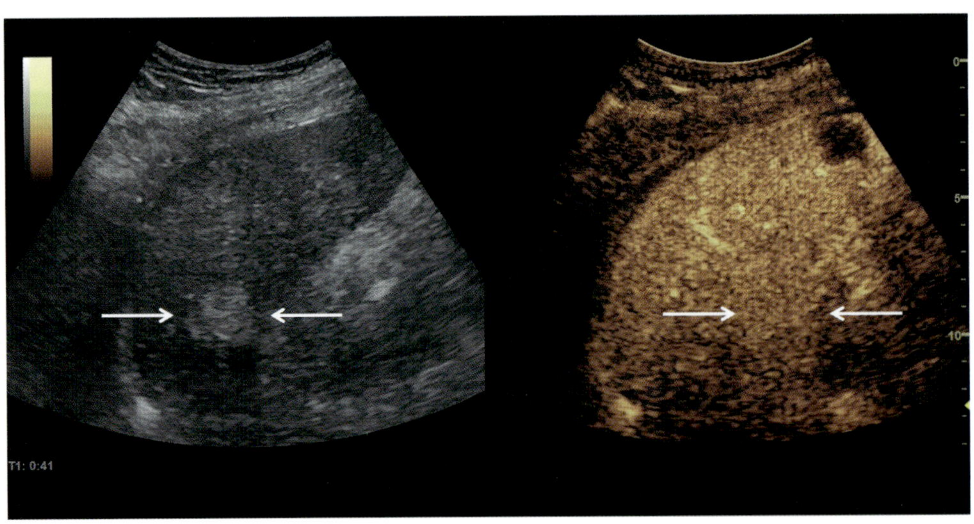

Fig. 7.40 An echogenic HCC tumor successfully treated with transarterial chemoembolization has no remaining vascularity. Nonetheless, pseudo-enhancement due to the echogenic tissue produces signal inside the tumor. (Courtesy Corinne Wessner, MS, RDMS, Thomas Jefferson University.)

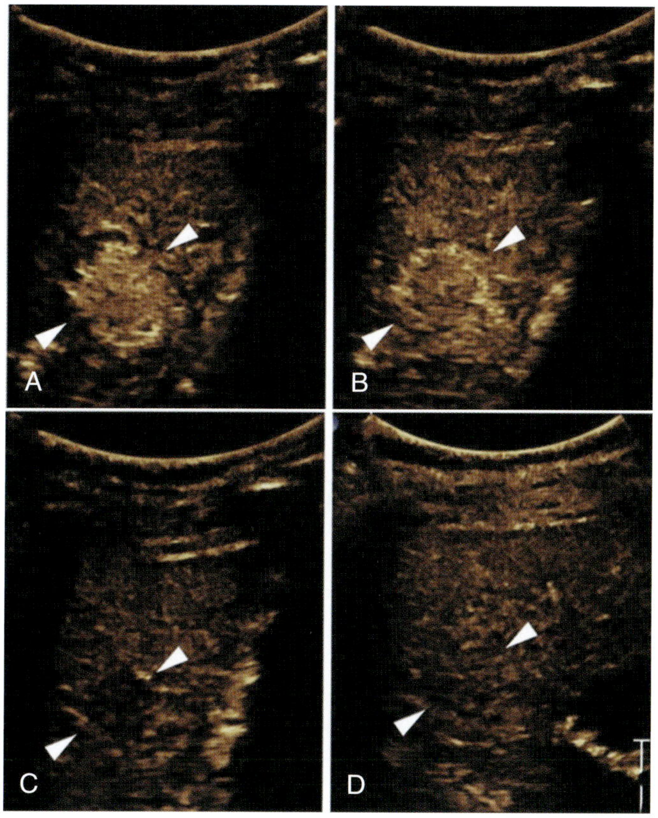

Fig. 7.41 An example of pseudo-washout with **A,** Early arterial phase of CEUS enhancement and **B**, late enhancement of a liver lesion (arrowheads) characteristic of HCC. **C,** However, at 70 s, atypical washout was encountered (arrowheads). **D,** A second injection of contrast with decreased frame rate (to reduce any unintentional bubble destruction) was performed showing the lesion to be iso-echoic at 70 s. (From Fetzer DT, Rafailidis V, Peterson C, Grant EG, Sidhu P, Barr RG. *Artifacts in contrast-enhanced ultrasound: a pictorial essay. Abdom Radiol (NY).* 43:977–997, 2018.)

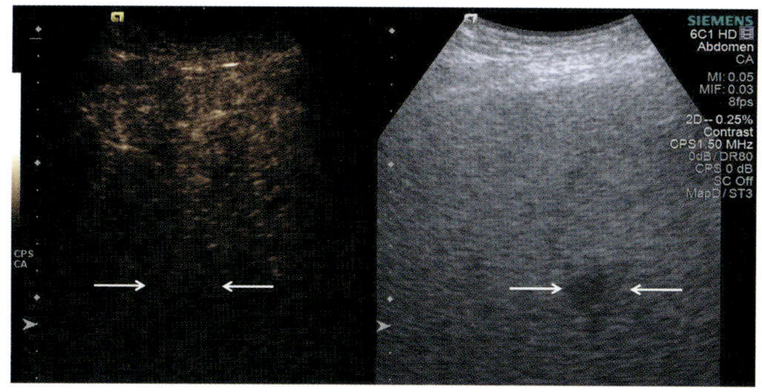

Fig. 7.42 Attenuation impeding a deep CEUS liver study. (Courtesy Corinne Wessner, MS, RDMS, Thomas Jefferson University.)

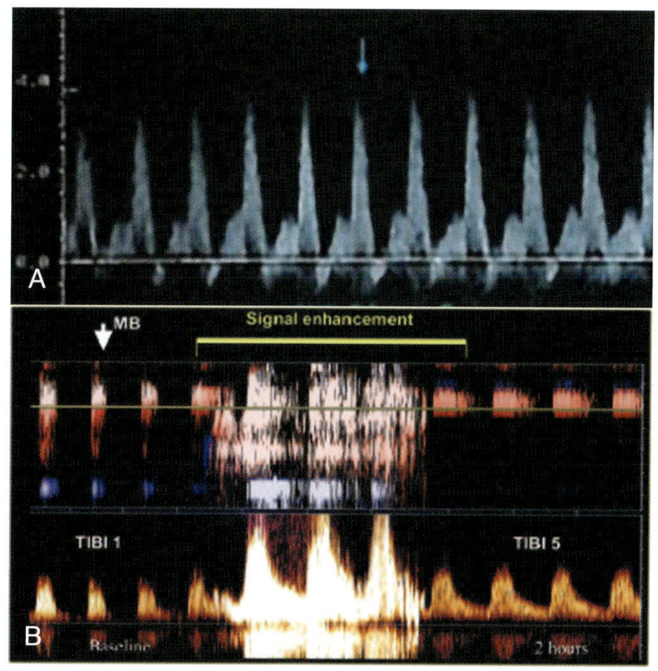

Fig. 7.43 **A,** Spectral Doppler waveform obtained during the arrival of an ultrasound contrast agent showing a steady increase in the measured Doppler shift (in kHz) associated with the peak systolic velocity. **B,** Microbubbles arriving in an occluded proximal left middle cerebral artery produce excessive and clearly artifactual enhancement before normal flow is reestablished. (**A**, from Forsberg F, et al. Artifacts in ultrasonic contrast agent studies. *J Ultrasound Med*, 13:357-365, 1994. **B**, From Molinas CA, et al. Microbubble administration accelerates clot lysis during continuous 2-MHz ultrasound monitoring in stroke patients treated with intravenous tissue plasminogen activator. *Stroke*, 37:425–429, 2006.)

same depths. If the level of enhancement is the same, then this is pseudo-washout and it should be ignored.

Attenuation

Attenuation-induced signal loss in the far field during CEUS studies tends to occur across the entire image, due to the microbubbles traversing the entire imaging plane. Localized shadowing or enhancement artifacts, as described for gray-scale imaging, are less common, and one should not expect any speckle reduction techniques to help in this situation. Moreover, CEUS-specific imaging techniques already involve multipulse firing and signal bandwidth manipulation (cf., Chapter 6), making the addition of speckle reduction approaches fraught with problems.

Unfortunately, there is not much one can do to reduce attenuation artifacts (especially in fatty livers; see Fig. 7.42) except increase the MI (and, thus, risk inducing near field signal loss through excessive bubble destruction) or decrease the imaging frequency. In general, it is important to be mindful with deeper lesions in CEUS examinations.

Spectral Doppler Velocity Measurements

In pulsed Doppler mode, injection of an ultrasound contrast agent markedly increases the displayed velocities seen in the

TABLE 7.3 Artifacts and Their Causes

Artifact	Cause
Comet tail	Reverberation
Grating lobe	Grating lobe
Mirror image	Multiple reflection
Refraction	Refraction
Reverberation	Multiple reflection
Slice thickness	Pulse width out of plane
Speckle	Interference
Speed error	Speed error
Range ambiguity	Finite speed of sound in tissue
Shadowing and general signal loss	High attenuation
Edge shadowing	Refraction or interference
Enhancement	Low attenuation
Focal enhancement	Focusing
Aliasing	Exceeding the Nyquist limit
Spectrum mirror	High Doppler gain
Near field signal loss	Microbubble destruction
Pseudo-enhancement	Highly echogenic tissue or excessive contrast dose
Pseudo-washout	Bubble signal decreasing over time
Spectral Doppler velocity increases	Limited dynamic range of the Doppler display

spectral display (see Fig. 7.43). This could be due to real flow with the Doppler shifts involving a limited number of red blood cells now becoming visible, due to contrast enhancement. Conversely, it could also be due to the limited dynamic range of the Doppler display and, hence, an artifact. There is a fine line between detecting real flow that was undetectable prior to the CEUS examination and the enhancement of the noise floor being interpreted as actual blood flow in the spectral display. This phenomenon may well be a combination of these two aspects, which in turn means the final display is impacted by artifacts and should be interpreted with care. This artifact is less of an issue these days as CEUS is used less often to save failed spectral Doppler exams.

This chapter has discussed several ultrasound imaging (including for CEUS) and flow artifacts, all of which are listed in Table 7.3, along with their causes. Most of these artifacts can cause confusion and error. However, shadowing and enhancement can be useful in interpretation and diagnosis, but this requires the operator to turn off any speckle reduction techniques. Artifacts seen in 2D imaging are also evidenced in 3D imaging, sometimes in unusual ways. All of these artifacts can hinder proper interpretation and diagnosis, and this must be avoided or handled properly when encountered. A proper understanding of artifacts and how to deal with them when they are encountered enables sonographers and physicians to avoid the pitfalls they can cause.

REVIEW

The following key points are presented in this chapter:

- The beam width perpendicular to the scan plane causes slice-thickness artifacts.
- Apparent fine-image details are not related directly to tissue texture but are a result of interference effects from a distribution of scatterers in the tissue, called speckle.
- Reverberation produces a set of equally spaced artifactual echoes distal to the real reflector.
- In the mirror-image artifact, objects that are present on one side of a strong reflector are displayed on the other side also.
- Refraction displaces echoes laterally.
- Propagation speed error and refraction can cause objects to be displayed in improper locations, with incorrect sizes, or both.
- Shadowing is caused by high-attenuation objects in the sound path.
- Refraction can also cause edge shadowing.
- Enhancement results from low-attenuation objects in the sound path.
- Aliasing occurs when the Doppler shift frequency exceeds one-half of the PRF (the Nyquist limit).
- Aliasing can be reduced or eliminated by using baseline shift, increasing the PRF or Doppler angle, reducing operating frequency, or using continuous-wave operation.
- CEUS introduces its own set of artifacts related to bubble destruction in the near field and excessive or incorrect depiction of enhancement.
- Spectral Doppler waveforms with CEUS result in a fine line between detecting additional real flow and the enhancement of the noise floor in the spectral display.

EXERCISES

Answers appear in the Answers to Exercises section at the back of the book.

1. The pulser of an instrument automatically reduces the PRF for deeper imaging to avoid the ___________ artifact.
   a. comet tail
   b. grating lobe
   c. mirror image
   d. range ambiguity

2. If an echo arrives 143 μs after the pulse that produced it was emitted, it should be located at a depth of ________ cm. If a second pulse was emitted 13 μs before the arrival of this echo, it will be placed incorrectly at a depth of ________ cm.
   a. 11, 1
   b. 14, 13
   c. 13, 14
   d. 13, 13
3. If the propagation speed in a soft tissue path is 1.60 mm/μs, a diagnostic instrument assumes a propagation speed too ____________ and will show reflectors too ____________ the transducer.
   a. high, close to
   b. high, far from
   c. low, close to
   d. low, far from
4. Mirror images can occur with only one reflector. True or false?
5. The most common artifact encountered in Doppler ultrasound is __________.
   a. aliasing
   b. range ambiguity
   c. spectrum mirror image
   d. location mirror image
   e. electromagnetic interference
6. Which of the following can reduce or eliminate aliasing?
   a. increased PRF
   b. increased Doppler angle
   c. increased operating frequency
   d. use of continuous wave mode
   e. more than one of the above
7. The fine texture in soft tissue indicates the excellent resolution that actually exists there. True or false?
8. The fact that a beam, as it scans through tissue, has some nonzero width perpendicular to the scan plane results in the ____________ artifact.
   a. mirror image
   b. range ambiguity
   c. slice thickness
   d. speed error
9. Which of the following can cause improper location of objects on a display? (More than one correct answer.)
   a. shadowing
   b. enhancement
   c. speed error
   d. mirror image
   e. refraction
   f. grating lobe
10. Refraction can cause shadowing. True or false?
11. The transducer face is one of the reflectors involved in reverberations in which illustration, Fig. 7.44,A or B?
12. Match these artifact causes with their result: (More than one correct answer.)

a. Reverberation:	1. Unreal structure displayed
b. Shadowing:	2. Structure missing on the display
c. Enhancement:	3. Structure displayed with improper brightness
d. Propagation speed error:	4. Structure improperly positioned
e. Refraction:	5. Structure improperly shaped

13. Reverberation results in added reflectors being imaged with equal ____________.
   a. depth
   b. separation
   c. width
   d. brightness
14. In reverberation, subsequent reflections are ____________ than previous ones.
   a. shallower
   b. brighter
   c. weaker
   d. stronger

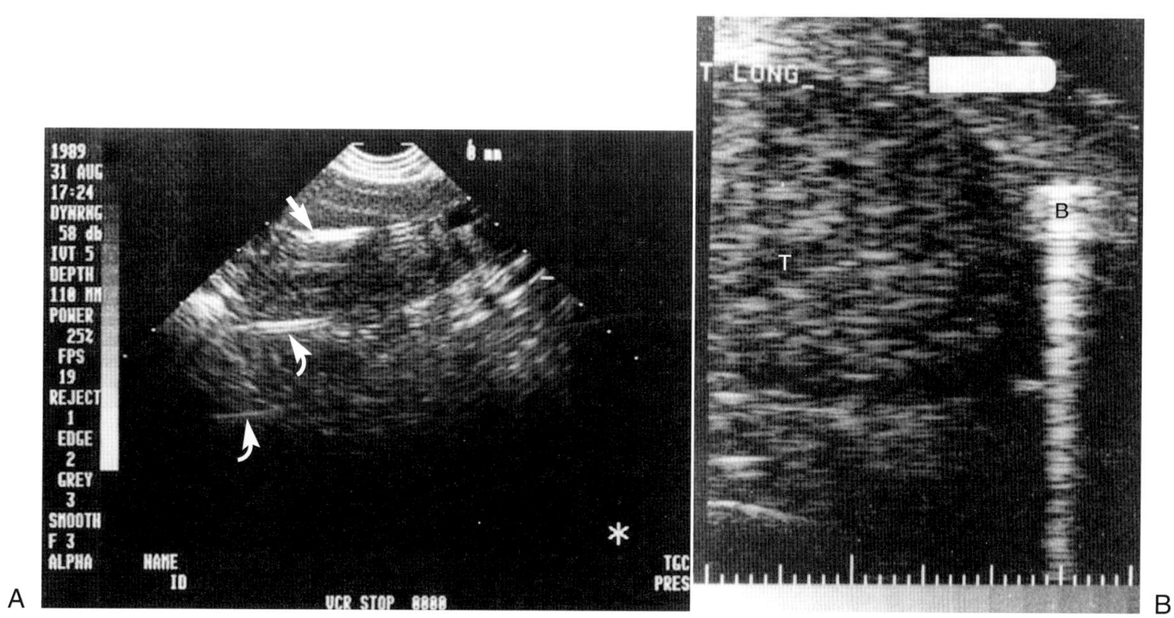

Fig. 7.44 A–B, Illustrations to accompany Exercise 11.

15. Enhancement is caused by a ____________.
    a. strongly reflecting structure
    b. weakly attenuating structure
    c. strongly attenuating structure
    d. refracting boundary
    e. propagation speed error
16. Which of the following can correct or eliminate aliasing?
    a. decreased PRF
    b. decreased Doppler angle
    c. increased operating frequency
    d. baseline shifting
    e. more than one of the above
17. Shadowing results in decreased echo amplitudes. True or false?
18. Propagation speed error results in improper ____________ position of a reflector on the display.
    a. lateral
    b. axial
19. To avoid aliasing, a signal voltage must be sampled at least ____________ time(s) per cycle.
    a. 1
    b. 2
    c. 3
    d. 4
    e. 5
20. If the highest Doppler-shift frequency present in a signal exceeds ______________ the PRF, aliasing will occur.
    a. one-tenth
    b. one-half
    c. two times
    d. five times
    e. ten times
21. When Doppler gain is set too high, which artifact is likely to occur?
    a. aliasing
    b. range ambiguity
    c. spectrum mirror image
    d. location mirror image
    e. speckle
22. Which artifact should be suspected if one observes twin gestational sacs when scanning through the rectus abdominis muscle?
    a. refraction
    b. reverberation
    c. speckle
    d. enhancement
23. Range ambiguity can occur in which of the following?
    a. imaging instruments
    b. duplex instruments
    c. pulsed-wave Doppler instruments
    d. color flow instruments
    e. all of the above
24. If the PRF is 4 kHz, which of the following Doppler shifts will cause aliasing?
    a. 1 kHz
    b. 2 kHz
    c. 3 kHz
    d. 4 kHz
    e. more than one of the above
25. If the PRF is 10 kHz, which of the following Doppler shifts will cause aliasing?
    a. 1 kHz
    b. 2 kHz
    c. 3 kHz
    d. 4 kHz
    e. none of the above
26. There is no problem with aliasing as long as the Doppler shifts are ____________ half the PRF.
    a. less than
    b. approximately equal to
    c. greater than
    d. all of the above
    e. none of the above
27. If Doppler shift is 2.6 kHz, no aliasing would result with a PRF of 10 kHz. True or false?
28. If there were a problem in Exercise 27, ____________ Doppler ultrasound could be used to avoid it.
    a. pulsed
    b. continuous wave
    c. color
    d. power
29. If red represents a positive Doppler shift and blue represents a negative one, what color is seen for normal flow toward the transducer? What color is seen for aliasing flow toward the transducer? What colors are seen for normal flow away and for aliasing flow away from the transducer?
    a. red, red, blue, blue
    b. red, blue, red, blue
    c. blue, red, blue, red
    d. red, blue, blue, red
30. When a pulse is emitted before all the echoes from the previous pulse have been received, which artifact occurs?
    a. mirror image
    b. range ambiguity
    c. slice thickness
    d. speed error
31. When a strong reflector is located in the scan plane, which of the following artifacts is likely to occur?
    a. aliasing
    b. range ambiguity
    c. spectrum mirror image
    d. location mirror image
    e. speckle
32. Increasing PRF to avoid aliasing can cause the following:
    a. baseline shift
    b. range ambiguity
    c. spectrum mirror image
    d. location mirror image
    e. speckle
33. Which of the following decreases the likelihood of range-ambiguity artifact?

a. decreasing operating frequency
b. decreasing PRF
c. decreasing Doppler angle
d. baseline shift
e. increasing pulser output

34. Range ambiguity produces which error in spectral-Doppler studies?
a. incorrect spectral peaks
b. incorrect gate location
c. intensity too high
d. intensity too low
e. all of the above

35. Range ambiguity produces which error in anatomic imaging?
a. range too long
b. range too short
c. intensity too high
d. Doppler shift too high
e. Doppler shift too low

36. If a pulse is emitted 65 μs after the previous one, echoes returning from beyond ___________ cm will produce range ambiguity.
a. 1
b. 2
c. 3
d. 4
e. 5

37. If the maximum imaging depth is 5 cm, the frequency is 2 MHz, and the Doppler angle is zero, what is the maximum flow speed that will avoid aliasing and range ambiguity?
a. 100 cm/s
b. 200 cm/s
c. 300 cm/s
d. 400 cm/s
e. 500 cm/s

38. Solving aliasing by decreasing operating frequency increases the possibility of range-ambiguity artifact. True or false?

39. If operating frequency is increased to decrease the possibility of range ambiguity (by increasing attenuation), the possibility of aliasing increases. True or false?

40. If a pulsed-wave Doppler sample volume is located at a depth of 8 cm, the sampled echoes arrive at what time following the emission of the pulse?
a. 25 μs
b. 50 μs
c. 75 μs
d. 104 μs
e. 117 μs

41. In Exercise 40, if the PRF is set at 11 kHz, a second gate would be located at what depth?
a. 1 cm
b. 2 cm
c. 3 cm
d. 4 cm
e. 5 cm

42. Connect the dots (samples) in Fig. 7.45 to determine the Doppler shift frequency. How many cycles are in each example?
a. ___________
b. ___________
c. ___________
d. ___________
e. ___________

43. The frequencies that were sampled in Exercise 42 are shown in Fig. 7.46. In which example(s) has aliasing occurred?

44. Which of the following instruments can produce aliasing?
a. continuous-wave Doppler
b. pulsed-wave Doppler
c. duplex
d. color Doppler
e. more than one of the above

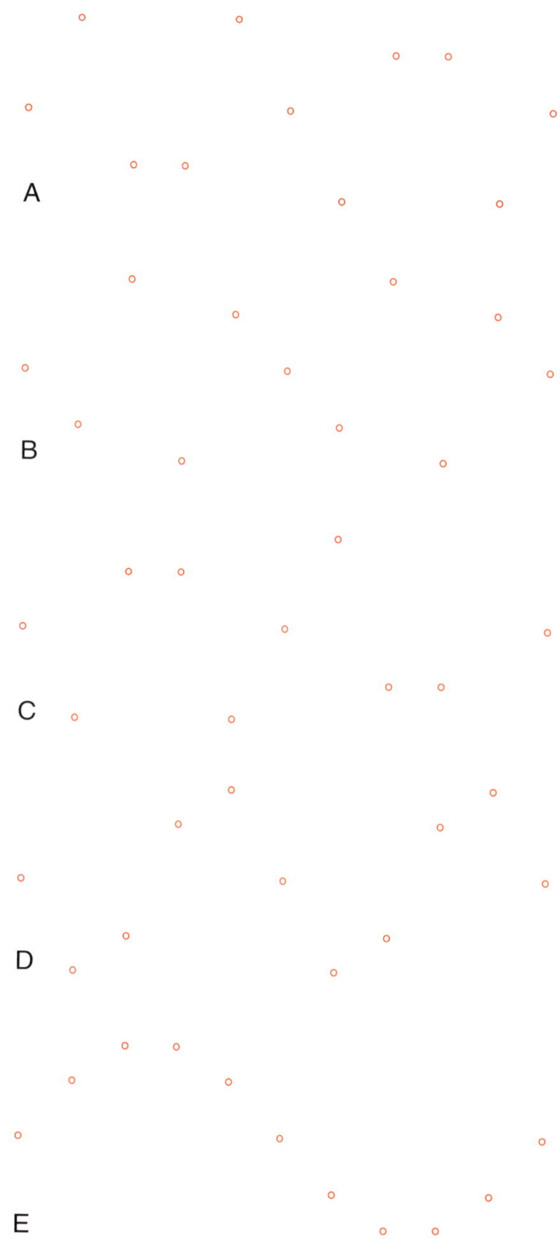

Fig. 7.45 **A–E**, Illustrations to accompany Exercise 42.

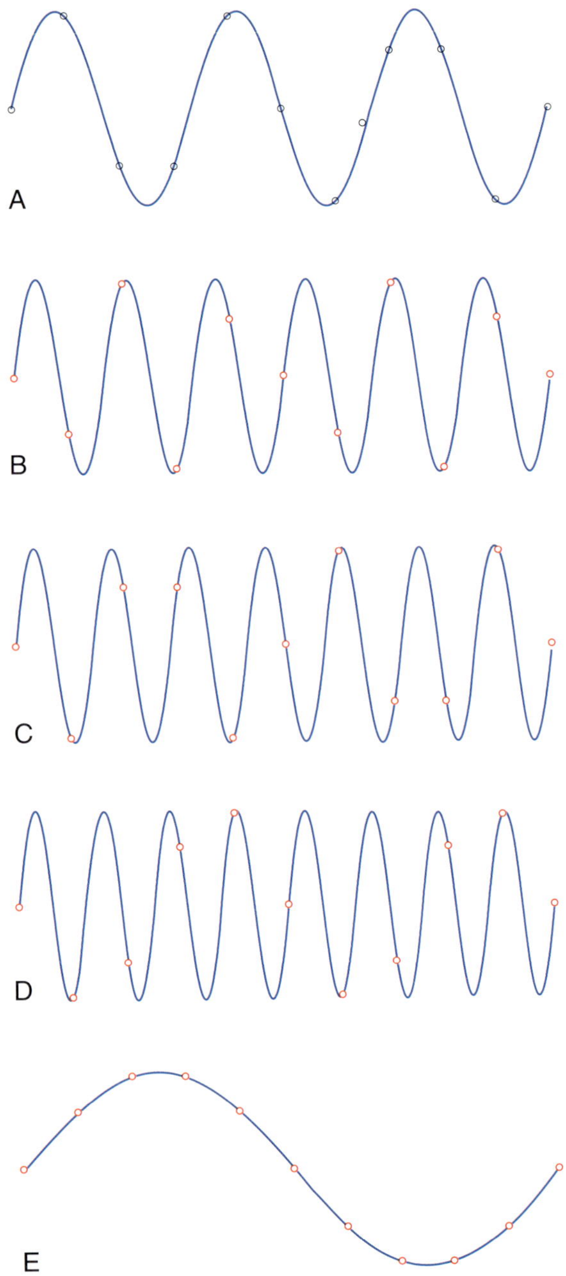

Fig. 7.46 A–E, Illustrations to accompany Exercise 43.

45. In Fig. 7.47, the solid line shows the Doppler shift. The dashed line shows the ______________ result of connecting samples of the shift. To avoid aliasing in this signal, at least __________ samples would be required.
 a. correct, 5
 b. correct, 10
 c. aliased, 5
 d. aliased, 10

46. In Fig. 7.48 (R, red; B, blue), assume the color bar shown in G and give the direction of blood flow (R for from right to the left; L for from left to the right) in each case.

47. Fig. 7.49 shows five regions of different colors in the flow. Match each of the following with the proper region.

a. _____	**1.** 90 degree Doppler angle
b. _____	**2.** Unaliased flow toward
c. _____	**3.** Unaliased flow away
d. _____	**4.** Aliased flow toward
e. _____	**5.** Aliased flow away

48. Which part of Fig. 7.50 shows a power Doppler display?
 a. A
 b. B
 c. C
 d. D

49. Referring to Fig. 7.50, B–D, what is the order of Fig. parts when they are arranged according to increasing flow speed?
 a. B, C, D
 b. D, C, B
 c. C, B, D
 d. B, D, C

50. What artifact appears in all parts of Fig. 7.50? What is the additional artifact that appears in Fig. 7.50,D?
 a. shadowing, aliasing
 b. aliasing, shadowing
 c. enhancement, shadowing
 d. enhancement, aliasing

51. At what MI values are microbubbles likely to start being destroyed resulting in which artifact?
 a. 0.2, near field enhancement
 b. 0.7, near field signal loss
 c. 0.4, near field signal loss
 d. 0.3, near field enhancement

52. Pseudo enhancement can be caused by _____ or _____.
 a. hypoechoic tissues, excessive contrast bubbles
 b. hyperechoic tissues, excessive contrast bubbles
 c. hypoechoic tissues, lack of contrast bubbles
 d. hyperechoic tissues, lack of contrast bubbles

53. Attenuation in CEUS examinations can be resolved by increasing the MI. True or false?

54. The Doppler shift increase in Fig. 7.43A is _____ which is _____.
 a. 1 kHz, trivial
 b. 25%, trivial
 c. 1 kHz, not trivial
 d. 33%, not trivial

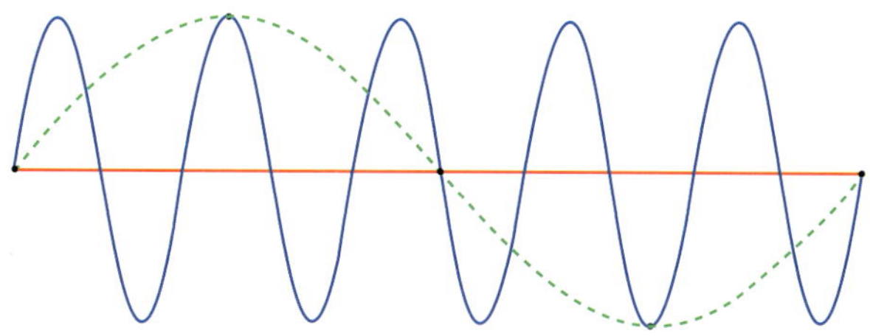

Fig. 7.47 Illustration to accompany Exercise 45.

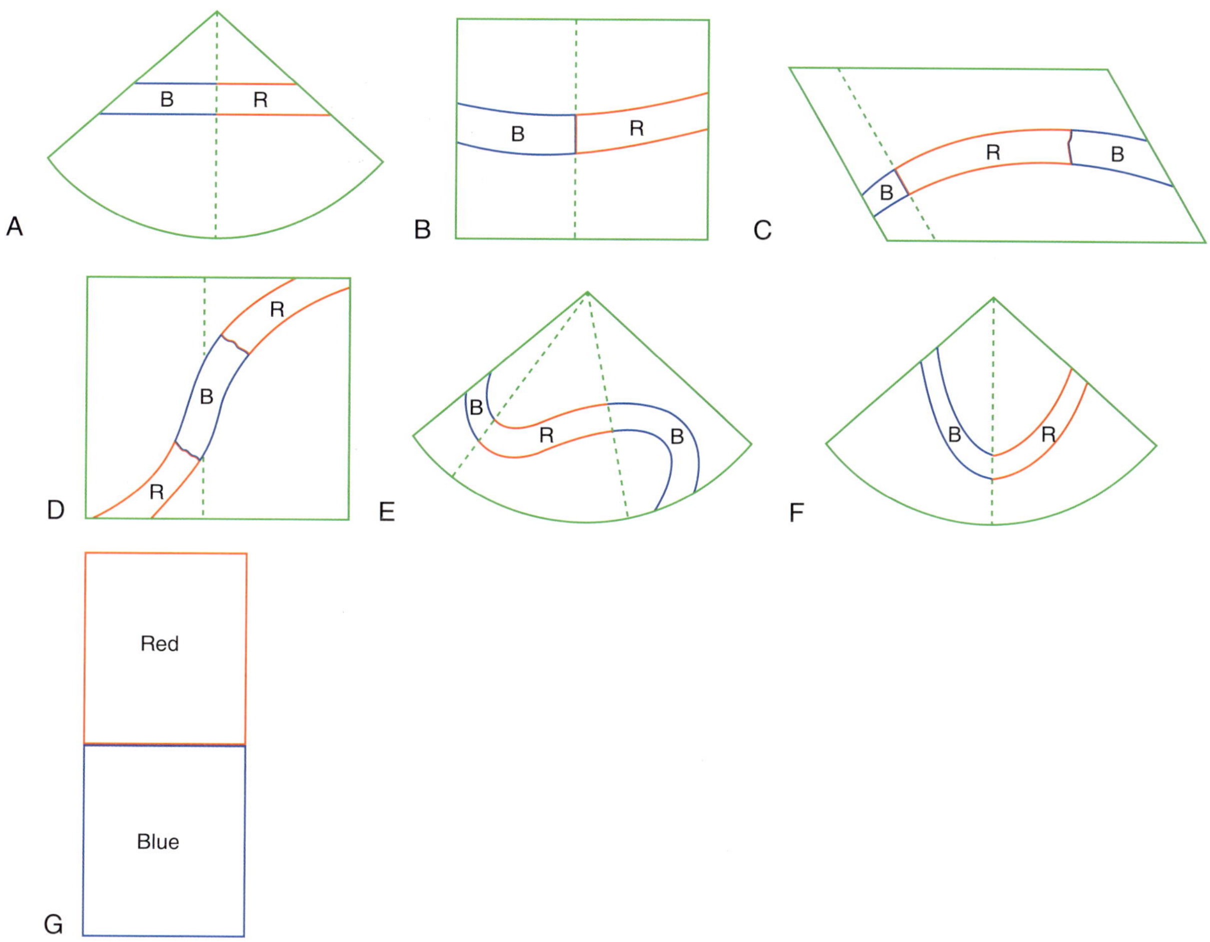

Fig. 7.48 A–G, Illustrations to accompany Exercise 46. (From Kremkau FW: Is it coming or going? Color flow interpretation, *J Vasc Technol* 18:365–366, 1994.)

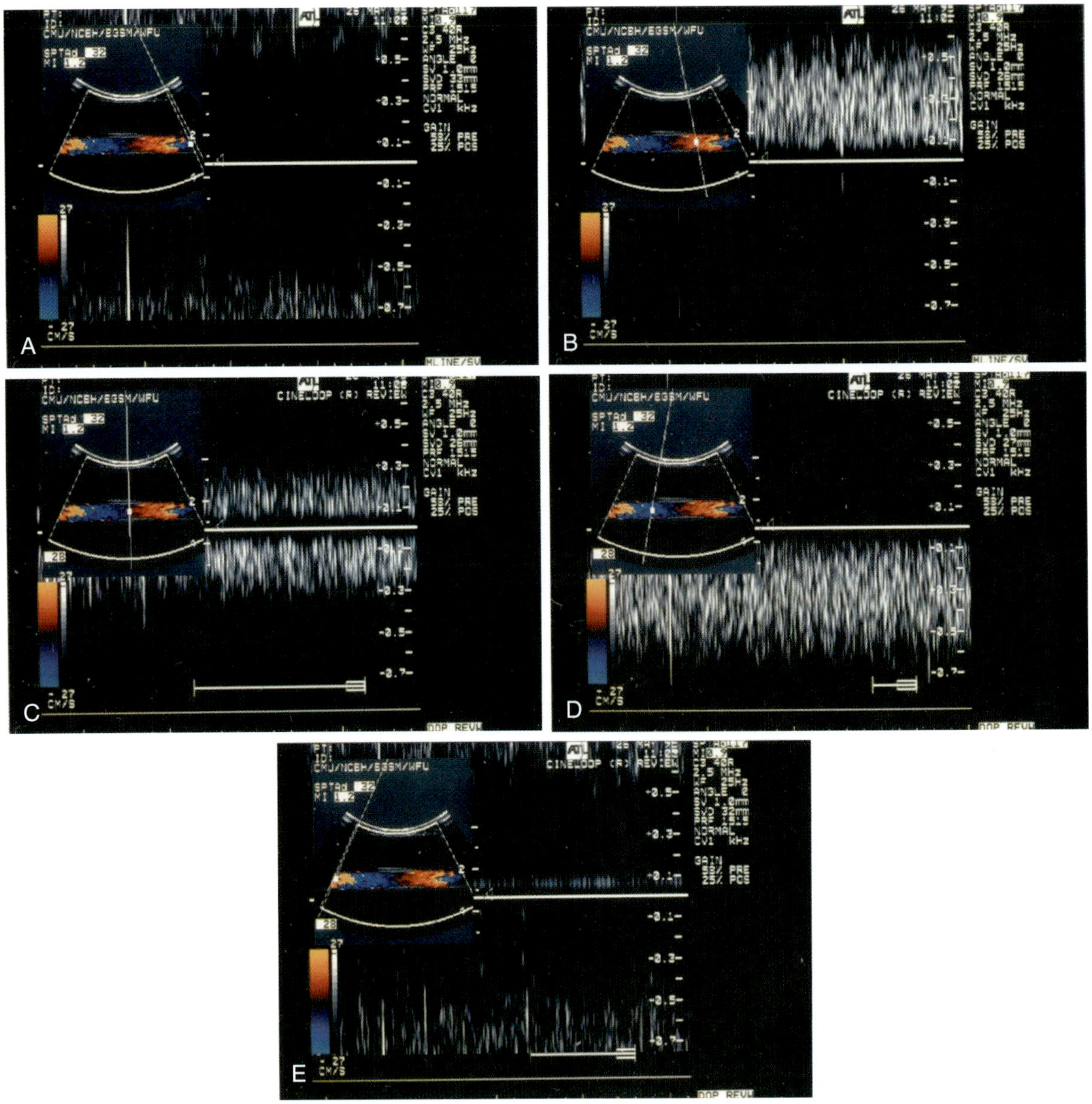

Fig. 7.49 **A–E**, Illustrations to accompany Exercise 47.

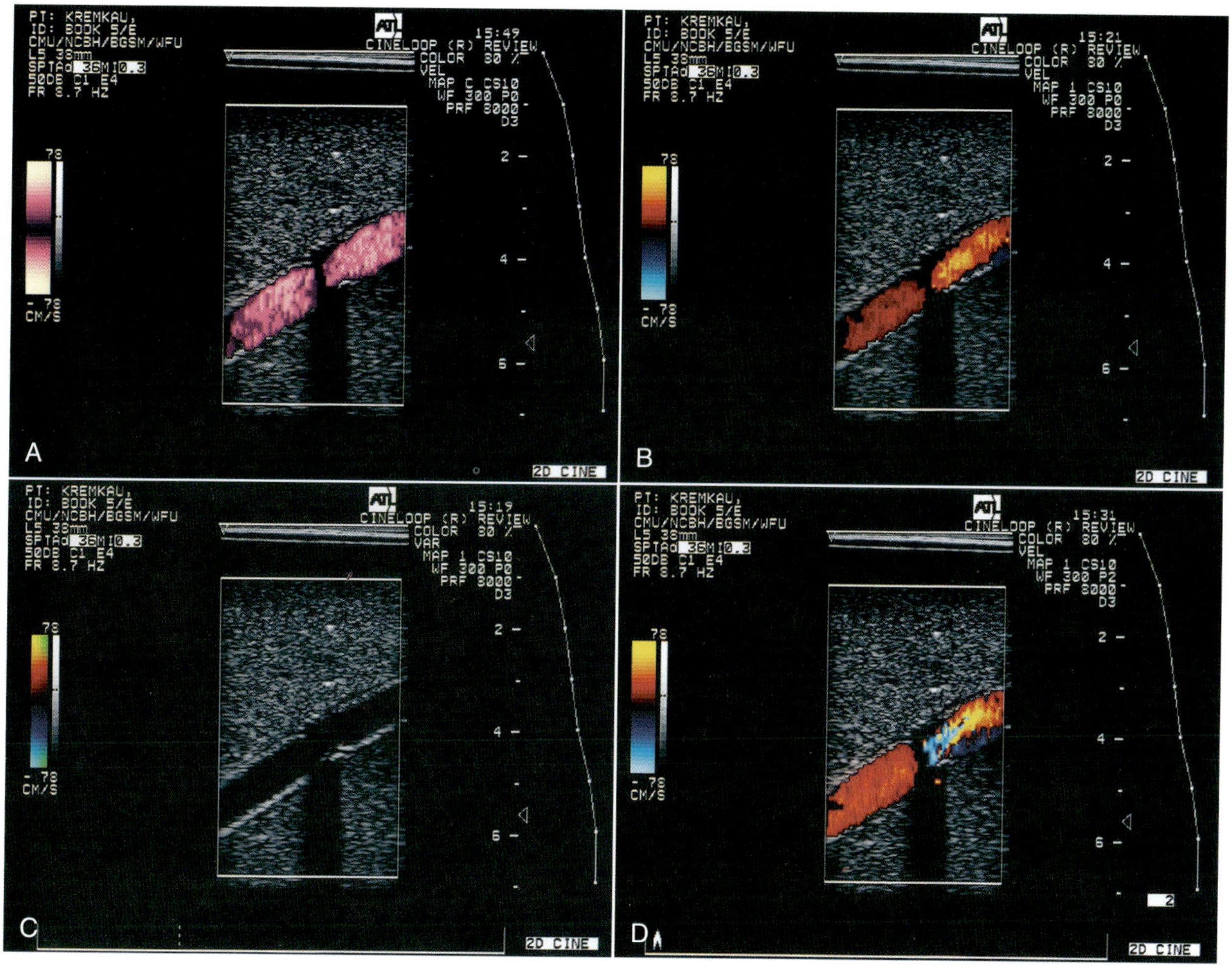

Fig. 7.50 A–D, Illustrations to accompany Exercises 48–50.

55. The key to understanding the CEUS attenuation artifact is to always compare the area of interest to normal tissue at the same depths. If the level of enhancement is the same, then it should be ignored. True or false?

8

Quality Assurance

LEARNING OBJECTIVES

After reading this chapter, the student should be able to do the following:

- Explain how to determine whether an ultrasound scanner is working properly.
- List the devices that are available to test various system performance characteristics.
- Compare a test object to a phantom.
- Describe how instrument output is measured.

CHAPTER OUTLINE

KEY TERMS

Hydrophone
Phantom
Quality assurance (QA)
Quality control
Test object

Now that we have covered the principles of grayscale and Doppler ultrasound and the artifacts that can (and occasionally do) occur, we turn to the performance of ultrasound systems. How are the performance characteristics of a modern digital ultrasound scanner and its acoustic outputs measured? What are the requirements and what are the practical implications?

Several devices (Fig. 8.1) are available to determine whether grayscale and Doppler ultrasound instruments are operating correctly and consistently. These devices can be divided into two groups:

1. Those that measure the acoustic output of the instrument. This group evaluates the beam former and the transducer acting together as a source of ultrasound. The acoustic output of a scanner is important when considering bioeffects, risk, and safety.
2. Those that test the operation of the instrument (anatomical imaging and flow evaluation performance). This group takes into account the operation of the entire instrument. Imaging and Doppler performance are important when evaluating a scanner as a diagnostic tool.

There are also specialty phantoms available, for example, for prostate scanning, biopsy training, or for evaluating elastography (phantoms with known stiffness for the background and possibly various inclusions).

PERFORMANCE MEASUREMENTS

Imaging performance is determined primarily by measuring the following parameters:

1. Monitor setup (on the scanner and the PACS system)
2. Image uniformity
3. Depth of penetration
4. Accuracy of distance measurements
5. Detail resolution
6. Contrast resolution
7. Time-gain-compensation
8. Dynamic range
9. Accuracy of spectral Doppler sample volume location
10. Accuracy of Doppler flow speed measurements

Among these parameters, items 1 to 3 or 4 are typically considered mandatory, while items 5 to 10 are (almost always) optional. Notice that this list does not include any mandatory Doppler performance tests.

Several devices are commercially available to test imaging performance. These devices fall into two categories: (1) tissue-equivalent **phantoms** and (2) **test objects**. Tissue-equivalent phantoms have some characteristics representative of tissues (such as scattering and attenuation properties); test objects do not. Some devices are combinations of the two (e.g., tissue-equivalent phantoms that contain resolution targets). The American Institute of Ultrasound in Medicine (AIUM) Practice Accreditation Program and the American College of Radiology Ultrasound Accreditation Program both require that routine **quality control** testing must occur regularly. The AIUM has published a manual on **quality assurance (QA)**, which is available for purchase.

A comprehensive QA program is comprised of daily tasks undertaken by instrument operators (i.e., sonographers and/or radiologists) as well as more infrequent testing conducted on a monthly or annual basis by a medical physicist, a biomedical engineer, or a sonographer with training in QA. Daily tasks are mainly focused on visible damage to the transducers or cables

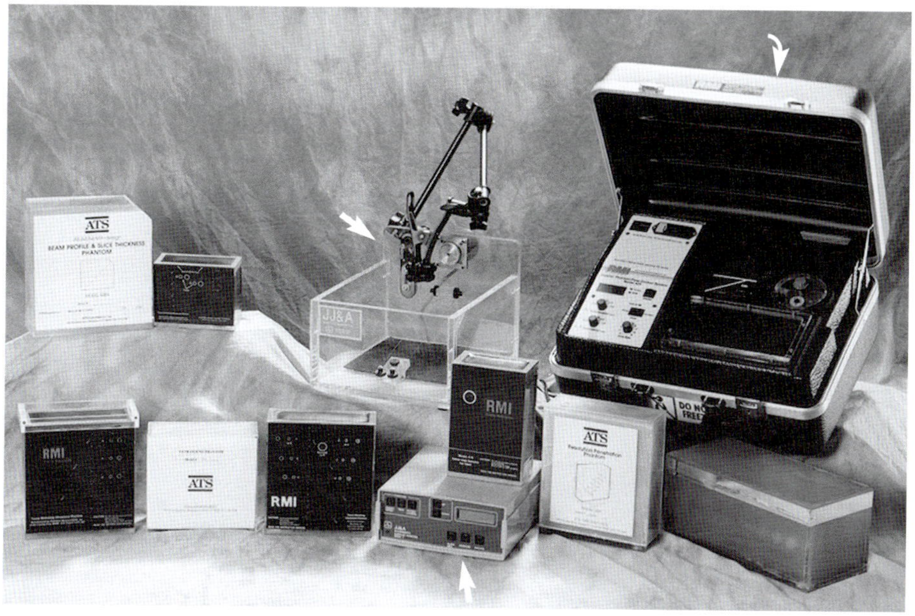

Fig. 8.1 Several test objects and phantoms. Those intended for Doppler applications are indicated by arrows. The other devices are used to evaluate imaging performance. Even though this is an older photo, it should be noted that all of these devices are still commercially available in 2025.

including element drop-out, while more infrequent assessments using phantoms (or test objects) evaluate image display and scanner (grayscale) performance.

Grayscale Tissue-Equivalent Phantoms and Test Objects

Tissue-equivalent phantoms are typically made of graphite-filled aqueous gels or urethane rubber materials. Graphite particles act as ultrasound scatterers in the materials. Graphite is the soft carbon that is used in pencils and as a lubricant. Attenuation and propagation speed in these materials are similar to those of soft tissue (i.e., around 0.5 dB/(cm MHz) and approximately 1540 m/s or 1.54 mm/μs). Tissue-equivalent phantoms typically contain echo-free (cystic) regions of various diameters and thin nylon lines (approximately 0.2 mm in diameter) to allow detail resolution and distance accuracy to be measured. Some phantoms contain cones or cylinders containing material of various scattering strengths (various graphite concentrations) that are hyperechoic or hypoechoic compared with the surrounding material. Figs. 8.2 to 8.5 show examples of several phantoms and the most common mandatory measurements performed in a QA program.

> Tissue-equivalent phantoms simulate tissue properties, allowing assessment of image uniformity and penetration as well as detail and contrast resolutions, dynamic range, and time-gain-compensation operation.

Test objects do not simulate tissue characteristics but do provide some specific measure of instrument performance (e.g., detail resolution or beam profiles); as such they are less versatile. The beam-profile slice-thickness test object (Fig. 8.6) contains a thin, scattering layer in an echo-free material. The object can be used to show beam width in the scan plane or perpendicular to it (section thickness). This is only relevant for traditional narrow transmit beam systems and is meaningless for broad transmit beam systems.

Doppler Tissue-Equivalent Phantoms and Test Objects

Tissue- and blood-mimicking phantoms are commercially available for the evaluation of Doppler instruments (Figs. 8.7 and 8.8). While these devices are useful for testing the ability to discriminate between different flow directions, the accuracy of sample volume location, and the accuracy of the measured flow speeds, they are not typically part of a modern QA program. Doppler flow phantoms pump a flowing blood-mimicking liquid around. They can be calibrated for speed and can produce pulsatile as well as reverse flow conditions.

These phantoms are calibrated with an electromagnetic flow meter or by fluid volume collection over time. Doppler test objects use a moving solid object (usually a string) for scattering the ultrasound but are rarely used these days. Refer to Fig. 5.25, which illustrates the use of a flow phantom in determining the accuracy of the gate location indicator on the grayscale display.

> Doppler flow phantoms enable calibration of speed measurements and the evaluation of spectral Doppler gate location and the penetration of spectral and color Doppler beams.

OUTPUT MEASUREMENTS

Several devices can measure the acoustic output of ultrasound instruments. These devices are used by engineers and physicists rather than by sonographers and radiologists. Only the

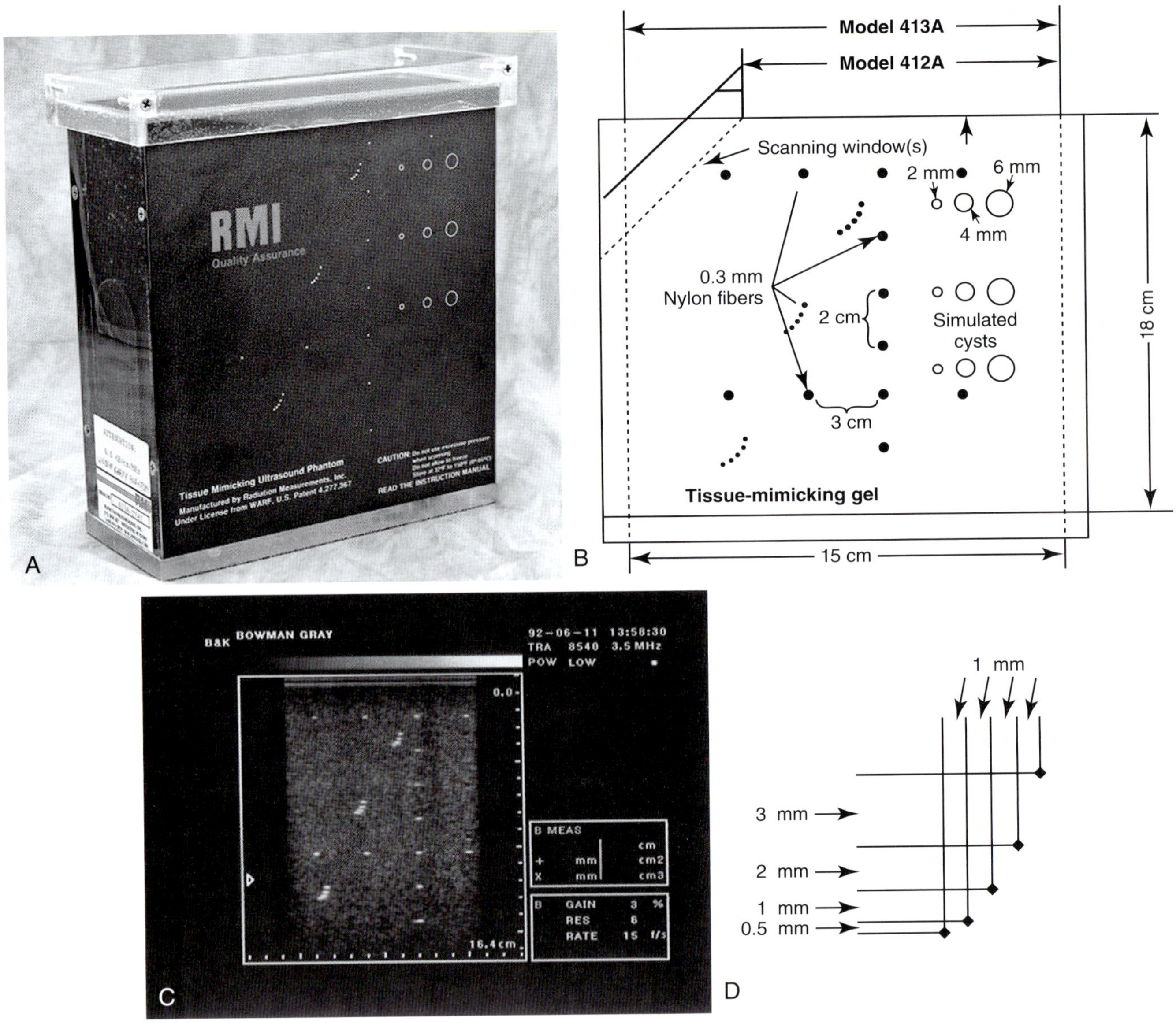

Fig. 8.2 A, A tissue-equivalent phantom containing groups of nylon lines and cystic regions of various sizes. **B,** Diagram detailing the construction of such a phantom. **C,** Scan of a phantom. **D,** Arrangement of the axial resolution line set in this phantom.

hydrophone is discussed here. The hydrophone is sometimes called a *microprobe*. It is used in two configurations (Figs. 8.9 and 8.10):

1. A small transducer element (with a diameter of ≤1 mm) mounted on the end of a hollow needle (i.e., a *needle hydrophone*)

A large piezoelectric membrane with small metallic electrodes centered on both sides (i.e., a *membrane hydrophone*)

Various construction approaches, not considered here, are used for hydrophones. Hydrophones receive sound reasonably well from all directions without altering the sound by their presence. In response to the varying sound pressures, they produce a varying voltage that can be displayed on an oscilloscope. This produces a picture from which period, pulse-repetition period, and pulse duration can be determined. From these quantities, frequency, pulse-repetition frequency, and duty factor can be calculated. Using a calibrated hydrophone (the relationship between measured voltage and acoustic pressure has been verified across the frequency bandwidth of the hydrophone using a reference standard), pressure amplitude may also be determined. In addition, wavelength, spatial pulse length, and intensities can be calculated as well.

With the use of hydrophones, acoustic pressure output levels have been measured, and intensities have been calculated for various diagnostic ultrasound instruments and transducers. Generally, grayscale imaging outputs are the lowest, and spectral Doppler outputs are the highest, with M-mode and color Doppler imaging outputs falling between the two.

> Needle and membrane hydrophones are used to measure pressure amplitude and period, from which several other acoustic pulse parameters can be calculated.

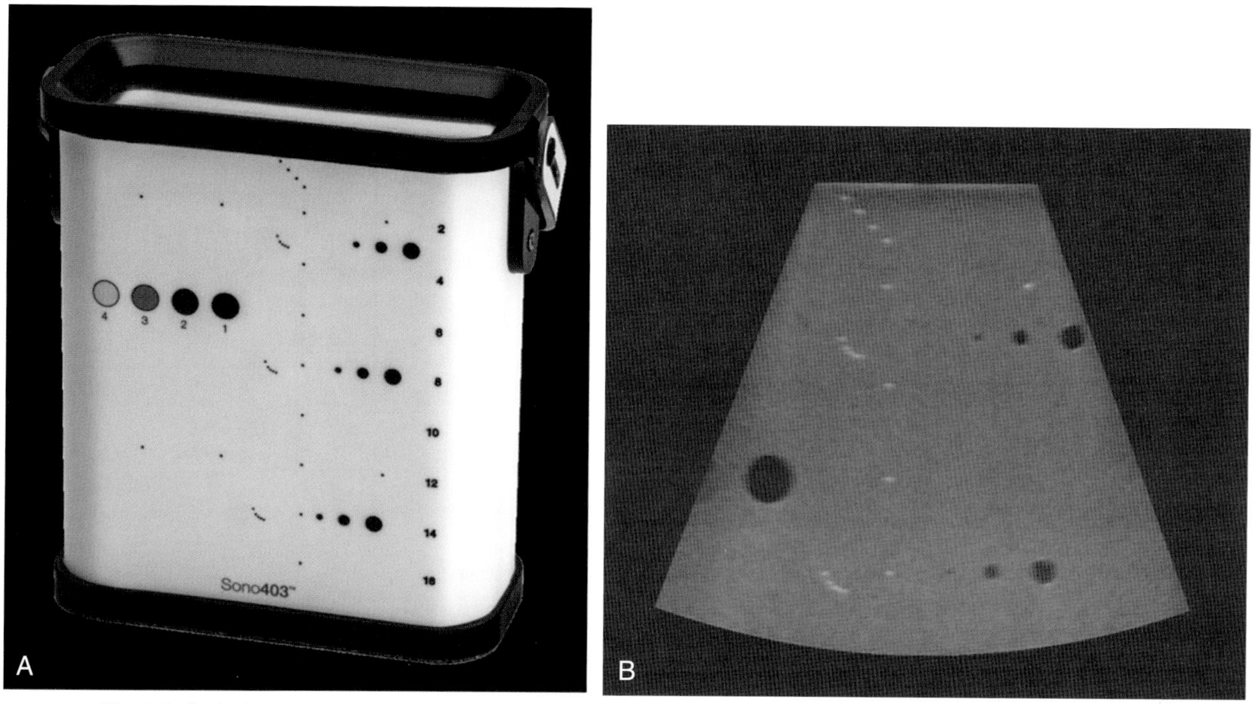

Fig. 8.3 **A,** A tissue-equivalent phantom containing nylon lines (for resolution and distance accuracy measurements), simulated cysts, and hyperechoic-simulated lesions of various sizes. **B,** Scan of this phantom. (Courtesy Sun Nuclear.)

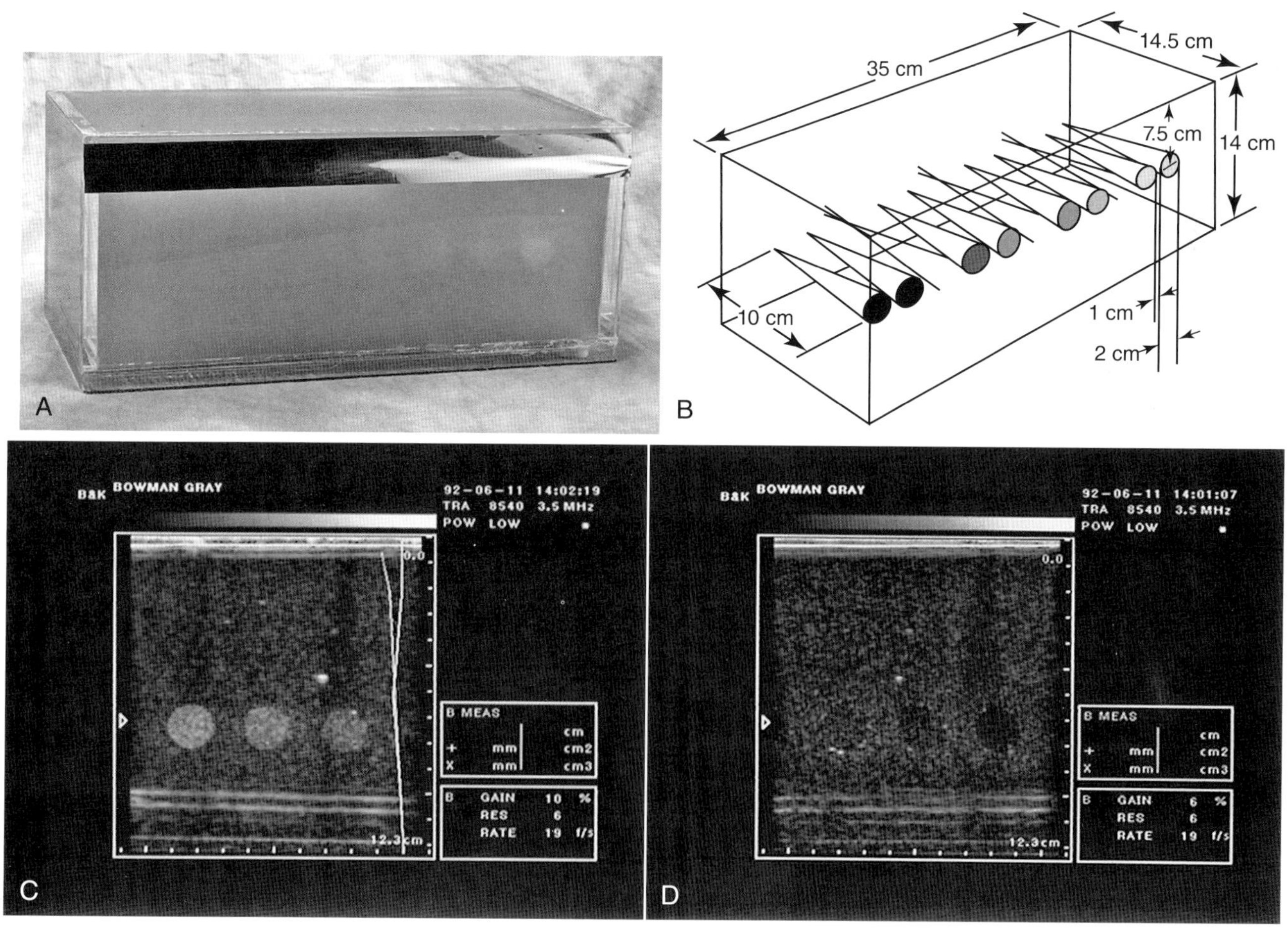

Fig. 8.4 **A,** A contrast-detail phantom containing cones of material of various echogenicities. **B,** Diagram detailing the construction of such a phantom. **C,** Scan of hyperechoic sections of phantom. **D,** Scan of hypoechoic sections of phantom.

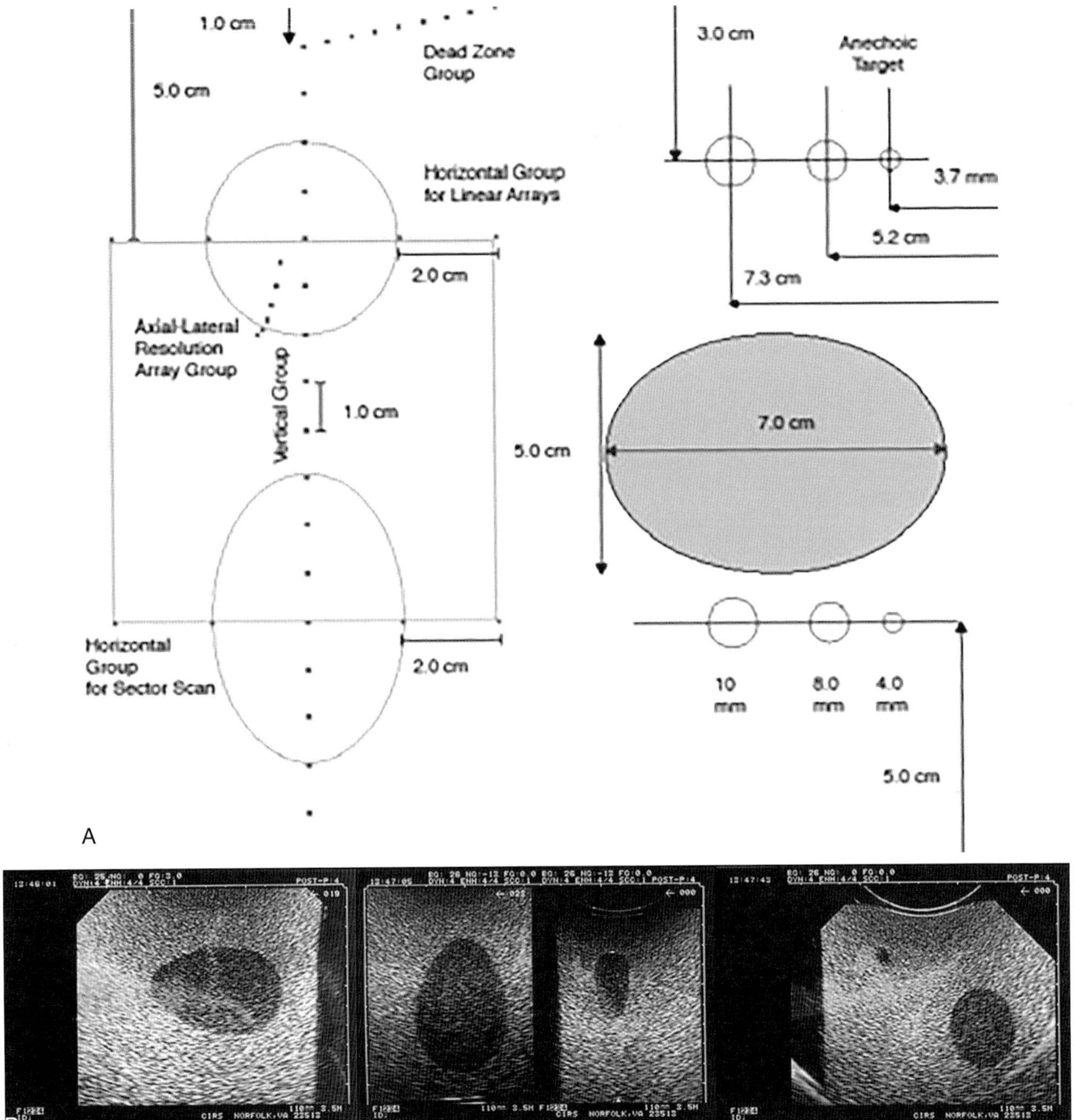

Fig. 8.5 **A,** Construction diagram for a 3D calibration phantom for the assessment of volumetric measurement accuracy. **B,** Images obtained by scanning a 3D calibration phantom. (**A,** Courtesy Sun Nuclear.)

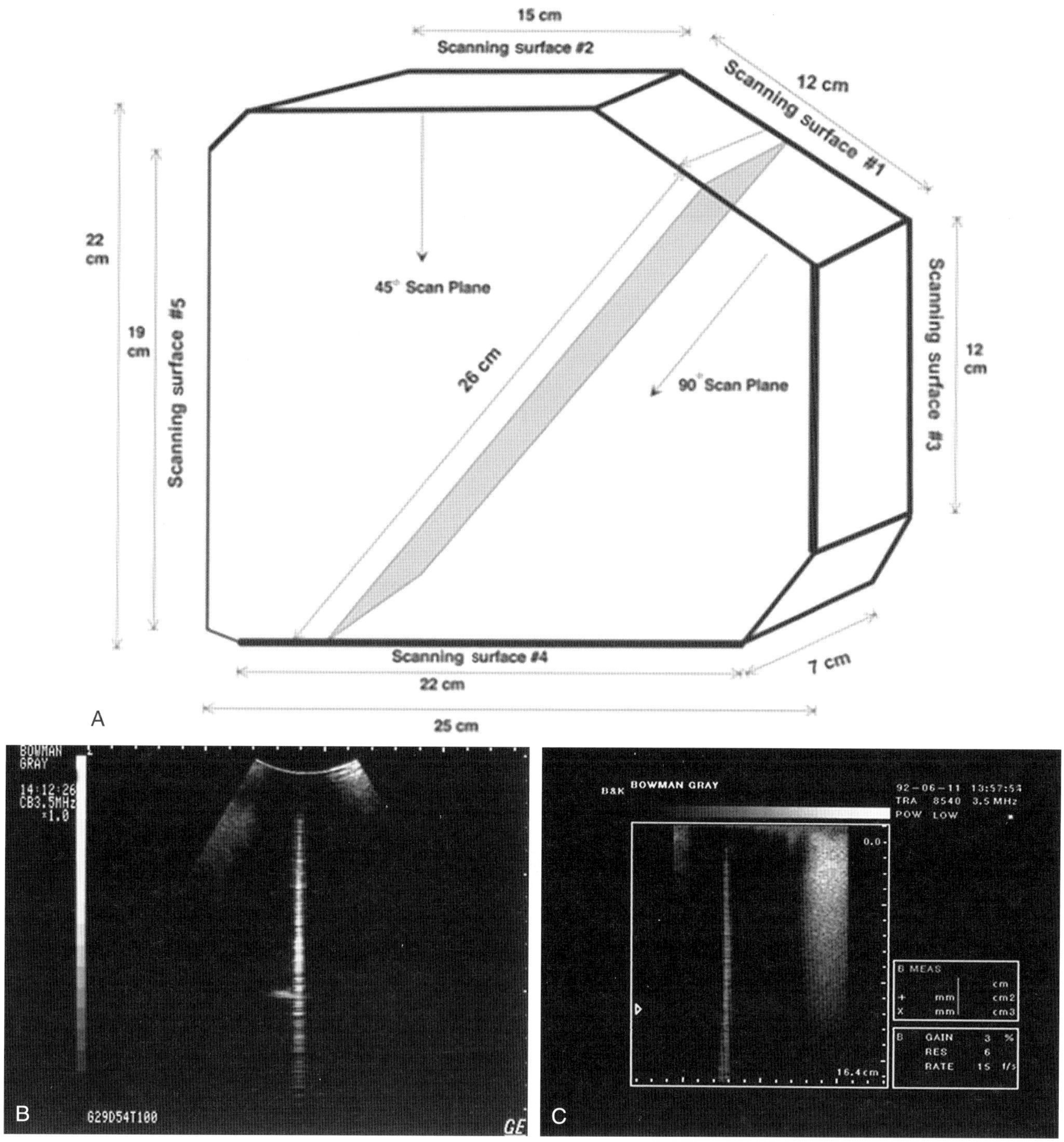

Fig. 8.6 **A,** Schematic of a beam profile and section thickness test object. It contains a thin, scattering layer in an anechoic material. This phantom is only useful for narrow transmit beam scanners. **B–C,** Scans of beam profiles. Shown in Figure 3.12, C is a beam profile obtained using this test object. (**A,** Courtesy Sun Nuclear.)

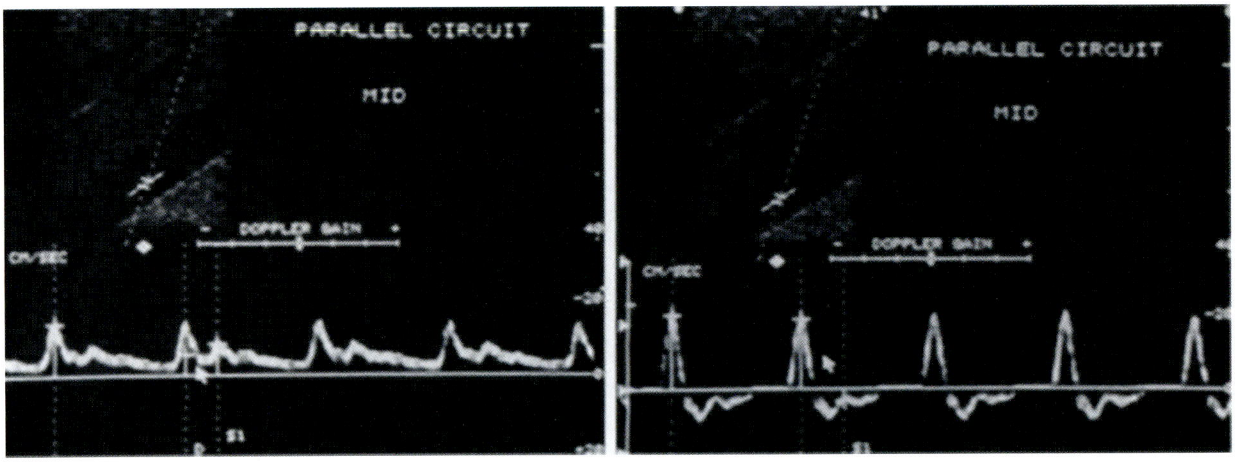

Fig. 8.7 Two examples of spectral displays from a pump operating in pulsatile mode. (From *Halpern EJ, et al: Effect of distal resistance on Doppler US flow patterns, Radiology 206:761–766, 1998.*)

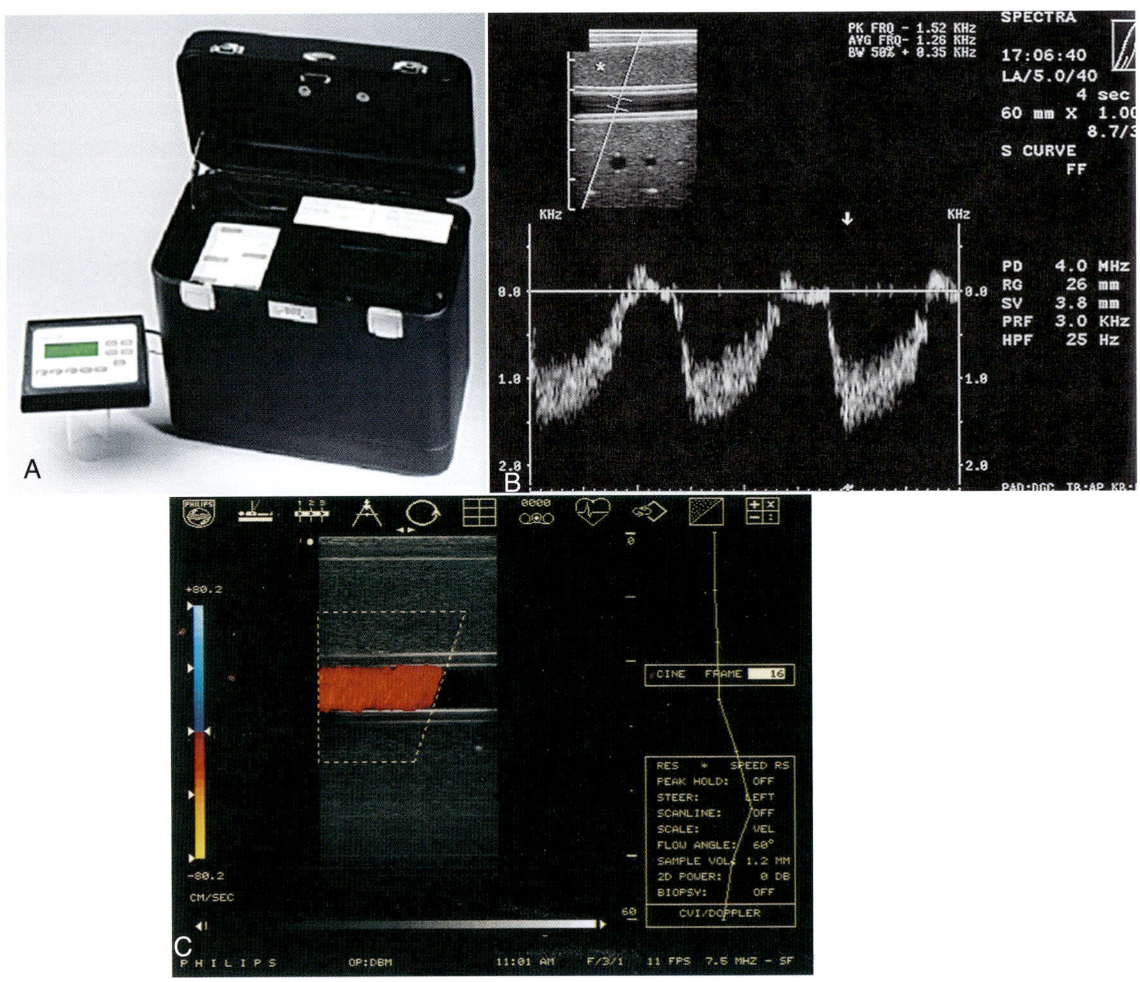

Fig. 8.8 **A,** Doppler flow phantom. **B,** Spectral display from a flow phantom. **C,** Color Doppler image from a flow phantom.

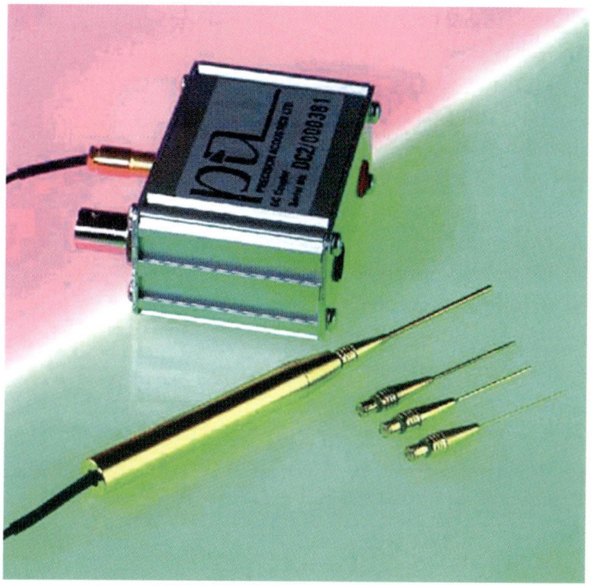

Fig. 8.9 A hydrophone consisting of a small transducer element mounted on the end of a needle.

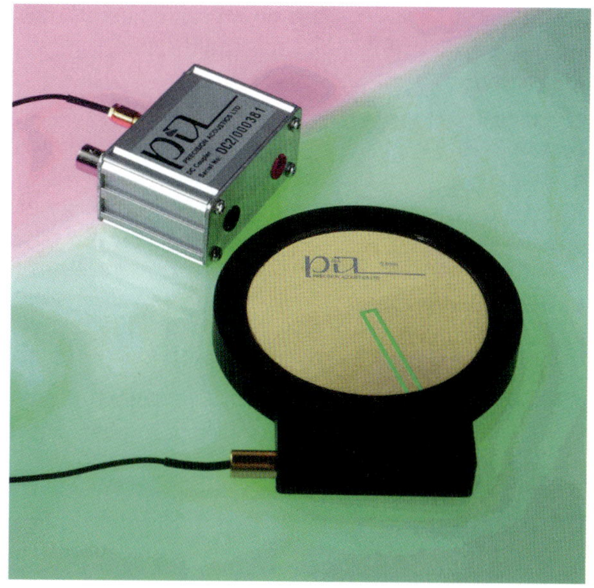

Fig. 8.10 A hydrophone consisting of a thin membrane with metal electrodes.

REVIEW

The following key points are presented in this chapter:

- Phantoms (and test objects) provide means for measuring monitor setup, image uniformity, depth of penetration, and the accuracy of distance measurements of ultrasound scanners.
- Other parameters such as detail resolution, compensation, sensitivity, and dynamic range can also be determined.
- Doppler flow phantoms are used to evaluate Doppler system performance.
- Hydrophones are used to measure the acoustic output of sonographic instruments.

EXERCISES

Answers appear in the Answers to Exercises section at the back of the book.

1. A tissue-equivalent ___________ has an attenuation of approximately 0.5 dB/(cm MHz) and a propagation speed of 1.54 mm/μs. A ___________ does not mimic tissue but provides a means for measuring some aspect of instrument performance.
   a. phantom, test object
   b. hydrophone, phantom
   c. transducer, phantom
   d. transducer, test object
2. Match the parameters measured with the items used (answers may be used more than once):
   1. nylon fibers
   2. attenuating scattering material
   3. simulated cysts
   4. hyperechoic- and hypoechoic-simulated lesions
   5. thin scattering layer
      a. axial resolution
      b. lateral resolution
      c. range accuracy
      d. caliper accuracy
      e. contrast resolution
      f. compensation
      g. sensitivity
      h. dynamic range
      i. beam profile
      j. section thickness
3. Match the parameters measured with the correlating types of observation modes (answers may be used more than once):
   1. gain settings
   2. deepest scattering material imaged
   3. fiber distances from the transducer or from each other on the display
   4. minimum spacing of separately displayed fibers
   5. lateral smearing of fibers
      a. axial resolution
      b. lateral resolution
      c. range accuracy
      d. caliper accuracy
      e. compensation
      f. sensitivity
      g. dynamic range
4. Test objects and phantoms are available commercially. True or false?
5. Test objects and phantoms can be used by the instrument operator. True or false?

6. A moving __________ test object can be useful in checking the accuracy of Doppler spectral displays.
   a. spectral
   b. string
   c. water
   d. fluid
7. A __________ phantom is useful in simulating physiologic __________ conditions for a Doppler instrument.
   a. tissue, flow
   b. flow, equilibrium
   c. tissue, equilibrium
   d. flow, flow
8. Which of the following is used for Doppler sensitivity measurements?
   a. cyst phantom
   b. profile test object
   c. string test object
   d. contrast phantom
   e. none of the above
9. Tissue-equivalent phantoms attempt to represent some acoustic property of __________.
   a. tissues
   b. blood
   c. cancer
   d. skin
10. The string test object measures volumetric flow rate. True or false?
11. With use of a hydrophone, which of the following can be measured or calculated? (There is more than one correct answer.)
    a. impedance
    b. amplitude
    c. period
    d. pulse duration
    e. pulse-repetition period
12. All hydrophones consist of a small element mounted on the end of a needle. True or false?
13. A needle hydrophone contains a small __________ element.
    a. transducer
    b. piezoelectric
    c. neither a nor b
    d. both a and b
14. Because of its small size, a hydrophone can measure spatial details of a sound beam. True or false?
15. A hydrophone __________.
    a. interacts with light
    b. produces a voltage
    c. measures intensity directly
    d. measures total energy
    e. none of the above
16. Match the items in column A with those in B and C (answers may be used more than once). (Note: Items in A can be calculated from B if C is known.)

    A.
    a. frequency: __________, __________
    b. pulse-repetition frequency: __________, __________
    c. duty factor: __________, __________
    d. wavelength: __________, __________
    e. spatial pulse length: __________, __________
    f. energy: __________, __________
    g. intensity: __________, __________

    B.
    1. wavelength
    2. period
    3. pulse-repetition period
    4. frequency
    5. energy
    6. power

    C.
    7. number of cycles in the pulse
    8. pulse duration
    9. propagation speed
    10. exposure time
    11. beam area
    12. nothing else

9

Safety Considerations

LEARNING OBJECTIVES

After reading this chapter, the student should be able to do the following:

- Explain what is known about bioeffects in cells, animals, and humans.
- Describe what is known about risk in the use of grayscale or Doppler ultrasound.
- Explain how an operator of an ultrasound scanner can implement the as low as reasonably achievable (ALARA) principle by minimizing patient exposure to ultrasound during scanning.

CHAPTER OUTLINE

KEY TERMS

ALARA
Cavitation
Contrast-enhanced ultrasound (CEUS)
Food and Drug Administration (FDA)
Inertial cavitation
Mechanical index
Nonthermal bioeffects
Output display standard (ODS)
Pulmonary capillary hemorrhage
Radiation force
Shear wave elastography (SWE)
Stable cavitation
Thermal bioeffects
Thermal index

In this chapter, we consider two important topics:

1. The bioeffects that can be caused by ultrasound
2. Risk and safety considerations in the use of diagnostic ultrasound scanners

Bioeffects are useful in the therapeutic applications of ultrasound and can be increased by the use of ultrasound contrast agents (under the right imaging settings). The main interest of this chapter is what is known about the bioeffects of ultrasound, and what that indicates about the safety or risk of diagnostic ultrasound. Knowing about the probability of damage or injury and under what imaging conditions this risk is maximized (to avoid those conditions) or minimized (to seek out those conditions), while still obtaining useful diagnostic information. In practice, this tends to be more of a balancing act between the two extremes.

BIOEFFECTS

The biologic effects and safety of diagnostic ultrasound have received considerable attention over the years. Review articles, meta-analyses, textbooks, and institutional documents have been published. Comprehensive, authoritative publications and official statements have been produced by the Bioeffects Committee of the American Institute of Ultrasound in Medicine (AIUM).

In this chapter, knowledge regarding reported bioeffects in cells, and experimental animals as well as with newer imaging modes such as **contrast-enhanced ultrasound (CEUS)** imaging and **shear wave elastography (SWE)** are reviewed. Moreover, the mechanisms of interaction between ultrasound and biologic cells and tissues, regulatory activities, epidemiology, risk and safety considerations, and elements of prudent practice will be described.

As with any diagnostic test, there may be some risk, that is, some possibility of damage or injury, with the use of diagnostic ultrasound. This risk, if known, must be weighed against the benefit of the diagnosis being sought. Knowing how to minimize the risk, even if the risk is unknown, is useful for every healthcare professional involved in diagnostic ultrasound examinations. Sources of information used in developing policy regarding the use of diagnostic ultrasound are outlined in Fig. 9.1, A. These sources include (1) bioeffects data from experimental systems, (2) output data from diagnostic instruments, and (3) knowledge and experience with regard to how the diagnostic information obtained is beneficial for patient management. Comparison of the first two components allows an assessment of risk, whereas the combination of the latter two components yields a determination of the benefit. It seems reasonable to assume that there is some risk (however small) in the use of diagnostic ultrasound, because ultrasound is a form of energy and has at least the potential to produce a biologic effect

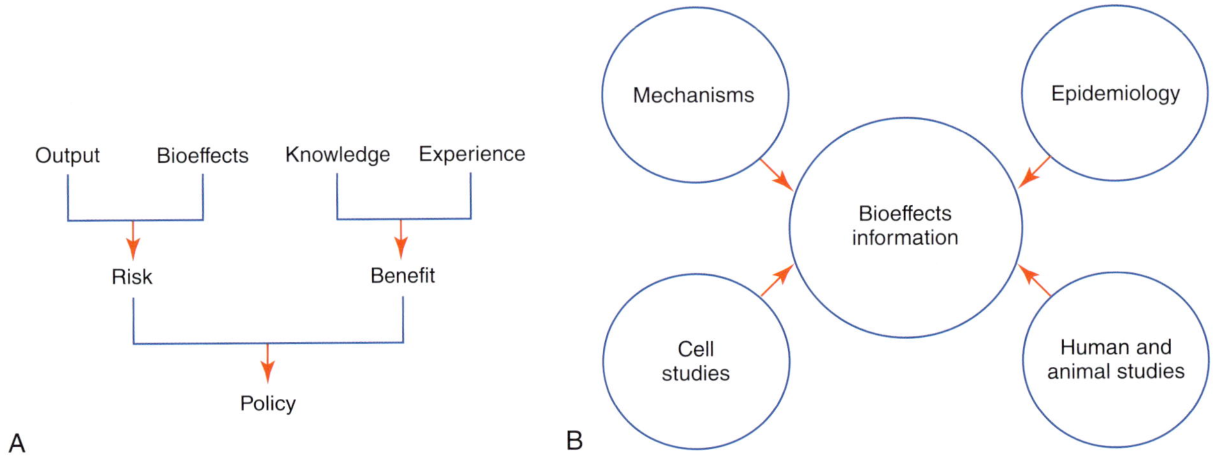

Fig. 9.1 A, Ultrasound risk and benefit information. Risk information comes from experimental bioeffects (including epidemiology) and instrument output data. Benefit information is derived from knowledge and experience in diagnostic ultrasound use and efficacy. Together, they lead to a policy on the prudent use of ultrasound imaging in medicine. **B,** Bioeffects information sources.

that could constitute risk. Even if this risk is so minimal that it is difficult to identify, prudent practice dictates that routine procedures be implemented to minimize risk, while allowing users to obtain the necessary information to achieve diagnostic benefits for patients. This is the ALARA (as low as reasonably achievable) principle of prudent scanning.

Our knowledge of bioeffects resulting from ultrasound exposure comes from several sources (see Fig. 9.1, B). These sources include experimental observations in cell suspensions and cultures as well as experimental animals; epidemiologic studies in human beings; and studies of interaction mechanisms including heating and cavitation in animals or humans (i.e., *in vivo*).

> Knowledge of bioeffects is important for the safe and prudent use of diagnostic ultrasound.

Cells

Because cells in suspension or culture are so different from those in the patient in a clinical environment, one should exercise the utmost restraint in extrapolating from in vitro results to clinical significance. Cellular studies are useful in determining mechanisms of interaction and guiding the design of experimental animal studies and epidemiologic studies. The AIUM issued the following statement (https://www.aium.org/resources/official-statements) on *in vitro* biological effects in 2019:

> *It is often difficult to evaluate reports of ultrasonically induced* in vitro *effects with respect to their clinical significance. An* in vitro *effect can be regarded as a real biological effect. However, the predominant physical and biological interactions and mechanisms involved in an* in vitro *effect may not pertain to the* in vivo *situation. ... Although [*in vitro *bioeffects] may have limited applicability to* in vivo *biological effects, such studies can disclose fundamental intercellular or intracellular effects of ultrasound. While it is valid for authors to place their results in context and to suggest further relevant investigations, reports which do more than that should be viewed with caution.*

Humans and Other Animals

In vivo experiments in animal models have reported effects such as fetal weight reduction, postpartum mortality, fetal abnormalities, tissue lesions, hind limb paralysis, blood flow stasis, wound repair enhancement, and tumor regression. However, many studies on fetal weight reduction in mice and rats have been performed, but all rat studies and several mouse studies yielded negative results. Focal lesion production is a well-documented bioeffect that has been observed over a wide range of intensity and exposure duration conditions (Fig. 9.2) but **ONLY** at more than 10× the Food and Drug Administration (FDA) limit for acoustic I_{SPTA} values (so >10× 720 mW/cm^2).

In 2019, the AIUM (https://www.aium.org/resources/official-statements) issued two statements on the biological effects of ultrasound in vivo; one general statement and one focused on tissues containing ultrasound contrast microbubbles. The former is quoted here in part:

> *Investigations involving laboratory mammals have contributed significantly to our understanding of ultrasonically induced biological effects in humans and the mechanisms that are most likely responsible. Adverse biological effects have been observed in some mammalian studies under conditions that may occur with diagnostic scanners.*

The mechanisms of action by which ultrasound could produce biologic effects can be divided into two groups: (1) heating (also called *thermal*) and (2) mechanical (also called *nonthermal*).

> Studies of *in vivo* bioeffects in animal models have established conditions under which thermal and nonthermal bioeffects occur. However, the translation of laboratory bioeffects findings to human clinical conditions is challenging.

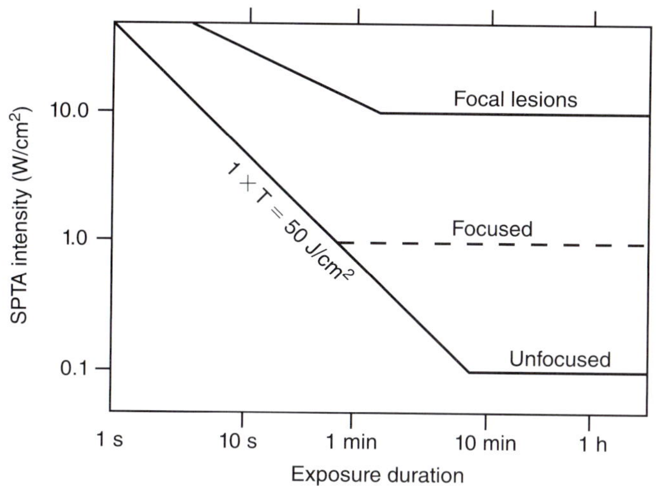

Fig. 9.2 Comparison of the minimum spatial peak-temporal average *(SPTA)* intensities required for ultrasonic bioeffects specified in the American Institute of Ultrasound in Medicine (AIUM) Statement on Mammalian Bioeffects. The minimum levels required for focal lesions also are shown in the figure for comparison. Note that logarithmic scaling has been used for the axes of this figure, so the horizontal lines are separated by factors of 10 in intensity. (From the American Institute of Ultrasound in Medicine: *Bioeffects and safety of diagnostic ultrasound*, 1993, Laurel.)

Heat

Attenuation is primarily caused by tissue absorption, that is, conversion of ultrasound to heat. Thus ultrasound can produce a temperature rise while it propagates through tissues , which in theory can produce **thermal bioeffects**. The extent of the temperature rise produced depends on the applied ultrasound intensity and frequency (because the absorption coefficient is approximately proportional to frequency) as well as on the degree of beam focusing and tissue perfusion. Heating increases when intensity or frequency is increased, which in turn means that heating effects decrease with increasing tissue depths because of the increased attenuation (that reduces the intensity at a given depth, especially at higher frequencies). Temperature rises are considered significant if they exceed 1.5°C. Intensities greater than a few hundred mW/cm^2 can produce such temperature rises. Absorption coefficients are higher in bone than they are in soft tissues, and bone heating, therefore, receives special consideration, particularly in the fetus.

Heating has been shown to be a consideration in some reports on bioeffects. Mathematic models have been developed for calculating temperature rises in tissues. Experimental measurements have shown somewhat reasonable agreement with these mathematical calculations (within a factor of 2). The biologic consequences of hyperthermia include fetal absorption or abortion, growth restriction, microphthalmia, cataract formation, abdominal wall defects, renal agenesis, palatal defects, reduction in brain waves, microencephaly, anencephaly, spinal cord defects, amyoplasia, forefoot hypoplasia, tibial and fibular deformations, and abnormal tooth genesis. Approximately 80 known biologic effects are attributed to hyperthermia. None have occurred at temperatures of less than 39°C. Above that, the occurrence of a biologic effect depends on temperature and exposure time. The 2021 AIUM Statement on Biological Effects of Ultrasound In Vivo (https://www.aium.org/resources/official-statements) indicates that even in fetal applications, temperature rises of 4°C will not induce adverse effects for dwell times at or below 2 minutes.

> Ultrasound is absorbed by tissue and thus produces a temperature rise. If critical time-temperature values are exceeded, tissue damage can occur (although this is very difficult to do in practice).

Mechanical

Nonthermal or mechanical **bioeffects** include **radiation force**, streaming, and cavitation. Radiation force is the force exerted by a sound beam, which can deform or disrupt cells. Radiation force can also cause flow in a fluid (i.e., streaming), which in turn can cause shear stresses that can also deform or disrupt cells. Some bioeffects observed in experimental animal studies have been attributed to these nonthermal mechanisms (that do not include cavitation).

So, what is **cavitation?** It is a phenomenon that may occur when a propagating sound wave of sufficiently high intensity interacts with gas bubbles within a liquid. Cavitation caused by ultrasound may produce gas bubbles spontaneously or may rely on gas bubbles already present in the liquid (such as gas microbubbles used as ultrasound contrast agents). There are two types of cavitation. **Stable cavitation** is the term used to describe bubbles that oscillate nonlinearly with the pressure variations of the sound wave, where the bubble expands more under lower pressures than it contracts under higher pressures. Local streaming and microjets can occur in the surrounding liquid in this situation, resulting in shear stresses on and membrane damage to endothelial cells and other cells in the vessel wall. **Inertial cavitation** occurs when bubble oscillations are so large that the bubble is destroyed (i.e., it collapses), which can produce shock waves with localized temperature increases (that can be extremely high) and even light emissions in clear liquids. Inertial cavitation has the potential for inducing significant bioeffects (which, obviously, can be destructive but which can also be exploited for therapy).

The AIUM (https://www.aium.org/resources/official-statements) issued two statements in 2021 regarding bubble-related biological effects in tissues. Thresholds for cavitation in soft tissue have been determined, and if there are no gas bubbles in the tissue, **mechanical index (MI)** values above 1.9 (i.e., outside the diagnostic range) are required to induce mechanical bioeffects. Bubble-related bioeffects (i.e., cavitation) depend on peak rarefactional pressure (Fig. 9.3) and frequency. Currently MI values above 0.3 to 0.4 are required for bioeffects to occur in bodily liquids.

> Cavitation can occur in tissues containing gas bubbles when using sufficient pressure amplitude and frequency. Tissue damage can result from cavitation.
>
> The clinical use of ultrasound contrast agents composed of gas microbubbles requires additional considerations. The presence of these bubbles decreases the acoustic pressure threshold for, and increases the severity of, cavitational bioeffects. Further details will be provided in the next section.

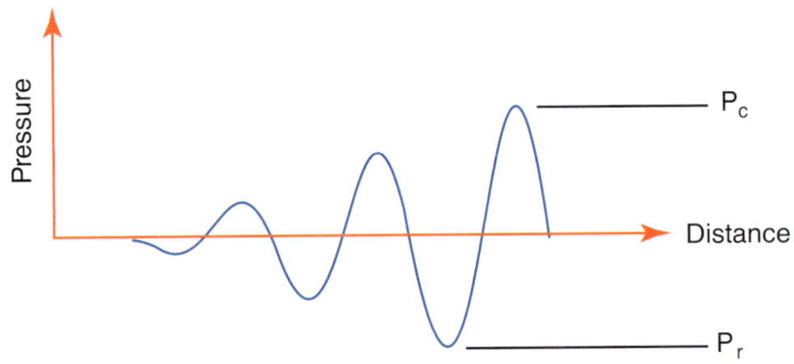

Fig. 9.3 Pressure versus distance for a three-cycle pulse of ultrasound. P_c, Peak compressional pressure; P_r, peak rarefactional pressure.

TABLE 9.1 Acoustic Output Exposure Limits for the 510(k) Process

Diagnostic Application	I_{SPTA} (mW/cm²)
Peripheral vessel	720
Cardiac	430
Ophthalmic	17
Fetal imaging and other[a]	94

[a]Abdominal, intraoperative, pediatric, small organ (breast, thyroid, testes), neonatal cephalic, adult cephalic.
I_{SPTA}, Spatial peak temporal average intensity.
From FDA: *Marketing clearance of diagnostic ultrasound systems and transducers guidance*, 2023.

SAFETY

The safety and risk associated with the use of diagnostic ultrasound rely on our current understanding of bioeffects, along with epidemiologic data and measured instrument output data, as well as the consideration of a number of special clinical circumstances. All of this leads to an approach to prudent use of diagnostic ultrasound imaging.

Instrument Outputs

Spatial peak temporal average (SPTA) intensity has most commonly been the quantity presented to describe instrument output. In general, grayscale imaging outputs are the lowest and outputs associated with spectral Doppler or SWE (essentially the push-pulse) are the highest, while M-mode and color Doppler operations fall somewhere between the two.

These output intensity measurements are usually made with hydrophones (see Chapter 8) located in the beam in a water bath. Attenuation in water is low compared with that in tissues, so an intensity at a comparable location within tissues would be considerably less than that in water. Accounting for the in vivo attenuation used to rely on mathematical tissue models, but nowadays it is much more common for scanners to estimate attenuation directly, as described in Chapter 6.

> Instrument output data are available that allow comparison with experimental conditions necessary for bioeffects to occur.

US Food and Drug Administration

Manufacturers are required to submit premarket notifications to the US *FDA* before marketing an ultrasound scanner for a specific application in the United States. The FDA then reviews this notification to determine whether the instrument is substantially equivalent, with regard to safety and effectiveness, to devices on the market before the enactment of the relevant act (in 1976). This is known as the 510(k) approval process, and if the device is determined to be substantially equivalent, the manufacturer may then market it for that application. Part of the FDA evaluation involves reviewing output data for the system, which then are compared with maximum values determined for the one pre-1976 system owned by the FDA at the time (Table 9.1).

To facilitate a parallel pathway to the 510(k) process for device approval, a voluntary **output display standard (ODS)** was developed by a joint committee involving the AIUM, the FDA, the National Electrical Manufacturers Association, and several other ultrasound-related professional societies in 1992. The ODS bypasses the limits in the 510(k) guide (i.e., Table 9.1) with the exception that an overall upper limit of 720 mW/cm² I_{SPTA} still applies in exchange for presenting output information on the display.

The ODS includes two indices that are displayed: thermal and mechanical (Fig. 9.4). The **thermal index (TI)** is defined as the transducer acoustic output power divided by the estimated power required to raise tissue temperature by 1°C. The estimated power calculation for the TI involves frequency, aperture, and intensity. There are three variations of the TI. The TIS (TI for soft tissues) applies when the beam travels through soft tissue and does not encounter bone. The TIB (TI for bone) applies for bone at or near the beam focus after passing through soft tissue. The TIC (TI for cranial tissues) applies when the transducer is close to bone. More specifics can be found in the AIUM statement of 2022 *Recommended Maximum Scanning Times for Displayed Thermal Index (TI)* Values (https://www.aium.org/resources/official-statements). The MI is equal to the peak rarefactional pressure (see Fig. 9.3) divided by the square root of the center frequency of the pulse:

$$MI = \frac{P_r}{\sqrt{f}}$$

where Pr is pressure amplitude (in MPa) and f is frequency (in MHz).

> The FDA regulates ultrasound scanners within the United States according to application and output intensities and/or TI and MI. Similar organizations exist across the world (e.g., the European Medicines Agency is involved in the regulatory process within the European Union).
>
> Today almost all cart-based ultrasound systems rely on the ODS pathway for FDA approval, while more application-specific devices (some point-of-care ultrasound [POCUS] systems for example) tend to use the 510(k) process.

Special Circumstances

CEUS imaging with gas microbubble–based contrast agents is a special situation when considering the safety aspects of ultrasound imaging. The presence of these bubbles decreases the

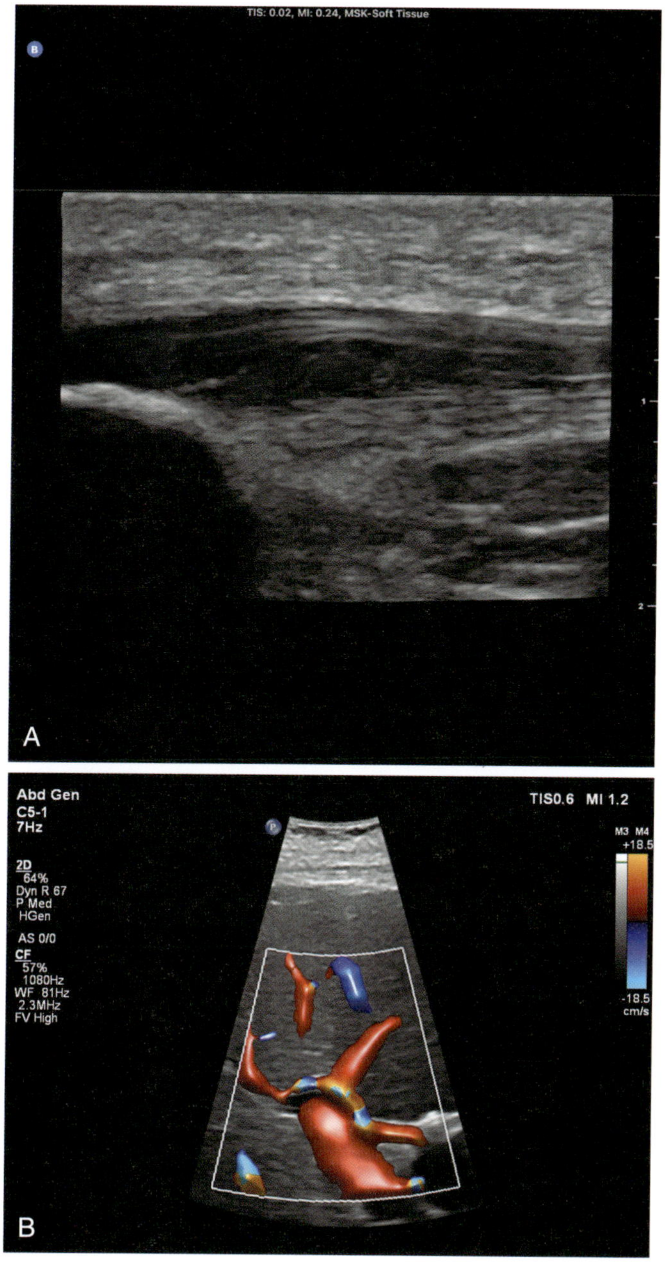

Fig. 9.4 **A,** Point-of-care ultrasound image of tendinosis of the patellar tendon showing thermal and mechanical indices (*arrows*). **B,** Example of color Doppler imaging of liver vessels with the thermal and mechanical indices displayed (*arrows*). (**A,** Courtesy Butterfly Network. **B,** Courtesy Philips Medical Systems.)

acoustic pressure threshold for inducing cavitation (Fig. 9.5). Above an MI of 0.4, premature ventricular contractions, microvascular leakage with petechiae, glomerular capillary hemorrhage, local cell killing, and other bioeffects from CEUS have been reported (and verified by other groups). The significance of such microscale bioeffects is not well established. Nonetheless, prudence indicates that CEUS at an MI above 0.4 should be weighed against the examination time and contrast agent dose required to obtain the necessary diagnostic information.

It should be mentioned that the CEUS bioeffect described above can be exploited for therapeutic applications by augmenting other treatments, such as temporarily opening the blood-brain barrier to allow larger drug molecules to pass through or changing tumor neovascularity to improve chemotherapy uptake (known as sonoporation) or increasing the radiation sensitivity of cancer cells.

Ocular ultrasound (i.e., of the eye) is a well-established clinical application, but dedicated ocular settings should be used to limit any thermal and mechanical bioeffects. If these settings are not available, limiting the acoustic output to the FDA-recommended maximum level (17 mW/cm^2; cf., Table 9.1) or below is strongly recommended. It is important to choose settings that reduce the acoustic output and limit the examination time—especially when performing Doppler examinations (spectral or color flow Doppler). Critically, the acoustic output of SWE is significantly higher than FDA guidelines for the eye (due to the push-pulse) and should not be used in regular clinical practice at this time.

Lung ultrasound has become an important tool for diagnosing a number of conditions including pneumonia, pulmonary edema, respiratory distress syndrome, COVID-19, and lung cancer. Lung ultrasound studies are particularly valuable in neonates being a POCUS examination and thus, avoiding ionizing radiation. **Pulmonary capillary hemorrhage** is a unique bioeffect associated with lung ultrasound, which was discovered more than 30 years ago in mice (and subsequently confirmed in a number of different species). Interestingly, lung ultrasound–induced pulmonary capillary hemorrhage cannot be explained by thermal or cavitational bioeffect mechanisms alone. Hence, the AIUM (https://www.aium.org/resources/official-statements) developed *Statement and Recommendations for Safety Assurance in Lung Ultrasound* in 2023 and strongly advocated for a neonatal lung ultrasound preset incorporating a limit of MI $\leq$ 0.3, which should be installed on all ultrasound systems that may be used in this application to reduce the risk of pulmonary capillary hemorrhage.

Epidemiology

Many epidemiologic studies have been conducted over decades focused in particular on obstetrical ultrasound (since the fetus would be more vulnerable than children and adults). No study to date has yielded repeatable and consistent evidence of any adverse bioeffect from diagnostic ultrasound. The AIUM (https://www.aium.org/resources/official-statements) developed the following *Conclusions Regarding Epidemiology for Obstetric Ultrasound* statement, which was last approved in 2022:

> *Based on the available epidemiologic data, there is insufficient justification to warrant conclusion of a causal relationship between diagnostic ultrasound and recognized adverse effects in humans. The epidemiologic evidence is based primarily on exposure conditions existing prior to 1992, the year in which maximum recommended levels of acoustic output for ultrasound machines were substantially increased for fetal/obstetric applications. Some older studies have reported effects of exposure to diagnostic ultrasound during pregnancy, such as low birth weight, delayed speech, dyslexia, and non-right-handedness. Other more recent*

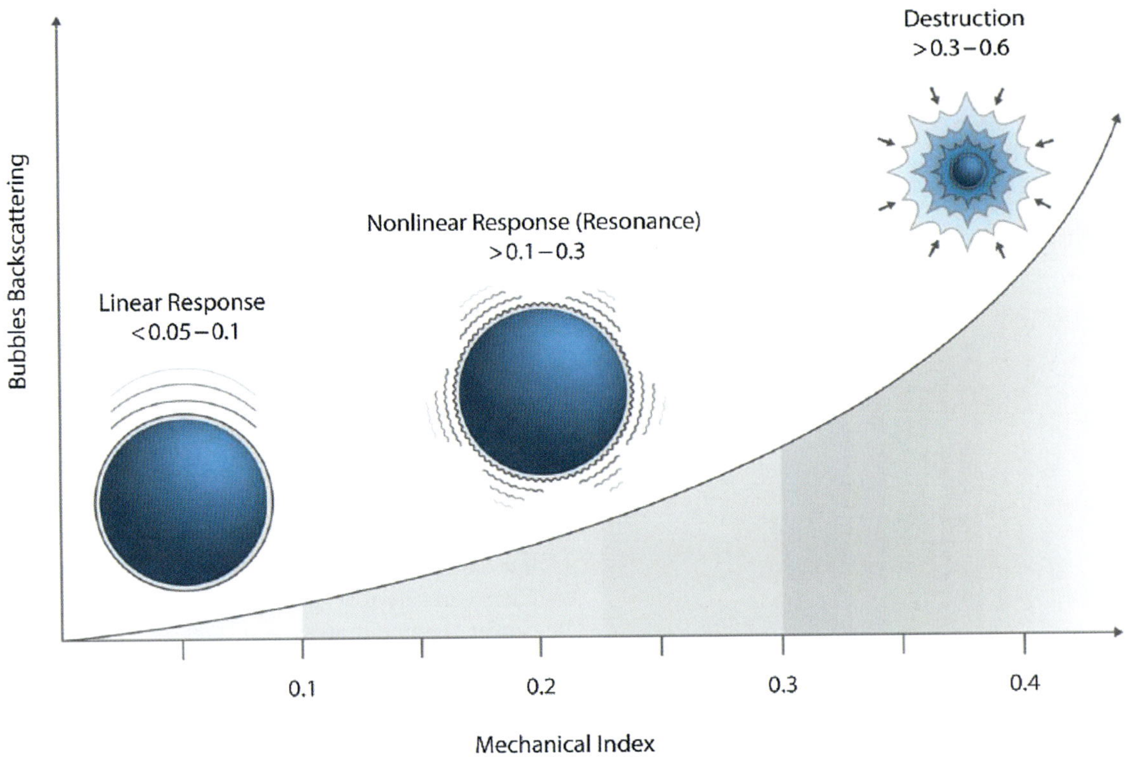

Fig. 9.5 Illustration of the approximate relationship between mechanical index values and contrast microbubble oscillations from the linear regime over stable to inertial cavitation. (From *Baun J: Contrast-enhanced ultrasound: a technology primer, J Diagn Med Sonogr 33(6):446–452, 2017.*)

studies have not demonstrated such effects. The absence of definitive epidemiologic evidence does not preclude the possibility of adverse effects of ultrasound in humans.

> Epidemiologic studies have not revealed any risk to the use of diagnostic ultrasound, although the absence of evidence does not completely eliminate the possibility of adverse bioeffects.

Table 9.2 shows the official statements of various professional societies regarding the risk associated with diagnostic ultrasound under different situations and exposure conditions.

Prudent Use

As discussed previously, epidemiologic studies have revealed no known risk associated with the use of diagnostic ultrasound. Biological effects (such as localized pulmonary bleeding) have been reported at diagnostically relevant exposures, but the clinical relevance of such effects is either not significant or is not yet known. Thus a comparison of instrument output data, adjusted for tissue attenuation, with experimental bioeffects data does not indicate any risk. We must be open, however, to the possibility that unrecognized risk may exist. Such risk, if it does exist, may have eluded detection up to this point because it is subtle or delayed or has incidence rates close to normal values. However, future larger studies might not reveal any bioeffects either, which strengthens the possibility that medical ultrasound imaging has no detectable risk.

In the meantime, with no known risk and with known benefit to ultrasound examinations, a conservative approach to imaging should nonetheless be adopted; that is, ultrasound imaging should be performed when medically indicated, with minimum exposure of the patient and/or fetus (Fig. 9.6). Exposure is limited by minimizing instrument output and exposure time during a study. Instrument outputs for spectral Doppler and SWE studies can be significantly higher than those for other applications. It thus seems most likely that the greatest potential for risk in ultrasound diagnosis (although no specific risk has been identified even in this case) is with fetal studies involving spectral Doppler or lung ultrasound. These studies involve potentially high-output intensities with stationary beams and a presumably more sensitive fetus. Consequently, a prudent and conservative approach to ultrasound safety is to assume that there may be unidentified risk, which should be minimized in medically indicated ultrasound studies by minimizing exposure time and output. This is known as the ALARA principle (see Fig. 9.6).

The AIUM (https://www.aium.org/resources/official-statements) issued a statement on the ALARA principle, which was last approved in 2020:

The potential benefits and risks of each examination should be considered. The as low as reasonably achievable (ALARA) principle should be observed when adjusting controls that affect the acoustic output and by considering both the transducer dwell time and overall scanning time.

TABLE 9.2 Conclusions of Various Medical Organizations Regarding Risk Under Different Ultrasound Imaging Conditions

	AIUM	WFUMB	EFSUMB	ASUM	ISUOG
B-mode	No contraindication, but prudent use	Diagnostic ultrasound can only be considered safe if used prudently	Same as WFUMB	Same as WFUMB	No contraindication
Doppler		Doppler modes can produce more tissue heating and hence higher TI values	Same as WFUMB	Use ALARA acoustic output and dwell time	Use only with clear indication
CEUS	At an MI above 0.4, use of CEUS should be weighed against the examination time and contrast agent dose required to obtain diagnostic information	Caution should be considered for CEUS in tissues where damage to microvasculature could have serious clinical implications, such as in the brain, the eye, and the neonate	Same as WFUMB	Same as WFUMB	
Exposure	Use minimum output and exposure time required to obtain diagnostic information (ALARA)	Users should adjust the machine controls to keep them as low as reasonably achievable (ALARA principle) without compromising the diagnostic value of the examination	Same as WFUMB	Same as WFUMB	Exposure time and acoustic output should be kept to the lowest levels consistent with obtaining diagnostic information
Mechanical effects	Possible with contrast agents but significance is uncertain	No mechanical effects have been demonstrated in humans, except when a microbubble contrast agent is present	Same as WFUMB	Same as WFUMB	
Thermal effects	No limits for TI ≤ 1.5 (see below for obstetric use)	Diagnostic levels of ultrasound are capable of producing temperature rises that may be hazardous to sensitive organs and the embryo/fetus	Same as WFUMB	Same as WFUMB	
First-trimester exposure	Do not use Doppler routinely. Keep TI ≤ 0.7	Endorses AIUM and ISUOG statements	Care should be taken to limit exposure time and the TI and MI to the minimum commensurate with an acceptable clinical assessment, particularly when the TI > 0.7	Same as WFUMB	Doppler ultrasound should not be used routinely. Keep TI ≤ 1.0 and exposure time as short as possible

ALARA, as low as reasonably achievable; *CEUS*, contrast-enhanced ultrasound; *MI*, mechanical index; *TI*, thermal index.
(Original concept D. Evans, PhD).

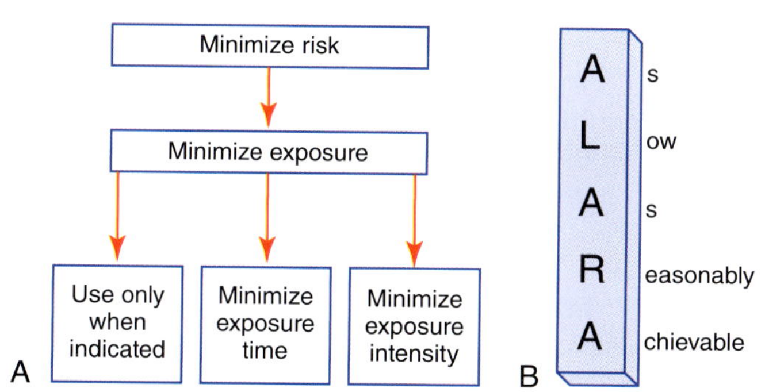

Fig. 9.6 Minimizing risk by minimizing exposure **(A)** is the cornerstone of the ALARA principle **(B)**.

The following recommendations should all be adhered to practice ALARA:

- Use the correct examination presets for medically indicated studies.
- Adjust the output power to the lowest available setting that still provides diagnostic image quality.
- Monitor the MI and TI.
- Remove the transducer when stationary imaging is not necessary to reduce dwell time (especially for sensitive areas such as the eye, the lung and intestines [being naturally gas filled], and fetal calcified structures [e.g., skull and spine]).

- Minimize scanning time, while still obtaining the required diagnostic information.

The AIUM has developed a number of additional official statements on the topic of prudent use of diagnostic ultrasound and ALARA (available at https://www.aium.org/resources/official-statements).

> Prudent practice of ultrasound imaging involves application of the ALARA principle. By requiring medical indication and by using minimum output and exposure time in diagnostic examinations, exposure and risk are minimized.
>
> It is difficult to make a firm statement about the clinical safety of diagnostic ultrasound. The experimental and epidemiologic bases for risk assessment are incomplete. However, much work has been done, and no evidence of clinical harm has been revealed. Patients should be informed that there currently is no basis for concluding that diagnostic ultrasound produces any harmful effects in patients. However, unobserved effects could be occurring and there are specific situations where risks will be higher (e.g., with the use of ultrasound contrast agents or when performing lung ultrasound or ophthalmic studies). Thus ultrasound should not be used indiscriminately. The AIUM Clinical Safety Statement forms an excellent basis for addressing any concerns. In practice, minimizing exposure time and output is prudent and the TI and MI can facilitate such an approach.

In more than six decades of use, there has been no report of injury to patients or operators caused directly by medical ultrasound equipment. Those working in the ultrasound community want to maintain that level of safety. Application-specific output limits and the user's knowledge of equipment controls and patient body characteristics (e.g., in ophthalmic or fetal lung ultrasound) should be taken into consideration to minimize exposure. As an alternative, the MI and TI provide users with information that can be applied specifically to the ALARA principle. These indices make it easier for the user to obtain the best image possible, while following the ALARA principle and thus maximizing the benefit-to-risk ratio.

REVIEW

The following key points are presented in this chapter:

- Mechanistic, in vitro, in vivo, and epidemiologic studies have revealed no known risk associated with current diagnostic ultrasound imaging practices.
- The AIUM has stated that there have been no independently confirmed, significant bioeffects reported to occur in mammalian tissues exposed to focused I_{SPTA} intensities below 1 W/cm^2. Furthermore, no risk has been identified with the use of diagnostic ultrasound in human beings.
- Because there is limited specific knowledge, a conservative approach is justified. Such an approach calls for diagnostic ultrasound to be used, with minimum exposure, when medical benefit is expected to be derived from the procedure.

EXERCISES

Answers appear in the Answers to Exercises section at the back of the book.

1. Heating depends most directly on ___________.
   a. SATA intensity
   b. SATP intensity
   c. SPTP intensity
   d. pressure
2. Conditions under which cavitation may occur are best described by ___________.
   a. SATA intensity
   b. SATP intensity
   c. SPTP intensity
   d. peak rarefactional pressure
3. Bioeffects have been observed in experimental animals with intensities greater than ___________.
   a. 100 mW/cm^{2}SPTA
   b. 1 W/cm^{2}SPTA
   c. 10 W/cm^{2}SPTA
   d. 1 mW/cm^{2}SPTP
   e. 10 mW/cm^{2}SPTP
4. Bioeffects have been observed in experimental animals with focused intensities greater than ___________.
   a. 100 mW/cm^{2}SPTA
   b. 1 W/cm^{2}SPTA
   c. 10 W/cm^{2}SPTA
   d. 1 mW/cm^{2}SPTP
   e. 10 mW cm^{2}SPTP
5. Focal lesions have been observed in experimental animals with intensities greater than ___________.
   a. 100 mW/cm^{2}SPTA
   b. 1 W/cm^{2}SPTA
   c. 10 W/cm^{2}SPTA
   d. 1 mW/cm^{2}SPTP
   e. 10 mW/cm^{2}SPTP
6. The available epidemiologic data are sufficient to make a final judgment on the safety of diagnostic ultrasound. True or false?
7. Exposure is minimized by using diagnostic ultrasound ___________.
   a. only when indicated
   b. with minimum intensity
   c. with minimum time
   d. all of the above
   e. none of the above
8. Which of the following is (are) used currently to indicate output on the display?
   a. percent
   b. decibel
   c. SPTA intensity
   d. mechanical index
   e. all of the above

9. Which of the following affect(s) exposure of a fetus?
   a. intensity at the transducer
   b. distance to the fetus
   c. frequency
   d. gain
   e. more than one of the above
   f. all of the above
10. There is no possible hazard involved in the use of diagnostic ultrasound. True or false?
11. Ultrasound should not be used as a diagnostic tool because of the bioeffects it can produce. True or false?
12. No independently confirmed, significant bioeffects in mammalian tissues have been reported at intensities below ___________.
   a. 10 W/cm^2 SPTP
   b. 100 mW/cm^2 SPTA
   c. 10 mW/cm^2 SPTA
   d. 10 mW/cm^2 SATA
   e. 1 mW/cm^2 SATP
13. Is there any known risk with the current use of diagnostic ultrasound? Yes or no?
14. Are there any bioeffects that ultrasound produces in small animals under experimental conditions? Yes or no?
15. Which of the following are mechanisms by which ultrasound can produce bioeffects? (More than one correct answer.)
   a. direction ionization
   b. absorption
   c. photoelectric effect
   d. cavitation
   e. Compton effect
16. Which of the following relates to heating?
   a. impedance
   b. sound speed
   c. absorption
   d. refraction
   e. diffraction
17. Which of the following end points is documented well enough in the scientific literature to allow a risk assessment for diagnostic ultrasound to be based on it?
   a. fetal weight
   b. sister-chromatid exchange
   c. fetal abnormalities
   d. carcinogenesis
   e. none
18. On which of the following end points has more than one epidemiologic study shown a statistically significant effect of ultrasound exposure?
   a. fetal activity
   b. birth weight
   c. fetal abnormalities
   d. dyslexia
   e. none
19. Which of the following acoustic parameters has (have) been documented in ultrasound epidemiologic studies published thus far?
   a. frequency
   b. exposure time
   c. intensity and pulsing conditions
   d. scanning patterns
   e. none
20. A device commonly used to measure the output of diagnostic ultrasound instruments is a(n) ___________.
   a. hydrophone
   b. optical interferometer
   c. Geiger counter
   d. photoelectric cell
   e. absorption radiometer
21. A typical output intensity (SPTA) for an ultrasound imaging instrument is ___________.
   a. 1540 W
   b. 13 kW/mm^2
   c. 3.5 MHz
   d. 1 mW/cm^2
   e. 2 dB/cm
22. Which of the following typically has the highest output intensity?
   a. fetal monitor Doppler
   b. duplex pulsed Doppler
   c. color Doppler imaging
   d. power Doppler imaging phased array, grayscale
   e. phased array, grayscale
23. As far as we know now, which of the following is the most correct and informative response to a patient's question, "Will this hurt me or my baby?"
   a. no
   b. yes
   c. We don't know.
   d. The risks are well understood, but the benefits always outweigh them.
   e. There is no known risk with ultrasound imaging as it is applied currently.
24. To minimize whatever risk there may be with ultrasound imaging, which of the following should be done? (More than one correct answer.)
   a. scan to produce pictures for the family album
   b. scan to determine fetal sex
   c. minimize exposure time
   d. scan for medical indication(s) only
   e. minimize exposure intensity
25. Which of the following controls affect instrument output intensity?
   a. dynamic range, compression
   b. transmit, output
   c. near gain, far gain
   d. overall gain
   e. slope, time gain compensation

26. Which of the following are correct for a duplex, pulsed-wave Doppler instrument? (More than one correct answer.)
    a. Tissue anywhere in the Doppler beam is exposed to ultrasound.
    b. Tissue anywhere in the imaging plane is exposed to ultrasound.
    c. Imaging intensities are higher than for conventional grayscale instruments.
    d. Doppler intensities are higher than for continuous wave fetal monitoring.
27. The tissue of greatest concern regarding bioeffects in an abdominal scan is the ___________.
    a. spleen
    b. pancreas
    c. liver
    d. kidney
    e. fetus
28. Would it be wise to substitute a duplex, pulsed-wave Doppler device for an inoperative fetal monitor for long-term (e.g., 2-hour) monitoring in labor?
    a. yes
    b. no
    c. depends on frame rate of the image
    d. depends on frequency of the Doppler beam
    e. depends on gate location
29. Which of the following is (are) likely to be exposed to ultrasound during a diagnostic study?
    a. patient
    b. sonographer
    c. radiologist
    d. observers in the room
    e. more than one of the above
30. No bioeffects have been observed in nonhuman mammalian tissues at thermal index values of less than ___________.
    a. 5
    b. 4
    c. 3
    d. 2
    e. 1
31. No bioeffects have been observed in nonhuman mammalian tissues at mechanical index values of less than ___________.
    a. 0.5
    b. 0.4
    c. 0.3
    d. 0.2
    e. 0.1
32. No bioeffects have been observed in nonhuman mammalian tissues at peak rarefactional pressure values (megapascals) of less than ___________.
    a. 0.5
    b. 0.4
    c. 0.3
    d. 0.2
    e. 0.1
33. ALARA is an abbreviation for ___________.
    a. as loud as reasonable allowable
    b. after leaving a red automobile
    c. acoustic lens and reverb analyzer
    d. am looking at right answer
    e. none of the above

10

To Conclude

CHAPTER OUTLINE

ARDMS SPI Examination Content Outline and JRC-DMS National Education Curriculum

Comprehensive Examination

Diagnostic medical ultrasound imaging (sonographic imaging) is a cross-sectional, 2D or 3D, anatomical, and/or flow imaging modality employing the pulse-echo principle (in the broadest sense possible). Pulses of ultrasound are generated by a transducer and are sent into the patient, where they produce echoes at organ boundaries and within tissues. These echoes return to the transducer, where they are detected and then presented on the display of an ultrasound scanner. Each pulse produces a series of echoes that are processed and displayed as one out of many physical scan lines making up the final anatomical image (traditional beamforming) or as a broad set of echoes across the transducer aperture that are processed again and again to produce the final image (virtual beamforming). If flowing blood or moving tissues produce echoes, a frequency change, called the *Doppler shift*, occurs. Doppler shifts provide motion information that can be presented in spectral form (audibly and/or as a displayed waveform) or as 2D, 3D, or 4D color Doppler flow maps.

Ultrasound is a mechanical sound wave (i.e., a wave of traveling acoustic variables that include pressure, density, and particle motion) with a frequency greater than 20 kHz. Ultrasound is described by frequency, period, wavelength, propagation speed, amplitude, intensity, and attenuation. Pulsed ultrasound is described by additional terms: pulse-repetition frequency (PRF), pulse-repetition period, pulse duration, duty factor, and spatial pulse length. Propagation speed and impedance are characteristics of the medium that are determined by density and stiffness. Attenuation increases with frequency and path length. Imaging depth decreases with increasing frequency. The average soft tissue propagation sound speed is 1540 m/s or 1.54 mm/μs, and the attenuation coefficient is approximately 0.5 dB/(cm MHz). When sound encounters boundaries between media with different impedances, part of the sound is reflected (the echo), and part is transmitted. With perpendicular incidence, if the two media have the same impedance, there is no reflection. With oblique incidence, the sound is refracted at a boundary between the media where propagation speeds are different. Incidence and reflection angles are always equal. Scattering occurs at rough media boundaries and within heterogeneous media. The range equation is used to determine distance to reflectors. Pulse-echo round-trip travel time is 13 μs/cm. The use of nonlinear harmonic echoes improves image quality, and ultrasound contrast agents made up of gas-filled microbubbles enhance echo generation and detection.

Ultrasound transducers convert electric energy to mechanical energy, and vice versa. They operate on the piezoelectric principle. The preferred operating frequency depends on element thickness. Axial resolution is equal to one-half of the spatial pulse length. Pulsed transducers have damping material to shorten the spatial pulse length for improved detail resolution. Transducers produce sound in the form of a few (at least one) and up to hundreds of beams with near and far zones. Lateral resolution is equal to the beam width (physical or virtual depending on the processing applied). Physical beam width is reduced by focusing to improve detail resolution, while the virtual beam is optimally focused at all locations throughout the image simultaneously. *Linear* and *curved* (or *convex*) are types of array construction, while *sequenced*, *phased*, and *vector* are types of array beam steering and scanning operations. Phasing also enables electronic focusing of physical scan lines (i.e., when using narrow transmit beams).

Ultrasound imaging systems are of the pulse-echo type. They use the strength, direction, and arrival time of received echoes to generate A-, B-, and M-mode displays. Imaging systems consist of the transducer, beam former, signal processor, image processor, and display. Beam formers direct and focus the transmitted beam through the imaged tissue cross section, amplify the received echo voltages, compensate for attenuation, and digitize the received echo voltages. Signal processors filter, detect, and compress echo signals. Image processors in narrow transmit beam systems convert scan-line signals to image formats, store images in digital form, and perform preprocessing and postprocessing on images, while in broad transmit beam systems the image processor performs high-speed, retrospective, computational, virtual beamforming bringing the entire image into focus and improving virtually every characteristic of ultrasound imaging. Preprocessing includes persistence, panoramic imaging, spatial compounding, and 3D acquisition. A mode shows echo amplitudes. B and M modes use a brightness display. M mode shows reflector motion in time. B mode scans show anatomical cross sections in grayscale through the scan plane. Image memories store echo amplitude information as numbers in the memory elements. Contrast resolution improves with increasing bits per pixel (layers of memory). Real-time imaging is the rapid sequential display of ultrasound images resulting in a moving presentation. Such imaging requires automatic, rapid, repeatable, sequential scanning of the sound beam through the tissue. This scanning is accomplished by electronic transducer arrays. Rectangular and sector display formats result from such scanning techniques. Displays are flat-panel liquid-crystal or LED displays. Instruments are usually connected to picture archiving and communication systems with options to connect peripheral devices (flash drives or other portable hard drives).

Blood is a liquid that flows through the vascular system under the influence of pulsatile pressure provided by the beating heart. Volume flow rate is proportional to pressure difference at the ends of a tube and inversely proportional to flow resistance. Flow resistance increases with viscosity and tube length and decreases (strongly) with increasing tube diameter. Seven (two temporal and five spatial) flow classifications include *steady, pulsatile, plug, laminar, parabolic, disturbed*, and *turbulent*. In a stenosis, flow speeds up, pressure drops (Bernoulli effect), and flow is disturbed. If flow speed exceeds a critical value, turbulence occurs. Pulsatile flow is common in arterial circulation. Diastolic flow, flow reversal, or both may occur in some locations within the arterial system. Fluid inertia and vessel compliance are characteristics that are important in determining flow with pulsatile driving pressure.

The Doppler effect is a change in frequency resulting from motion. In most medical ultrasound applications, the motion is that of blood flow in circulation. The *change* in frequency of the returning echoes with respect to the emitted frequency is called the *Doppler shift*. For flow toward the transducer, the Doppler shift is positive; for flow away, it is negative. The Doppler shift depends on the speed of the scatterers of sound, the angle between their direction and that of the sound propagation, and the operating frequency of the Doppler system. A moving scatterer of sound produces a double Doppler shift. Greater flow speeds and smaller Doppler angles produce larger Doppler shifts but not stronger echoes. Higher operating frequencies produce larger Doppler shifts. Typical ranges of flow speeds (10–300 cm/s), Doppler angles (30–60 degrees), and operating frequencies (2–18 MHz) yield Doppler shifts in the range of 100 Hz to 20 kHz for vascular studies. In echocardiography, in which zero angle and speeds of a few meters per second can be encountered, Doppler shifts can be as high as 30 kHz.

Doppler-capable instruments make use of the Doppler shift to yield information regarding motion and flow. Continuous-wave (CW) operation provides motion and flow information without depth selection capability. Pulsed-wave (PW) Doppler operation provides the capability of selecting a depth from which Doppler information is received. Spectral analysis provides quantitative information on the distribution of received Doppler-shift frequencies that result from the distribution of scatterer velocities (speeds and directions) encountered. In addition to audible output, visual presentation of flow spectral waveforms is possible in Doppler operation. Combined (duplex) operation that uses real-time grayscale ultrasound and CW or PW Doppler is standard on most scanners. The Doppler spectrum is generated by the range of scatterer velocities encountered by the ultrasound beam. The Doppler spectrum is derived electronically using the fast Fourier transform and is presented on the display as Doppler shift versus time, with brightness indicating power. Flow conditions at the site of measurement are indicated by the width of the spectrum; spectral broadening may indicate disturbed and turbulent flow or an artifact. Flow conditions downstream, particularly distal flow resistance, are indicated by the relationship between peak systolic and end diastolic flow velocities. Various indexes for quantitatively presenting this information have been developed.

Color flow imaging (color Doppler or power Doppler) acquires Doppler-shifted echoes from a cross section of tissue scanned by the ultrasound beam(s). These echoes then are presented in color and are superimposed on the grayscale anatomical image of stationary structures. The flow echoes are assigned colors according to the selected color map. Red, orange, yellow, blue, cyan, and white indicate positive or negative Doppler shifts (i.e., approaching or receding flow). Several pulses (the number is called *ensemble length*) are needed to generate a color scan line (or frame in broad transmit beam systems). Color controls include gain, color map selection, persistence, ensemble length, color/gray priority, scale (PRF), baseline shift, wall filter, and color window angle, location, and size (it should be noted that in practice, more and more of these parameters are inaccessible to the end user). Color Doppler mode is pulsed and subject to the same limitations—Doppler angle dependence and aliasing—as spectral operation. Power Doppler displays encode the strength of the Doppler shifts into a sensitive presentation of flow information that is angle and aliasing independent.

Axial resolution is determined by spatial pulse length, whereas lateral resolution is determined by beam width in narrow transmit beam systems. The beam width perpendicular to the scan plane causes section thickness artifacts. Apparent resolution close to the transducer is not related directly to tissue texture but is a result of interference effects from a distribution of scatterers in the tissue (speckle). Reverberation produces a set of equally spaced artifactual echoes distal to the real reflector. Refraction displaces echoes laterally. In the mirror-image artifact, objects that are present on one side of a strong reflector are displayed on the other side as well. Shadowing is caused by high-attenuation objects in the sound path. Enhancement results from low-attenuation objects in the sound path. Propagation speed error and refraction can cause objects to be displayed in improper locations or incorrect sizes or both. Refraction can also cause edge shadowing. Artifacts that can occur with Doppler ultrasound include aliasing, range ambiguity, color-Doppler image mirroring, and spectral trace mirroring. Aliasing is the most common artifact. Aliasing occurs when the Doppler-shift frequency exceeds one-half the PRF (the Nyquist limit). Aliasing can be reduced or eliminated by increasing the PRF or Doppler angle, shifting the baseline, reducing operating frequency, or switching to CW operation.

Phantoms and test objects provide means for measuring the detail and contrast resolutions, distance accuracy, compensation, penetration, and dynamic range of diagnostic ultrasound instruments. Hydrophones are used to measure the acoustic output of ultrasound systems.

Guidelines and Official Statements from experts associated with the American Institute of Ultrasound in Medicine (AIUM) have concluded that no independently confirmed, significant bioeffects have been reported to occur in mammalian tissues exposed to focused spatial peak-temporal average intensities of less than 1 W/cm^2. Furthermore, no risk has been identified with the use of diagnostic ultrasound in human beings. Because there is limited specific knowledge, a conservative approach is justified; that is, diagnostic ultrasound should be used, with minimum exposure, when medical benefit is expected to be derived from the procedure (the ALARA [as low as reasonably achievable] principle).

ARDMS SPI EXAMINATION CONTENT OUTLINE AND JRC-DMS NATIONAL EDUCATION CURRICULUM

The complete, detailed American Registry for Diagnostic Medical Sonograph (ARDMS) *Sonography Principles and Instrumentation* (SPI) Examination Content Outline is available at https://www.ardms.org/wp-content/uploads/pdf/SPI-Examination-Content-Outline-V24.1.pdf.

A brief version of the outline is shown here with relevant chapters in this book indicated:

- Perform Ultrasound Examinations, 23% (see Chapters 2, 4, and 6)
- Manage Ultrasound Transducers, 7% (see Chapter 3)
- Optimize Sonographic Images, 26% (see Chapters 4, 6, and 7)
- Apply Doppler Concepts, 34% (see Chapters 5–7)
- Provide Clinical Safety & Quality Assurance, 10% (see Chapters 8 and 9)

The Joint Review Committee on Education in Diagnostic Medical Sonography (JRC-DMS) National Education Curriculum is available at https://jrcdms.org/pdf/NECCommonCurricula.pdf.

The topics listed under Sonographic Physics and Instrumentation are shown here with relevant chapters in this book indicated:

- Basic Principles and Wave Analysis (see Chapters 1 and 2)
- Propagation of Acoustic Waves Through Tissues (see Chapter 2)
- Sonographic Transducers and Sound Beams (see Chapter 3)
- Principles of Pulse-Echo Imaging (see Chapters 4 and 6)
- Hemodynamic and Doppler Imaging (see Chapters 5 and 6)
- Sonographic Instrumentation (see Chapters 4–6)
- Artifacts (see Chapter 7)
- Quality Assurance/Quality Control of Sonographic Instruments (see Chapter 8)
- Bioeffects and Safety (see Chapter 9)

COMPREHENSIVE EXAMINATION

Answers appear in the Answers to Exercises section at the back of the book.

This comprehensive examination applies only to traditional narrow transmit beam operations. For questions applicable to broad transmit beams, see the appropriate sections in Chapters 4 and 5.

1. Which of the following frequencies is in the ultrasound range?
   a. 15 Hz
   b. 15 kHz
   c. 15 MHz
   d. 17,000 Hz
   e. 17 km
2. The average propagation speed in soft tissues is ____________.
   a. 1.54 mm/μs
   b. 0.501 m/s
   c. 1540 dB/cm
   d. 37.0 km/min
   e. 1 to 10 km/min
3. The propagation speed is greatest in ____________.
   a. lung
   b. liver
   c. bone
   d. fat
   e. blood
4. Which of the following has a significant dependence on frequency in soft tissues?
   a. propagation speed
   b. density
   c. stiffness
   d. attenuation
   e. impedance
5. The frequencies used in diagnostic ultrasound imaging ____________.
   a. are much lower than those used in Doppler measurements
   b. determine imaging depth in tissue
   c. determine detail resolution
   d. all of the above
   e. b and c
6. An echo from reflector at 5cm depth arrives at the transducer ____________ μs after pulse emission.
   a. 13
   b. 154
   c. 65
   d. 5
   e. 77
7. A small (relative to the wavelength) reflector is said to ____________ an incident sound beam.
   a. focus
   b. speculate
   c. scatter
   d. shatter
   e. amplify

8. Which of the following determines the operating frequency of an ultrasound transducer?
   a. element diameter
   b. element thickness
   c. speed of sound in tissue
   d. element impedance
   e. all of the above
9. The fundamental operating principle of medical ultrasound transducers is ___________.
   a. Snell's law
   b. Doppler law
   c. magnetostrictive effect
   d. piezoelectric effect
   e. impedance effect
10. The axial resolution of a transducer is primarily determined by ___________.
   a. spatial pulse length
   b. the near-field limit
   c. the transducer diameter
   d. the acoustic impedance of tissue
   e. density
11. The lateral resolution of a transducer is primarily determined by ___________.
   a. spatial pulse length
   b. the near-field limit
   c. the aperture
   d. the acoustic impedance of tissue
   e. applied voltage
12. Increasing frequency ___________.
   a. improves resolution
   b. increases penetration
   c. increases refraction
   d. a and b
   e. a and c
13. Ultrasound bioeffects ___________.
   a. do not occur
   b. do not occur with diagnostic instruments
   c. are not confirmed below a spatial peak-temporal average intensity of 100 mW/cm^2
   d. b and c
   e. none of the above
14. Diagnostic ultrasound frequency range is mainly ___________.
   a. 2–10 MHz
   b. 2–10 kHz
   c. 2–25 MHz
   d. 5–15 kHz
   e. none of the above
15. What determines the lower and upper limits of frequency range useful in diagnostic ultrasound?
   a. resolution and penetration
   b. intensity and resolution
   c. intensity and propagation speed
   d. scattering and impedance
   e. impedance and wavelength
16. Reverberation causes us to think there are reflectors that are too great in ___________.
   a. impedance
   b. attenuation
   c. range
   d. size
   e. number
17. A flat-panel display is composed of a backlighted rectangular matrix of thousands of ___________ display elements.
   a. plasma
   b. television
   c. LED
   d. liquid-crystal
   e. c or d
18. In an ultrasound imaging instrument, a flat-panel display may be used as a ___________.
   a. pulser
   b. digitizer
   c. memory
   d. display
   e. preprocessor
19. The compensation (time gain compensation) control ___________.
   a. compensates for machine instability in the warmup time
   b. compensates for attenuation
   c. compensates for transducer aging and the ambient light in the examining area
   d. decreases patient examination time
   e. none of the above
20. An image processor changes signals from ___________ to ___________ format.
   a. grayscale, color
   b. radio frequency, amplitude
   c. B-mode, M-mode
   d. scan line, image
   e. none of the above
21. Enhancement is caused by a ___________.
   a. strongly reflecting structure
   b. weakly attenuating structure
   c. strongly attenuating structure
   d. frequency error
   e. propagation speed error
22. Echo intensity is represented in image memory by ___________.
   a. positive charge distribution
   b. a number
   c. electron density of the display writing beam
   d. a and c
   e. all of the above
23. Which of the following is (are) performed in a signal processor?
   a. filtering
   b. detection
   c. compression
   d. all of the above
   e. none of the above

24. Increasing the PRF ___________.
   a. improves detail resolution
   b. increases maximum unambiguous depth
   c. decreases maximum unambiguous depth
   d. both a and b
   e. both a and c
25. Attenuation is corrected by ___________.
   a. demodulation
   b. desegregation
   c. decompression
   d. compensation
   e. remuneration
26. What must be known to calculate distance to a reflector?
   a. attenuation, speed, density
   b. attenuation, impedance
   c. attenuation, absorption
   d. travel time, speed
   e. density, speed
27. Which of the following improve(s) sound transmission from the transducer element into the tissue?
   a. matching layer
   b. Doppler effect
   c. damping material
   d. coupling medium
   e. a and d
28. Lateral resolution is improved by ___________.
   a. damping
   b. pulsing
   c. focusing
   d. reflecting
   e. absorbing
29. Axial resolution is improved by ___________.
   a. damping
   b. pulsing
   c. focusing
   d. reflecting
   e. absorbing
30. An image memory divides the cross-sectional image into ___________.
   a. frequencies
   b. bits
   c. pixels
   d. binaries
   e. wavelengths
31. In general, as a reflector approaches a transducer at constant speed, the positive Doppler-shift frequency ___________.
   a. increases
   b. decreases
   c. remains constant
   d. b or c
   e. none of the above
32. A reduction in vessel diameter produces a(n) ___________.
   a. increase in flow resistance
   b. decrease in area
   c. increase in flow speed
   d. decrease in flow speed
   e. all of the above
33. Which of the following increases vascular flow resistance?
   a. decreasing vessel length
   b. decreasing viscosity
   c. decreasing vessel diameter
   d. decreasing pressure
   e. decreasing flow speed
34. The Doppler effect occurs as ___________.
   a. leukocytes move through plasma
   b. erythrocytes move through plasma
   c. erythrocytes move through serum
   d. blood moves relative to the vessel wall
   e. all of the above
35. When a reflector is moving toward the transducer, ___________.
   a. propagation speed increases
   b. propagation speed decreases
   c. the Doppler shift is positive (higher frequency)
   d. the Doppler shift is negative (lower frequency)
   e. none of the above
36. Doppler sample volume is determined by ___________.
   a. beam width
   b. pulse length
   c. frequency
   d. amplifier gate length
   e. all of the above
37. Doppler-shift frequencies ___________.
   a. are generally in the audible range
   b. are usually higher than 1 MHz
   c. can be applied to a loudspeaker
   d. a and b
   e. a and c
38. The quantitative presentation of frequencies contained in echoes is called ___________.
   a. preamplification
   b. digitizing
   c. optical encoding
   d. spectral analysis
   e. all of the above
39. The Doppler frequency shift is caused by ___________.
   a. relative motion between the transducer and the reflector
   b. the patient shivering in a cool room
   c. a high transducer frequency and real-time scanner
   d. small reflectors in the transducer beam
   e. changing transducer thickness
40. The Doppler effect is a change in ___________.
   a. intensity
   b. wavelength
   c. frequency
   d. all of the above
   e. b and c
41. The Doppler shift is zero when the angle between the sound direction and the movement (flow) direction is ___________ degrees.
   a. 30
   b. 60
   c. 90
   d. 45
   e. none of the above

42. Duplex Doppler presents ___________.
a. anatomical (structural) data
b. physiological (flow) data
c. impedance data
d. more than one of the above
e. all of the above

43. The Doppler-shift frequencies are usually in a relatively narrow range above 20 kHz. True or false?

44. Continuous-wave sound is used in ___________.
a. all ultrasound imaging instruments
b. only bistable instruments
c. all Doppler instruments
d. some Doppler instruments
e. some M-mode instruments

45. An advantage of continuous-wave Doppler over pulsed Doppler is ___________.
a. depth information
b. bidirectionality
c. no aliasing
d. b and c
e. all of the above

46. In color-Doppler instruments, hue can represent ___________.
a. sign (+ or −) of Doppler shift
b. flow direction
c. magnitude of the Doppler shift
d. amplitude of the Doppler shift
e. all of the above

47. The Doppler effect for a scatterer moving toward the sound source causes the scattered sound (compared with incident sound) received by the transducer to have ___________.
a. increased intensity
b. decreased intensity
c. increased impedance
d. increased frequency
e. decreased impedance

48. Duplex Doppler operation includes ___________.
a. pulsed-wave Doppler
b. continuous-wave Doppler
c. B-scan imaging
d. dynamic imaging
e. more than one of the above

49. If the Doppler shifts from normal and stenotic arteries are 4 and 10 kHz, respectively, for which will there be aliasing with a PRF of 7 kHz?
a. normal artery
b. stenotic artery
c. both
d. neither

50. The signal processor in a Doppler system compares the ___________ of the output with the returning echo voltage from the transducer.
a. wavelength
b. intensity
c. impedance
d. frequency
e. all of the above

51. In the Doppler equation that follows, which can normally be ignored?
a. $f_D = \frac{2fv}{(c - v)}$
b. v in the denominator
c. v in the numerator
d. f
e. D
f. b and c

52. For which of the following is the reflected frequency less than the incident frequency?
a. advancing flow
b. receding flow
c. perpendicular flow
d. laminar flow
e. all of the above

53. Doppler ultrasound can measure flow speed in the ___________.
a. heart
b. veins
c. arterioles
d. capillaries
e. a and b

54. Which of the following are fluids?
a. gas
b. liquid
c. solid
d. a and b
e. all of the above

55. The mass per unit volume of a fluid is called its ___________.
a. resistance
b. viscosity
c. kinematic viscosity
d. impedance
e. density

56. The resistance to flow offered by a fluid is called ___________.
a. resistance
b. viscosity
c. kinematic viscosity
d. impedance
e. density

57. Viscosity divided by density is called ___________.
a. resistance
b. viscosity
c. kinematic viscosity
d. impedance
e. density

58. If the following is increased, flow increases.
a. pressure difference
b. pressure gradient
c. resistance
d. a and b
e. all of the above

59. Flow resistance depends most strongly on ________.
a. vessel length
b. vessel radius
c. blood viscosity
d. all of the above
e. none of the above

60. Proximal to, at, and distal to a stenosis, ___________ must be constant.
a. laminar flow
b. disturbed flow
c. turbulent flow
d. volume flow rate
e. none of the above

61. Added forward flow and flow reversal in diastole are results of ___________ flow.
a. volume
b. turbulent
c. laminar
d. disturbed
e. pulsatile

62. A broad spectrum indicates ___________ flow.
a. pulsatile
b. laminar
c. constant
d. turbulent
e. a and b

63. While diameter at a stenosis decreases, the following pass(es) through a maximum.
a. flow speed at the stenosis
b. flow speed proximal to the stenosis
c. volume flow rate
d. Doppler shift at the stenosis
e. a and d

64. The Doppler shift (in kHz) for 4 MHz, 50 cm/s, and 60 degrees is ___________.
a. 0.5
b. 1.0
c. 1.3
d. 2.6
e. 5.0

65. Physiologic flow speeds can be as much as ___________% of the propagation speed in soft tissues.
a. 0.01
b. 0.3
c. 5
d. 10
e. 50

66. Which Doppler angle yields the greatest Doppler shift?
a. −90
b. −45
c. 0
d. 45
e. 90

67. Doppler-shift frequency does not depend on ___________.
a. amplitude
b. flow speed
c. operating frequency
d. Doppler angle
e. propagation speed

68. The Fourier transform technique is not used in color Doppler operation because it is not ___________ enough.
a. slow
b. fast
c. bright
d. cheap
e. none of the above

69. Which of the following on a color Doppler display is (are) presented in real time?
a. grayscale anatomy
b. flow direction
c. Doppler spectrum
d. a and b
e. all of the above

70. For a 5 MHz instrument and a 60 degree Doppler angle, a 100 Hz filter eliminates flow speeds below ___________ cm/s.
a. 1
b. 2
c. 3
d. 4
e. 5

71. For a 7.5 MHz instrument and a 0-degree Doppler angle, a 100 Hz filter eliminates flow speeds below ___________ cm/s.
a. 1
b. 2
c. 3
d. 4
e. 5

72. The functions of a Doppler detector include ___________.
a. amplification
b. phase quadrature detection
c. demodulation
d. all of the above
e. none of the above

73. A later amplifier gate time means a(n) ___________ sample volume depth.
a. earlier
b. shallower
c. deeper
d. stronger
e. none of the above

74. The Doppler shift is typically ___________ the source frequency.
a. one-thousandth
b. one-hundredth
c. one-tenth
d. 10 times
e. 100 times

75. Approximately ___________ pulses are required to obtain one line of color-Doppler information.
a. 1
b. 10
c. 100
d. 1000
e. 1,000,000

76. There are approximately ___________ samples per line on a color-Doppler display.
    a. 2
    b. 20
    c. 200
    d. 2000
    e. 2,000,000
77. Which of the following Doppler operations can produce aliasing?
    a. continuous wave
    b. pulsed
    c. duplex
    d. color
    e. more than one of the above
78. For normal flow in a large vessel, a ___________ range of Doppler-shift frequencies is received.
    a. narrow
    b. broad
    c. steady
    d. disturbed
    e. all of the above
79. Doppler signal power is proportional to ___________.
    a. the volume flow rate
    b. flow speed
    c. the Doppler angle
    d. cell density
    e. more than one of the above
80. Stenosis affects ___________.
    a. peak systolic flow speed
    b. end diastolic flow speed
    c. spectral broadening
    d. window
    e. all of the above
81. Spectral broadening is a ___________ of the spectral trace.
    a. vertical thickening
    b. horizontal thickening
    c. brightening
    d. darkening
    e. horizontal shift
82. While stenosis is increased, ___________ increase(s).
    a. vessel diameter
    b. systolic Doppler shift
    c. diastolic Doppler shift
    d. spectral broadening
    e. more than one of the above
83. Flow reversal in diastole (normal flow) indicates ___________.
    a. stenosis
    b. aneurysm
    c. high distal flow resistance
    d. low distal flow resistance
    e. more than one of the above
84. How many fast Fourier transforms are performed per second on a spectral display?
    a. 3
    b. 10
    c. >100
    d. >700
    e. 17,000
85. Each fast Fourier transform appears on a spectral display as a ___________.
    a. dot
    b. circle
    c. horizontal line
    d. vertical line
    e. none of the above
86. Hue is ___________.
    a. color seen
    b. light frequency
    c. brightness
    d. mix with white
    e. more than one of the above
87. A component not included in CW Doppler operation is a(n) ___________.
    a. loudspeaker
    b. wall filter
    c. oscillator
    d. demodulator
    e. range gate
88. On a spectral display, amplitude is indicated by ___________.
    a. brightness
    b. horizontal position
    c. vertical position
    d. b and c
    e. none of the above
89. Doppler shift can change because of changes in ___________.
    a. velocity
    b. speed
    c. direction
    d. frequency
    e. all of the above
90. A gate-open time of 10 ms corresponds to a sample volume length (millimeters) of ___________.
    a. 10.0
    b. 7.7
    c. 3.8
    d. 3.3
    e. 2.0
91. Sample volume width is determined by ___________.
    a. gate-open time
    b. pulse duration
    c. pulse-repetition frequency
    d. pulse-repetition period
    e. beam width

92. What problem(s) is (are) encountered if the pulse-repetition frequency is 10 kHz, sample volume is located at a depth of 10 cm, and the Doppler shift is 4 kHz?
   a. aliasing
   b. mirror image
   c. refraction
   d. range ambiguity
   e. more than one of the above
93. What problem(s) is (are) encountered if the pulse-repetition frequency is 10 kHz, sample volume is located at a depth of 5 cm, and the Doppler shift is 6 kHz?
   a. aliasing
   b. mirror image
   c. refraction
   d. range ambiguity
   e. more than one of the above
94. What problem(s) is (are) encountered if the pulse-repetition frequency is 10 kHz, sample volume is located at a depth of 10 cm, and the Doppler shift is 6 kHz?
   a. aliasing
   b. mirror image
   c. refraction
   d. range ambiguity
   e. more than one of the above
95. The functions of a color Doppler signal processor include ___________.
   a. amplification
   b. phase quadrature detection
   c. demodulation
   d. autocorrelation
   e. all of the above
96. If all cells in a vessel were moving at the same constant speed, the spectral trace would be a ___________ line.
   a. thin horizontal
   b. thick horizontal
   c. thin vertical
   d. thick vertical
   e. none of the above
97. Power Doppler imaging displays ___________.
   a. are independent of Doppler angle
   b. are more sensitive than Doppler-shift displays
   c. are independent of aliasing
   d. show uniform flow presentations
   e. all of the above.
98. For a physiologic flow speed, a 5 MHz beam could produce a Doppler shift of about ___________.
   a. 5 kHz
   b. 5 MHz
   c. 5 Hz
   d. depends on the mode (continuous wave or pulsed wave)
   e. none of the above
99. Spectral analysis is performed in a Doppler instrument ___________.
   a. electronically
   b. mathematically
   c. acoustically
   d. mechanically
   e. more than one of the above
100. The Doppler shift is proportional to ___________.
   a. the volume flow rate
   b. flow speed
   c. the Doppler angle
   d. cell density
   e. more than one of the above
101. Which of the following can be used to evaluate the performance of a Doppler instrument?
   a. contrast detail phantom
   b. string test object
   c. flow phantom
   d. b and c
   e. all of the above
102. Place the following instruments in general order of increasing acoustic output: (1) spectral Doppler, (2) B mode, and (3) color Doppler.
   a. 1, 2, 3
   b. 2, 3, 1
   c. 3, 1, 2
   d. 3, 2, 1
   e. 2, 1, 3
103. If operating frequency is 5 MHz, Doppler angle is 60 degrees, pulse-repetition frequency is 9 kHz, and the Doppler shift is 2 kHz, what problem is encountered if the angle is changed to zero?
   a. aliasing
   b. range ambiguity
   c. mirror image
   d. refraction
   e. none
104. When angle correction is applied in color Doppler, the Nyquist limits (in cm/s) on the color map ___________.
   a. increase
   b. decrease
   c. do not change
   d. are irrelevant
   e. are ambiguous
105. When angle correction is applied in color Doppler, the Nyquist limits (in kHz) on the color map ___________.
   a. increase
   b. decrease
   c. do not change
   d. are irrelevant
   e. are ambiguous
106. Flow is ___________ if it appears red on a color Doppler imaging display.
   a. approaching
   b. receding
   c. turbulent
   d. disturbed
   e. undetermined (depends on color map)
107. Two different colors in the same vessel indicate ___________.
   a. flow reversal
   b. sector scan
   c. vessel curvature
   d. aliasing
   e. any of the above

108. Which of the following increase(s) the amount of color appearing in a vessel?
a. increased color gain
b. increased wall filter
c. increased priority
d. increased pulse-repetition frequency
e. more than one of the above

109. Which of the following decrease(s) the amount of color appearing in a vessel?
a. increased wall filter
b. increased pulse-repetition frequency
c. increased ensemble length
d. baseline shift
e. more than one of the above

110. Which of the following on a color Doppler display is (are) presented as a two-dimensional, cross-sectional display?
a. grayscale anatomy
b. flow direction
c. Doppler spectrum
d. a and b
e. all of the above

111. Comparing gray with white is an example of ___________.
a. hue
b. luminance
c. saturation
d. b and c
e. all of the above

112. Comparing red with green is an example of ___________.
a. hue
b. luminance
c. saturation
d. b and c
e. all of the above

113. There are about ___________ frames per second produced in color Doppler mode.
a. 10
b. 20
c. 40
d. 80
e. more than one of the above

114. The autocorrelation technique yields ___________.
a. the mean Doppler shift
b. a sign of the Doppler shift
c. a spread around the mean (variance)
d. all of the above
e. none of the above

115. Increasing ensemble length ___________ color sensitivity and accuracy and ___________ frame rate.
a. improves, increases
b. degrades, increases
c. degrades, decreases
d. improves, decreases
e. none of the above

116. Which control can be used to help with clutter?
a. wall filter
b. gain
c. baseline shift
d. pulse-repetition frequency
e. smoothing

117. Doubling the width of a color window produces a(n) ___________ frame rate.
a. doubled
b. quadrupled
c. unchanged
d. halved
e. quartered

118. Steering the color window to the right or left changes the ___________.
a. frame rate
b. pulse-repetition frequency
c. Doppler angle
d. Doppler shift
e. more than one of the above

119. Lack of color in a vessel may be attributed to ___________.
a. low color gain
b. low wall filter setting
c. small Doppler angle
d. low baseline shift
e. more than one of the above

120. Which control(s) can help with aliasing?
a. wall filter
b. gain
c. smoothing
d. pulse-repetition frequency
e. more than one of the above

121. Pulse duration is the ___________ for a pulse to occur.
a. space
b. time
c. delay
d. pressure
e. reciprocal

122. Spatial pulse length equals the number of cycles in the pulse multiplied by ___________.
a. period
b. impedance
c. beam width
d. resolution
e. wavelength

123. If pulse duration is 1 ms and the pulse-repetition period is 100 ms, duty factor is ___________ %.
a. 1
b. 10
c. 50
d. 90
e. 100

124. The attenuation of 5 MHz ultrasound in 4 cm of soft tissue is ___________.
a. 5 dB/cm
b. 10 dB
c. 2.5 MHz/cm
d. 2 cm
e. 5 dB/MHz

125. If the maximum value of an acoustic variable in a sound wave is 10 units and the normal (no sound) value is 7 units, the amplitude is ___________ units.
a. 1
b. 3
c. 7
d. 10
e. 17

126. Impedance equals propagation speed multiplied by ___________.
a. density
b. stiffness
c. frequency
d. attenuation
e. path length

127. Which of the following cannot be determined from the others?
a. frequency
b. amplitude
c. intensity
d. power
e. beam area

128. For perpendicular incidence, in medium 1, density equals 1 and propagation speed equals 3; in medium 2, density equals 1.5 and propagation speed equals 2. What is the intensity reflection coefficient?
a. 0
b. 1
c. 2
d. 3
e. 4

129. For perpendicular incidence, if the intensity transmission coefficient is 96%, what is the intensity reflection coefficient?
a. 2%
b. 4%
c. 6%
d. 8%
e. 10%

130. The colors presented in power Doppler imaging represent the ___________ of the spectrum.
a. mean Doppler shift
b. variance
c. area
d. angle
e. all of the above

131. For oblique incidence and a medium 2 speed that is equal to twice the speed of medium 1, the transmission angle will be about ___________ times the incidence angle.
a. 0.5
b. 17
c. 2
d. 4
e. 5

132. The range equation describes the relationship of ___________.
a. reflector distance, propagation time, and sound speed
b. distance, propagation time, and reflection coefficient
c. number of cows and sheep on a ranch
d. propagation time, sound speed, and transducer frequency
e. dynamic range and system sensitivity

133. Axial resolution in a system equals ___________.
a. four times the spatial pulse length
b. the ratio of reflector size to transducer frequency
c. the maximum reflector separation expected to be displayed
d. the minimum reflector separation expected to be displayed
e. spatial pulse length

134. In soft tissue, two boundaries that generate reflections are separated in axial distance (depth) by 1 mm. With a two-cycle pulse of ultrasound, the minimum frequency that will axially resolve these boundaries is ___________ MHz.
a. 1.0
b. 2.0
c. 3.0
d. 4.0
e. 5.0

135. Transducers operating properly in pulse-echo imaging systems have a quality factor of approximately ___________.
a. 1 to 3
b. 7 to 10
c. 25 to 50
d. 100
e. 500

136. Which of the following quantities varies most with distance from the transducer face?
a. axial resolution
b. lateral resolution
c. frequency
d. wavelength
e. period

137. The near-zone length for an unfocused, 5 MHz, circular transducer with a diameter of 13 mm is greater than that for a 5 MHz transducer with a diameter of ___________.
a. 19 mm
b. 15 mm
c. 9 mm
d. depends on impedance
e. none of the above

138. If the near-zone length of an unfocused transducer that is 13 mm in diameter extends (in soft tissue) 6 cm from the transducer face, at which of the following distances from the face can the lateral resolution be improved by focusing the sound from this transducer?
  a. 13 cm
  b. 8 cm
  c. 3 cm
  d. 9 cm
  e. none of the above
139. The lateral resolution of an ultrasound system depends on ___________.
  a. the aperture
  b. the transducer frequency
  c. the speed of sound in soft tissue
  d. the memory and the display
  e. all of the above
140. Which of the following is a characteristic of a medium through which sound is propagating?
  a. impedance
  b. intensity
  c. amplitude
  d. frequency
  e. period
141. Which of the following cannot be determined from the others?
  a. frequency
  b. period
  c. amplitude
  d. wavelength
  e. propagation speed
142. For perpendicular incidence, if the impedances of two media are the same, there will be no _________.
  a. inflation
  b. reflection
  c. refraction
  d. calibration
  e. b and c
143. What is the transmitted intensity if the incident intensity is 1 and the impedances are 1.00 and 2.64?
  a. 0.2
  b. 0.4
  c. 0.6
  d. 0.8
  e. 1.0
144. Increasing the intensity produced by the transducer _________.
  a. is accomplished by increasing pulser voltage
  b. increases the sensitivity of the system
  c. increases the possibility of biologic effects
  d. all of the above
  e. none of the above
145. If the propagation speeds of two media are equal, incidence angle equals ___________.
  a. the reflection angle
  b. the transmission angle
  c. the Doppler angle
  d. a and b
  e. b and c
146. If no reflection occurs at a boundary, it always means that media impedances are equal in the case of ___________.
  a. perpendicular incidence
  b. oblique incidence
  c. refraction
  d. a and b
  e. b and c
147. Increasing spatial pulse length ___________.
  a. accompanies increased transducer damping
  b. is accompanied by decreased pulse duration
  c. improves axial resolution
  d. all of the above
  e. none of the above
148. Select the correct order of increasing sound propagation speed.
  a. gas, solid, liquid
  b. solid, liquid, gas
  c. gas, liquid, solid
  d. liquid, solid, gas
  e. solid, gas, liquid
149. What is the wavelength of a 1 MHz ultrasound pulse in tissue with a propagation speed of 1540 m/s?
  a. 1×10^6m
  b. 1.54 mm
  c. 1540 m
  d. 1.54 cm
  e. 0.77 cm
150. What is the spatial pulse length for two cycles of ultrasound having a wavelength of 2 mm?
  a. 4 cm
  b. 4 mm
  c. 7 mm
  d. 1.5 mm
  e. 3 mm
151. Increased damping produces ___________.
  a. increased bandwidth
  b. shorter pulses
  c. decreased efficiency
  d. all of the above
  e. none of the above
152. If no refraction occurs as an oblique sound beam passes through the boundary between two materials, what is unchanged as the boundary is crossed?
  a. impedance
  b. propagation speed
  c. intensity
  d. sound direction
  e. b and d
153. If the spatial average intensity in a beam is 1 W/cm^2 and the transducer is 5 cm^2 in area, what is the total acoustic power?
  a. 1 W
  b. 2 W
  c. 3 W
  d. 4 W
  e. 5 W

154. How does the propagation speed in bone compare with that in soft tissue?
   a. lower
   b. the same
   c. higher
   d. cannot say unless soft tissue is specified
   e. b and c
155. Attenuation along a sound path is a decrease in ________.
   a. frequency
   b. amplitude
   c. intensity
   d. b and c
   e. impedance
156. A focused transducer that is 13 mm in diameter has a lateral resolution at the focus of better than (i.e., smaller than) ________.
   a. 26 mm
   b. 13 mm
   c. 6.5 mm
   d. depends on frequency
   e. none of the above
157. An important factor in the selection of a transducer for a specific application is the ultrasonic attenuation of tissue. Because of this attenuation, a 7.5 MHz transducer generally should be used for ________.
   a. imaging deep structures
   b. imaging superficial structures
   c. imaging deep and shallow structures
   d. imaging adult intracranial structures
   e. all of the above
158. A real-time scan ________.
   a. consists of many frames produced per second
   b. depends on how short a time the sonographer takes to make a scan
   c. is made only between 8 a.m. and 5 p.m.
   d. yields a grayscale image, whereas other scans yield only an M-mode display
   e. none of the above
159. Which of the following is determined by the pulser in an instrument?
   a. amplitude
   b. pulse-repetition frequency
   c. length of time required for a pulse to reach a specific reflector and return to the instrument
   d. more than one of the above
   e. none of the above
160. If the power at the output of an amplifier is 1000 times the power at the input, the gain is ________.
   a. 60 dB
   b. 30 dB
   c. 1000 dB
   d. 1000 volts
   e. none of the above
161. The dynamic range of an ultrasound system is defined as ________.
   a. the speed with which an ultrasound examination can be performed
   b. the range over which the transducer can be manipulated
   c. the ratio of the maximum to the minimum intensity that can be displayed
   d. the range of pulser voltages applied to the transducer
   e. none of the above
162. The display generally will have a dynamic range ________ than other portions of the ultrasound instrument.
   a. larger
   b. smaller
163. The number 30 in the binary system is ________.
   a. 0110
   b. 1110
   c. 1001
   d. 1111
   e. none of the above
164. An ultrasound scanner that can represent 64 shades of gray would require an 8-bit memory. True or false?
165. Imaging systems consist of a beam former, display, and ________ and ________ processors.
   a. beam, digitizer
   b. image, amplifier
   c. signal, pulser
   d. amplifier, digitizer
   e. signal, image
166. Phased arrays involve the sequential switching of a small group of elements along the array. True or false?
167. For a two-cycle pulse of 5 MHz in soft tissue, the axial resolution is ________ mm.
   a. 0.1
   b. 0.3
   c. 0.5
   d. 0.7
   e. 0.9
168. Postprocessing is the process of assigning numbers to be placed in the memory. True or false?
169. The minimum displayed axial dimension of a reflector is approximately equal to ________.
   a. the beam diameter
   b. half the beam diameter
   c. twice the beam diameter
   d. the spatial pulse length
   e. half the spatial pulse length
   f. twice the spatial pulse length
170. The minimum displayed lateral dimension of a reflector is approximately equal to ________.
   a. the beam diameter
   b. half the beam diameter
   c. twice the beam diameter
   d. the spatial pulse length
   e. half the spatial pulse length
   f. twice the spatial pulse length

171. M-mode recordings have ____________ dimension(s).
  a. two spatial
  b. one spatial and one temporal
  c. one Doppler and one temporal
  d. one Doppler and one spatial
  e. b and c

172. Nonlinear propagation of ultrasound in tissue generates ____________.
  a. speckle
  b. attenuation
  c. harmonics
  d. refraction
  e. reverberations

173. The operation in the signal processor that reduces noise is ____________.
  a. filtering
  b. time gain compensation
  c. scan conversion
  d. compression
  e. detection

174. The binary number 01001 is ____________ in the decimal system.
  a. 1
  b. 3
  c. 5
  d. 7
  e. 9

175. Reflectors may be added to the display because of ____________.
  a. reverberation
  b. propagation speed error
  c. enhancement
  d. oblique reflection
  e. the Doppler shift

176. If the propagation speed in a soft tissue path is 1.60 mm/μs, a diagnostic instrument assumes a propagation speed too ____________ and will show reflectors too ____________ the transducer.
  a. high, close to
  b. high, far from
  c. low, close to
  d. low, far from
  e. none of the above

177. The reflector information that can be obtained from an M-mode display includes ____________.
  a. distance and motion pattern
  b. transducer frequency, reflection coefficient, and distance
  c. acoustic impedance, attenuation, and motion pattern
  d. all of the above
  e. none of the above

178. Increasing gain generally produces the same effect as ____________.
  a. decreasing attenuation
  b. increasing compression
  c. increasing rectification
  d. both b and c
  e. all of the above

179. A grayscale display shows ____________.
  a. gray color on a white background
  b. reflections with one brightness level
  c. a white color on a gray background
  d. a range of reflection amplitudes or intensities
  e. none of the above

180. Electric pulses from the pulser are applied through the delays and transmit/receive switch to the ____________.
  a. pulser
  b. transducer
  c. demodulator
  d. display
  e. memory

181. Peak detection is part of ____________.
  a. amplipression
  b. rejection
  c. a and b
  d. compression
  e. amplitude demodulation

182. Multiple focus is not used with color-Doppler instruments because of ____________.
  a. ensemble length
  b. wall filter
  c. priority
  d. low frame rate
  e. a and d

183. If the gain of an amplifier is reduced by 3 dB and input power is unchanged, the output power of the amplifier is ____________ what it was before.
  a. equal to
  b. twice
  c. one-half
  d. greater than
  e. none of the above

184. If gain was 30 dB and output power is reduced by one-half, the new gain is ____________ dB.
  a. 15
  b. 60
  c. 33
  d. 27
  e. none of the above

185. If four shades of gray are shown on a display, each twice the brightness of the preceding one, the brightest shade is ____________ times the brightness of the dimmest shade.
  a. 2
  b. 4
  c. 8
  d. 16
  e. 32

186. The dynamic range displayed in Exercise 185 is ____________ dB.
  a. 100
  b. 9
  c. 5
  d. 2
  e. 0

187. Phantoms with nylon lines measure ____________.
a. resolution
b. pulse duration
c. spatial average-temporal average intensity
d. wavelength
e. all of the above

188. Which of the following may be used to measure acoustic output?
a. hydrophone
b. optical encoder
c. 100 mm test object
d. all of the above
e. none of the above

189. Real-time imaging is made possible by ____________.
a. preprocessors
b. single-element transducers
c. grayscale display
d. transmit/receive switches
e. arrays

190. Gain and attenuation are usually expressed in ____________.
a. decibels
b. decibels per centimeter
c. centimeters
d. centimeters per decibel
e. none of the above

191. Grayscale display requires ____________.
a. array transducers
b. cathode-ray storage tubes
c. more than one bit per pixel
d. b and c
e. all of the above

192. With which of the following is time represented on one axis?
a. B mode
b. B scan
c. M mode
d. a la mode
e. none of the above

193. Analog voltages occur at the output of the ____________.
a. beam former
b. transducer
c. signal processor
d. display
e. a and b

194. Digital signals occur at the output of the ____________.
a. beam former
b. transducer
c. signal processor
d. display
e. a and c

195. Which of the following produce(s) a rectangular image format?
a. vector array
b. convex array
c. phased array
d. linear array
e. all of the above

196. The piezoelectric effect describes how ____________ is converted into ____________ by a ____________.
a. electricity, an image, display
b. incident sound, reflected sound, boundary
c. ultrasound, electricity, transducer
d. ultrasound, heat, tissue
e. none of the above

197. Propagation speed in soft tissues ____________.
a. is directly proportional to frequency
b. is inversely proportional to frequency
c. is directly proportional to intensity
d. is inversely proportional to intensity
e. none of the above

198. Power Doppler imaging indicates (with color) the ____________ of flow.
a. presence
b. direction
c. speed
d. character
e. more than one of the above

199. While frequency is increased, ____________.
a. wavelength increases
b. a three-cycle ultrasound pulse decreases in length
c. imaging depth decreases
d. propagation speed decreases
e. b and c

200. Focusing ____________.
a. improves lateral resolution
b. improves axial resolution
c. increases beam width in the focal region
d. shortens pulse length
e. increases duty factor

GLOSSARY

All of the key terms that were listed at the beginning of the individual chapters are compiled and defined here. More detailed and complete compilations of terminology are available, e.g., in American Institute of Ultrasound in Medicine: *Recommended ultrasound terminology*, ed 4, Laurel, MD, 2019.

A

A mode Mode of operation in which the display presents echo amplitude versus depth (used in ophthalmology).

absorption Conversion of sound to heat.

acoustic Having to do with sound.

acoustic radiation force impulse imaging (ARFI) Quantifying and/or imaging tissue stiffness by transmitting a long push-pulse to generate and then track the shear displacements of the slower propagating shear wave.

acoustic variables Pressure, density, and particle vibration; sound wave quantities that vary in space and time.

ALARA As low as reasonably achievable. The principle that it is prudent to obtain diagnostic information with the least amount of energy exposure to the patient as possible.

aliasing Improper Doppler information obtained in spectral or color Doppler modes when the true Doppler shift exceeds one-half the pulse-repetition frequency.

amplification The process by which small values (e.g., small voltages) are increased to larger ones.

amplifier A device that accomplishes amplification.

amplitude Maximum variation of an acoustic variable or voltage.

amplitude modulation A multipulse CEUS technique designed to suppress fundamental echoes and retain the nonlinear echoes (from contrast microbubbles) to improve CEUS image quality. Two pulses are transmitted with one being half the amplitude of the other and the returned echoes from this pulse are scaled up and subtracted from the other pulse echoes.

analog Related to a procedure or system in which data are represented by proportional, continuously variable, and physical quantities (e.g., electric voltage).

analog-to-digital converter (ADC) A device that converts voltage amplitude to a number.

anechoic Echo-free.

aperture Size of a transducer element (for a single-element transducer) or group of elements (for an array).

apodization Nonuniform (i.e., involving different voltage amplitudes) driving of elements (or weighing of echo responses) in an array to reduce grating lobes.

array A transducer assembly containing several (up to thousands) of piezoelectric elements.

artificial intelligence A computer algorithm for intelligent assessment of the input information. In ultrasound imaging AI is being used to evaluate images and provide guidance on scan planes, biopsies and tissue characterization (e.g., assessing breast lesions as more or less likely to be benign or malignant).

attenuation Decrease in amplitude and intensity with distance as a wave travels through a medium.

attenuation coefficient Attenuation per centimeter per MHz of wave travel; typical value is 0.5 dB/(cm MHz).

attenuation imaging Quantitative estimation and display of tissue attenuation coefficients.

autocorrelation A rapid technique, used in most color flow Doppler instruments, to obtain mean Doppler-shift frequency or amplitude (or intensity or power or energy).

axial In the direction of the transducer axis (sound travel direction).

axial resolution The minimum reflector separation along the sound path that is required to produce separate echoes (i.e., to distinguish between two reflectors).

B

B color A form of postprocessing that assigns colors, rather than gray level, to different echo strengths.

B flow Using coded excitation to produce grayscale imaging of blood flow.

B mode Mode of operation in which the display presents a spot of appropriate brightness for each echo received by the transducer.

B scan A B-mode image that represents an anatomical cross section through the scanning plane.

Bandpass filter A digital filter that passes a range of frequencies (its bandwidth) and rejects those above and below the acceptance bandwidth.

backscatter Sound scattered back in the direction from which it originally came.

bandwidth Range of frequencies contained in an ultrasound pulse; range of frequencies within which a material, device, or system can operate.

baseline shift Movement of the zero Doppler-shift frequency or zero flow speed line up or down on a spectral display.

beam Region containing continuous wave sound; region through which a sound pulse propagates.

beam former The part of an instrument that accomplishes electronic beam scanning, apodization, steering, focusing, and aperture with arrays.

Bernoulli effect Pressure reduction in a region of high-flow speed.

bistable Having two possible states (e.g., on or off, white or black, and one or zero).

bit Binary digit; one or zero.

broad transmit beam imaging A few (as low as one) unfocused or minimally focused beams of ultrasound are transmitted through the anatomical cross-section to be imaged, but they do not produce a one-for-one correspondence between transmitted pulse and displayed scan line. Instead, all the echo information from throughout the imaged cross section is collected, and then a massive computational process determines the location and strength of each echo at each given location in the anatomy. This approach is used in newer, more sophisticated instruments and produces improved image quality compared with traditional narrow beam scanners. (See also *grayscale image* and *narrow transmit beam imaging.*)

C

capacitive micromachined ultrasound transducer See *CMUT.*

Cardiac strain imaging An echocardiographic technique that provides information regarding contraction and relaxation strain and strain rate information for the myocardium of the beating heart.

cavitation Production and/or dynamics of bubbles in a sound field.

channel A single one- or two-way path for transmitting electric signals or digital numbers, in distinction from other parallel paths; an independent transmission delay line and transducer element path; an independent reception transducer element, amplifier, analog-to-digital converter, and delay line path.

cine loop Sequential display of all the frames stored in memory at a controllable frame rate.

clutter Noise in the Doppler signal that generally is caused by high-amplitude, Doppler-shifted echoes from the heart or vessel walls or other slow-moving structures in the body.

CMUT capacitive micromachined ultrasound transducer that contains miniature elements that are comprised of two electrically conducting layers facing each other; one of which is fixed and the other of which is a flexible membrane.

coded excitation A sophisticated form of transmission in which the driving voltage pulses have intrapulse variations in amplitude, frequency, and/or phase.

color Doppler display The presentation of two-dimensional, real-time Doppler shift information in color superimposed on a real-time, grayscale, anatomical, cross-sectional image. Flow directions toward and away from the transducer (i.e., positive and negative Doppler shifts) are presented as different colors on the display.

comet tail A series of closely spaced reverberation echoes.
compensation Equalization of received echo amplitude differences caused by different attenuations for different reflector depths; also called *depth gain compensation* or *time gain compensation*.
compliance Distensibility; nonrigid stretchability of vessels.
composite Combination of a piezoelectric ceramic and a nonpiezoelectric polymer.
compounding Averaging of frames that depict the anatomy from different aspects. See also *frequency compounding* (i.e., averaging over different frequencies) and *spatial compounding* (i.e., averaging over different angles).
compression Reduction in differences between small and large amplitudes. Region of high density and pressure in a compressional wave.
constructive interference Combination of only positive or only negative pressures.
continuous wave (CW) A wave in which cycles repeat indefinitely; not pulsed.
continuous-wave (CW) Doppler A Doppler device or procedure that uses continuous-wave ultrasound.
contrast agent A suspension of microbubbles introduced into circulation to enhance the contrast between anatomical structures and the blood, thereby improving imaging.
contrast enhanced ultrasound (CEUS) Imaging of an ultrasound contrast agent to enhance the echo strength between anatomical structures and the blood, thereby improving imaging.
contrast-specific imaging Any CEUS imaging mode that is specifically designed to depict nonlinear microbubble signals and suppress linear (i.e., tissue) echoes. For example, *contrast harmonic imaging.*
contrast resolution Ability of a grayscale display to distinguish between echoes of slightly different intensities.
convex array Curved or curvi linear array.
Cosine (*cos*) The cosine of angle A in Fig. C.1 is the length of side b divided by the length of side c.
coupling medium A gel used to eliminate the air between a transducer and the skin thus providing a good sound path to couple ultrasound pulses into a patient.
cross-talk Leakage of strong signals in one direction channel of a Doppler receiver into the other channel; can produce the spectral Doppler mirror-image artifact.
crystal Element.
Curie point Temperature at which an element material loses its piezoelectric properties.
cycle One complete variation of an acoustic variable.

D

damping Material attached to the rear face of a transducer element to reduce pulse duration; the process of pulse duration reduction.
decibel (dB) Unit of power or intensity ratio; the number of decibels is 10 times the logarithm (to the base 10) of the power or intensity ratio.
deep learning A specific form of AI. (See also *artificial intelligence.*
demodulation Detection.
density Mass divided by volume.
depth gain compensation (DGC) See *time gain compensation.*
destructive interference Combination of both positive and negative pressures.
detail resolution The ability to image fine detail and to distinguish closely spaced reflectors. (See also *axial resolution* and *lateral resolution.*)
detection Conversion of voltage pulses from radio frequency to video form or digital numbers. Also called *demodulation, amplitude detection*, and *envelope detection.*
digital Related to a procedure or system in which data are represented by numeric digits.
digital-to-analog converter (DAC) A device that converts a number to a proportional voltage amplitude.
disk A thin, flat, and circular object.
display A device that presents a visual image derived from voltages or digital numbers received from an image processor.
disturbed flow Flow that cannot be described by straight, parallel streamlines.
Doppler angle The angle between the sound beam and the flow direction.
Doppler effect A change in frequency caused by reflector motion.
Doppler equation The mathematical description of the relationship between the Doppler shift, frequency, Doppler angle, propagation speed, and reflector speed (typically the velocity of the moving blood).
Doppler shift Reflected frequency minus incident frequency; the change in frequency caused by motion.
Doppler spectrum The range of frequencies present in Doppler-shifted echoes.
Doppler ultrasound Doppler ultrasound modes include the detection, quantification, and evaluation of tissue motion and specifically blood flow by using the Doppler effect with ultrasound imaging.
duplex instrument An ultrasound instrument that combines grayscale ultrasound with pulsed wave (PW) Doppler and, possibly, continuous wave (CW) Doppler.
duty factor Fraction of time that pulsed ultrasound is on.
dynamic aperture Aperture that increases with increasing focal length (to maintain constant focal width).
dynamic focusing Continuously varying focusing on reception that corrects for the increasing depth of the transmitted pulse as it travels.
dynamic range Ratio (in decibels) of largest to smallest power that a system can handle; ratio of the largest to smallest intensity of echoes encountered.

E

echo Reflection (in this context of sound).
eddies Regions of circular flow patterns present in turbulence.
elastography Imaging tissue stiffness by tracking movement under mechanical stress.
element The piezoelectric component of a transducer assembly.
elevational resolution The detail resolution in the direction perpendicular to the scan plane. It is equal to the section thickness and is the source of section thickness artifact in narrow transmit beam systems.
energy Capability of doing work.
enhancement Increase in echo amplitude from reflectors that lie behind a weakly attenuating structure or from an ultrasound contrast agent.
ensemble length Number of pulses used to generate one color flow Doppler scan line.

F

far zone The region of a sound beam in which the beam diameter increases as the distance from the transducer increases; also called *far field* or *Fraunhofer zone.*
fast Fourier transform (FFT) Very fast, digital computer implementation of the Fourier transform, which is a mathematical technique for obtaining a (Doppler) frequency spectrum.
filter An electrical circuit or software implemented digital filter that passes frequencies within a defined range and eliminates frequencies outside of this range.
flat-panel display A backlighted rectangular matrix of thousands of liquid-crystal display (LCD) or light emitting diodes (LED) elements that presents images.
flow To move in a stream; volume flow rate.
fluid A material that flows and conforms to the shape of its container; a gas or liquid.
focal length Distance from a focused transducer to the center of a focal region or to the location of the spatial peak intensity.
focal region Region of minimum beam diameter and area.
focal zone Length of the focal region.
focus The concentration of the sound beam into a smaller beam area than would exist otherwise.
Food and Drug Administration (FDA) The regulatory body within the federal government responsible for approving medical devices and drugs such as ultrasound scanners and contrast agents.
four-dimensional (4D) imaging Three-dimensional (3D) imaging performed over time; see *three-dimensional (3D) imaging.*
fractional bandwidth Bandwidth divided by the operating frequency.
frame A single image produced by one complete scan of the sound beam.
frame rate Number of frames of echo information stored and/or displayed each second.

freeze Constant display of one of the frames in memory.
frequency Number of cycles per second.
frequency compounding Averaging of frames that depict the anatomy from a collection of different bandpass filters, i.e., averaging over different frequencies. (See also *compounding.*)
frequency spectrum The range of Doppler shifted frequencies present in the returning echoes.
fundamental frequency The primary (transmitted) frequency in a collection of frequencies that can include odd and even harmonics and subharmonics.
fusion imaging The real time and synchronous presentation of ultrasound images together with cross-sectional images from CT, MRI, or PET in the same anatomical imaging plane.

G

gain Ratio (in decibels) of amplifier output to input electric power or digital values.
gate A device that allows only echoes from a selected depth (i.e., arrival time) to pass.
graphics processing unit (GPU) An electronic device that rapidly performs digital calculations to accelerate the creation of images. A GPU includes 1000 to 10,000 processing cores running in parallel in order to reach 10 to 100 trillion operations per second.
grating lobes Additional weaker beams of sound traveling out in directions different from the primary beam as a result of the multielement structure of transducer arrays. Are not encountered in modern scanners.
grayscale Range of brightnesses (gray levels) between white and black.
grayscale image An ultrasound image showing echoes as visible dots, where the brightness of each dot corresponds to the echo strength, producing an of the anatomical location of the echo-generating structures.

H

harmonics Frequencies that are even and odd multiples of another, commonly called the *fundamental* or *operating frequency.*
hertz (Hz) Unit of frequency, one cycle per second; unit of pulse repetition frequency, one pulse per second.
high sensitive Doppler New Doppler flow modes with high sensitivity to slow flow in small vessels by use of advanced adaptive clutter suppression techniques. This information is displayed at high frame rates as a color overlay image (although grayscale maps of flow are also available).
hue The color perceived based on the frequency of light. It is used to indicate the relative velocity or power of the Doppler shifted echoes in color flow Doppler imaging (i.e., in color Doppler and power Doppler imaging)
hydrophone A small transducer element mounted on the end of a narrow tube/needle; a piezoelectric membrane with small metallic electrodes.
hypoechoic Having relatively weak echoes. Opposite of hyperechoic (having relatively strong echoes).

I

image A reproduction, representation, or imitation of the physical form of a person or thing.
image former The part of a scanner using broad transmit beams that acquires the echo information from the signal processor, performs the retrospective, virtual-beam computations and sends the results to the display.
image memory The part of the image processor where echo information is stored in image format.
image processor An electronic device that digitally manipulates and prepares images for visual presentation.
impedance Density multiplied by the sound propagation speed.
incidence angle Angle between incident sound direction and a line perpendicular to the boundary of a medium.
inertia Resistance to acceleration.
inertial cavitation This phenomenon occurs when nonlinear bubble oscillations are so large that the bubble is destroyed (i.e., it collapses), which can produce shock waves with localized temperature increases.
instrument An electronic system that electrically drives a transducer, receives returning echoes, and presents them on a visual display as an anatomical image, Doppler spectrum, or color-Doppler presentation.
intensity Power divided by area.
intensity reflection coefficient Reflected intensity divided by incident intensity; the fraction of incident intensity reflected.
intensity transmission coefficient Transmitted intensity divided by incident intensity; the fraction of incident intensity transmitted into the second medium.
interference Combinations of positive and/or negative pressures.
intravenous (IV) In a vein (as in contrast agents are injected into a vein).

K

kiloHertz (kHz) One thousand Hertz (i.e., 1000 Hz).

L

laminar flow Flow in which fluid layers slide over each other in a smooth, orderly manner, with no mixing between layers.
lateral Perpendicular to the direction of sound travel.
lateral gain control Gain controls that enable different gain values to be applied laterally across an image to compensate for differing attenuation values in different anatomical regions.
lateral resolution Minimum reflector separation perpendicular to the sound path that is required to produce separate echoes (i.e., to distinguish between the two reflectors).
lead zirconate titanate (PZT) A ceramic piezoelectric material.
lens A curved material that focuses a sound or light beam.
linear Adjectival form of *line.*
linear array Array made of rectangular elements arranged in a straight line.
linear scan/image An anatomical image presented in a rectangular format.
linear phased array Linear array operated by applying voltage pulses to all elements, but with small time differences (phasing) to direct ultrasound pulses out in various directions. The phasing can also be used for focusing.
longitudinal wave Wave in which the particle motion is parallel to the direction of wave travel (compressional wave).
luminance Brightness of a presented hue and saturation.

M

M mode A brightness presentation (grayscale or colorized) of changing reflector position (motion) versus time (used in echocardiography).
machine learning A specific form of AI. (See also *artificial intelligence.*
matching layer Material attached to the front face of a transducer element to reduce the reflections at the transducer/air interface (i.e., the surface of the transducer).
mechanical index An indicator of nonthermal mechanical activity; equal to the peak rarefactional pressure (derated by 0.3 dB/(cm MHz) divided by the square root of the center frequency of the pulse bandwidth.
medium Material through which a wave travels.
megaHertz (MHz) One million Hertz.
microbubbles Small (typically <10 μm), gas-filled bubbles used as ultrasound contrast agents.
mirror image An artifactual grayscale, color flow, or spectral Doppler signal appearing on the opposite side (from the real structure or flow) of a strong reflector.

N

narrow transmit beam imaging Many (hundreds) of focused beams of ultrasound are transmitted through the anatomical cross-section to be imaged. Positional information is determined by knowledge of the direction of the pulse when it enters the patient and by measurement of the time it takes for each echo to return to the transducer. Knowledge of the sound speed ensures a one-to-one correspondence between the pulse echo transmission and the displayed scan line. (See also *grayscale image* and *broad transmit beam imaging.*)
natural focus The narrowing of a sound beam that occurs with an unfocused flat transducer element.
near field signal loss The destruction of contrast microbubbles in the near field during CEUS.
near zone The region of a sound beam in which the beam diameter decreases as the distance from the transducer increases; also called *near field* or *Fresnel zone.*

nonlinear propagation Sound propagation in which the propagation speed depends on pressure causing the wave shape to change and higher as well as lower harmonics to be generated.
nonthermal bioeffects Mechanical effects on biological tissue caused by e.g., radiation force, streaming, and cavitation that can deform or disrupt cells. Also known as mechanical bioeffects. (See also *radiation* and *cavitation*.)
Nyquist limit The Doppler frequency above which aliasing occurs; one-half of the pulse repetition frequency.

O

oblique incidence Sound direction that is not perpendicular to media boundaries.
operating frequency Preferred (maximum efficiency) frequency of operation of a transducer. (See also *resonance frequency*.)
output display standard (ODS) This FDA approval pathway bypasses the limits in the 510(k) guide with the exception that an overall upper limit of 720 mW/cm² I_{SPTA} still applies in exchange for presenting output information on the display. (See also *mechanical index* and *thermal index*.)

P

panoramic imaging The extension of the field of view beyond the normal limits of a transducer scan plane.
parabolic flow Laminar flow with a profile in the shape of a parabola.
penetration Imaging depth.
period Time per cycle.
perpendicular Geometrically related by 90 degrees.
perpendicular incidence Sound direction that is perpendicular to the boundary between media.
persistence Averaging sequential frames together.
phantom Tissue-equivalent device that has characteristics that are representative of tissues (e.g., scattering, propagation speed, and attenuation).
phase quadrature Two signals differing by one-fourth of a cycle.
phased array An array that steers and focuses the beam electronically (with short time delays).
phased linear array Linear array with phased focusing added for phased steering of pulses to produce a parallelogram-shaped display. (See also *vector array*.)
physical beam The transmitted beam used to form a scan line. A concept mainly used in narrow transmit beam systems (as opposed to a virtual beam).
picture archiving and communications system (PACS) A system for electronically communicating images and associated information to workstations and devices external to the ultrasound scanner and the examining room.
piezoelectricity Conversion of mechanical pressure to electric voltage.
pixel Picture element; the unit into which imaging information is divided for storage and display in a digital scanner.
plug flow Flow with all fluid portions traveling with the same flow speed and direction.
point of care ultrasound (POCUS) Refers to clinicians (typically not radiologists) performing studies at the bed-side (in the ER or in the OR), at a sporting event, among underserved and/or inaccessible communities or just anywhere else where patients can be found and quick decision making based on ultrasound imaging is required.
poise Unit of viscosity.
Poiseuille equation The mathematical description of the dependence of volume flow rate on pressure, vessel length and radius, and fluid viscosity.
postprocessing Image processing done after storage in the memory.
power Rate at which work is done; rate at which energy is transferred.
Power Doppler display Color flow Doppler display in which colors are assigned according to the strength (amplitude, power, intensity, and energy) of the Doppler shifted echoes.
preprocessing Signal and image processing accomplished before storage in the memory.
pressure Force divided by the area in a medium.
priority The grayscale echo strength below which color-coded Doppler information is shown preferentially on a display (also known as *write priority*).
probe Transducer assembly.
propagation Progression or travel.
propagation speed Speed at which a wave moves through a medium.
pseudo enhancement An artifact when the region of interest of a CEUS examination contains highly echogenic tissue or when an excessive amount of contrast has been administrated, it is possible that area will appear as enhanced.
pseudo-washout An artifact when the internal vascularity of a lesion or other area of interest appear to washout over time, but in reality, it is the contrast signal decreasing over time.
pulsatile flow Flow that accelerates and decelerates with each cardiac cycle.
pulse A brief excursion of a quantity from its normal value; a few cycles.
pulse duration Interval of time from beginning to end of a pulse.
pulsed Doppler A Doppler device or procedure that uses pulsed-wave ultrasound (also known as *pulsed wave [PW] Doppler*).
pulse-echo principle Ultrasound imaging in which pulses are reflected and used to produce a display. Also referred to as the *pulse echo technique*.
pulse-echo technique See *pulse echo principle*.
pulse inversion A multipulse CEUS technique designed to suppress fundamental echoes and retain the nonlinear echoes (from contrast microbubbles) to improve CEUS image quality. Two pulses are transmitted with one being 180 degrees out of phase with the other. The returned echoes from this pulse are added to echoes from the other pulse to cancel out linear (i.e., fundamental) signals.
pulse-repetition frequency (PRF) Number of pulses per second.
pulse-repetition period Interval of time from the beginning of one pulse to the beginning of the next.
pulsed ultrasound Ultrasound produced in pulsed form by applying electric pulses or voltages of one or a few cycles to the transducer.

Q

quality assurance (QA) Regularly performed testing program to verify the performance characteristics of a given ultrasound scanner has not deteriorated over time.
quality control (QC) See *quality assurance*.
quantitative ultrasound Deriving quantitative information related to the underlying acoustic properties of different tissues. (See also *attenuation imaging*.)

R

radiation force The force exerted by a sound beam on an absorber or a reflector.
radio frequency (RF) Voltages representing echoes in cyclic form.
range ambiguity An artifact produced when echoes are placed too close to the transducer because a second pulse was emitted before they were received from the first pulse.
range equation Relationship between round-trip pulse travel time, propagation speed, and distance to a reflector.
range gating Selection of the depth from which echoes are accepted based on echo arrival time.
rarefaction Region of low density and pressure in a compressional wave.
rayl Unit of impedance.
real-time Imaging with a rapid frame sequence display (as a rule of thumb: a frame rate >10 Hz).
real-time display A display that, with a sufficient frame rate (typically >10 Hz), appears to image moving structures or a changing scan plane continuously.
reflection Portion of sound returned from a media boundary; echo.
reflection angle Angle between the reflected sound direction and a line perpendicular to the media boundary.
reflector Media boundary that produces a reflection; reflecting surface.
refraction Change of sound direction pf travel when passing from one medium to another.
refresh rate The number of times each second that information is sent from the image memory to the display. The number of times per second that a computer monitor redraws the information found in the memory.
resistance Pressure difference divided by volume flow rate for steady flow.

resolution The ability to distinguish echoes in terms of space, time, or strength (called *detail, temporal,* and *contrast resolutions,* respectively).
resonance frequency Preferred (maximum efficiency or response) frequency of operation of a transducer. (Also called *operating frequency.*)
reverberation Multiple reflections.

S

sample volume The anatomical region from which PW Doppler echoes are accepted
saturation The amount of hue present in a mix with white.
scan line A line produced on a display that represents ultrasonic echoes returning from the body. A narrow transmit beam ultrasound image is composed of many such lines.
scanhead Transducer assembly.
scanning The sweeping of a sound beam through the anatomy to produce an image.
scatterer An object that scatters sound in many directions because of its small size or its surface roughness.
scattering Diffusion or redirection of sound in several directions upon encountering a particle suspension or a rough surface.
sector A geometric figure bounded by two radii and the arc of the circle included between them.
sector scan/image An anatomical image presented in a pie slice–shaped format.
sensitivity Ability of an imaging system to detect weak echoes.
shadowing Reduction in echo amplitude from reflectors that lie behind a strongly reflecting or attenuating structure.
shear wave A sound wave in which the particle motion is perpendicular to the direction of wave travel, also called a *transverse wave.*
shear wave elastography Imaging tissue stiffness by transmitting a long push-pulse to generate and then track the shear displacements of the slower propagating shear wave, which are depicted as a color overlay on the anatomical grayscale image. Quantitative values in kPa or m/s are obtained.
side lobes Weaker beams of sound traveling out from a single element in directions different from those of the primary beam. Rarely encountered in clinical practice.
signal Information-bearing voltages in an electric circuit; an acoustic, visual, electric, or other conveyance of information in analog or digital format. The physical representation of a message or information.
signal processor An electronic device that manipulates signals (analog or digital) in preparation for appropriate presentation of information contained in them.
slice thickness Thickness of the scanned tissue volume perpendicular to the scan plane; also called *section thickness.*
sonography Medical two-dimensional, cross-sectional, and three-dimensional volumetric anatomical and flow imaging using ultrasound.
sound Traveling wave of acoustic variables.
sound beam The region of a medium that contains virtually all of the sound produced by a transducer.
source An emitter of ultrasound; a transducer.
spatial compounding Averaging of frames that view the anatomy from different angles. (See also *compounding.*)
spatial pulse length Length of a pulse in space (e.g., in mm).
speckle The granular appearance of images and spectral displays that is caused by the interference of echoes from the distribution of scatterers in tissue.
spectral analysis Separation of frequencies in a Doppler signal for display as a Doppler spectral waveform; the application of the Fourier transform to determine the frequency components present in a Doppler signal.
spectral broadening The widening of the Doppler spectrum; i.e., the increase in the range of Doppler shifted frequencies present that occurs because of a broadened range of flow velocities encountered by the sound beam. This occurs for disturbed and turbulent flow pr can be an artifact caused by the limited beam width.
spectral Doppler display The presentation of quantitative Doppler information in a waveform of Doppler shifts (in kHz or cm/s) versus time. Visual display of a Doppler spectrum.
specular reflection Reflection from a large (relative to wavelength), flat, and smooth boundary.
speed error Propagation speed that is different from the assumed value (1.54 mm/μs).
stable cavitation The phenomenon where bubbles oscillate nonlinearly and they expand more under lower pressures than they contract under higher pressures resulting in local streaming, microjets, shear stresses, and membrane damage to exposed cells.
stenosis Narrowing of a vessel lumen.
stiffness Property of a medium; applied pressure divided by the fractional volume change produced by the pressure.
strain The increase or decrease of the length of a segment of a material, subjected to a stress, divided by its original length.
streamline A line representing the path of motion of a particle of fluid.
strength Nonspecific term referring here to amplitude or intensity.
stress A force per unit area applied to a material that compresses or stretches it.

T

temporal resolution Ability to distinguish closely spaced events in time; improves with increased frame rate.
test object A device without tissue-like properties that is designed to measure some characteristic of an imaging system.
thermal bioeffects As ultrasound is absorbed by tissue, the temperature rises. If critical time-temperature values are exceeded, tissue damage can occur (very difficult to do in practice).
thermal index An indicator of thermal mechanism activity (estimated temperature rise); a value equal to transducer acoustic output power divided by the estimated power required to raise tissue temperature by 1°C.
three-dimensional (3D) imaging Scanning through many adjacent 2D cross-sections to form a 3D volume of echo information, which can then be processed and displayed as multiple simultaneous 2D images or as 3D volumes of the anatomy and/or flow within it.
time gain compensation (TGC) Equalization of echo amplitude differences caused by different attenuations for different reflector depths; also called *depth gain compensation.*
time intensity curves Mapping changes in echo strength (due to contrast enhancement) as a function of time.
tissue Doppler imaging An echocardiographic technique that provides a quantitative evaluation of myocardial tissue motion (by displaying the low velocity, high amplitude signals from the heart muscle itself). There are both spectral (i.e., pulsed wave) and color tissue Doppler imaging (TDI) modes available.
tissue harmonic imaging A technique for improving image quality by transmitting pulses at a given fundamental frequency into the body, but then receiving echoes at double that frequency to form the displayed images.
transducer A device that converts energy from one form to another. For ultrasound imaging the conversion is from mechanical to electrical energy and *vice versa.*
transducer assembly Transducer element(s) with damping and matching materials assembled within a case or housing.
transient elastography Imaging tissue stiffness by tracking tissue movement induced by mechanical stress from the sonographer pushing on the transducer.
transmission angle Angle between the transmitted sound direction and a line perpendicular to the media boundary.
transverse wave A sound wave in which the particle motion is perpendicular to the direction of wave travel, also called a *shear wave.*
turbulence Random, chaotic, multidirectional flow of a fluid with mixing between layers; flow that is not laminar.
two-dimensional (2D) imaging Producing cross-sectional scans (or "slices" or "imaging planes") through the anatomy.

U

ultrasound Sound having a frequency greater than what humans can hear, that is, greater than 20 kHz.

ultrasound computed tomography Attempts to solve the acoustic inverse problem that arises when collecting echoes from 360° around an object. It is now possible to produce simultaneous images mapping speed of sound, attenuation, reflection (acoustic impedance) and/or stiffness in the female breast.

ultrasound transducer A device that converts electric energy to ultrasound energy, and *vice versa*.

V

variance The square of the standard deviation; one of the outputs of the autocorrelation process; a measure of spectral broadening (i.e., spread around the mean).

vector array Linear phased array that emits pulses from different starting points and (by phasing) in different directions.

virtual beam An imaginary beam (as opposed to a physical ultrasound beam) that describes the result of retrospective, computed beam forming. The virtual beam can be imagined in transmission or reception form.

virtual beam forming Computational, retrospective beam forming that is accomplished by high-speed, computational post-processing graphics processing units (GPUs), which calculates how echoes from different origination locations arrive at the elements across the transducer aperture in different sequences depending on the distance and direction of travel. This information varies with transmission and reception, and can be used to sort out what arrived when from each pixel location in order to form the final image associated with broad transmit beam systems.

virtual reception beam An imaginary reception beam that can be thought of as determining the echo produced at each pixel location in the image when using a broad transmit beam system.

virtual transmission beam An imaginary laser-thin transmitted ultrasound beam that can be thought of as producing excellent detail resolution throughout the image that is accomplished with retrospective, computed beam forming (i.e., in a broad transmit beam scanner).

viscosity Resistance of a fluid to flow.

volume imaging Three-dimensional (3D) or near real time four-dimensional (4D) imaging.

volumetric flow rate Volume of fluid passing a point per unit of time (i.e., per second or minute).

W

wall filter A filter (typically digital although older analog filters do exist) that passes frequencies above a set level and eliminates strong, low-frequency Doppler shifts from pulsating heart or vessel walls or tissue motion (i.e., clutter).

wave Traveling variation of one or more quantities.

wavelength Length of a single cycle in space (e.g., in mm).

window An anechoic region appearing beneath Doppler frequencies or velocities presented in a Doppler spectral waveform display.

Y

Young's modulus A measure of the hardness (stiffness) of a material. It is the ratio of the applied stress to the resulting strain in a material subjected to the stress.

ANSWERS TO EXERCISES

CHAPTER 1

1. d
2. a
3. a
4. c
5. c
6. d
7. a
8. b
9. c
10. a
11. c
12. a
13. b
14. d
15. d
16. b
17. d
18. d
19. a
20. c
21. a
22. d
23. c
24. e
25. b

CHAPTER 2

1. b
2. d
3. c
4. d
5. d
6. b
7. a
8. a
9. c
10. c
11. b
12. a
13. a
14. d
15. d
16. b
17. d
18. c
19. c
20. b
21. a
22. c
23. d (fastest in solids)
24. b
25. a
26. d (mechanical, longitudinal, or compressional)
27. b
28. d (determined by the medium)
29. b
30. a (information or energy)
31. c
32. True
33. c
34. d
35. c
36. d
37. c
38. d
39. True
40. True
41. a
42. c
43. b
44. d
45. b
46. b
47. b
48. c
49. b
50. c
51. a 1 (100%)
52. a
53. b (Soft tissue propagation speed is 1.54 mm/μs; wavelength is 0.3 mm.)
54. c (Period is 0.2 μs; soft tissue is irrelevant.)
55. d (1000 pulses per second; 1/1000 second from one pulse to the next)
56. a (0.04%)
57. d
58. e (50,000)
59. c
60. a
61. a
62. b
63. d
64. a (also W/cm2)
65. d
66. c
67. b
68. a
69. d
70. d
71. a
72. c
73. b
74. a
75. d

76. c
77. a
78. a
79. d
80. c
81. False (Attenuation = absorption + scattering)
82. True
83. b
84. b (Attenuation is 8 dB, and intensity ratio is 0.16.)
85. d (Attenuation is 80 dB, and intensity ratio is 0.00000001.)
86. c (0.5×7.5 MHz $\times$ 0.8 cm = 3 dB)
87. a
88. c
89. d
90. d
91. True, for perpendicular incidence
92. d (difference in numerator; sum in denominator)
93. b
94. a
95. c
96. d
97. True
98. d
99. a
100. False
101. a
102. c
103. True
104. b
105. a
106. b
107. d
108. a
109. False
110. False
111. b
112. d (<20 MHz in many applications)
113. c
114. d
115. c
116. a
117. e
118. True
119. True
120. False, in general (only true near the transducer)
121. b, c, e, f
122. True (axial resolution 0.3 mm)
123. d
124. c

CHAPTER 3

1. a
2. d
3. b
4. c
5. d
6. a
7. b
8. c
9. d
10. b
11. d
12. a
13. d
14. b
15. e
16. d
17. a
18. False
19. False
20. Back
21. Front
22. c
23. a
24. f (a, b, c)
25. d
26. a
27. c
28. No (because these frequencies are outside the bandwidth [4.5 to 5.5 MHz])
29. No (because these frequencies are outside the 2.5 MHz bandwidth [3.75 to 6.25 MHz]). 3 and 7 MHz requires a bandwidth of 4 MHz.
30. a
31. b
32. a
33. c
34. c
35. a
36. b
37. False (can focus only in the near zone)
38. c
39. d (all of the above)
40. False (See Fig. 3.12.)
41. a
42. a
43. d
44. a (the lateral dimension in the scan plane)
45. c
46. d
47. a, 1; b, 2; c, 1
48. b
49. c
50. a, e
51. b, c, d
52. c
53. d
54. b
55. d
56. a, 4; b, 3; c, 2; d, 1
57. a, d
58. a, 10; b, 0.15; c, 14; d, 6.5; e, 13; f, 14
59. c

60. b
61. d
62. d (frequency not needed)
63. a (size not needed)
64. True
65. False
66. d
67. True
68. False
69. a, 1, 2, 3; b. 2; c. 2; d. 1
70. e
71. a
72. b, c, d
73. c
74. b
75. d
76. a, 1; b, 4; c, 3; d, 5; e, 2

CHAPTER 4

1. b
2. a
3. a (A minimum echo reception time of 130 μs is required.)
4. d
5. a, 2; b, 4; c, 5; d, 1; e, 3
6. c
7. b
8. a
9. b
10. d
11. a
12. b
13. b
14. c
15. False
16. c
17. c
18. c
19. a
20. d
21. c
22. d
23. d
24. c
25. d
26. a, 6; b, 9; c, 10; d, 13; e, 14
27. a (43/32)
28. c (45/64)
29. a, 5; b, 3; c, 2; d, 6; e, 1; f, 4
30. e
31. a, 4; b, 5; c, 6; d, 7; e, 8
32. e
33. c
34. e
35. a
36. c (0 and 1)
37. d
38. a
39. a, 3; b, 7; c, 8; d, 5; e, 4; f, 2; g, 1; h, 6
40. c
41. b
42. a, 5; b, 10; c, 3; d, 1; e, 9; f, 2; g, 8; h, 7; i, 4; j, 6
43. a, 1 (0); b, 1 (1); c, 3 (101); d, 4 (1010); e, 5 (11001); f, 5 (11110); g, 6 (111111); h, 7 (1000000); i, 7 (1001011); j, 7 (1100100)
44. a, 3 (111); b, 4 (1111); c, 2 (11); d, 9 (111111111); e, 10 (1111111111); f, 6 (111111); g, 8 (11111111); h, 1 (1); i, 7 (1111111); j, 5 (11111)
45. a, 1 (0, 1); b, 2 (00, 01, 10, 11); c, 3 (000, 001, 010, 011, 100, 101, 110, 111); d, 4; e, 4; f, 5; g, 5; h, 6; i, 7; j, 7
46. a
47. c
48. d
49. a
50. d
51. a, 1; b, 2; c, 2; d, 2
52. b
53. b
54. True ($10 \times 1 \times 100 \times 30 = 30{,}000 < 77{,}000$)
55. c
56. a
57. a
58. b
59. d
60. c
61. b
62. c
63. b
64. d
65. a
66. b
67. d
68. b
69. b
70. a
71. d
72. d
73. a
74. a
75. a
76. b
77. b
78. c
79. d
80. c
81. b
82. a
83. False
84. d
85. b
86. a
87. b
88. c
89. a

90. d
91. a
92. a
93. a
94. b; e (a, c, d)
95. b
96. d
97. b
98. e (approaching the focus)
99. d
100. b
101. c
102. d
103. b
104. a
105. a
106. d
107. c
108. b
109. a
110. b
111. a
112. c
113. False
114. True
115. True
116. a
117. c

CHAPTER 5

1. a, c, d, e, g, h
2. c
3. a, b, f
4. c
5. b
6. b
7. d
8. c
9. a
10. a
11. b
12. d
13. b
14. d
15. c
16. d
17. b
18. b
19. e
20. e
21. e
22. c
23. d
24. b
25. b
26. a
27. d
28. a
29. b
30. a
31. a
32. e
33. e
34. b
35. d
36. e
37. d
38. d
39. d
40. b
41. c
42. d
43. d
44. b
45. b (The Doppler shift is cut in half.)
46. c (There is no Doppler shift at 90 degrees.)
47. d
48. a
49. a
50. c
51. c
52. c
53. c
54. d
55. e
56. b
57. d
58. False
59. e
60. a
61. a
62. False
63. False
64. e (b, c, d)
65. False (Remember the Doppler angle.)
66. c
67. a
68. b
69. d
70. c
71. c
72. a
73. d
74. b
75. b
76. True (Power Doppler displays have no angle dependence.)
77. No
78. False
79. b
80. e (a, b, or c)
81. False
82. False (It can also mean aliasing or changing Doppler angle.)
83. False (Remember the Doppler angle.)

84. b
85. b
86. a and c
87. a, b, c
88. d
89. a
90. b
91. d
92. c
93. b, c
94. e (c and d)
95. b
96. e
97. False
98. e
99. a
100. e (a, b, c, d)
101. False
102. c

CHAPTER 6

1. b (Remember attenuation is a function of the tissue not the beam)
2. e
3. a
4. c
5. c
6. c
7. b
8. e
9. a
10. d
11. c
12. b
13. d
14. d
15. c
16. a
17. d
18. c
19. d
20. c
21. c
22. d
23. c
24. d
25. a

CHAPTER 7

1. d
2. a
3. c (assumes 1.54 mm/μs, lower than the actual speed)
4. False
5. a
6. e (a, b, d)
7. False (This is the display of the interference pattern [speckle] of scattered sound from the distribution of scatterers within the ultrasound pulse in the tissue.)
8. c (also called section thickness)
9. c, d, e, f
10. True (edge shadowing)
11. Fig. 7.44A and B, shows a comet-tail artifact originating as reverberations within a structure.
12. a, 1; b, 2, 3; c, 3; d, 4, 5; e, 4, 5
13. b
14. c
15. b
16. d
17. True
18. b
19. b
20. b
21. c
22. a (double image)
23. e
24. e (c and d)
25. e
26. a
27. True
28. b
29. d
30. b
31. d
32. b
33. b
34. b
35. b
36. e
37. c
38. True (less attenuation, greater penetration, later echoes)
39. True (Doppler shift increases with increasing frequency.)
40. d
41. a
42. a, 3; b, 4; c, 3; d, 2; e, 1
43. b, c, d
44. e (b, c, d)
45. d
46. a, R (Color changes at a 90-degree angle because scan lines go in different directions. They are heading upstream on the right and downstream on the left.); b, L (Vessel curvature causes flow to be away from the transducer on the left and toward the transducer on the right.); c, R (The blue area at right is aliasing.); d, L (The blue in the center is aliasing.); e, L; f, L (The color changes because the vessel is curved; flow is away from the transducer on the left and toward the transducer on the right.)
47. a, 4; b, 2; c, 1; d, 3; e, 5
48. a
49. c
50. a
51. c.
52. b

53. false (since this just produce other artifacts)
54. d
55. false

CHAPTER 8

1. a
2. a, 1, 3; b, 1, 3; c, 1; d, 1; e, 4; f, 2; g, 2; h, 2; i, 5; j, 5
3. a. 4; b. 5; c. 3; d. 3; e. 1; f. 2; g. 1, 2
4. True
5. True
6. b
7. d
8. e
9. a
10. False
11. b, c, d, e
12. False
13. d
14. True
15. b
16. a, 2, 12; b, 3, 12; c, 3, 8; d, 4 or 2, 9; e, 1, 7; f, 6, 10; g, 6, 11

CHAPTER 9

1. a
2. d
3. a
4. b
5. c
6. False
7. d
8. e
9. e (a, b, c)
10. False
11. False
12. b
13. No
14. Yes
15. b and d
16. c
17. e
18. e
19. e
20. a
21. d
22. b
23. e
24. c, d, e
25. b
26. a, b, d
27. e (pregnancy possibility in fertile female)
28. b
29. a
30. d
31. b
32. b
33. e

CHAPTER 10

After each answer is the chapter number in which the subject is discussed. Most answers also have explanatory comments.

1. c. Ultrasound is sound of frequency greater than 20 kHz (0.02 MHz). (Chapter 2)
2. a. Propagation speeds in soft tissues are in the range of approximately 1.4 to 1.6 mm/μs Answer c is not in speed units. (Chapter 2)
3. c. Solid; high stiffness. (Chapter 2)
4. d. Propagation speed and impedance increase only slightly with frequency. (Chapter 2)
5. e. (Chapters 2 and 3)
6. c. Round-trip travel time is 13 μs/cm. (Chapter 2)
7. c. Scattering occurs with rough surfaces and with heterogeneous media (made up of small particles relative to the wavelength). Large, flat, smooth surfaces produce specular reflections. (Chapter 2)
8. b. The operating frequency of a transducer is such that its thickness is equal to one-half of the wavelength in the transducer element material. (Chapter 3)
9. d. Transducer elements expand and contract when a voltage is applied; conversely, when returning echoes apply pressure to the element, a voltage is generated. (Chapter 3)
10. a. Axial resolution is equal to one-half of the spatial pulse length. (Chapter 2)
11. c. Lateral resolution is equal to beam width. Beam width depends on the aperture (size of the element or group of elements generating the beam). (Chapters 2 and 3)
12. a. Penetration decreases with increasing frequency, and frequency has no effect on refraction. (Chapters 2 and 3)
13. c. This is part of the American Institute of Ultrasound in Medicine's *Statement on Mammalian In Vivo Ultrasonic Biological Effects*. (Chapter 9)
14. c. Frequencies lower than this range do not provide the needed resolution, whereas frequencies higher than this range do not allow for adequate penetration for medical purposes. Frequencies higher than 25 MHz are used for some superficial applications. (Chapters 2 and 3)
15. a. See answer to question 14. (Chapters 2 and 3)
16. e. Reverberation adds additional reflectors on the display that are deeper than the true ones. (Chapter 7)
17. e. (Chapter 4)
18. d. (Chapter 4)
19. b. (Chapter 4)
20. d. (Chapter 4)
21. b. (Chapter 7)
22. b. (Chapter 4)
23. d. (Chapter 4)
24. c. Pulse repetition frequency has no direct effect on detail resolution. (Chapters 4 and 7)
25. d. (Chapter 4)
26. d. Distance equals one-half of the speed multiplied by the round-trip time. (Chapter 2)
27. e. The matching layer improves sound transmission by reducing the reflection at the transducer-skin boundary. The coupling medium improves it by removing the air layer between the transducer and the skin. (Chapter 3)

28. c. (Chapter 3)
29. a. (Chapter 3)
30. c. (Chapter 4)
31. d. If the transducer is in the path of the reflector, answer c is correct because the Doppler angle is zero. If this is not the case, then b is correct because the Doppler angle will increase (decreasing the Doppler shift) while the reflector approaches. (Chapter 5)
32. e. The diameter referred to can be the entire vessel diameter or the diameter of a small portion of it (stenosis). For the former, d is correct. For the latter, c is correct at the stenosis. In either case, both a and b are correct. (Chapter 5)
33. c. Poiseuille equation shows that resistance increases with increasing vessel length, increasing fluid viscosity, or decreasing vessel diameter. (Chapter 5)
34. d. The blood cells move along with the plasma, not through it. (Chapter 5)
35. c. Propagation speed is determined by the medium, not by motion. (Chapters 2 and 5)
36. e. (Chapter 5)
37. e. (Chapter 5)
38. d. Spectral comes from spectrum, referring to color spectrum. A prism is an optical spectrum analyzer that breaks down white light into its component colors. (Chapter 5)
39. a. (Chapter 5)
40. e. If frequency changes, wavelength also changes. (Chapters 2 and 5)
41. c. (Chapter 5)
42. d. Answers a and b are correct. Anatomic data are provided by the real-time B scan, and physiologic data are provided from the pulsed Doppler sample volume. (Chapter 5)
43. False. Physiologic Doppler-shift frequencies are usually in the audible frequency range. (Chapter 5)
44. d. All imaging instruments and some Doppler instruments use pulsed ultrasound. (Chapter 4)
45. c. (Chapter 5)
46. e. (Chapter 5)
47. d. (Chapter 5)
48. e. They include pulsed Doppler (and sometimes continuous-wave Doppler) and dynamic B-scan imaging. (Chapter 5)
49. c. Both Doppler shifts exceed one-half of the pulse repetition frequency. (Chapter 5)
50. d. (Chapter 5)
51. a. This is because physiologic speeds (v) are small compared with the speed of sound (c) in tissues. (Chapter 5)
52. b. (Chapter 5)
53. e. Arterioles and capillaries are too small. (Chapter 5)
54. d. (Chapter 5)
55. e. (Chapter 5)
56. b. (Chapter 5)
57. c. (Chapter 5)
58. d. This is the Poiseuille law. Increasing resistance decreases flow. (Chapter 5)
59. b. It depends on radius to the fourth power. (Chapter 5)
60. d. This is the continuity rule. (Chapter 5)
61. e. (also the results of distensible vessels) (Chapter 5)
62. d. (Chapter 5)
63. e. See Figure 5.8. (Chapter 5)
64. c. (assuming a reflector moving at 50 cm/s) (Chapter 5)
65. b. (that is, about 5 m/s) (Chapter 5)
66. c. (smaller angle, larger cosine, larger shift) (Chapter 5)
67. a. (Chapter 5)
68. e. Spectrum is not needed; it cannot be displayed in a pixel. (Chapter 5)
69. d. The spectrum can be shown in addition to the color-Doppler display. (Chapter 5)
70. c. (Chapter 5)

$$v = \frac{77 \times 0.100}{(5 \times 0.5)} = 3.08$$

71. a. (Chapter 5)

$$v = \frac{77 \times 0.100}{7.5} = 1.03$$

72. d. (Chapter 5)
73. c. (13 μs of delay per centimeter of depth) (Chapter 5)
74. a. This is because flow speeds are typically one-thousandth the speed of sound in tissues (i.e., Doppler shits in kHz vs. imaging in MHz). (Chapter 5)
75. b. The range is about 4 to 32. (Chapter 5)
76. c. The range is about 40 to 400. (Chapter 5)
77. e. Any pulsed operation (b, c, d) can. (Chapter 5)
78. a. This is called near-plug flow. (Chapter 5)
79. d. (Chapter 5)
80. e. A stenosis generally increases a, b, and c and decreases d. (Chapter 5)
81. a. (that is, a widening of the spectrum) (Chapter 5)
82. e. Items b, c, and d are increased; a is decreased. (Chapter 5)
83. c. The blood flows back out of the high-impedance vascular bed during the low-pressure portion of the cardiac cycle. (Chapter 5)
84. c. (Chapter 5)
85. d. (Chapter 5)
86. e. (a resulting from b) (Chapter 5)
87. e. (Chapter 5)
88. a. (gray level or sometimes color) (Chapter 5)
89. e. (a = b + c) (Chapter 5)
90. b. (Chapter 5)
91. e. Items a and b determine sample volume length. (Chapter 5)
92. d. Echoes from the sample volume arrive after another pulse is emitted. (Chapter 5)
93. a. The shift exceeds the Nyquist limit (5 kHz). (Chapter 5)
94. e. (a and d) (Chapter 5)
95. e. (Chapter 5)
96. a. (Chapter 5)
97. e. (Chapter 5)
98. a. Because physiologic flow speeds are about one-thousandth the ultrasound propagation speed (1540 m/s), Doppler shifts are about one-thousandth the operating frequency. (Chapter 5)
99. e. (a and b) (Chapter 5)
100. b. (also proportional to the *cosine* of the Doppler angle) (Chapter 5)
101. d. Item a is for grayscale instruments. (Chapter 5)
102. b. (Chapter 7)

103. e. Shift increases to 4 kHz, which is still less than the Nyquist limit (4.5 kHz). (Chapter 5)
104. a. A nonzero Doppler angle increases calculated equivalent flow speed. (Chapter 5)
105. c. The Nyquist limit is still one-half of the pulse-repetition frequency. (Chapter 5)
106. e. (Chapter 5)
107. e. (Chapters 5 and 7)
108. e. (a and c) (Chapter 5)
109. e. (a and b; c increases the amount of color) (Chapter 5)
110. d. Item c is not strictly part of the color flow display. Also, it is not a cross-sectional display but rather a frequency-versus-time presentation. (Chapter 5)
111. b. White is brighter than gray. (Chapter 5)
112. a. Red and green are different hues, representing different light wave frequencies. (Chapter 5)
113. e. (a, b, c; about 5 to 50 frames per second are displayed) (Chapter 5)
114. d. (Chapter 5)
115. d. (Chapter 5)
116. a. The wall filter removes the lower-frequency clutter Doppler shifts. (Chapter 5)
117. d. (twice as many scan lines per frame) (Chapter 5)
118. e. Items c and d change because the scan line (pulse path) orientation changes. (Chapter 5)
119. a. Items b and c increase the amount of color. (Chapter 5)
120. d. Increasing pulse repetition frequency increases the Nyquist limit, reducing aliasing. (Chapter 5)
121. b. (Chapter 2)
122. e. The wavelength is the length of each cycle in a pulse. (Chapter 2)
123. a. Duty factor is pulse duration divided by pulse-repetition period. (Chapter 2)
124. b. The attenuation coefficient of 5-MHz ultrasound is approximately 2.5 dB/cm. The attenuation coefficient multiplied by the path length yields the attenuation (in decibels). Only answer b is given in attenuation (decibel) units. (Chapter 2)
125. b. Amplitude is the maximum amount that an acoustic variable varies from the normal value (in this case, 10 − 7 = 3 units). (Chapter 2)
126. a. (Chapter 2)
127. a. Amplitude, intensity, power, and beam area are related to one another. If two of these are known, the others can be found. Frequency is independent of these. All four of them can be known, and yet frequency remains undetermined. (Chapter 2)
128. a. Impedance 1 equals 3, which equals impedance 2; thus there is no reflection. (Chapter 2)
129. b. If 96% of the intensity is transmitted, 4% is reflected because what is not reflected is transmitted (i.e., the two must add up to 100%). (Chapter 2)
130. c. (Chapter 5)
131. c. If the second speed is twice the first speed, then the transmission angle is approximately twice the incidence angle. (Chapter 2)
132. a. Reflector distance x speed x time. (Chapter 2)
133. d. If reflectors are separated by less than the axial resolution, they are not separated on the display. (Chapter 2)
134. b. Axial resolution is equal to one-half the spatial pulse length. Spatial pulse length is equal to the number of cycles in the pulse multiplied by wavelength. Wavelength is equal to propagation speed divided by frequency. For 1 MHz, wavelength is 1.54 mm, spatial pulse length is 2×1.54, and axial resolution is 1.54 mm, so two reflectors separated by 1 mm would not be resolved. For 2 MHz, the resolution is 0.77, and the reflectors would be resolved. (Chapter 2)
135. a. For highly damped transducers, the quality factor (Q) is approximately equal to the number of cycles in the pulse. (Chapter 3)
136. b. Beam width changes with distance from transducer, and thus so does lateral resolution. (Chapter 2)
137. c. Near-zone length increases with transducer diameter so that the only transducer that would have a shorter near-zone length would be a transducer of smaller diameter. (Chapter 3)
138. c. Focusing can be accomplished only in the near zone of a beam. (Chapter 3)
139. e. Answers a, b, and c affect the beam. Resolution of the *system* is also affected by the electronics of the instrument. (Chapters 2 and 3)
140. a. All the others are characteristics of the sound. (Chapter 2)
141. c. Frequency, period, wavelength, and propagation speed are related to one another. However, all four of these can be known, and yet the amplitude is undetermined. (Chapter 2)
142. e. For perpendicular incidence, there is no refraction. For equal impedances, there is no reflection. (Chapter 2)
143. d. (Chapter 2)

$$IRC = \left(\frac{2.64 - 1.00}{2.64 + 1.00}\right)^2 = \left(\frac{1.64}{3.64}\right)^2 = (0.45)^2 = 0.2$$

For an intensity reflection coefficient (IRC) of 0.2 and an incident intensity of 1, the reflected intensity is 0.2, and the transmitted intensity is 0.8. (Chapter 2)

144. d. (Chapters 4 and 9)
145. d. Incidence angle always equals the reflection angle. For equal propagation speeds, incidence angle equals the transmission angle as well. (Chapter 2)
146. a. For oblique incidence, it is possible to have no reflection, even if the media impedances are unequal. (Chapter 2)
147. e. Increased transducer damping decreases the spatial pulse length. Increasing spatial pulse length is accompanied by increased pulse duration and degraded axial resolution. (Chapters 2 and 3)
148. c. (Chapter 2)
149. b. Wavelength is equal to propagation speed divided by frequency. (Chapter 2)
150. b. Spatial pulse length is equal to wavelength multiplied by the number of cycles in the pulse. (Chapter 2)
151. d. (Chapter 3)
152. e. No refraction means that there is no change in sound direction. This is a result of no change in propagation

speed (i.e., equal propagation speeds on both sides of the boundary). (Chapter 2)

153. e. If there is 1 W in each square centimeter of area, then there are 5 W in 5 cm2 of area. (Chapter 2)
154. c. Speeds in solids are higher than in liquids. Soft tissue behaves acoustically as a liquid (as it is mostly water). (Chapter 2)
155. d. (Chapter 2)
156. c. An unfocused 13 mm transducer has a beam width of 6.5 mm at the near-zone length. Focusing would reduce the lateral resolution below this value (i.e., improve it). (Chapters 2 and 3)
157. b. A 7.5 MHz transducer can image to a depth of only 5–7 centimeters in tissue. (Chapter 2)
158. a. The other answers make little sense. (Chapter 4)
159. d. (a and b) (Chapter 4)
160. b. For each 10 dB, there is a factor of 10 increase in power. (Chapter 4)
161. c. (Chapter 4)
162. b. (Chapter 4)
163. e. Decimal numbers greater than 15 require at least five bits in a binary number. The number 30 in binary is 11110. (Chapter 4)
164. False. Sixty-four shades require a 6-bit memory. (Chapter 4)
165. e. (Chapter 4)
166. False. This is a description of a linear array rather than a phased array. (Chapter 3)
167. b. (Chapter 2)

$$AR = \tfrac{1}{2} SPL = 0.5 \times n \times c/f = \left(\tfrac{1}{2}\right)(2)(1.54/5) = 0.3$$

168. False. Postprocessing is the assignment of display brightness to numbers coming out of memory. (Chapter 4)
169. e. (Chapter 2)
170. a. (Chapter 2)
171. b. In M mode, echo depth is displayed as a function of time. (Chapter 4)
172. c. (Chapter 2)
173. a. (Chapter 4)
174. e. (1 + 8 = 9) (Chapter 4)
175. a. (Chapter 7)
176. c. The instrument assumes a speed of 1.54 mm/μs. Echoes will arrive sooner because of their higher propagation speed and will be placed closer to the transducer than they should be. (Chapters 2 and 7)
177. a. (Chapter 4)
178. a. Increasing gain or decreasing attenuation increases echo intensity. (Chapters 2 and 4)
179. d. (Chapter 4)
180. b. (Chapters 3 and 4)
181. e. (Chapter 4)
182. e. Multiple pulses per scan line (ensemble length) are required for color-Doppler imaging. More pulses per scan line for multiple foci would make the frame rate unacceptably low. (Chapter 5)
183. c. A reduction of 3 dB is a 50% reduction. (Chapter 4)
184. d. See answer to Exercise 183. (Chapter 4)
185. c. (Chapter 4)
186. b. A factor of 8 is three doublings (i.e., 3 + 3 + 3 dB). (Chapter 4)
187. a. (Chapter 8)
188. a. (Chapter 8)
189. e. (Chapter 3)
190. a. (Chapters 2 and 4)
191. c. (Chapter 4)
192. c. (Chapter 4)
193. e. Transmission output side (to the transducer) of a beam former is analog. (Chapters 3 and 4)
194. e. Reception output side of a beam former (to the signal processor) is digital. (Chapter 4)
195. d. (Chapter 3)
196. c. (Chapter 3)
197. e. Propagation speed is independent of frequency and intensity. (Chapter 2)
198. a. (Chapter 5)
199. e. (Chapter 2)
200. a. (Chapter 3)

APPENDIX A

Lists of Symbols

TABLE A.1 Listed by Symbol

Symbol	Represents
A	area
a	attenuation
a_p	aperture
AR	axial resolution
c	propagation speed
cos	cosine
c_s	Shear wave propagation speed
c_t	element propagation speed
d	diameter; distance to reflector; distance from transducer
DF	duty factor
d_f	focal beam diameter
E	Young's modulus of elasticity
f	frequency
f_D	Doppler-shift frequency
fl	focal length
f_o	operating frequency
f_{NL}	Nyquist limit frequency
FR	frame rate
f_R	received (echo) frequency
f_T	transmit frequency
FR_m	maximum frame rate
I	intensity
I_i	incident intensity
I_r	reflected intensity
IRC	intensity reflection coefficient
I_t	transmitted intensity
ITC	intensity transmission coefficient
L	path length; tube length
LPF	lines per frame
LR	lateral resolution
MI	mechanical index
n	number of cycles per pulse; number of foci; ensemble length
P	power
p	pressure amplitude
PD	pulse duration
pen	penetration
PRF	pulse-repetition frequency
PRP	pulse-repetition period
Q	volumetric flow rate
R	flow resistance
r	radius
SPL	spatial pulse length
T	period
th	element thickness
TI	thermal index
v	flow speed, scatterer speed
v_a	average flow speed
w_b	beam width
z	impedance
ΔP	pressure difference; pressure drop
α	attenuation coefficient
ν	viscosity
θ_D	Doppler angle
θ_i	incidence angle
θ_r	reflection angle
θ_t	transmission angle
λ	wavelength
ρ	density

TABLE A.2 Listed by Parameter

Parameter	Represented by
aperture	a_p
area	A
attenuation	a
attenuation coefficient	α
average flow speed	v_a
axial resolution	AR
beam width	w_b
cosine	cos
density	ρ
diameter	d
distance from transducer	d
distance to reflector	d
Doppler angle	θ_D
Doppler-shift frequency	f_D
duty factor	DF
element propagation speed	c_t
element thickness	th
ensemble length	n
flow resistance	R
flow speed	v
focal beam diameter	d_f
focal length	fl
frame rate	FR
frequency	f
impedance	z
incidence angle	θ_i
incident intensity	I_i
intensity	I
intensity reflection coefficient	IRC
intensity transmission coefficient	ITC
lateral resolution	LR
lines per frame	LPF
maximum frame rate	FR_m
mechanical index	MI
number of cycles per pulse	n
number of foci	n
Nyquist limit frequency	f_{NL}
operating frequency	f_o
path length	L
penetration	pen
period	T
power	P
pressure amplitude	p
pressure difference	ΔP
pressure drop	ΔP
propagation speed	c
pulse duration	PD
pulse-repetition frequency	PRF
pulse-repetition period	PRP
radius	r
received (echo) frequency	f_R
reflected intensity	I_r
reflection angle	θ_r
scatterer speed	v
spatial pulse length	SPL
thermal index	TI
transmission angle	θ_t
transmitted frequency	f_T
transmitted intensity	I_t
tube length	L
viscosity	ν
volumetric flow rate	Q
Wavelength	λ
Young's modulus	E

APPENDIX B

Compilation of Equations

For convenient reference, the essential equations in this book (i.e., not from Advanced Concepts) are compiled here.

Chapter 2

$$T\,(\mu s) = \frac{1}{f(MHz)}$$

$$\lambda\,(mm) = \frac{c\,(mm/\mu s)}{f(MHz)}$$

$$PRP(ms) = \frac{1}{PRF(kHz)}$$

$$PD\,(\mu s) = n \times T\,(\mu s)$$

$$DF = \frac{PD\,(\mu s)}{PRP\,(\mu s)} = \frac{PD\,(\mu s) \times PRF\,(kHz)}{1000\,(KHz/(MHz)}$$

$$I\,(mW/cm^2) = \frac{P\,(mW)}{A\,(cm^2)}$$

$$a\,(dB) = \alpha(dB/(cm\,MHz)) \times L(cm) \times f(MHz)$$

$$a\,(dB) = \tfrac{1}{2}(dB/cm\,MHz) \times f\,(MHz) \times L\,(cm)$$

$$z\,(rayls) = \rho\,(kg/m^3) \times c\,(m/s)$$

$$IRC = \frac{I_r(W/cm^2)}{I_i(W/cm^2)} = \left[\frac{(z_2 - z_1)}{(z_2 + z_1)}\right]^2$$

$$ITC = \frac{I_t(W/cm^2)}{I_i(W/cm^2)} = 1 - IRC$$

$$\theta_i(degrees) = \theta_r(degrees)$$

$$d\,(mm) = \tfrac{1}{2}[c\,(mm/\mu s) \times t\,(\mu s)]$$

$$AR\,(mm) = \frac{SPL(mm)}{2}$$

$$LR\,(mm) = w_b(mm)$$

Chapter 3

$$f_o(MHz) = \frac{c_t(mm/\mu s)}{2 \times th\,(mm)}$$

Chapter 4

$$pen\,(cm) \times PRF\,(kHz) \le 77\,(cm/ms)$$

$$PRF\,(Hz) = n \times LPF \times FR\,(Hz)$$

$$pen\,(cm) \times n \times LPF \times FR(Hz) \le 77{,}000\ cm/s$$

Chapter 5

$$Q(mL/s) = \frac{\Delta P(Pa)}{R(kg/m\text{-}s)}$$

$$R(g/cm^4\text{-}s) = 8 \times L(cm) \times \frac{\vartheta(kg/m\text{-}s)}{\pi \times r^4(cm^4)}$$

$$Q\,(mL/s) = \frac{\Delta P(Pa) \times \pi \times d^4(cm^4)}{128 \times L(cm) \times \vartheta(kg/m\text{-}s)}$$

$$\Delta P = \tfrac{1}{2}\rho(v_2^2 - v_1^2)$$

$$\Delta P \sim 4(v_2)^2$$

$$f_D(kHz) = f_R(kHz) - f_T(kHz) = f_D(kHz) \times \frac{2 \times \upsilon\,(cm/s)}{c\,(cm/s)}$$

$$v(cm/s) = \frac{77(cm/ms) \times f_D(kHz)}{f_T(MHz)}$$

$$f_D(kHz) = \frac{f_T(kHz) \times 2 \times \upsilon(cm/s) \times \cos\theta}{c(cm/s)}$$

$$\upsilon(cm/s) = \frac{77(cm/ms) \times f_D(kHz)}{f_T(MHz) \times \cos\theta}$$

$$FR_m(Hz) = \frac{77{,}000\,(cm/s)}{pen(cm) \times LPF \times n}$$

Chapter 6

$$c_s = [E/3\rho]^{1/2}$$

Chapter 7

$$f_{NL} = \frac{PRF}{2} \text{ (in kHZ)}$$

Chapter 9

$$MI = \frac{P_r}{\sqrt{f}}$$

APPENDIX C

Mathematics Review

Algebra and trigonometry are used in the discussion of ultrasound and Doppler principles. Logarithms are involved in decibels, and binary numbers are involved in digital electronics. Mathematic concepts that are applicable to the material in this book are reviewed in this appendix. Relevant aspects of algebra, trigonometry, logarithms, scientific notation, binary numbers, units, and statistics are covered.

First, we review some mathematic terminology. In algebraic equations such as:

$$x + y = z$$

$$x - y = z$$

x and y are called *terms.* Terms are connected with each other by addition or subtraction. With addition, the result is called the *sum.* With subtraction, the result is called the *difference.*

In the equations,

$$x \times y = z$$

$$\frac{x}{y} = z$$

x and y are called *factors.* Factors are connected with each other by multiplication or division. When multiplied, the result is called the *product.* When divided, the result is called the *quotient.*

The inverse or reciprocal of x is 1/x, sometimes described as "one over" x.

Algebra

Transposition of quantities in algebraic equations is accomplished by performing identical mathematical operations on both sides.

Example C.1

For the equation,

$$x + y = z$$

transpose to get x alone (solve for x). To do this, subtract y from both sides:

$$x + y - y = z - y$$

Because $y - y = 0$, the left-hand side of the equation is

$$x + y - y = x + 0 = x$$

so that

$$x = z - y$$

Example C.2

For the equation,

$$x - y = z$$

solve for x. Add y to both sides:

$$x - y + y = z + y$$

$$x + 0 = z + y$$

$$x = z + y$$

Example C.3

For the equation,

$$xy = z$$

solve for x. Divide both sides by y:

$$\frac{xy}{y} = \frac{z}{y}$$

Because $y/y = 1$

$$\frac{xy}{y} = x(1) = x$$

and

$$x = \frac{z}{y}$$

Example C.4

For the equation,

$$\frac{x}{y} = z$$

solve for x. Multiply both sides by y:

$$\left(\frac{x}{y}\right)y = zy$$

$$x(1) = zy$$

$$x = zy$$

Example C.5

Using some numbers, and combining the previous examples, consider the equation

$$\left(\frac{5x + 3}{2}\right) - 3 = 1$$

and solve for x. First, add 3 to both sides:

$$\left(\frac{5x + 3}{2}\right) - 3 + 3 = 1 + 3$$

$$\frac{5x + 3}{2} = 4$$

Multiply by 2:

$$\left(\frac{5x+3}{2}\right)\times 2 = 4\times 2$$

$$5x+3=8$$

Subtract 3:

$$5x+3-3=8-3$$

$$5x=5$$

Divide by 5:

$$x=1$$

Substitution of the answer into the original equation shows that the equality is satisfied and the answer is correct:

$$\left[\frac{5(1)+3}{2}\right]-3=1$$

$$\left(\frac{8}{2}\right)-3=1$$

$$4-3=1$$

$$1=1$$

Example C.6

For the equation,

$$c=f\times\lambda$$

solve for wavelength. Divide by frequency:

$$\frac{c}{f}=\frac{f\times\lambda}{f}$$

$$\frac{c}{f}=\lambda$$

Example C.7

If the intensity reflection coefficient (IRC) is 0.1 and the reflected intensity (I_r) is 5 mW/cm², find the incident intensity (I_i), given that

$$IRC=\frac{I_r}{I_i}$$

Multiply by incident intensity:

$$IRC\times I_i=\frac{I_r}{I_i}\times I_i$$

Divide by IRC:

$$\frac{IRC\times I_i}{IRC}=\frac{I_r}{IRC}$$

$$I_i=\frac{I_r}{IRC}=\frac{5\text{ mW/cm}^2}{0.1}=50\text{ mW/cm}^2$$

Example C.8

If the IRC is 0.01 and the impedance for medium 1 (z_1) is 4.5, find the medium 2 impedance (z_2), given that

$$IRC=\left(\frac{z_2-z_1}{z_2+z_1}\right)^2$$

Take the square root of each side:

$$RC^{1/2}=\frac{z_2-z_1}{z_2+z_1}$$

Multiply by the sum of z_2 and z_1:

$$IRC^{1/2}\times(z_2+z_1)=(z_2-z_1)$$

Add z_1:

$$IRC^{1/2}\times(z_2+z_1)+z_1=z_2$$

Subtract $IRC^{1/2}\times z_2$:

$$(IRC^{1/2}\times z_1)+z_1=z_2-(IRC^{1/2}\times z_2)$$

$$z_1(1+IRC^{1/2})=z_2(1-IRC^{1/2})$$

Divide by $(1-IRC^{1/2})$ and interchange sides of the equation:

$$z_2=z_1\left[\frac{(1+IRC^{1/2})}{(1-IRC^{1/2})}\right]$$

$$=4.5\left[\frac{1+(0.01)^{1/2}}{1-(0.01)^{1/2}}\right]$$

$$=4.5\left(\frac{1+0.1}{1-0.1}\right)=4.5\left(\frac{1.1}{0.9}\right)=4.5(1.22)=5.5$$

Trigonometry

If the sides and angles of a right triangle ("right" means one of the angles equals 90 degrees) are labeled as in Fig. C.1, the sine of angle A (sin A), the cosine of angle A (cos A), and the tangent of angle A (tan A) are defined as follows:

$$\sin A=\frac{\text{length of side a}}{\text{length of side c}}$$

$$\cos A=\frac{\text{length of side b}}{\text{length of side c}}$$

$$\tan A=\frac{\text{length of side a}}{\text{length of side b}}$$

Example C.9

If the lengths of the sides a, b, and c are 1, $\sqrt{3}$, and 2, respectively, what are sin A and cos A?

$$\sin A=\frac{1}{2}=0.5$$

$$\cos A=\frac{\sqrt{3}}{2}=0.87$$

If the sine or cosine is known, angle A may be found using a calculator or a table such as Table C.1.

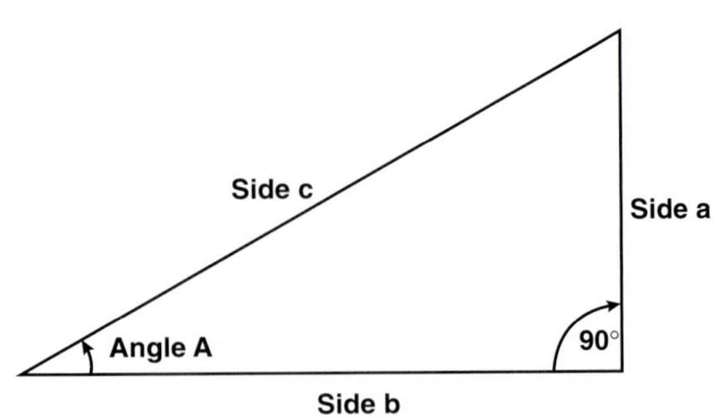

Fig. C.1 If the sides and angles of a right triangle are labeled as in this figure, the cosine of angle A (cos A) is equal to the length of side b divided by the length of side c. Sine A is equal to the length of side a divided by the length of side c.

Example C.10

If sin A is 0.5, what is A? From Table C.1, A = 30 degrees.

Example C.11

If cos A is 0.87, what is A? From Table C.1, A = 30 degrees.

If angle A is known, sin A or cos A may be found by using a calculator or a table such as Table C.1.

Example C.12

If A = 45 degrees, what are the sin A and cos A? From Table C.1, sin A = 0.71 and cos A = 0.71.

Logarithms: The logarithm to the base 10 (log) of a number is equal to the number of tens that must be multiplied together to result in that number. More generally, the logarithm is the power to which 10 must be raised to give a particular number.

Example C.13

What is the logarithm of 1000? To obtain 1000, three tens must be multiplied together:

$$10 \times 10 \times 10 = 1000$$

Three tens then yield the logarithm (log) of 1000.

$$\log 1000 = 3$$

The logarithm of the reciprocal of a number is equal to the negative of the logarithm of the number.

Example C.14

What is the logarithm of 0.01?

$$0.01 = \frac{1}{100}$$

$$\log 100 = 2$$

$$\log 0.01 = \log \frac{1}{100} = -2$$

Decibels are quantities that result from taking 10 times the logarithm of the ratio of two powers or intensities.

Example C.15

Compare the following two powers in decibels: power 1 = 1 W; power 2 = 10 W.

$$10\log\left(\frac{\text{power 1}}{\text{power 2}}\right) = 10\log\left(\frac{1}{10}\right) = 10(-\log 10) = 10(-1) = -10\text{ dB}$$

Power 1 is 10 dB less than power 2, or power 1 is 10 dB below power 2. Also,

$$10\log\left(\frac{\text{power 2}}{\text{power 1}}\right) = 10\log\left(\frac{10}{1}\right) = 10(\log 10) = 10(1) = 10\text{ dB}$$

TABLE C.1 Trigonometric Functions

Angle (°)	Sine	Cosine	Tangent
0	0	1.00	0
30	0.50	0.87	0.58
45	0.71	0.71	1.00
60	0.87	0.50	1.73
90	1.00	0	∞

Note: The symbol ∞ indicates infinity or indeterminate; that is, dividing by zero can be executed an unlimited number of times.

Power 2 is 10 dB more than power 1, or power 2 is 10 dB above power 1.

Example C.16

An amplifier has a power output of 100 mW when the input power is 0.1 mW. What is the amplifier gain in decibels?

$$\text{amplifier gain (dB)} = 10\log\left(\frac{\text{power out}}{\text{power in}}\right)$$

$$= 10\log\left(\frac{100}{0.1}\right) = 10\log 1000 = 10(3) = 30\text{ dB}$$

Example C.17

An electric attenuator has a power output of 0.01 mW when the input power is 100 mW. What is the attenuation of the attenuator in decibels?

$$\text{attenuator attenuation (dB)} = -10\log\left(\frac{\text{power out}}{\text{power in}}\right)$$

$$= -10\log\left(\frac{0.01}{100}\right) = -10\log\left(\frac{1}{10000}\right)$$

$$= -10(-\log 10{,}000)$$

$$= -10(-4) = 40\text{ dB}$$

The first minus sign is used in the equation to give the attenuation as a positive number. If the minus number had not been used, the "gain" of the attenuator would have been calculated and would have turned out to be −40 dB. A gain of −40 dB is the same as an attenuation of 40 dB.

Example C.18

Compare intensity 2 with intensity 1; intensity 1 = 10 mW/cm^2; intensity 2 = 0.01 mW/cm^2.

$$10\log\left(\frac{\text{intensity 2}}{\text{intensity 1}}\right) = 10\log\left(\frac{0.01}{10}\right)$$

$$= 10\log\left(\frac{1}{1000}\right) = 10(-\log 1000)$$

$$= 10(-3) = -30\text{ dB}$$

Intensity 2 is 30 dB less than or below intensity 1.

Example C.19

As sound passes through a medium, its intensity at one point is 1 mW/cm^2 and at a point 10 cm farther along is 0.1 mW/cm^2. What are the attenuation and attenuation coefficient? (See Chapter 2.)

$$\text{attenuation (dB)} = 10\log\left(\frac{\text{intensity at second point}}{\text{intensity at first point}}\right)$$

$$= -10\log\left(\frac{0.1}{1}\right) = -10\log\left(\frac{1}{10}\right)$$

$$= -10(-\log 10) = -10(-1) = 10\text{ dB}$$

See Example C.17 for comment on the first minus sign. The attenuation coefficient is the attenuation (dB) divided by the separation between the two points:

$$\text{attenuation coefficient (dB/cm)} = \frac{\text{attenuation (dB)}}{\text{separation (cm)}}$$

$$= \frac{10\text{ dB}}{10\text{ cm}} = 1\text{ dB/cm}$$

Example C.20

Show by example that log x^2 is equal to 2 log x.

Let x = 5.

Then log x = 0.70 and 2 log x = 1.40.

Thus x = 5^2 = 25 and log 25 = 1.40.

Example C.21

Power and intensity are proportional to amplitude squared. A power or intensity ratio expressed in decibels is calculated using the definition.

$$10\log\left(\frac{\text{power 1}}{\text{power 2}}\right)$$

This is equivalent to

$$20\log\left(\frac{\text{amplitude 1}}{\text{amplitude 2}}\right)$$

as seen with the following values:

Amplitude 1 = 4

Amplitude 2 = 3

Power 1 = 4^2 = 16

Power 2 = 3^2 = 9

$$\text{power ration (dB)} = 10\log\left(\frac{\text{power 1}}{\text{power 2}}\right)$$

$$= 10\log\left(\frac{16}{9}\right) = 2.5$$

$$\text{amplidute ration (dB)} = 20\log\left(\frac{\text{amplitude 1}}{\text{amplitude 2}}\right)$$

$$= 20\log\left(\frac{4}{3}\right) = 2.5$$

Table C.2 lists various values of power or intensity ratio with corresponding decibel values of gain or attenuation.

Some authors put output or end-of-path values in the numerator of the equation used for calculating decibels. If the numerator value is less than the denominator value (e.g., attenuation), a negative decibel value is calculated. For example, if the input and output powers for an electrical attenuator were 2 W and 1 W, respectively, the result is −3 dB; that is, this attenuator has −3 dB of gain. In this book, only positive decibel values are considered with clarification regarding whether attenuation or gain is considered. In this example, the result would be given as 3 dB of attenuation.

TABLE C.2 Decibel Values of Attenuation or Gain for Various Values of Power or Intensity Ratio

Decibel Gain or Attenuation	Attenuation	Gain
1	0.79	1.3
3	0.50	2.0
6	0.25	4.0
10	0.10	10.0
30	0.001	1000
100	0.0000000001	10,000,000,000

The ratio is output power or intensity divided by input power or intensity.

Scientific Notation

Scientific notation uses factors of 10, expressed in exponential form, to shorten the expression of very large or very small numbers. For example, 1,540,000 mm/s can be expressed as 1.54×10^6. In the expression x^y, x is called the base and y is called the exponent. When multiplying factors in scientific notation, the exponents are added. When dividing, the exponents are subtracted.

Example C.22

$$\frac{(1.54\times10^6\ \text{mm/s})\times(3.60\times10^3\ \text{s/hr})}{(1.61\times10^6\ \text{mm/mile})} = 3.44\times10^3\ \text{mph}$$

Here, the multiplication result is 5.54×10^9. Then the division by 1.61×10^6 yields 3.44×10^3.

Binary Numbers

The use of digital memories in ultrasound scanners presents a need for understanding the binary numbering system. Digital (computer) memories and data processors use binary numbers in carrying out their functions because they contain electronic components that operate in only two states, off (0) and on (1).

Binary digits (bits) consist of only zeros and ones, represented by the symbols 0 and 1. As in the decimal numbering system, with which we are so familiar, other numbers must be represented by moving these symbols to different positions (columns). In the decimal system, where there are 10 symbols (0 through 9), there is no symbol for the number 10 (9 is the largest number for which there is a symbol). To represent 10 in symbolic form, the symbol for one is used, moving it to the second (from the right) column. A zero is placed in the right column to clarify this so that 10 is, symbolically, 10. The symbol for one has been used in such a way that it no longer represents one, but rather 10.

A similar procedure is used in the binary numbering system. The symbol 1 represents the largest number (one) for which there is a symbol in the system. To represent the next number (2), the same thing is done as in the decimal system; that is, the symbol 1 is placed in the next column to represent the number 2. Columns in the two systems represent values as follows:

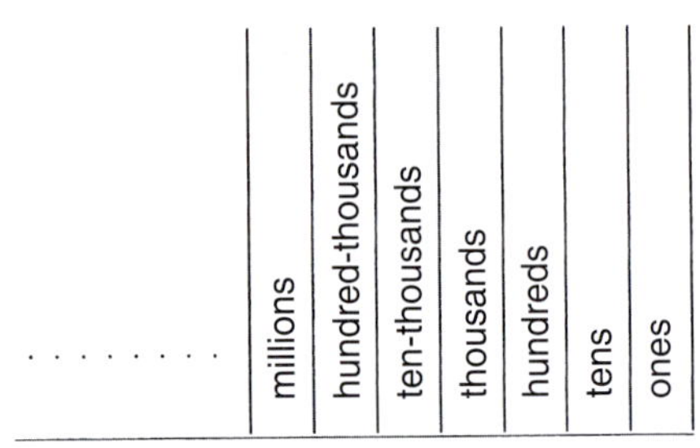

Decimal

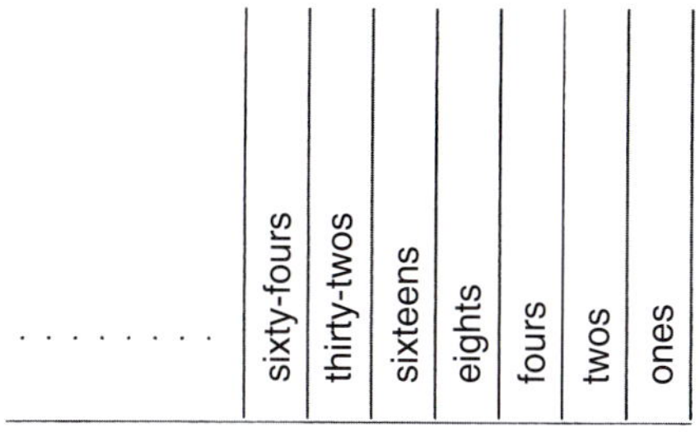

Binary

In the decimal system, each column represents 10 times the column to the right. In the binary system, each column represents two times the column to the right.

The decimal number 1234 represents (reading from right to left) four ones, three tens, two hundreds, and one thousand; that is, 4 + 30 + 200 + 1000 = 1234. Likewise, the decimal number 10,110 represents zero ones, one ten, one hundred, zero thousand, and one ten thousand. The binary number 10110 represents zero ones, one two, one four, zero eights, and one sixteen, or 0 + 2 + 4 + 0 + 16 = 22 in decimal form. This represents a straightforward way of converting a number from the binary system to the decimal system.

Example C.23

Convert the binary number 101010 to decimal form. This number represents 0 + 2 + 0 + 8 + 0 + 32, or 42 in decimal form.

To convert a number from decimal to binary form, one must successively subtract the largest possible multiples of 2, which are the binary column values, in succession from the decimal number.

Example C.24

Convert the decimal number 60 to binary form:

a. Can 64 be subtracted from 60? No. (Enter 0 in the 64 column of the binary number.)
b. Can 32 be subtracted from 60? Yes. (Enter 1 in the 32 column.) 60 – 32 = 28 (the difference)
c. Can 16 be subtracted from 28? Yes. (Enter 1 in the 16 column.) 28 – 16 = 12 (the difference)
d. Can 8 be subtracted from 12? Yes. (Enter 1 in the 8 column.) 12 – 8 = 4 (the difference)
e. Can 4 be subtracted from 4? Yes. (Enter 1 in the 4 column.) 4 – 4 = 0 (the difference)
f. Can 2 be subtracted from 0? No. (Enter 0 in the 2 column.)
g. Can 1 be subtracted from 0? No. (Enter 0 in the 1 column.)

Therefore the decimal 60 equals 0111100 in the binary system. As in the decimal system, we normally drop leading zeroes, that is, those to the left of the first nonzero digit. The result is 111100. To check this answer, convert it back to decimal form. This number, 111100, reading from the right, represents 0 + 0 + 4 + 8 + 16 + 32, or 60 in decimal form.

TABLE C.3 Binary and Decimal Number Equivalents

Decimal	Binary	Decimal	Binary
0	000000	32	100000
1	000001	33	100001
2	000010	34	100010
3	000011	35	100011
4	000100	36	100100
5	000101	37	100101
6	000110	38	100110
7	000111	39	100111
8	001000	40	101000
9	001001	41	101001
10	001010	42	101010
11	001011	43	101011
12	001100	44	101100
13	001101	45	101101
14	001110	46	101110
15	001111	47	101111
16	010000	48	110000
17	010001	49	110001
18	010010	50	110010
19	010011	51	110011
20	010100	52	110100
21	010101	53	110101
22	010110	54	110110
23	010111	55	110111
24	011000	56	111000
25	011001	57	111001
26	011010	58	111010
27	011011	59	111011
28	011100	60	111100
29	011101	61	111101
30	011110	62	111110
31	011111	63	111111

Table C.3 lists the binary forms of the decimal numbers 0 to 63. Numbers 64 to 127 would have one additional digit and so forth with higher multiples of 2.

Units

Units for the physics and acoustics quantities discussed in this book are presented in this section. They are drawn primarily from the international system of units (SI).

Table C.4 lists units for the quantities discussed in this book. Table C.5 gives equivalent units. Table C.6 lists prefixes for units, and Table C.7 gives conversion factors between common units.

In algebraic equations involving these units, the units for the quantity solved for are determined by manipulation of the units for the other quantities in the equation.

TABLE C.4 Units and Unit Symbols for Physics and Acoustic Quantities

Quantity	Unit	Unit Symbol or Abbreviation
Acceleration	meter/second^2	m/s^2
Angle	degree	°
Area	meter^2	m^2
Attenuation	decibel	dB
Attenuation coefficient	decibel/meter	dB/m
Beam area	meter^2	m^2
Current	Ampere	A
Density	kilogram/meter^3	kg/m^3
Displacement	meter	m
Doppler shift	Hertz	Hz
Energy	Joule	J
Force	Newton	N
Frequency	Hertz	Hz
Gain	decibel	dB
Heat	Joule	J
Impedance	rayl	—
Intensity	Watt/meter^2	W/m^2
Mass	kilogram	kg
Period	seconds	s
Power	Watt	W
Pressure	Newton/meter^2	N/m^2
Propagation speed	meter/second	m/s
Pulse duration	seconds	s
Pulse-repetition frequency	Hertz	Hz
Pulse-repetition period	seconds	s
Resistance	Ohm	Ω
Spatial pulse length	meter	m
Speed	meter/second	m/s
Stiffness	Newton/meter^2	N/m^2
Temperature	degrees Kelvin	K
Time	seconds	s
Velocity	meter/second	m/s
Voltage	volts	V
Volume	meter^3	m^3
Wavelength	meter	m
Work	Joule	J

Example C.25

Determine the unit for frequency in the equation

$$\text{frequency} = \frac{\text{propagation speed (m/s)}}{\text{wave length (m)}}$$

The units on the right-hand side of the equation are

$$\frac{\text{m/s}}{\text{m}} = \frac{1}{\text{s}}$$

TABLE C.5 Equivalent Units for Physics and Acoustics Quantities

Unit Given in Table C.4	Equivalent Unit	Equivalent Unit Abbreviation
Hertz	1/second	1/s
Joule	Newton-meters	N-m
Joule	Watt-seconds	W-s
Rayl	kilogram/meter^2-second	kg/m^2-s
Newton	kilogram-meter/second^2	kg-m/s^2
Newton/meter	Pascal	Pa
Watt	Joule/second	J/s

TABLE C.6 Unit Prefixes

Prefix	Factor[a]	Symbol or Abbreviation
mega	1,000,000	M
kilo	1000	k
centi	0.01	c
milli	0.001	m
micro	0.000001	μ

[a]Factor is the number of unprefixed units in a unit with the prefix. For example, there are 1000 Hz in 1 kHz, and there is 0.001 m in 1 mm.

TABLE C.7 Conversion Factors Among Common Units

To Convert	From	To	Multiply by
Area	m^2	cm^2	10,000
	cm^2	m^2	0.0001
Displacement	m	mm	1000
	m	cm	100
	m	km	0.001
	mm	m	0.001
	mm	km	0.000001
	km	mm	1,000,000
Frequency	Hz	kHz	0.001
	Hz	MHz	0.000001
	kHz	MHz	0.001
	MHz	kHz	1,000
	kHz	Hz	1000
	MHz	Hz	1,000,000
Intensity	W/cm^2	W/m^2	10,000
	W/cm^2	kW/m^2	10
	W/cm^2	mW/cm^2	1000
	W/m^2	W/cm^2	0.0001
	W/m^2	mW/cm^2	0.1
	W/m^2	kW/m^2	0.001
Speed	m/s	km/s	0.001
	km/s	m/s	1000
	km/s	mm/μs	1

From Table C.5, it can be found that

$$\frac{1}{s} = Hz$$

Therefore the frequency unit is Hertz.

Example C.26

Determine the unit for frequency in the equation

$$\text{frequency} = \frac{\text{propagation speed (m/s)}}{\text{wavelength (mm)}}$$

The units on the right-hand side of the equation are

$$\frac{m/s}{mm}$$

From Table C.6, it can be found that 1 mm equals 0.001 m, so that

$$\frac{m/s}{0.001m} = 1000 1/s$$

and from Tables C.5 and C.6,

$$1000\ 1/s = 1000\ Hz = 1\,kHz$$

Therefore, the frequency unit is kiloHertz. To convert a frequency given in kiloHertz to megaHertz, multiply by 0.001. To convert a frequency given in kiloHertz to Hertz, multiply by 1000.

Example C.27

Determine the unit for intensity in the equation

$$\text{intensity} = \frac{\text{power(W)}}{\text{area(cm}^2)}$$

The units on the right-hand side of the equation are W/cm^2; therefore, the intensity unit is watts per centimeter squared.

Example C.28

Determine the unit for impedance in the equation

$$\text{impedance} = \text{density(kg/m}^3) \times \text{propagation speed (km/s)}$$

The units on the right-hand side of the equation are

$$kg/m^3 \times km/s$$

From Table C.6,

$$kg/m^3 \times km/s = kg/m^3 \times 1000\ m/s = 1000\ kg/m^2 \cdot s$$

From Table C.5,

$$1000\ kg/m^2 \cdot s = 1000\ \text{rayls}$$

From Table C.6,

$$1000\ \text{rayls} = 1\,\text{krayl}$$

Therefore, the impedance unit is kilorayl. Because this is uncommon, it would be better to keep the result in rayls.

TABLE C.8 Definitions of Numbers in Groups Tested

Test Result	Disease	Nondiseased	Total
Positive	TPV	FPV	TP
Negative	FNV	TNV	TN
Total	TD	TND	TOT

A positive test indicates disease. A negative test indicates disease free. *FNV* (false-negative value), the number of diseased persons testing negative; *FPV* (false-positive value), the number of nondiseased persons who tested positive; *TD*, the total number of diseased persons; *TN*, the total number of persons testing negative; *TND*, the total number of nondiseased persons; *TNV* (true-negative value), the number of disease-free persons testing negative; *TOT*, the total number of persons in the study; *TP*, the total number of persons testing positive; *TPV* (true-positive value), the number of diseased persons (in the study) testing positive.

Statistics

Several concepts are used in evaluating the usefulness of diagnostic tests. These tests can be qualitative, as in the case of interpreting an anatomic image, or they can be quantitative, as with Doppler flow values. Diagnoses are positive and negative; that is, the test indicates the presence or absence of disease. Table C.8 defines the various groups involved in testing for disease.

The sensitivity (SENS) of a test is the proportion of those having the disease (TD) who test positive (TPV):

$$SENS = \frac{TPV}{TD}$$

The specificity (SPEC) of a test is the proportion of those who are disease free (TND) who test negative (TNV):

$$SPEC = \frac{TNV}{TND}$$

The positive predictive value (PPV) of a test is the proportion of all positive (TP) test results that are correct, that is, the number of true positive results (TPV):

$$PPV = \frac{TPV}{TP}$$

The positive predictive value is the probability that a person who tests positive actually has the disease.

The negative predictive value (NPV) of a test is the proportion of all negative (TN) test results that are correct, that is, the number of true negative results (TNV):

$$NPV = \frac{TNV}{TN}$$

The negative predictive value is the probability that a person who tests negative is actually disease free.

The accuracy (ACC) of a test is the proportion of all tests in the study (TOT) that have the correct result

$$ACC = \frac{(TPV + TNV)}{TOT}$$

Example C.29

Given the following table, calculate TD, TND, TP, TN, TOT, SENS, SPEC, PPV, NPV, and ACC.

Test Result	Disease	Nondiseased	Total
Positive	8	2	TP
Negative	5	85	TN
Total	TD	TND	TOT

Test Result	Disease	Nondiseased	Total
Positive	8	2	10
Negative	5	85	90
Total	13	87	100

$$\text{SENS} = \frac{8}{13} = 0.62$$

$$\text{SPEC} = \frac{85}{87} = 0.98$$

$$\text{PPV} = \frac{8}{10} = 0.80$$

$$\text{NPV} = \frac{85}{90} = 0.94$$

$$\text{ACC} = \frac{(8+85)}{100} = 0.93$$

EXERCISES

1. Solve each of the following for x:
   a. $x + y + 2 = z$
   b. $x - y = z - 1$
   c. $2xy = z$
   d. $\frac{x}{y} = 3z$
   e. $\frac{(x+5)}{4} - 2 = 4$
   f. $\frac{(3x+3)}{2} - 2 = 4$
2. Solve each of the following for the quantity with the asterisk:
   a. propagation speed = frequency* × wavelength
   b. $\text{intensity} = \frac{\text{power}}{\text{beam area}^*}$
   c. $\text{period} = \frac{1}{\text{frequency}^*}$
3. The age of an ultrasound instrument is equal to 3 times its age 3 years from now minus 3 times its age 3 years ago. What is its present age?
4. Let

$$y + x = \tfrac{1}{2}(7y - 3x)$$

   a. Subtract 2x from both sides so that

$$y - x = \tfrac{1}{2}(7y - 3x) - 2x$$

   b. Divide both sides by (y – x):

$$\frac{(y-x)}{(y-x)} = \frac{(7y-3x)}{2(y-x)} - \frac{2x}{(y-x)}$$

   c. Combine right side into single fraction:

$$\frac{(y-x)}{(y-x)} = \frac{(7y-3x-4x)}{2(y-x)} = \frac{7(y-x)}{2(y-x)}$$

   d. Multiply both sides by 2:

$$2\left[\frac{(y-x)}{(y-x)} = 7\frac{(y-x)}{(y-x)}\right]$$

   Therefore 2 = 7. What went wrong?
5. If side a, b, and c in Figure C.1 have lengths of 3, 4, and 5, respectively, then sin A is ____________ and cos A is____________.
6. If angle A is 90 degrees, sin A is ____________ and cos A is ____________.
7. If sin A is 0.17, angle A is ____________ degrees.
8. If cos A is 0.94, angle A is ____________ degrees.
9. Give the logarithms of the following numbers:
   a. 10 ____________
   b. 0.1 ____________
   c. 100 ____________
   d. 0.001 ____________
10. One watt is ____________ dB below 100 W.
11. One watt is ____________ dB above 100 mW.
12. If the input power is 1 mW and the output is 10,000 mW, the gain is ____________ dB.
13. If the input power is 1 W and the output is 100 mW, the gain is ____________ dB. The attenuation is ____________ dB.
14. If the intensities of traveling sound are 10 mW/cm² and 0.1 mW/cm² at two points 5 cm apart, the attenuation between the two points is ____________ dB. The attenuation coefficient is ____________ dB/cm.
15. If an amplifier has a gain of 33 dB, the ratio of output power to input power is ____________. (Use Table C.2.)
16. If an attenuator has an attenuation of 26 dB, the ratio of output power to input power is ____________. (Use Table C.2.)
17. If the intensity at the start of a path is 3 mW/cm² and the attenuation over the path is 13 dB, the intensity at the end of the path is ____________ mW/cm². (Use Table C.2.)
18. If the output of a 22-dB gain amplifier is connected to the input of a 24-dB gain amplifier, the total gain is ____________ dB. The overall power ratio is ____________. (Use Table C.2.)
19. If a 17-dB attenuator is connected to a 14-dB amplifier, the net gain is ____________ dB. The net attenuation is ____________ dB. For a 1 W input, the output is ____________ W. (Use Table C.2.)
20. In binary numbers, how many symbols are used? ____________

21. The term binary digit commonly is shortened into the single word ___________.
22. Each binary digit in a binary number is represented in memory by a memory element, which, at any time, is in one of ___________ states.
23. Match the following: Column in a binary number hgfedcba:
    a. ___________
    b. ___________
    c. ___________
    d. ___________
    e. ___________
    f. ___________
    g. ___________
    h. ___________

    Decimal number represented by a 1 in the column:
    1. 64
    2. 32
    3. 1
    4. 16
    5. 8
    6. 128
    7. 2
    8. 4
24. The binary number 10110 represents zero ones, one two, one four, zero eights, and one sixteen, that is, $0 + 2 + 4 + 0 + 16 = 22$. What decimal number is represented by the binary number 11001? ___________
25. The decimal number 13 is made up of one one, zero twos, one four, and one eight ($8 + 4 + 0 + 1 = 13$). The decimal number, therefore, is represented by the binary number ___________.
26. Match the following:

a. 1 ___________	1. 0001111
b. 5 ___________	2. 0011001
c. 10 ___________	3. 0001010
d. 15 ___________	4. 0110010
e. 20 ___________	5. 0000001
f. 25 ___________	6. 1100100
g. 30 ___________	7. 0101000
h. 40 ___________	8. 0011110
i. 50 ___________	9. 0010100
j. 100 ___________	10. 0000101

27. How many binary digits are required in the binary numbers representing the following numbers?
    a. 0 ___________
    b. 1 ___________
    c. 5 ___________
    d. 10 ___________
    e. 25 ___________
    f. 30 ___________
    g. 63 ___________
    h. 64 ___________
    i. 75 ___________
    j. 100 ___________
28. Match the following: Largest decimal number that can be represented by a binary number with this many bits:

a. 7 ___________	1. 1
b. 15 ___________	2. 2
c. 3 ___________	3. 3
d. 511 ___________	4. 4
e. 1023 ___________	5. 5
f. 63 ___________	6. 6
g. 255 ___________	7. 7
h. 1 ___________	8. 8
i. 127 ___________	9. 9
j. 31 ___________	10. 10

29. How many bits are required to store numbers representing each number of different gray shades?
    a. 2 ___________
    b. 4 ___________
    c. 8 ___________
    d. 15 ___________
    e. 16 ___________
    f. 25 ___________
    g. 32 ___________
    h. 64 ___________
    i. 65 ___________
    j. 128 ___________
30. The unit of frequency in the equation

$$\text{frequency} = \frac{\text{propagation speed(km/s)}}{\text{wavelength(mm)}}$$

    is ___________. To convert frequency in this unit to frequency in kiloHertz, multiply by ___________.
31. A frequency of 50 kHz is equal to ___________ MHz and ___________ Hz.
32. A speed of 1.5 mm/ms is equal to ___________ km/s, ___________ m/s, ___________ cm/s, and ___________ mm/s.
33. If the frequency is 2 MHz and

$$\text{period} = \frac{1}{\text{frequency}}$$

    the period is ___________ ms, ___________ ms, or ___________ s.
34. Mass is given in units of ___________.
    a. megaHertz
    b. kilogram
    c. degrees Kelvin
    d. Watt
    e. none of the above
35. Displacement is given in ___________.
    a. megaHertz
    b. decibel
    c. Ohm
    d. meter
    e. all of the above
36. Attenuation is given in ___________.
    a. decirayl
    b. deciWatt
    c. decibel
    d. decimeter
    e. deciHertz

37. Given the following table, calculate TD, TND, TP, TN, TOT, SENS, SPEC, PPV, NPV, and ACC.

Test Result	Disease	Nondiseased	Total
Positive	80	20	TP
Negative	50	850	TN
Total	TD	TND	TOT

38. Solve the following for x and y:

$$x + y = 1 \quad x - y = 2$$

ANSWERS

1. a. z − y − 2; b. y + z − 1; c. z/2y; d. 3yz; e. 19; f. 3
2.
   a. $\frac{\text{propagation speed}}{\text{wavelength}}$
   b. $\frac{\text{power}}{\text{intensity}}$
   c. $\frac{1}{\text{period}}$
3. 18
4. Division by zero is what went wrong. Note that

$$y + x = \frac{1}{2}(7y - 3x)$$

yields

$$2(y + x) = 7y - 3x$$
$$2y + 2x = 7y - 3x$$
$$5x = 5y$$
$$x = y$$

so that dividing by (y 2 x) is dividing by zero (not allowed in algebra).

5. 0.6, 0.8
6. 1, 0
7. 10
8. 20
9. a, 1; b, −1; c, 2; d, −3
10. 20
11. 10
12. 40
13. −10, 10
14. 20, 4
15. 2000
16. 0.0025
17. 0.15
18. 46; 40,000
19. −3, 3, 0.50
20. Two (0, 1)
21. Bit
22. Two (off, on)
23. a, 3; b, 7; c, 8; d, 5; e, 4; f, 2; g, 1; h, 6
24. 25
25. 1101
26. a, 5; b, 10; c, 3; d, 1; e, 9; f, 2; g, 8; h, 7; i, 4; j, 6
27. a, 1 (0); b, 1 (1); c, 3 (101); d, 4 (1010); e, 5 (11001); f, 5 (11110); g, 6 (111111); h, 7 (1000000); i, 7 (1001011); j, 7 (1100100)
28. a, 3 (111); b, 4 (1111); c, 2 (11); d, 9 (111111111); e, 10 (1111111111); f, 6 (111111); g, 8 (11111111); h, 1 (1); i, 7 (1111111); j, 5 (11111)
29. a, 1 (0, 1); b, 2 (00, 01, 10, 11); c, 3 (000, 001, 010, 011, 100, 101, 110, 111); d, 4; e, 4; f, 5; g, 5; h, 6; i, 7; j, 7
30. MegaHertz, 1000
31. 0.05; 50,000
32. 1.5; 1500; 150,000; 1,500,000
33. 0.5, 0.0005, 0.0000005
34. b
35. d
36. c
37.

Test Result	Disease	Nondiseased	Total
Positive	80	20	100
Negative	50	850	900
Total	130	870	1000

$$SENS = \frac{80}{130} = 0.62$$

$$SPEC = \frac{850}{870} = 0.98$$

$$PPV = \frac{80}{100} = 0.80$$

$$NPV = \frac{850}{900} = 0.94$$

$$ACC = \frac{(80 + 850)}{1000} = 0.93$$

38. x = +3/2

    y = −1/2

    Insertions of these values into the original equations verifies their correctness.

INDEX

Note: Page numbers followed by "f" refer to illustrations; page numbers followed by "t" refer to tables; page numbers followed by "b" refer to boxes.